# EXPERIMENTAL SENSORY PSYCHOLOGY

# EXPERIMENTAL SENSORY PSYCHOLOGY

Edited by Bertram Scharf
Northeastern University

George S. Reynolds, Consulting Editor
University of California, San Diego

Scott, Foresman and Company    Glenview, Illinois
Dallas, Tex.    Oakland, N.J.    Palo Alto, Cal.    Tucker, Ga.    Brighton, England

## ACKNOWLEDGMENTS

*The authors would like to thank all sources for the use of their material. The credit lines for copyrighted materials appearing in this work are placed in the Reference section following each chapter. These pages are to be considered an extension of the copyright page.*

Library of Congress Catalog Card Number: 74-79320
ISBN: 0-673-05428-4

Printed in the United States of America.

*Dedicated to S. S. Stevens (1906–1973) Teacher, Colleague, Friend*

# PREFACE

This book is about seeing, hearing, tasting, smelling, and feeling. Designed for undergraduate and graduate students, it explains what the sensory systems do, and how a response depends on the stimulus and the observer. What is the dimmest light one can just barely see, and how does that minimum, or threshold, depend on the wavelength of the stimulus, its duration, size, background, and so forth? How is threshold intensity affected by the state of the observer—by the size of his pupil, by how much light he was just exposed to, by which part of his eye is being stimulated? What is the relation between loudness and sound intensity, and how is the relation affected by stimulus variables such as frequency, duration, complexity, and background noise, or by observer variables such as preceding exposure to noise, sensitivity, instructions? The answers to these questions are obtained in the laboratory where the experimenter can precisely control the stimulus and carefully define and limit the observer's response. This book deals primarily with those answers and how they are obtained in the laboratory—hence, the word *experimental* in the book's title.

*Experimental Sensory Psychology* is concerned not only with responses, stimuli, and the state of the observer, but also with the sensory organs and nervous systems that must function in order for an observer to make a response to a stimulus. We are keenly interested in the possible physiological mechanisms that underlie our sensory capacities. For example, to what extent is the ability to distinguish among salty, sweet, sour, and bitter flavors based on different kinds of taste receptors on the tongue? Does the finding that humans respond very differently to slow and fast vibratory stimuli on the skin mean that we have one receptor system for low-frequency vibration and a separate one for high-frequency vibration?

All such questions about the capacities and mechanisms of the five senses are treated in four separate chapters on audition, cutaneous sensation, olfaction and taste, and vision, each by a psychologist who is an active researcher specializing in the sensory system he has written about.

These specialized chapters are preceded by two chapters that look at all the senses. Chapter 2, Psychophysics, deals with the basic theoretical and methodological problems in sensory psychology, and describes the procedures for measuring the observer's ability to detect the presence of a stimulus or changes in a stimulus, as well as for scaling sensory magnitude. Chapter 3, General Biology of Sensory Systems, deals with basic physiological structures and mechanisms, such as the neuron, the synapse, receptor action, which are common to all the senses. That chapter also treats each sensory system separately, giving basic information essential to the understanding of succeeding chapters on sensory psychology. The introductory chapter tells what sensory psychology is about and how it is related to modern physiology, why sensory psychology is so important, and how it sprung from the philosophical concerns and physiological research of the nineteenth century.

This book, which was originally conceived by Dr. George S. Reynolds of the University of California at San Diego, was designed primarily for the undergraduate student in an experimental psychology course. With the help of John Amacker, John Cox, Joanne Elliott, George Jacobson, and Linda Peterson at Scott, Foresman we have pursued that original goal, and at the same time have tried to make the book useful for undergraduate and graduate courses on sensation or sensory processes. Our goal has been to give readers a basic understanding of the human senses and sufficient knowledge to help them carry out meaningful experiments in sensory psychology.

As editor of the volume, any success I may have had I owe largely to my years of studying, discussing, and arguing with S. S. Stevens, the man who almost single-handedly freed psychophysics from its century-long concentration on thresholds by showing how to measure sensory magnitude. I also thank my four coauthors for their long patience and continued cooperation as our project approached completion. We have written and rewritten nearly every sentence in this book, trying to achieve the homogeneity of style and level so often missed in multiauthored volumes, trying to make difficult data and concepts clear to the beginner. Our readers will decide how well we have succeeded in our goals.

B. S.

## ABOUT THE AUTHORS

### Thomas S. Brown

Professor Brown received his doctorate at Catholic University of America in 1962. He spent two years as a predoctoral fellow in the laboratory of H. Enger Rosvold at the National Institute of Mental Health, and followed this with a one-year postdoctoral fellowship in the laboratory of W. Ross Adey at the University of California at Los Angeles. He was director of the Neuropsychology Laboratory at Michael Reese Hospital in Chicago before joining the Psychology Department at DePaul University, where he holds the rank of Professor. He has published research in several areas and, in recent years, his work has examined behavioral changes resulting from hippocampal ablations. Another current research interest centers on the effects of early alcoholism.

### Leo Ganz

Professor Ganz received his doctorate from Austin H. Riesen at the University of Chicago in 1959 and did postdoctoral research with Lorrin A. Riggs at Brown University. Since then he has been a member of the Psychology Department at the University of California at Riverside, at New York University, and since 1967 at Stanford University. He is a member of the Society for Neurosciences and the Association for Research in Vision and Ophthalmology. He has published research articles and book chapters in the areas of perception, the development of perception, and the neurophysiological basis of perception.

### Bertram Scharf

Professor Scharf received his doctorate with S. Smith Stevens at Harvard University in 1958. Since then he has been a member of the Psychology Department at Northeastern University, except for leaves spent at the Technische Hochschule in Stuttgart, Germany, the Royal Ear, Nose, and Throat Hospital in London, the Institute for Sensory Research at Syracuse University, and most recently the Physiological Institute of the University of Helsinki. A Fellow of the Acoustical Society of America, he has published articles and book chapters mostly on hearing, but also on vision and touch. He is a coeditor of a memorial volume dedicated to S. S. Stevens.

### Joan Gay Snodgrass

Professor Snodgrass received her Ph.D. in psychology in 1966 from the University of Pennsylvania, with R. Duncan Luce. Since that time, she has been a member of the faculty of New York University. Her major research interests are in the areas of reaction time, storage and retrieval processes in visual long- and short-term memory, pattern recognition, and esthetics. She is presently working on a statistics book and a book on art and psychology.

### Ronald T. Verrillo

Professor Verrillo received his doctorate in psychology at the University of Rochester in 1958. He is coauthor of a book on the determinants of personal adjustment in blind adolescents which resulted from early research concerning the measurement of attitudes toward blindness. Since 1957 he has been at Syracuse University, where he is now Professor of Sensory Science in the Institute for Sensory Research. He spent a sabbatical year in the Department of Human Anatomy at Oxford University where he wrote, with Graham Weddell, a chapter on the neuroanatomy of pain. Although his primary research interest is cutaneous sensation, he has also published in the fields of vision and hearing. He is a member of the Acoustical Society of America, the Psychonomic Society, the Society for Neuroscience, and other professional societies.

## CONTENTS

# EXPERIMENTAL SENSORY PSYCHOLOGY

# 1

# INTRODUCTION

**Bertram Scharf**
**Northeastern University**

Human beings are bombarded constantly by myriad forms of physical energy—light, sound, air pressure, odors, temperature gradients, movement of clothing, gravity, radio waves, cosmic radiation, and so forth. We are aware of some of these forms of energy and can respond to them because we have sensory organs like the eye, ear, and nose which are highly sensitive to particular forms of energy. The simple responses evoked by simple forms of energy and how these responses depend on the stimulus and the subject are essentially the basic concerns of sensory psychology. How these relationships are measured under controlled laboratory conditions constitutes the major emphasis of the psychological study of sensation.

## THE SCOPE OF SENSORY PSYCHOLOGY

How dim is the dimmest star you can see? How much louder is the roar of a passing jet than the rumble of a trailer truck? These two kinds of questions represent nearly the whole content area of sensory psychology, for the first question concerns *thresholds* and the second question concerns *sensory magnitudes*. Thresholds are the limits of our sensory capacities—the dimmest light we can see, the softest sound we can hear, the lightest touch we can feel, the weakest odor we can smell, the mildest flavor we can taste. Besides these *absolute* thresholds, sensory psychology is concerned with *difference* thresholds, or *just noticeable differences*, that is, the smallest change in a light or sound or other stimulus that a person can detect. The measurement of absolute and difference thresholds under a great variety of conditions constitutes a large part of sensory psychology.

Almost all the rest of the field of sensory psychology is concerned with the measurement of sensory magnitude, which is the perceived or subjective strength of a stimulus such as a light or sound or odor. The concern is mostly not with absolute magnitude, but with relative magnitude: How much sweeter are 2 grams of sugar than 1 gram, or how much warmer is water at 90° than at 80°? Sensory magnitude depends not only on how much of a stimulus is presented to the observer, but also on what kind of stimulus is presented. For example, the sweetness of a gram of cane sugar is quite different from that of a gram of saccharin; a red light bulb and a yellow light bulb do not appear equally bright even though the two bulbs may be of equal physical intensity.

So, the study of sensory magnitude involves both finding out about the subjective impressions, or magnitudes, produced by different amounts of the same kind of stimulus (same sweetener or same color light) and finding out about the subjective magnitudes produced by different kinds of a stimulus (different sweeteners or different colored lights).

The study of both thresholds and sensory magnitudes depends on behavioral responses—verbal or motor—by an intact organism, most often by a human being. Thresholds can be measured with or without verbal instructions, but words are almost always used with humans in order to facilitate matters. To date, however, there is no nonverbal way of measuring sensory magnitude in nonhuman subjects.

This volume, then, is mostly about how we measure thresholds and sensory magnitudes in human beings and about the results obtained. The measurement procedures are often subsumed under the term *psychophysics*; coined by Gustav Fechner in the middle of the nineteenth century, psychophysics referred more generally to the relation between mind and body, between sensation and stimulus, and so in its orginal sense is congruent with the phrase *sensory psychology* as it is used here (see Chapter 2 for further discussion).

Although sensory psychology primarily deals with the input to a subject in the form of a stimulus and the output from the subject in the form of a behavioral response, sensory psychology is also deeply concerned with the events that occur between the input and output. Physiological data from the sensory organs (eye, ear, tongue, etc.) and from the sensory nervous systems are used whenever possible to elucidate the relations between stimuli and responses. Accordingly, this book is not only about psychophysical procedures and results, but also about the physiological (and psychological) interpretation of the interactions between stimulus and subject that lead to the obtained results.

The most important physiological event common to every sensory system is *sensory transduction*, which is the conversion of stimulus energy into neural energy. Without transduction, a stimulus cannot elicit a response, for every behavioral response is mediated via the nervous system. Transduction takes place within the receptor cells of the sensory organs, which, in effect, introduce the stimulus into the nervous system: They take energies which they are especially adapted to handle (for example, light to the eye, sound to the ear, and so on) and change those stimulus energies into a form of neural energy usable by the nervous system. Yet we know little about just how a stimulus, any stimulus, is transduced. We do know a great deal, however, about what happens to a stimulus in the sensory organs (especially in the eye and ear) before transduction, and we also know something about what happens in the sensory nervous systems after transduction.

As mentioned earlier, the sensory psychologist applies physiological data about sensory organs and the nervous system to the interpretation and understanding of measured stimulus-response relations. By definition, sensory psychologists themselves do not collect the physiological data. They perform "dry" experiments, using intact observers who make conscious responses. Sensory physiologists and physiological psychologists perform the "wet" experiments. They surgically invade the organism (which is almost always an animal), going inside the sensory organ or nervous system to tap limited mechanical, chemical, or electrical (the most usual) responses which can be correlated with stimulus properties. (Humans can be subjected to certain physiological procedures that do not require surgical intervention, such as the external measurements of electrical responses from the brain, called evoked potentials, or from the eye and ear, but such measurements still belong to the domain of sensory physiology.)

## THE BROAD GOALS OF SENSORY PSYCHOLOGY

### Sensation, not perception

Sensory psychology is a highly abstract approach to behavior. Simple stimuli and responses are substituted for the complex stimuli and responses of everyday life. Instead of trees, music, steaks, perfumes, and velvets, the sensory psychologist typically uses artificial stimuli like spots of light, pure tones (similar to the notes on a piano), sugar solutions, single odorants, and calibrated sandpapers. Responses are of the type, "I hear it," or "I don't hear it," "Solution A is sweeter than solution B," "This sheet of sandpaper feels twice as rough as that sheet of sandpaper." Even the simplest of these responses does require the subject to make a complex decision. And asking a subject to judge, for example, the roughness of paper requires that he ignore other properties of the paper such as hardness, temperature, and size. As soon as a human being is asked to make voluntary responses, the experiment becomes complex no matter how simple the stimuli and how restricted the responses. Despite this complexity, the intent of the experiment is to study a circumscribed aspect of a subject's experience produced by a simple stimulus.

Such experimental procedures and intentions are often contrasted with those employed in the study of perception. In studying perception the stimulus situation is often inherently complex; in studying sensation it is made as simple as possible. In perception the concern is with objects; in sensation stimulus properties are isolated and abstracted as much as possible from objects. In perception meaning is often a critical variable; in sensation every effort is made to avoid the attachment of meaning or significance to the sensory experience. Problems in perception include perceptual illusions (why does the moon appear larger when near the horizon than when on the meridian?), size constancy (why do objects look the same size no matter how far from the observer?), speech perception (how are the sounds of speech put together by the auditory system?).

Presented in this manner the distinction between sensation and perception may be clear, but in fact there is much overlap between the two. The distinction is semantic and therefore arbitrary. Some psychologists, like Gibson (1966), propose that all sensation is part of perception and that the sensory systems are true perceptual systems by which "an organism can take account of its environment and cope with objective facts [p. 6]."

## Functional relationships

This book takes a different, reductionist approach to sensation. First of all, it is felt, we must find out how simple stimulus properties are handled by each sensory system. Over and over again in this volume *functional relationships* will appear, either in the form of mathematical equations or X-Y plots. These functional relationships show how a response variable (e.g., the correct detection of a threshold stimulus or the numerical estimate of sensation magnitude) or a response-determined stimulus variable (e.g., the intensity at threshold or the temperature at which one substance feels as warm as another substance) is quantitatively related to a stimulus variable controlled by the experimenter. For example, the threshold or minimum energy needed to detect a light is plotted as a function of the wavelength of the light. The threshold intensities are determined by the subject's responses (e.g., the light intensity at which he reports seeing the light on 50 percent of the trials), and the wavelength is manipulated by the experimenter. Or the loudness of a sound is plotted against the physical intensity of a sound. The loudness value is based entirely on, for example, a numerical estimate by the subject and the intensity is varied by the experimenter. To a large extent, that is what sensory psychology is about, whether dealing with thresholds or sensory magnitude—a mapping out of functional relationships between response variables (the dependent variable) and stimulus variables (the independent variable) under a variety of controlled conditions. Students of perception are seldom able to specify the stimulus precisely enough to permit this kind of quantification. The functional relationships represent laws of behavior, invariant, unchanging relations between stimuli and responses; they comprise the major achievements and basic subject matter of sensory psychology.

## The relevance of sensory psychology

What purposes do such functional relationships serve? First and foremost, they tell us about lawful relationships in the world. And that is what science is all about, the uncovering of invariant, constant relationships, sometimes called laws. These functional relationships also guide us in understanding the implications of sensory physiological data and in the search for new physiological data.

The discoveries in sensory psychology have far-reaching practical applications as well. Indeed, much of the best research on hearing has been done in telephone laboratories, work in vision in the laboratories owned by photographic or lamp manufacturers, work on taste in the laboratories of food manufacturers, and so forth. Facts about how our sensory systems work are essential in designing the optimal color television system, or telephone network, or food mixture, as well as in lighting a room or fighting noise and odor pollution.

The other major use of the information gathered by sensory psychologists is in the diagnosis and treatment of sensory defects. Many of the common auditory and visual tests are based on techniques developed in the laboratory. This is especially true of the more sophisticated tests used in localizing, in the auditory system, the cause of impaired hearing or, in the visual system, the cause of blurred vision. Sensory psychologists also provide the data needed in alleviating sensory defects through devices such as hearing aids for the deaf and eyeglasses for the visually impaired. Furthermore, sensory data help guide corrective surgical operations. They are also essential in making possible the use of alternative sensory channels for getting around in the world, as in teaching the deaf to speak by means of visual stimuli or giving the blind information about their surroundings via pulses to the skin or sounds to the ear. Often what seems esoteric and difficult in sensory psychology is of great actual or potential practical importance.

## BRIEF HISTORICAL BACKGROUND OF SENSORY PSYCHOLOGY

Sensory psychology is as old as man's queries about himself. The Greeks and Romans posed questions and suggested answers about how we gain knowledge of the world around us. Some of their theories seem bizarre today, like the suggestion by ancient philosophers that the eye emits particles which mix with an emanation from the seen object to produce visual sensations. On the other hand, Aristotle's division of the senses into seeing, hearing, feeling, smelling, and tasting is still the basic way we categorize the senses. Modern sensory psychology—the study of thresholds and sensory magnitudes and the search for functional relationships—did not, however, begin until the nineteenth century with the work of E. H. Weber (1795–1878) and G. T. Fechner (1801–87). Fechner, the father of psychophysics, developed the methods that were used in finding out most of what we now know about sensory thresholds and equivalencies (subjective matches of sensory magnitude between dissimilar stimuli, such as between lights of different color). Wilhelm Wundt (1832–1920), who is sometimes called the father of experimental psychology, devoted much of his laboratory's work, the first psychology laboratory in the world, to the study of dark adaptation, color vision, sound perception, reaction time in the various senses, and other sensory topics.

Fechner and Wundt and many other nineteenth-century investigators did "dry" sensory psychology, working exclusively with human beings who made voluntary responses. Johannes Müller (1801–58) and H. von Helmholtz (1821–94) did "wet" sensory physiology, and Helmholtz discovered much of what we know about the basic functioning of the eye and ear. Among twentieth-century physiologists, G. von Békésy (1899–1972) greatly extended our understanding of the ear, and R. Granit (1900–), H. K. Hartline (1903–), and G. Wald (1906–) did the same for the eye. (All four men have received Nobel Prizes for their discoveries in sensory physiology.) The oustanding psychologist of the twentieth century to work on the senses was S. S. Stevens (1906–73), who spawned modern psychophysics by shifting the emphasis from the measurement of thresholds to the measurement of sensory magnitude. (Chapter 2 deals in some detail with the history of psychophysics.)

The key concept of sensory transduction, discussed earlier, first became clear in the twentieth century. This concept plus the knowledge gained about the nervous system in general has required a new approach to the age-old mind-body problem. It was this problem that Fechner tried to resolve in the nineteenth century, and which Stevens, among others, tried to dissolve in the twentieth. Neither Fechner nor Stevens succeeded; the basic question of what is meant by sensation and how it is related to mind remains with us, unsolved. The next section briefly reviews the history of the problem and relates it to modern sensory psychology.

### Mind-body dualism

Psychologists along with physiologists and philosophers of the nineteenth century usually made a clear distinction between mind and body. They inherited this dualism from Descartes via John Locke, Thomas Reid, and most of the other important philosophers of the seventeenth and eighteenth centuries. Mind was viewed as unextended, intangible, and unitary. Body was viewed as extended, that is, covering definable space, tangible, and composed of numerous discrete parts including skin, nerves, bones, and so forth. Body, part of the mechanical world of matter, made contact through the nerves with mind; the external world of body and matter was represented in mind as sensations. The Cartesian notion was that minuscule movements of objects around us are impressed on the nerves either directly via the skin or indirectly through the air. The nerves then transmit these movements and impress them on the soul, located somewhere in the brain, where they are experienced as sensations. According to this doctrine, stimulus movement or, in contemporary terms, stimulus energy remains the same right up to the point in the brain where contact is made with the soul or mind. Aristotle had treated the problem in somewhat the same manner, without referring to nerves. Generally, the notion seemed to prevail that within the body some aspect of the stimulus is propagated—form, according to Aristotle; motion, according to Descartes. David Hartley in 1749 suggested that the motion is vibratory and presented his theory of miniature vibrations, or *vibratiuncles*. As late as 1764, the Scottish philosopher Thomas Reid wrote of the inability of "anatomists or philosophers . . . to discover the nature and effects of [light], whether it produces a vibration in the nerve [Hartley's proposal], or the motion of some subtile fluid contained in the nerve [Descartes' proposal], or something different from either . . . [p. 146]."

### Sensory transduction

Not until around 1800 did the physiologists make it clear that the sensory organs do not transmit properties of the stimulus in the same form in which they arrive at the receptor. As we have already noted, the receptors transduce stimulus energy into nerve energy. Each organ is adapted to transduce a particular kind of stimulus energy—the eye, electromagnetic (light) energy; the ear, acoustic energy; the nose and tongue, chemical energy; the skin, mechanical, thermal, and chemical energy.

Of course, energy is actually transduced in the receptor cells of each sensory organ, which constitute only a small portion of the organ (see Chapter 3). Each whole sensory organ, however, is adapted to handle incoming energy efficiently and rapidly, thus permitting transduction to take place optimally. The particular kind of energy that a sensory organ handles best is called the *adequate stimulus*.

The concept of sensory transduction seemed to make little impression on the outlook of the nineteenth-century psychologists, who continued to differentiate between mind and body, limiting body to the same material world as objects. Their dualist position was mostly that of *psychophysical parallelism*: Mind parallels events in the body but does not interact with those events. (Descartes had believed that mind and body interact, but in the nineteenth century that view was mostly supplanted by the view that mind and body operate only in parallel.) It took a long time before psychologists were able and willing to incorporate into their thinking the idea that the interface between the outer world and inner organism is not in the brain but in the body's periphery, in the sensory organs where transduction takes place. Yet this concept made obsolete the distinction between mental and bodily processes. There is no essential difference between neural functions and other physiological functions. Sensory receptors transduce physical stimulus energy into another, very different form of energy whose effects can be spread throughout the nervous system and thence to the motor system. The philosophical dilemma of how the mind obtains knowledge about the material world could be bypassed when it became clear that the living organism operates with its own forms of electrochemical energy whose very organization may be the essence of consciousness and self-awareness. The organism, human and animal alike, could be seen as a unitary whole in which a stimulus triggers neural processes that lead to a series of other neural processes resulting in a response. The role of mind in this series becomes uncertain. Coupled with the failure of nineteenth-century psychology to solve the riddle of the mind (and the press for practical contributions from psychology to deal with the individual in mass society—contributions in the form of tests, therapies, educational procedures, advertising, etc.), this uncertainty led at the beginning of the twentieth century to the behaviorists' total rejection of introspection, of mind, and of the notion of sensation as an internal, personal event.

### Sensation as a discriminative response

An important goal of behaviorism was to redefine sensation and rid psychology of *introspection*, the method used in the nineteenth century and the early part of the twentieth century to study sensation. The subject "perceived within himself" and analyzed the subjective experience evoked by a stimulus, attempting to describe every facet of the experience. A good example is from a classic paper by E. G. Boring (1916) on the sensations he felt after a severed nerve in his left arm began to regenerate: ". . . sensations were felt in the lower arm. These sensations were of a pressury kind. There was perhaps slight pain; but the complex was almost completely one of pressures—deep and superficial. It is very much like a 'drawing-up' cramp without the pain, or like pins-and-needles without the pricks or tingle [p. 32]."

The behaviorists opposed this type of introspection because only the subject had access to what he was reporting, namely, the sensations in the mind. Why, they asked, deal with mind and sensation, which are internal events admittedly observable only by the introspecting subject, when one could deal with the later part of the sequence of neural events, that is, the response, which is observable to all? Introspection could at best give a glimpse of one part in the chain of stimulus-evoked events. By 1930 introspection had been discarded and, indeed, sensation and perception were getting little attention from American psychology. The goal of scientific psychology was no longer the study of mind but of behavior. Indeed, Watson's (1913) program for psychology was to predict and control behavior. Sensation and perception had not been discarded, but redefined as responses observable to all, rather than subjective events observable only to the introspecting subject. Nevertheless, the emphasis was on learning, on the modification of behavior. After all, it didn't really seem to matter what intervened between the stimulus and the response, so long as stimuli could be so manipulated as to allow the prediction and eventual control of responses.

Avoiding all reference to subjective experience, the behaviorists defined sensation as a discriminative response to a stimulus: If the subject can respond differently to each of two different stimuli, then the stimuli must evoke different sensations. By this definition, one need not ask the subject to say anything about the content of his experience—he has only to respond, usually verbally, sometimes manually. Indeed, the tendency has been to ignore the sensation as such. However, the response itself depends on intervening events. No matter how difficult to grasp intuitively, the fact remains that stimuli are transduced. Sensation refers to those events intervening within the observer between transduction and response. These events can be studied directly by the physiologist, but only in bits and pieces since he looks at only one part of the system at a time, often a part as minute as a single neuron. The psychologist looks at the response to which these events give rise, and from the nature of the response can infer much about the totality of the events.

Paradoxically, the early behaviorist approach to sensation amounted to a continuation of Cartesian dualism, of the distinction between mind and body. Behaviorism did not deny the possibility of subjective experience and consciousness, but treated them as irrelevant to the correlation between stimulus and response. The mind was left to reign in its own invisible world, while the body was observed responding to physical events. The concept of sensory transduction ought to have made this kind of dualism untenable. The only possible dualism in these matters is between neural events and stimulus events. Once stimulus events were shown to trigger neural changes in the sensory organs and nervous system, then mind could be viewed as an aspect of those same neural processes.

Sensation presents a special problem to the modern experimental psychologist. Rejecting any sort of introspection as a tool for analyzing and studying sensation, the behaviorists ignored the possibility of the subject making even simple reports about internal events and left us with only the discriminative response. If the presentation of a stimulus is followed by a constant change in the organism's behavior, or if the organism makes a different response to each of two different stimuli, then sensation has occurred. But the behaviorist identifies the sensation with the response, verbal or motor. Had the behaviorist admitted that the response implies a sensation, he would have still had to define sensation and probably been forced to reopen the whole question of mental events.

Identifying sensation with a discriminative response is hardly a sharp enough definition. All kinds of things, animate and inanimate, animal and vegetable, multicelled and single celled, make discriminative responses. A photocell responds to varying amounts of light by producing different amounts of electric current. A plant's direction of growth alters in response to a change in the source of its light. An amoeba moves toward or away from various chemicals. Defining sensation as a response was an attempt to rid psychology of the notion of sensation as an internal experience, which was the way philosophers had been viewing sensation for several thousand years, most explicitly since Descartes.

Despite behaviorism, sensation and response continue to be distinguished in the two major developments in psychophysics in the middle of the twentieth century, Stevens' formulation of the power law and signal detection theory. Sensation is viewed as an internal event which serves as the basis for a response by the subject, human or animal. The subject doesn't have to be able to talk about this internal event. Obviously, a cat or rat cannot; but even a human does not experience stimuli as something happening inside, but as external lights, sounds, and odors. Our inference about sensation does not depend on the subject's report. Between the stimulus and the response lies an organism whose complex nervous system distinguishes it from a photocell or an amoeba. Just how complex the apparatus intervening between stimulus and response must be in order to permit the sensational inference is not clear. That the human's nervous system is complex enough is clear. Associated with the complexity of the nervous system in which the stimulus is handled in the form of neural energy is the plasticity of the response. Whereas the photocell's response is limited to a single mode, animals and humans have a large number of possible response forms. To distinguish discriminative responses by photocells and amoebas from those by higher animals, we must include in the definition of sensation reference to the transduction of energy and the ensuing physiological events.

For sensation to take place, a stimulus must impinge on a sensory organ of a living organism, where it is transduced into neural energy and directed to an intact central nervous system. Given these structures, a discriminative response then implies sensation; physiological changes in the sensory organ and in the central nervous system must have mediated between stimulus and response. Since these conditions are met, for example, by the sleeping man who swats the feather applied to his arm, we must add a further condition. The physiological responses to the stimulus must occur in such a manner as to give the organism an opportunity to choose among a number of possible responses. (Choice need not imply free choice.)

What we are left with, then, is that a sensation is a complex of physiological events in an organized nervous system, which is triggered by a stimulus, and about which the organism can report by a discriminative response, verbal or motor. The response (aside from reflexes), however, must be under control of the intact organism, implying that the organism can choose whether and how to respond. To study sensation we need know nothing about the intervening physiological events in order to discover invariant relations between the stimuli and the reported sensation.

**Response or report?**

There are difficulties which are inherent in ascribing existential status to sensation as an internal event. The only way to observe these events, given present technology and understanding of the nervous system, is by the subject's report, which may be verbal or nonverbal. One issue surrounding the report of a perceptual experience is whether it should be treated as a report or as a response. Natsoulas (1967) has discussed this distinction. Depending on how one treats the subject's response, the interpretation of an experiment can be quite different. The problem is the old one of whether to accept subjective experience as proper scientific material. Up to now, we have been arguing that sensation precedes or is concomitant with most perceptual responses. Accordingly, the response can always or nearly always be treated as a report about the sensation.

The view that a response to a stimulus may be treated as a report about a sensation is attacked usually on two grounds. First, as such, it is a report about a private event to which only the reporter, the subject, has access. Second, this treatment seems to postulate a little man inside the head who sits watching what goes on and then reports about it. Proponents of the first objection do not deny that every response to a stimulus is preceded by sensory transduction. They claim that psychology need only correlate stimulus with response and should not concern itself with intervening variables such as sensation. However, a stimulus may give rise to a great variety of different responses, depending partly on instructions, partly on past experience, and so on. Nevertheless, analysis of these differing responses may reveal an invariant intermediary that correlates well with certain aspects of the subject's reports and with the experimenter's own experience when presented with the same stimulus. In psychophysical and perceptual studies, very often experiments are designed so as to elicit different kinds of responses to the same stimuli. Referred to as *converging operations*, such procedures allow the experimenter to compare one set of responses with another to see if there is some constant intermediary, the sensation, between the nearly invariant stimulus and the highly variable responses. For example, in one kind of experiment the subject may be asked to judge loudness either by assigning numbers to sounds or by adjusting the intensity of one tone until it sounds as loud as another. When both procedures measure the same internal event, then two tones which have been set equally loud are assigned the same numbers. Loudness, a property of a sensation, is assumed to be the invariant quantity that permits agreement between quite different procedures.

The objection that treating responses to stimuli as reports about internal events is like postulating a little man, a *homunculus*, who reports what the big man is doing and feeling, is almost irrelevant. Clearly, higher organisms have developed central processors into which a variety of information feeds from all parts of the body, including the sensory organs. The central processor uses this information to respond appropriately to its environment, internal as well as external. Although the central processor is only a part of the same system as the rest of the neural and physiological structures that constitute the organism, it nevertheless is capable of reporting ongoing or earlier events in other parts of the system. The functioning organism is a sequential process into which we can tap at various stages by instructions or experimental conditions. That the central processor, which is designed to organize and evaluate the incoming information, can also report verbally about that information is not surprising. After all, some behaviorists have claimed that thinking is subvocal speech. All the sensory psychologist does is ask the subject to think a little louder.

One could discuss interminably these mainly philosophical issues concerning dualism and transduction. Much of the basic controversy, however, has been put aside, not in a manner satisfactory to the rigorous philosopher, but well enough to permit a vast collection of data about sensation both before and after the advent of behaviorism. The following sections on the law of specific nerve energies and the attributes of sensation trace briefly the history of two other, better-defined problems in sensory psychology.

### Law of specific nerve energies

Acceptance of the concept of transduction in the early 1800s led to the empirical problem of how the properties of the stimulus are reflected in the nervous system. Stated in contemporary terms, the problem was how the nervous system codes the physical, external energy changes. First, however, there was the question of how the various senses were kept apart in the subject if all stimuli—sounds, lights, odors, tastes, etc.—were converted into similar kinds of nervous energy.

The first comprehensive and systematic attempt to handle these problems was Müller's *law of specific nerve energies*. Müller (1838) introduced the ten principles that constitute his law by pointing out that what is perceived "is indeed merely a property or change of condition of our nerves [in Herrnstein & Boring, 1965, p. 27]." He stated this more formally in his eighth principle: "The immediate objects of the perception of our senses are merely particular states induced in the nerves . . . [p. 33]." Whereas Descartes had in effect allowed the stimulus right into the brain, conducted there by the animal spirits along the nerves, Müller banished the stimulus to the sensory organ and gave the nerves their own particular states. So it was not the dichotomy between stimulus and sensation that was new, but the dichotomy between neural activity and stimulus.

Müller's main concern was the problem of sensory differentiation. He pointed out, as had Descartes some 200 years earlier (Descartes, 1638), that regardless of how stimulated, a nerve from a given sensory organ gives rise to the sensation corresponding to that organ. Pressure on the eye or an electrical pulse, as well as light, may give rise to seeing. On the other hand, depending on which sensory organ is stimulated, a given stimulus, such as a strong pressure or an electric current, gives rise to different sensations. Briefly, the nature of the sensation evoked by a stimulus depends on which sensory organ is stimulated and not how. Müller interpreted this fact as showing that a sensory organ transduces stimuli into energy peculiar to the particular nerve serving that organ. In other words, he surmised that each sensory system responds to stimuli in a different way, and that these differences tell us whether we are hearing, seeing, tasting, and so on. (Only much later, early in the twentieth century, did evidence refuting this hypothesis become available. In fact, all nerves fire in the same way by sending discrete pulses through the axons, as described in Chapter 3.)

Although he seemed to favor the view that the various nerves differed in themselves, Müller did equivocate, including in his seventh principle the following statement: "Either the nerves themselves may communicate impressions different in quality to the sensorium [brain], which in every instance remains the same; or the vibrations of the nervous principle may in every nerve be the same and yet give rise to the perception of different sensations in the sensorium, owing to the parts of the latter with which the nerves are connected having different properties [Herrnstein & Boring, 1965, p. 33]." Müller thus left open the possibility that the difference between, for example, seeing and hearing may depend primarily on which part of the brain is excited. For example, when the ear is stimulated, it in turn excites one part of the brain which is distinct from the part that is excited when the eye is stimulated.

Much earlier, Descartes (1638) came closer to the correct notion of brain localization as the basis for sensory differentiation. But he came to that notion from a false conception of nerve transmission. Descartes thought that animal spirits (which were "a certain very subtle wind, or rather a very quick and pure flame") conveyed the motions of the stimulus to the brain where sensation took place. The nerves only served to transmit the wind or flame whose motion would duplicate that of the stimulus. Since the same stimulus could give rise to different sensations depending on which sensory organ it excited, differences in the various sensations could not depend on properties peculiar to the different sensory nerves; the differences must depend on the places in the brain where the nerves terminate. Lacking the concept of transduction, Descartes came closer to the truth than did Müller for whom transduction proved to be somewhat misleading on this score.

After its formulation by Müller, probably the most respected physiologist of his time, the doctrine of the specificity of nerve function became current. Still, it was more than 20 years after Müller (1838) codified his law and nearly 50 years after Bell (1811) first alluded to the same ideas before Helmholtz (1860) resurrected Thomas Young's (1802) theory of three visual fibers corresponding to the three primary colors (see Chapter 7). Helmholtz (1863) carried the doctrine to an extreme when he suggested that each of the many thousands of pitches in hearing is mediated by its own neural fiber.

## Modern concepts of stimulus coding

Müller's law of specific nerve energies stated that the kind of sensory experience evoked by a stimulus depends not on the stimulus but on which part of the nervous system is activated. Müller limited himself, however, to distinguishing among the five major senses. Helmholtz later tried to explain how different kinds of a single type of stimulus to the same sensory organ leads to different sensory experiences, specifically how different wavelengths of light produce different colors and how different tonal frequencies produce different pitches. Today, we should say that both Müller and Helmholtz were wrestling with the problem of how stimuli are coded in the nervous system. How are stimulus properties like size, wavelength, sound frequency, chemical composition, temperature, and so forth represented in the nervous system? Put another way, how is information about a stimulus represented in the nervous system?

This problem is the central problem of empirical sensory physiology. When Müller and Helmholtz tackled the problem, relatively little was known about how nerves and neurons function. Since their time, it has been discovered that all neurons operate according to the all-or-none principle: Each neuron transmits a series of discrete but identical impulses (see Chapter 3). Consequently, the ways in which neural activity can code stimulus properties are severely limited. Nevertheless, we can distinguish at least four major codes, depending on (1) which neurons are activated, (2) the quantity of neural activity, (3) the temporal patterning of the nerve impulses, and (4) combinations of neurons that together form distinctive patterns of neural activity. These possible codes are by no means mutually exclusive; the nervous system may use all of them. Nor are they the only possible codes. They are, however, the simplest codes and receive much attention in this book.

### *Place code*

The place code is the heart of the law of specific nerve energies even though Müller was not sure whether the ultimate sensation depended on the kind of neural activity that reached the brain or on which part of the brain was activated. He was sure that which nerves a stimulus initially excites determine whether the result is seeing, hearing, smelling, tasting, or feeling. The place theory seemed to receive additional support when at the end of the nineteenth century it became clear that all neurons do the same thing, namely, pass along discrete impulses.

The place theory has worked well for sensory continua in which quality rather than quantity is the basic dimension, continua like color, pitch, auditory localization, line orientation. As described in Chapters 3 and 4, much evidence has accumulated to show that as a sound's frequency changes, different parts of the inner ear are maximally stimulated, and consequently, different sections of the auditory nerve are maximally excited. The experimental findings accord closely with Helmholtz' original place theory of pitch perception. Similarly, the eye has three different kinds of light-sensitive elements each of which responds best to lights of different wavelengths. (Again, Helmholtz was essentially correct.) Thus for both pitch and color, the sensory systems signal changes in the stimulus by responding maximally with different receptors (or combinations of receptors) and, therefore, with different neurons.

Evidence for a place code is found also at higher levels of the nervous system, not just at the receptors. For auditory localization, a place code appears to operate among those neurons which receive inputs from the two ears. Sounds arriving from one direction in space affect one group of neurons more than other groups; sounds from a different direction affect maximally another group of neurons. In seeing, line orientation appears to be coded at a still higher neural level. Located in the visual cortex are neurons that respond best to a line presented at one angle but hardly at all to the same line turned 90°.

Clearly, different neurons or groups of neurons can signal different stimulus properties and stimulus changes. And so place of excitation is an important, perhaps the most important, basis for stimulus coding in the nervous system. However, the place theory cannot account for all sensory phenomena. Even in hearing, the place theory of pitch perception leaves unexplained many data described in Chapter 4. Furthermore, for two of sensory psychology's major concerns, absolute threshold and sensory magnitude, place theory seems of little importance; quantity rather than locus of neural activity seems to be the basic stimulus code.

*Quantity of neural activity*

The notion is simple. The greater the activity elicited by a stimulus in the nervous system, the more easily it is detected or, once above threshold, the greater its sensory magnitude. Neural activity increases when more neurons fire and when they fire more often, thus yielding a larger total number of nerve impulses per second. Loudness, for example, is "usually attributed to the number of nerve impulses per second traversing the auditory nerve [Davis, 1959, p. 583]." But increasing stimulus intensity does not always result in more neural activity. Inhibitory mechanisms may reduce the neural response, even as stimulus magnitude increases. In the visual system, for example, increasing light intensity to the eye may result in a decrease in neural firing rate, not an increase (De Valois, Jacobs, & Jones, 1962). (The reader who may be uneasy at the idea that a reduction in neural activity could result in a stronger sensation should recall that although the image on the retina is upside down we do not see the world as upside down.)

*Temporal codes in the nervous system*

As noted, increased stimulus intensity usually causes neurons to fire more rapidly (at least over a limited range of stimulus intensities). Other changes in a stimulus may also alter the firing rate or the time intervals between successive nerve impulses. In the auditory system, the frequency of a tonal stimulus is often duplicated in the frequency of firing of individual neurons (see Chapter 4). More generally, in all the sensory systems, the longer a stimulus lasts, the slower each neuron's firing rate becomes; this decrease over time is called adaptation. On the whole, however, little is yet known about the relation between stimulus events and temporal patterns in the nervous system.

*Multineuron firing patterns*

Groups of fibers may be so orchestrated by the nature of incoming stimuli that their combined pattern of firing—that is, particular neurons firing in particular sequences—could serve as a cue to stimulus properties. Such codes have been suggested for taste and smell (see Chapter 3) as well as for pain (see Chapter 6).

Place, quantity, time, and pattern are four commonly proposed codes of stimulus properties, but neurons, once excited, function as complex networks that include feedback loops at most stages of the nervous system; neurons at a given level may inhibit each other (lateral inhibition) and neurons at a higher level in the nervous system may inhibit neurons at lower levels (efferent inhibition). The simple stimulus codes we have been discussing may turn out to play but a small role in the overall complexities of the sensory nervous systems.

*A modern psychophysical parallelism*

In a way, the search for neural events that mirror stimulus events is a contemporary form of the psychophysical parallelism of the nineteenth century. Instead of mind in parallel with body, the nervous system (body) is viewed as in parallel with, or correlated with, the stimulus. Unlike the inaccessible mind, both the physiological events of the body and the properties of the stimuli are observable and accessible. The basic assumption is that for every stimulus change to which an organism can respond there must be a parallel change in the nervous system. If a subject can discriminate blue from green, then something during and after sensory transduction must reflect the change from a blue stimulus to a green stimulus. As noted earlier and as shown in greater detail in later chapters of this book, sensory physiologists have uncovered many neural changes that parallel stimulus changes. Slowly but surely we are nearing solutions to the problem of stimulus coding in the nervous system.

While these strides are made in solving what may be called the body-stimulus problem, the classical mind-body problem remains as controversial as ever. We seem no closer to understanding how information in the nervous system is brought into awareness; we don't know with which neural events our sensory and perceptual experiences correspond. Perhaps the problems of awareness and personal experience will turn out, as the behaviorists claim, to be pseudoproblems, problems created by semantic ambiguities. However that may be, let us stress once again that the philosophical mind-body problem and even the physiological body-stimulus problem are of secondary importance to the working sensory psychologist. Of more immediate importance, for example, is the problem that seems first to have become apparent in the nineteenth century concerning the attributes of sensation.

**Attributes of sensation**

Although sensations are supposed to be simple, they can almost always be broken down still further into a number of properties, or *attributes*. A colored disc has hue, brightness, and saturation, as well as spatial extent, shape, distance, duration, and so on. A subject can make judgments about any one of these aspects, and so must be told which aspect to report on. For example, if you want to know when two tones at different frequencies are equally loud, you may ask the subject to adjust the intensity of one of them until it sounds as loud as the other. But how do you know that "equally loud" means the same thing to the subject as to you or as to other subjects? Perhaps he sets the tones to seem equally large in size (for sounds do have volume) or equally far away. Or if you want two lights to be set to be equal in saturation (richness of color), how can you know that the subject is not matching with respect to hue?

Külpe in the late nineteenth century suggested that a given sensory attribute can be distinguished from all others if it can be *independently varied* while the other attributes remain unchanged. (He also stressed that the attribute is inseparable from the sensation.) This principle means that the loudness of a tone can be changed while its pitch, volume, and other attributes are held constant. In fact, however, the principle doesn't work. In the auditory example, a subject does not report that only loudness changes while the other attributes remain fixed, since the stimulus changes necessary to vary loudness also affect other attributes. If, for example, intensity is increased, loudness will increase, but at the same time volume and density will change. Now, if both intensity and frequency are changed in an attempt to keep volume and density constant while loudness varies, the subject will report changes in pitch owing to the frequency changes. No combination of frequency and intensity changes will allow the subject to report changes only in loudness and in no other aspect of the sound.

**Independent invariance**

Stevens (1934) suggested that one attribute can be distinguished from all others if it can be kept constant while the others are varied. According to the principle of *independent invariance*, it is possible to manipulate a stimulus so that only one attribute is invariant. If a second purported attribute also remains invariant, then that other attribute differs from the first in name only. Using this guide, Stevens was able to eliminate several candidates for attribute status in hearing. For example, whenever the subject adjusted the intensity and frequency of a tone so as to keep "brightness" constant while changing loudness and pitch, he made the same adjustments as when he kept "density" constant. Brightness and density are therefore different names for the same attribute.

The combinations of intensity and frequency at which density is always the same map out a *constant-density function* when intensity is plotted as a function of frequency. This function is shown in Figure 1.1 along with the *constant-loudness*,

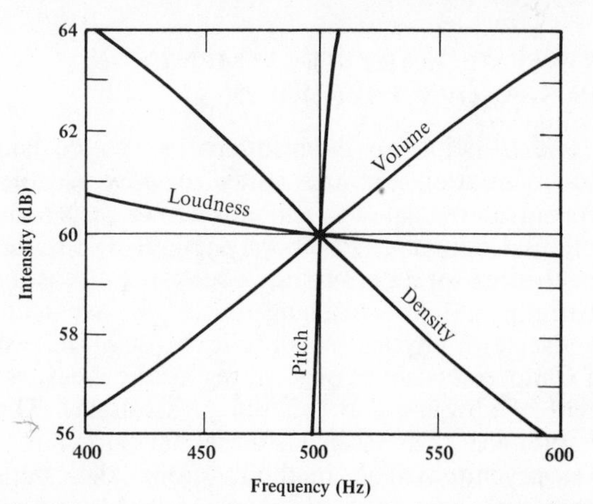


**Figure 1.1** Constancy functions for four tonal attributes. The standard tone has a frequency of 500 Hz and an intensity of 60 dB. Each curve gives the combinations of intensities and frequencies at which the given attribute remains constant. (From Stevens, 1934.)

*constant-pitch*, and *constant-volume functions*. According to the density function, the subject judged a 64-decibel, 405-Hertz tone as being equal in density to a 60-dB, 500-Hz tone and also to a 56-dB, 595-Hz tone (see Chapter 4 for explanation of these units of measurement). In other words, all these combinations of intensity and frequency lie on the constant-density curve. For loudness to be constant, the subject required the 405-Hz tone to be set to 60.5 dB and the 595-Hz tone to 59.5 dB. Thus when density was judged equal, loudness was not equal. Similarly, volume and pitch have very different curves from density, so that only density remained constant or invariant when intensity and frequency were varied along the constant-density curve. Each of the other attributes was invariant when the tone was varied in the way indicated by the appropriate curve. Stevens' subjects could generate only four different curves corresponding to four different attributes of pure tones. If intensity and frequency were varied along a fifth curve, different from any of the four in Figure 1.1, then no sensory attribute would remain invariant. Hence, there are only four independent attributes of pure tones whose intensity and frequency are varied.

Boring (1937) generated a set of constant-sensation curves for a light stimulus. Brightness, hue, and saturation are the three attributes that can be held independently invariant by the appropriate manipulation of a light's wavelength and intensity.

## CONTEMPORARY TREATMENT OF SENSORY PSYCHOLOGY

The principle of independent invariance laid the foundation for the study of how sensory attributes are related to stimulus variables. Nearly half of Chapter 2, Psychophysics, discusses the procedures for determining a scale for a sensory attribute and for matching that subjective scale to a scale of physical magnitude. Most of the rest of Chapter 2 is about procedures for the measurement of absolute and difference thresholds. The chapter also reviews the historical development of the psychophysical methods from the mid-nineteenth century until today. Thus this second chapter presents much that is basic to all of sensory psychology, for it tells how experiments on every aspect of sensory psychology are carried out, what their rationale is, and what theories stand behind them.

As has been repeatedly emphasized, sensory psychology attempts to incorporate physiological data about the sensory organs and the nervous system. The twentieth century has seen a huge increase in those data, much of it still to be assimilated and made meaningful. The third chapter is therefore about the biology of the sensory systems. It gives the basic information on the nervous system in general, and then on each of the sensory systems in turn. No attempt is made there to relate the physiology of the sensory systems to the results of psychophysical measurements. Instead, the basis is laid for understanding the many physiological references and interpretations that appear in later chapters.

After the general treatments of methodology and biology, the five senses as understood in contemporary sensory psychology are treated in four separate chapters. Each chapter deals with the problem of defining the stimulus, classifies the sensory attributes, provides the information on thresholds and sensory magnitude—how they are measured in the specific sensory system and what factors affect them. As in every mature science, many of the problems so important during the development of the field—in this instance, the mind-body problem, the definition of sensation, introspection, independent invariance, scales of measurement, and so on—seem to have evaporated. This is so because scientists adopt certain norms, a way of looking at problems, and then set about obtaining the facts as best they can. And if the assumptions that underlie the search lead to interesting and valid data, then the arguments about those assumptions are all but forgotten. Hence, this book is mostly about the facts of sensory psychology, and about how those facts were collected and analyzed in hearing, feeling, tasting, smelling, and seeing.

# REFERENCES

**Bell, C.** *Idea of a new anatomy of the brain: Submitted for the observation of his friends.* London: Privately printed, 1811.

**Boring, E. G.** On how the discrimination of two points may be mediated by deep sensibility. *Quarterly Journal of Experimental Physiology*, 1916, **10**, 1–95.

**Boring, E. G.** Isochromatic contours. *American Journal of Psychology*, 1937, **49**, 130–34.

**Davis, H.** Excitation of auditory receptors. In J. Field (Ed.), *Handbook of physiology:* Section 1. *Neurophysiology*. Vol. 1. Baltimore: Williams & Wilkins, 1959. Pp. 565–613.

**Descartes, R.** *La dioptrique*. Leiden, 1638.

**De Valois, R. L., Jacobs, G. H., & Jones, A. E.** Effects of increments and decrements of light on neural discharge rate. *Science*, 1962, **136**, 986–88.

**Fechner, G. T.** *Elemente der Psychophysik*. Leipzig: Breitkopf und Härtel, 1860. (Translated by H. Adler, New York: Holt, Rinehart & Winston, 1966.)

**Gibson, J. J.** *The senses considered as perceptual systems*. Boston: Houghton Mifflin, 1966.

**Hartley, D.** *Observations on man, his frame, his duty, and his expectations*. London, 1749.

**Helmholtz, H. von.** *Handbuch der physiologischen Optik*. Vol. II. Leipzig. 1860. (Translated by J. P. C. Southall, *Helmholtz' treatise on physiological optics*. Vol. II. Rochester, N.Y.: Optical Society of America, 1924–25.)

**Helmholtz, H. von.** *Die Lehre von den Tonempfindungen*. Brunswick, 1863. (Translated by A. J. Ellis, *Sensations of tone*. New York: Dover, 1954.)

**Herrnstein, R. J., & Boring, E. G.** *A source book in the history of psychology*. Cambridge, Mass.: Harvard University Press, 1965.

**Müller, J.** *Handbuch der Physiologie des Menschen für Vorlesungen*. Vol. II. Coblenz, 1838.

**Natsoulas, T.** What are perceptual reports all about? *Psychological Bulletin*, 1967, **67**, 247–72.

**Reid, T.** *An inquiry into the human mind on the principles of common sense*. Edinburgh, 1764.

**Stevens, S. S.** The attributes of tones. *Proceedings of the National Academy of Sciences*, 1934, **20**, 457–59.

**Watson, J. B.** Psychology as the behaviorist views it. *Psychological Review*, 1913, **20**, 158–77.

**Young, T.** On the theory of light and colours. *Philosophical Transactions of the Royal Society of London*, 1802, **92**, 18–21.

# 2

# PSYCHOPHYSICS

**Joan Gay Snodgrass**
**New York University**

> Tarzan of the Apes paused to listen and to sniff the air. Had you been there you could not have heard what he heard, or had you you could not have interpreted it. You could have smelled nothing but the mustiness of decaying vegetation, which blended with the aroma of growing things.
>
> The sounds that Tarzan heard came from a great distance and were faint even to his ears; nor at first could he definitely ascribe them to their true source, though he conceived the impression that they heralded the coming of a party of men. . . .
>
> As the distance closed between him and those he went to investigate, his keen ears cataloged the sound of padding, naked feet and the song of native carriers as they swung along beneath their heavy burdens.

Edgar Rice Burroughs (1929, pp. 8–9) thus describes in *Tarzan at the Earth's Core* the responses of a remarkable subject whom the modern psychophysicist would be pleased to study.

Tarzan's first responses, as described by Burroughs, were those we refer to as *detection* and *discrimination*: He detected sounds and smells which at first he could not recognize, and he discriminated the faint smells of the column of men from that of decaying vegetation. His second responses were those we classify as *recognition*. As the distance between him and the column of men decreased, he was able to recognize the sounds of padding, naked feet and the songs of the native carriers. And if we can assume that he made judgments of the distance separating him from the column of men, his final responses would be those we call *scaling*. These are illustrations of the four types of responses—detection, discrimination, recognition, and scaling—that concern psychophysics.

*Psychophysics* is a group of methodologies, developed and refined over the last one hundred years, for measuring the effect of some aspect of a stimulus on some aspect of an observer's response. The word *psychophysics* owes its derivation to the attempt to measure the relation between the psychological and the physical. Traditionally, psychophysics has been concerned with stimuli for which relatively unambiguous physical measures exist, such as lights of given intensities or tones of fixed

Much of the organization and many of the concepts of this chapter were developed through conversations with A. Charles Catania. I am indebted to both Professor Catania and to Professor R. Duncan Luce for the many constructive suggestions and comments they made on an early draft of this chapter.

frequencies. Certain well-defined responses to these stimuli are measured to determine whether the subject detects the presence of the stimulus, knows what the stimulus is, can determine whether it differs from a second stimulus, or can judge how much it differs. The first question, whether the stimulus is there, is the problem of detection; the second question, what the stimulus is, is the problem of recognition; the third question, whether the stimulus is different from a second stimulus, is the problem of discrimination; and the fourth question, how different this stimulus is from that one, is the problem of scaling. Psychophysical measurements are often summarized in a function that relates psychological magnitudes to physical magnitudes of stimuli—the *psychophysical function*. Psychological magnitude is the subjective intensity of sensation evoked by a stimulus.

Despite the emphasis on physical stimulus measurement, some of the most interesting applications of psychophysical methods have been to stimuli for which no obvious physical measures exist. Suppose one wants to measure the degree of perceived complexity of some randomly constructed figures. Presumably, certain physical characteristics of these figures determine their perceived complexity, but it is not clear which ones are important, or how the subject combines them. The psychophysicist might ask subjects to scale the complexity of the figures, and then look for those physical characteristics of the figures that show the largest correlation with the subjects' judgments. In this manner, psychophysical methods may be used to discover the physical measure most appropriate for the attribute under study—in this case, complexity.

What, however, if the attribute were the degree of excellence of the music of various composers? One could ask knowledgeable people, such as musicians, to rate the excellence of the composers' music, and from these responses construct a psychological scale for excellence of music. However, it seems unlikely that any physical measure of the music would be lawfully related to the excellence scale. This last case is an example of *psychological scaling*, which concerns scaling of stimuli, objects, or events for which no physical measure presently exists or is likely to exist; *psychophysical scaling* is scaling of stimuli, objects, or events for which physical measures do exist.

Psychophysical responses may take a number of different forms. In detection, discrimination, and recognition, the subject makes one of several discrete responses to each stimulus presentation. In detection, it is one of two responses: Yes, I detect the stimulus, or No, I do not detect the stimulus. In discrimination, the response may be either one of two—the second of two stimuli is greater or less than the first—or one of three—the second stimulus is greater than, equal to, or less than the first. In recognition, the set of responses is usually the same size as the set of stimuli, so that the response may be one of $n$ responses, where $n$ represents number of stimuli. In all these cases, the experimenter's most usual response measure is *estimated response probability*, defined as the number of responses of type $R$ made to stimulus $S$, divided by the total number of responses made to stimulus $S$.

In scaling, responses may be *discrete*, as in *category scaling* in which the subject categorizes each stimulus into one of $n$ categories, or responses may include a very large undefined set, as in *magnitude scaling* in which the subject assigns any positive number to each stimulus presentation. Here, the measure used is not response probability, but the mean or median response to each stimulus. In category scaling, the categories are assigned numbers, which are then averaged.

One can determine not only which response a subject makes to a stimulus, but also how long it takes him to make that response. The measure of response time is usually referred to as *reaction time* or *response latency*. Although reaction time can be considered a type of psychophysical response, the reaction-time experiment developed historically as an area apart from psychophysics until the early 1900s, when Cattell (1902) suggested that reaction time, rather than response probability, be used to measure subjective stimulus differences.

Subjects in a psychophysical experiment need not be humans. Animals may be trained to make one response in the presence of a stimulus and to make a different response in its absence. These responses, which correspond to saying yes and no in a detection experiment, are established in animals by training with appropriate reinforcement contingencies. Blough (1956) has used such a procedure to study the course of dark adaptation in the pigeon. Responses corresponding to those of discrimination or recognition may similarly be conditioned in animals.

It is less obvious how to train animals to emit responses indicating magnitude of stimulus differences or ratios; in humans we take advantage of well-established number habits in order to scale stimuli, while no such response repertoire exists for animals. However, advances have been made in the use of scaling responses in animals (e.g., Catania, 1970; Herrnstein & van Sommers, 1962).

## HISTORY OF PSYCHOPHYSICS AND REACTION TIME

Because of its one-hundred-year history and its quantitative approach to response data, psychophysics is considered one of the most exact and least mentalistic disciplines in psychology. However, its founder, Gustav Theodor Fechner (1801–87), had something quite different in mind when he developed his theories. Fechner, a physicist turned philosopher, was disturbed by science's materialistic view of man and the universe. Fechner's mission was to develop a philosophy that viewed the universe in terms of its consciousness as well as its matter. To this end, he argued for the mental life of plants and, more important for psychology, developed methods to relate mind to matter. Specifically, he proposed a way of relating an increase in the physical intensity of a stimulus to the corresponding increase in mental intensity.

Because Fechner knew that a scientific world committed to materialism would be convinced of his philosophy only by empirical results, he set out to develop methods of empirically measuring psychological responses to physical stimuli and of treating the results mathematically. He developed the three classical psychophysical methods, used them in experiments in different sense modalities, and from the results of his experiments and those of others derived the law bearing his name, which gives the form of the psychophysical function. The publication in 1860 of his book, *Elemente der Psychophysik,* describing his researches, marks the founding of psychophysics.

Fechner's three methods—the method of limits, the method of constant stimuli, and the method of adjustment—dealt with the measurement of thresholds, both the *absolute threshold* (detection) and the *difference threshold* (discrimination). The absolute threshold is defined as the magnitude of the stimulus that is detected 50 percent of the time. The difference threshold is defined as the magnitude of the difference betweeen two stimuli that is detected 50 percent of the time.

The second great contributor to psychophysics was Wilhelm Wundt (1832–1920). Generally regarded as the founder of experimental psychology, Wundt set up the first formal psychological laboratory in 1879 in Leipzig. Out of his laboratory came a voluminous amount of experimental research which he eventually published in his own journal, the *Philosophische Studien.* Wundt believed that the study of a living system from the outside is physiology, but the study of the system from the inside is psychology. Thus his psychology was based on study from the inside, or *introspection.* His students used introspection to analyze perceptions into individual components or sensations, to analyze and time mental processes, and to analyze attention and emotion. Wundt's experiments on the timing of mental events hold an important place in the history of reaction time. But before considering these experiments, we will return to the late eighteenth century to examine the beginnings of the reaction-time experiment.

The reaction-time experiment was born in the astronomer's observatory rather than in the psychologist's laboratory. In 1796, Maskelyne, the head astronomer at the Greenwich observatory, dismissed his assistant, Kinnebrook, because the latter was found to have observed the transit of stars almost a second later than his superior. At that time, astronomers employed what was known as the eye-and-ear method for recording the exact instant of a star's transit across one of the parallel cross wires of the reticle of the telescope. The task of the observer was to record, to the nearest tenth of a second, the time a particular star crossed a particular cross wire of the telescope.

Boring (1950) describes the eye-and-ear method as follows:

> The observer looked at the clock, noted the time to a second, began counting seconds with the heard beats of the clock, watched the star cross the field of the telescope, noted and "fixed in mind" its position at the beat of the clock just before it came to the critical wire, noted its position at the next beat after it had crossed the wire, estimated the place of the wire between the two positions in tenths of the total distance between the positions, and added these tenths of a second to the time in seconds that he had counted for the beat before the wire was reached [p. 135].

Although this was an exceedingly complicated judgment, it was supposed to be accurate to within one- or two-tenths of a second, so that an error as large as Kinnebrook's was intolerable.

There the matter rested until Bessel, the astronomer at Königsberg, noticed an account of the Kinnebrook affair in an astronomical journal of that day. Bessel decided to determine whether such discrepancies in personal observation times might exist between more practiced observers. Accordingly, in 1820 he compared his transit times with those of another astronomer, Walbeck, at the observatory at Königsberg. Bessel found, much to his astonishment, that he observed transit times to be more than a second earlier, on the average, than did Walbeck. In light of this large discrepancy between two highly practiced observers, Bessel compared himself with other astronomers at every opportunity and repeatedly found differences in observation times. There seemed no way of compensating for this error by making changes in the observational technique, for each astronomer was convinced that it would be impossible for him to observe differently. Instead, Bessel was led to develop a computational correction for the discrepancies known as the *personal equation*, whereby every astronomer's observations could be related, in terms of personal error, to every other.

The development of the chronograph around 1850 provided a more accurate means of recording star transits and, more important for psychology, of measuring the *absolute error* of observation. The chronograph had one pen for recording time in seconds on a continuously moving roll of paper. The observer pressed a key at the instant of star transit, causing a second pen to make a mark on the paper. The transit time was then read from the chronograph record. To measure the absolute error, an artificial star was produced whose transit time was known, and the time of the observer's key-press could be compared with the true transit time.

Two types of experiments were carried out—the first concerned with synchronous responding and the second with what we now call reaction time. In the first, the observer was instructed to respond at the instant the star crossed the cross wire; in the second, the observer was instructed to wait until the star was bisected by the cross wire and then respond. Sometimes he was prevented from anticipating by having the portion of the field to the left of the cross wire covered, so that he saw the star only when it emerged on the other side. The second type of judgment, reaction time, was found to be less variable than synchronous responding.

The astronomers soon found that errors of observation could be reduced and almost eliminated by more automatic ways of recording star transits, and the problem of measuring observation errors was taken up by the early psychologists. They focused on two problems: judgments of simultaneity between two sense modalities, studied via the *complication experiment,* and reaction time, the problem we now consider.

The first use of the simple reaction-time experiment is usually attributed to Hermann von Helmholtz (1821–94), a physicist and a physiologist who contributed a great deal to our knowledge of sensation and perception. In 1850, Helmholtz conceived the idea of using reaction time to measure the speed of nerve conduction. By stimulating the skin with electric shock at various parts of the body and measuring the time between stimulation and a motor response, he calculated the speed of human nerve transmission to be about 60 meters per second. However, because the times were so variable, and because sometimes the reaction times were faster to stimulation of parts of the body farther from the brain than those closer to the brain, he eventually abandoned the method and the figure. (Helmholtz' measurements of the conduction time in the motor nerves of the frog were more consistent and have since been confirmed.)

It also became clear that reaction time was sensitive to a number of other variables, such as stimulus intensity, sensitivity of the stimulated part to the stimulus, the relationship of the stimulated part to the required response, and so forth. Furthermore, the simple reaction time was so long and so variable that it obviously could not reflect a simple redirection of the nerve impulse from sensory to motor nerves, but must include considerable central processing time.

To exploit the possibility of timing central processes by the reaction-time method, the Dutch physiologist Donders (1818–89) devised several situations, differing in the complexity of the inferred mental processes, and attempted to time these processes. The first was that of simple reaction time, in which a single response is required for a single stimulus. He called this the *a-reaction* and assumed its time was the sum of stimulus-input, central processing, and motor response times. He saw no way to disentangle the separate times of these three processes.

He next introduced discrimination and motor choice into the simple-reaction-time situation by presenting several different stimuli and having the subject respond to each of them with a different motor response. He called this the *b-reaction;* today we call it *choice reaction time.*

Finally, Donders attempted to eliminate response choice from the b-reaction by presenting several different stimuli, but having the subject respond to only one of them with a single motor response. He called this the *c-reaction.* Thus, the a-reaction involves the simplest processes, the b-reaction the most complex, and the c-reaction the next most complex. Donders lettered the responses in the order in which they were investigated in his laboratory, rather than in order of increasing complexity. By assuming that each of the situations involves the insertion of the process not included in the simpler situation, he proceeded to time mental processes by subtracting the time for the simpler response from that for the more complex one. Thus, b − a = discrimination time, and b − c = response-choice time.

The validity of this subtraction method rests on obtaining reliable and positive differences between pairs of responses, and on certain assumptions about the inserted processes. Some of these assumptions were questioned by Wundt, who argued that the c-reaction included both discrimination and choice, since the subject had to choose between responding and not responding. In order to eliminate choice completely, Wundt developed the *d-reaction.* Several stimuli were presented and the subject made the same response to each one, but only after he had identified the stimulus. Wundt felt that the difference between a and d times would yield discrimination time, uncontaminated by choice.

However, as with Donders' reactions, the validity of the d-reaction is based on finding a reliable positive difference between d- and a-reactions. Although early results were encouraging, it was soon found that for many subjects the two times were almost equal. Other workers pointed out that there was no way to ascertain whether the subject had in fact identified the stimulus before responding, since he made the same motor response to all stimuli. Eventually, the d-reaction fell into disrepute, and the whole subtraction method was abandoned.

Despite the failure of the subtraction method, the simple or a-reaction and the choice or b-reaction have been useful as psychophysical responses. As we shall see, choice reaction times bear a logical and coherent relationship to stimulus differences, and simple reaction times are lawfully related to stimulus intensity.

Having briefly reviewed the history of psychophysics and reaction time, we next describe the psychophysical methods separately under two major headings: Thresholds and Scaling. The threshold section considers detection and discrimination and describes Fechner's three classical psychophysical methods, as well as two modern methods. The scaling section considers the problem of recognition, redefined as nominal scaling, and ordinal, interval, and ratio scaling. Recognition is a relatively new problem area in psychology and as such uses somewhat distinct methodologies and data analyses. The scaling of subjective intensity on an interval or ratio scale was the problem Fechner thought he solved by using the data of discrimination to measure indirectly the magnitude of sensation. In the scaling section, Fechner's indirect method is contrasted with the direct method of magnitude estimation. The role of reaction time as a psychophysical response measure is discussed in each section.

## THRESHOLDS

The environment surrounding us is replete with stimuli of which we are not commonly aware. The ticking of the watch on our wrist is usually inaudible to us, although if we bring the watch to our ear we can easily hear its ticking. This is an example of an absolute threshold, which we have exceeded by moving the source of the sound close to our ear. On the dark background of a midnight sky, the faint light of the stars is visible, but when the background is brightened by the sun, the light of the stars is no longer noticeable. This is an example of a difference threshold, which changes with changes in background. We go into a supermarket and pick up one melon and then another, in the attempt to identify the heavier one. Or we might smell them in succession and attempt to pick the one with the more desirable aroma. Whether we can tell them apart accurately or not depends on our difference thresholds for weight and for smell. The older term for threshold is *limen,* from which such terms as *subliminal perception* are derived.

Modern psychophysicists view detection and discrimination as virtually identical. This modern view maintains that in both detection and discrimination there is a background to which an increment is added: In detecting the ticking of a watch, the background is incidental noise in the room and internal noise within the observer generated by random neural activity; in the case of the stars, it is the dark night or bright daylight sky plus the internal noise.

The classical methods, on the other hand, treat absolute and difference thresholds as separate processes, and measure them with separate procedures. Determining the difference thresholds by one of the classical methods is illustrated not by the star problem, but by the problem of picking the heavier or more odorous melon, or determining whether the oboe player in a symphony orchestra played the same note twice in a row. In detection a single stimulus is presented against some sort of background (whether introduced by the experimenter or assumed to be an intrinsic part of the observer), while in discrimination two stimuli, distinct either temporally or spatially, are presented and the two stimuli are compared by the observer with respect to some attribute.

### Detection

There are two questions in detection. The first, an empirical one, is What are the limits of sensitivity of man? The second, a theoretical one, is What accounts for these limits?

The answer to the first question is that man is not infinitely sensitive. The eye, for example, is sensitive to only a very narrow band of the total spectrum of electromagnetic radiation, and within that band of visible light energy are regions of energy large enough to measure but not large enough to see.

In answer to the second question, the concept of a threshold or barrier imposed by some physiological limit has traditionally been invoked to account for the lower limit of sensitivity. However, the threshold is a statistical rather than an *all-or-none* phenomenon. If a stimulus is presented a number of times at the same fixed intensity near threshold, on some proportion $p$ of the trials a subject will report a sensation, and on the rest of the trials he will report no sensation. There is no single intensity below which he never reports a sensation and above which he always reports one. In the classical psychophysical methods, the intensity at which $p = 0.5$ is taken as the absolute threshold. The three classical methods are the method of limits, the method of constant stimuli, and the method of adjustment.

#### *The method of limits*

The method of limits (also known as the *method of minimal changes*) was favored by Wundt because the subject knew the order in which the stimuli were presented and could thereby concentrate on his perception. The subject reports either yes he perceives the stimulus or no he does not in response to each stimulus presentation. In the *ascending* method of limits, the stimulus intensity is set far enough below the absolute threshold so that it is never detected, and it is then increased in small steps until the subject detects the stimulus. In the *descending* method of limits, the stimulus intensity is set far enough above the threshold so that it is always detected, and it is decreased in small steps until the subject no longer detects it. The threshold on each ascending series is the midpoint between the intensity that elicited the last no response and the intensity that elicited the first yes response. On each descending series, it is the midpoint between the last yes and the first no response. For example, if on a descending series the subject says yes at an intensity of 6 and no at an intensity of 5, his threshold on that series is 5.5; if on an ascending series the subject says no at an intensity of 6 and yes at an intensity of 7, his threshold is 6.5. Typically, ascending and descending series are alternated, and the mean of the thresholds of all the series is taken as an estimate of the absolute threshold.

Because of the systematic nature of the method, the subject knows that the stimulus intensity is being either increased or decreased on every trial. Although Wundt believed this to be an advantage, others have criticized the method on exactly that ground. Knowing the stimulus-presentation schedule, the subject may commit one of two errors: the error of *habituation,* a tendency to continue reporting that he perceives the stimulus in a descending series (or reporting that he does not in an ascending series); or the error of *expectation,* a tendency to change his response from yes to no (or vice versa) after a certain number of stimulus presentations. Whether these two types of errors cancel each other out can be determined by comparing the mean threshold or limen for the ascending series (*AL*) to its value for the descending series (*DL*). If the AL is greater than the DL, the error of habituation is probably greater than the error of expectation. If the DL is greater than the AL, then the converse is probably true.

The staircase method introduced by von Békésy (1960) is a modified method of limits. In this method, used mostly in hearing experiments (see Chapter 4), the subject is presented a repeated stimulus (generally a pure tone) which automatically decreases in intensity whenever he presses a button signifying that he hears the tone, and increases in intensity when he fails to press the button. The method is widely used to track the threshold as a function of frequency. This is accomplished by slowly increasing the frequency of the tone during the threshold determinations.

*The method of constant stimuli*

The method of constant stimuli differs from the method of limits in that stimulus intensities are presented randomly rather than in a regular order. Several stimulus intensities are selected in the vicinity of the absolute threshold so that the stimulus at the lowest intensity is never detected and the stimulus at the highest intensity is always detected. The stimuli are presented at least ten times at each intensity in a random order; thus the subject has no idea which intensity will be presented on a given trial. The relevant data from such an experiment are the proportion of trials ($p$) on which the subject reported detecting the stimulus at each intensity. The psychometric function, a plot of $p$ against stimulus intensity, summarizes the data.

Figure 2.1 represents a hypothetical psychometric function for visual detection, in which a normal ogive (the cumulative of the normal distribution) has been fitted to the data points. The absolute threshold is taken as that stimulus intensity for which $p = 0.5$, which in this example is approximately 9.4. Usually, for no intensity does the subject respond yes on exactly 50 percent of the trials. The threshold is then located by linear interpolation between the closest point below 50 percent and the closest one above 50 percent. Other, more elegant statistical methods are also available (see Guilford, 1954, Chapter 6).

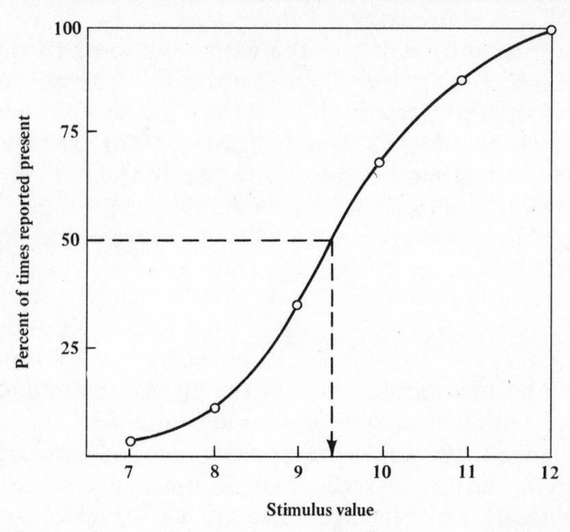


**Figure 2.1** A hypothetical psychometric function for absolute detection. The value of the absolute threshold, indicated by the arrow, is found graphically to be approximately 9.4. (From Underwood, 1966.)

*The method of adjustment*

The third classical method is the method of adjustment, also called the *method of average error.* In contrast to the other two methods, the subject, rather than the experimenter, controls the stimulus. The subject is given some device, such as a knob, for controlling stimulus intensity, which he adjusts until he just barely perceives the stimulus. This is a difficult judgment since, as we have seen, the threshold is a statistical, not an all-or-none, phenomenon. For this reason, the method of adjustment is rarely used to determine the absolute threshold. Indeed, it was developed specifically to compare two stimuli and is important in measuring discrimination.

## Discrimination

In the typical discrimination experiment, two stimuli in temporally or spatially discrete positions are presented, and the subject's task is to say whether the second or *variable* stimulus is greater than, equal to, or less than the first or *standard* stimulus. In some experiments no equality judgment is permitted.

The two quantities of interest are the *point of subjective equality (PSE),* the value at which the variable is perceived to be equal to the standard, and the value of the *just noticeable difference (jnd)* between the standard and the variable. The jnd, or *difference limen (DL),* is defined as that difference which is noticed 50 percent of the time. The method of calculating the jnd depends on which of the three classical psychophysical methods is used to collect the data.

*The method of limits*

A task in temporal discrimination is used to illustrate the method of limits. The subject is presented a first stimulus of constant duration, called the standard, and a second stimulus of variable duration, called the variable. He then indicates whether the variable appears shorter than, equal to, or longer than the standard. For ascending trials, the variable is initially set at a value that

**Table 2.1 Example of the Determination of the DL for Temporal Discrimination by the Method of Limits (Standard = 0.4 sec; ↓ = Ascending Trial; ↑ = Descending Trial)**

| Variable (sec) | Trials | | | | | | | | | | | | | | | |
|---|---|---|---|---|---|---|---|---|---|---|---|---|---|---|---|---|
| | ↓ | ↑ | ↓ | ↑ | ↓ | ↑ | ↓ | ↑ | ↓ | ↑ | ↓ | ↑ | ↓ | ↑ | ↓ | ↑ |
| .20 | < | | | | | | | | | | | | | | | |
| .24 | < | | | | < | | < | | < | | | | < | | < | |
| .28 | < | | < | | < | | < | | < | | | | < | | < | |
| .32 | < | | < | < | = | < | < | < | < | | < | < | < | | = | |
| .36 | < | < | < | = | = | = | = | = | = | < | = | = | = | < | = | < |
| .40 | = | = | = | = | > | = | > | = | = | = | = | = | > | = | > | = |
| .44 | > | > | > | > | | > | | > | > | > | > | = | | > | | > |
| .48 | | > | | > | | > | | > | | > | | > | | > | | > |
| .52 | | | | > | | | | > | | > | | > | | | | |
| .56 | | | | > | | | | | | | | > | | | | |
| PSE | .40 | .40 | .40 | .38 | .34 | .38 | .36 | .38 | .38 | .40 | .38 | .40 | .36 | .40 | .34 | .40 |
| $L_u$ | .42 | .42 | .42 | .42 | .38 | .42 | .38 | .42 | .42 | .42 | .42 | .46 | .38 | .42 | .38 | .42 |
| $L_l$ | .38 | .38 | .38 | .34 | .30 | .34 | .34 | .34 | .34 | .38 | .34 | .34 | .34 | .38 | .30 | .38 |

| | | | | | |
|---|---|---|---|---|---|
| Mean $L_u$ | .412 | Mean $L_l$ | .350 | Mean PSE | .381 |
| (descending) | .425 | (descending) | .360 | Mean DL | .031 |
| (ascending) | .400 | (ascending) | .340 | CE | −.019 |

always produces a "shorter than" response from the subject and is increased in small steps through a range of durations eliciting "equal to" responses until the first "longer than" response is elicited. The opposite order is followed in the descending trials. A typical data sheet for the method of limits in temporal discrimination is shown in Table 2.1.

As illustrated in Table 2.1, the sequence is terminated whenever the subject shifts from a judgment of equality to one of inequality. Typically, ascending trials are alternated with descending trials. The *upper difference limen* ($L_u$) is the mean stimulus duration at which the subject changes from equality to longer judgments across all trials, and the *lower difference limen* ($L_l$) is the mean value at which the subject changes from equality to shorter judgments across all trials. Both the PSE and the jnd may be calculated from the $L_u$ and the $L_l$. The jnd is computed as half the difference between the $L_u$ and the $L_l$, or

$$\text{jnd} = \frac{L_u - L_l}{2}. \qquad [1]$$

The PSE is the midpoint between the $L_u$ and the $L_l$, or

$$\text{PSE} = \frac{L_u + L_l}{2}. \qquad [2]$$

The difference between the PSE and the standard (the standard is sometimes also referred to as the *point of equality,* or *PE*) is called the *constant error (CE).* The sign of the constant error indicates the direction of the error, since CE is defined as PSE − PE. In the example in Table 2.1, a negative CE was obtained.

The initial value of the variable is varied from trial to trial so that the subject will not be able to anticipate when equality between the variable and the standard is reached. In Table 2.1, for example, the first stimulus duration to be presented on a given trial was chosen by randomly picking a point 1, 2, or 3 steps beyond the $L_u$ or $L_l$ on the preceding trial.

### *The method of constant stimuli*

This method differs from the method of limits in that the value of the variable stimulus is not changed on each presentation in a systematic order, either increasing or decreasing, but in a random order. (As indicated earlier, the two methods differ in the same way when they are used to measure the absolute rather than the difference threshold.) Originally, the subject made the same three judgments as in the method of limits: judgments of less than, equal to, and greater than. This procedure yields three psy-

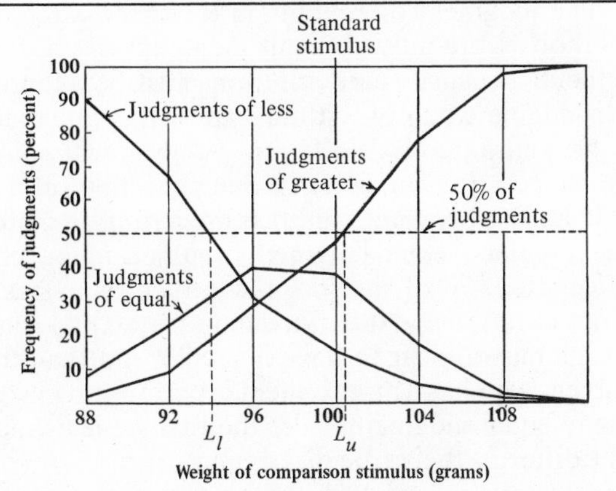


**Figure 2.2** Psychometric functions for the three-category method of constant stimuli for weight discrimination for a standard of 100 grams. The vertical dashed lines represent the upper difference limen ($L_u$) and lower difference limen ($L_l$). (From Boring, Langfeld, & Weld, 1935.)

chometric functions: one for the proportion of less-than judgments, one for the proportion of greater-than judgments, and one for the proportion of equal judgments. The proportion is plotted as a function of the magnitude of the variable. Figure 2.2 presents these psychometric functions for lifted weights. The standard weighed 100 grams.

The jnd is determined as follows: The $L_l$ is that weight judged less than the standard 50 percent of the time (94 grams in Figure 2.2) and the $L_u$ is that weight judged greater than the standard 50 percent of the time (100.5 grams). Then

$$\text{jnd} = \frac{L_u - L_l}{2} = 3.25 \text{ grams,}$$
$$\text{PSE} = \frac{L_u + L_l}{2} = 97.25 \text{ grams, and}$$
$$\text{CE} = \text{PSE} - \text{PE} = -2.75 \text{ grams.} \quad [3]$$

In this example, which is typical of experiments on lifted weights and loudness of tones, there is a negative constant error. Phenomenologically, this means that when two physically equal weights are picked up in succession, the second tends to appear heavier. This type of CE, involving temporally distinct stimuli, is called a *negative time-order error*. It is negative not because the CE has a negative sign, but because the first stimulus, which was the standard in this example, was judged of lesser magnitude than the second, when the two were physically equal. If the variable were presented prior to the standard, then the functions on the graph would be displaced to the right, and a positive CE would result. However, since the judged magnitude of the first stimulus would still seem to have decreased over time, the error would still be considered a negative time-order error.

Early in the history of psychophysics, the negative time-order error was ubiquitous, occurring particularly for loudness and lifted weights. An early theory which predicted that the time-order error would always be negative was Kohler's *sinking trace theory* (Guilford, 1954). According to this theory, intensities of memory traces decay with time: At the time of judgment, the observer compares an old weak memory trace produced by the first stimulus with a fresh strong trace produced by the second stimulus, and decides that the second stimulus is greater than the first even though the second may be physically equal to or less than the first.

The sinking trace theory predicts that as the interval between the standard and variable increases, the size of the negative time-order error should increase. This prediction was verified by Kohler, who found positive time-order errors for intervals below about 3 seconds and increasingly negative ones for intervals longer than 3 seconds. However, several other factors, such as the magnitude of the standard, the range of variable stimuli, experience with the situation, and nature of the background stimuli affect the direction and magnitude of the time-order error. The time-order error is positive for small magnitude standards, zero for some intermediate standard (called the *indifference point*), and negative for large standards. This dependence of the time-order error on absolute magnitude of stimuli has been observed for weights, loudnesses, and time intervals. The range of variable stimuli is also important. Increasing the upper range of the set of variable stimuli increases the value of the indifference point.

An experiment by Needham (1935) illustrates both the effect of the time interval between the standard and the variable, and the effect of the magnitude of the standard. Subjects made discriminations of loudnesses of pure tones under the three-category method of constant stimuli. Four standards were presented, in random order, ranging in 10-decibel steps from 30 to 60 dB above threshold, and were followed by the variable stimulus after intervals of 1, 3, or 6 seconds. The five variables paired with each standard differed from it by +2 dB, +1 dB, and 0 dB. Figure 2.3 (see next page) plots a measure of the time-order error, *D* percent (the number of "weaker" judgments

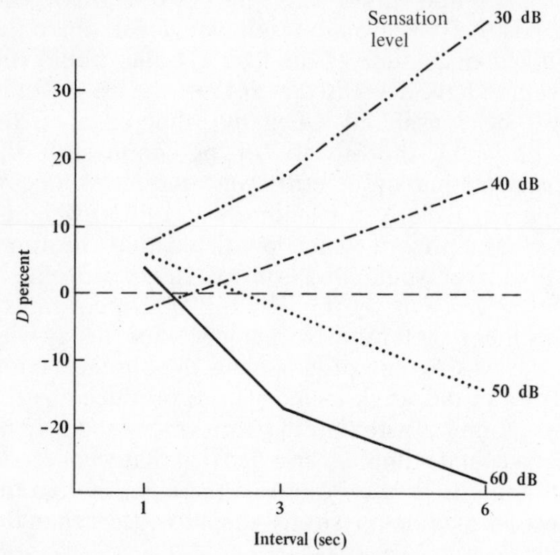

**Figure 2.3** Magnitude of the time-order error (in $D$ percent) as a function of standard-variable time interval for various values of the standard. $D$ percent $= (W - L)/N$, where $W$ is the number of "weaker" judgments, $L$ is the number of "louder" judgments, and $N$ is the total number of judgments for that condition. (From Needham, 1935.)

minus the number of "louder" judgments divided by the total number of responses), against time interval with the sensation level (see Chapter 4) of the standard as the parameter. Points above the 0 $D$-percent line indicate a positive time-order error and those below, a negative error. Louder standards produced negative time-order errors and weaker standards produced positive time-order errors, and the effect increased with the time interval. Clearly these results cannot be accounted for by the sinking trace theory, and so alternative explanations are required.

One such explanation has been proposed by Bartlett (1939) and is very similar to Helson's (1964) theory of *adaptation level.* Bartlett's hypothesis is that the *image* or memory trace of the first stimulus regresses toward the central value of all the stimuli in the experiment. Thus standards of low magnitude are enhanced in memory and therefore lead to a positive time-order error; high-magnitude standards are decreased in memory and lead to a negative time-order error. If it is also assumed that the regression to the mean increases as the time interval between the standard and variable becomes longer, then Bartlett's hypothesis can account for the findings of Needham and other investigators.

The judgment of equality in the three-category method is the most difficult judgment of all. It is difficult because some criterion must be adopted for judging when two stimuli are equal, and there is no guarantee that different subjects will adopt the same criterion, or even that the same subject will continue to maintain the same criterion. Since the number of equal judgments a subject makes can affect the size of the jnd, the subject who has a strict criterion and therefore makes few equal judgments may appear to have a smaller jnd than the subject who has a more lenient criterion and makes many equal judgments. Yet the two subjects may not differ in their true discriminatory ability. This uncertainty is reduced in the *forced-choice procedure,* which restricts the subject to only two categories—greater and less. It is assumed that when the variable and the standard appear equal, the subject will judge the variable greater on 50 percent of the trials. A single psychometric function, plotting the proportion of greater responses against the magnitude of the variable, summarizes the data. The jnd, as in the method of limits, is $(L_u - L_l)/2$, and the PSE is defined as the value at which the variable elicits 50 percent greater responses.

A psychometric function generated by the two-category method is shown in Figure 2.4. The $L_u$ is the value of the variable that elicits 75 percent longer responses, and the $L_l$, the value that elicits 25 percent longer responses.

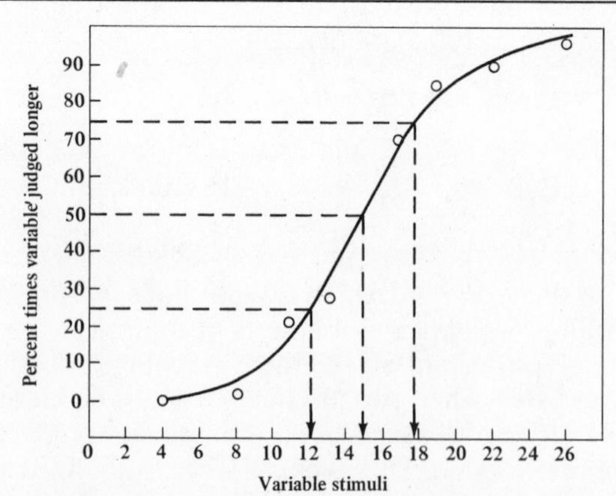


**Figure 2.4** Psychometric function for the forced-choice procedure for a standard of 15. The middle arrow indicates the PSE, the arrow on the left indicates the $L_l$, and the arrow on the right indicates the $L_u$. Since the PSE = 15, the CE is zero in this example. (From Underwood, 1966.)

*The method of adjustment*

The subject's task in this method is to adjust the magnitude of the variable stimulus until it appears to be equal to the standard. He does this repeatedly; the mean of the distribution of his adjustments is defined as the PSE, and the semi-interquartile range (one-half the difference between the 75th and the 25th percentiles) is defined as the jnd. In the older psychophysical literature, the semi-interquartile range is referred to as the *probable error*.

The method of adjustment is used primarily to measure the PSE rather than the jnd. Its use as a measure of the jnd has been questioned on several grounds. First, the judgments include not only variability in sensations, but variability from the motor responses made by the subjects. Second, Kellogg (1929) found that the jnd's from this method were poorly correlated with those from the method of constant stimuli and were more variable from day to day than were those from the method of constant stimuli.

Most so-called matching tasks are one version or another of the method of adjustment. An example is *heterochromatic matching,* in which subjects adjust the intensity of one hue to match the intensity of a second hue. Another example is the adjustment of a vertical line so that it appears as long as a horizontal line. In both cases, the PSE is of paramount importance, and often the variability of the judgments is of little or no interest.

## Empirical vs. theoretical approaches to thresholds and reaction time

There are two distinct approaches to an analysis of threshold and reaction-time data. The first approach is empirical. The psychologist is concerned with the threshold or the reaction time (RT) as an index of the effect of a stimulus. For example, the experimenter might be interested in the absolute thresholds for different wavelengths of light as a measure of the relative sensitivity of the observer to these wavelengths. Or he might be interested in choice RTs to various differences in wavelengths as a measure of the discriminability of two wavelengths.

From the empirical viewpoint, it is appropriate to collect threshold data with any of the methods described previously, as long as the subject uses the same criteria to respond to each of the stimuli. Similarly, the investigator using choice RT need not know the correct theoretical distribution of reaction times in order to use mean RT as a meaningful measure, unless the distribution is such that one measure of central tendency would be more appropriate than another.

In taking the theoretical approach, on the other hand, the investigator analyzes the empirical data in order to discover the underlying judgmental process involved in thresholds or reaction times. Often a theory for the underlying process is proposed which is consonant with present empirical facts and which predicts the form of the data when certain experimental manipulations are carried out.

Sometimes, as we shall see, detection theories prescribe quite different methodologies for collecting data. Basically, a theory of detection makes two assumptions: one about the way stimulus energy is transformed into internal sensation or response, and the second about the way the internal response is transformed into a recordable judgment. Theories of reaction time are primarily concerned with predicting the form of the reaction-time distribution and usually do not specify the experimental procedure for collecting RT data.

## Theories of thresholds

*The classical theory*

The concepts on which classical theory depend originated with Fechner (1860) and were further developed by Cattell (1893), Jastrow (1888), and Urban (1910). The latter's *phi-gamma hypothesis* forms the basis for the classical theory of detection. As previously noted, theories of detection start with assumptions about three continua: *stimulus*, *internal response,* and *judgment*. The three continua proposed by the classical theory are shown in Figure 2.5.

The stimulus continuum is assumed to be fixed; that is, the stimulus is assumed not to vary in its physical parameters from trial to trial. However, the internal response continuum is assumed to be variable. Each physically constant stimulus is assumed to produce a normally distributed response distribution, thus giving rise to a series of overlapping distributions. The threshold, $T$, is a fixed point within these overlapping distributions.

The subject's judgment continuum is usually assumed to correspond exactly to his response continuum; that is, the subject is assumed to judge the stimulus present whenever it exceeds his threshold and to judge it absent whenever it does

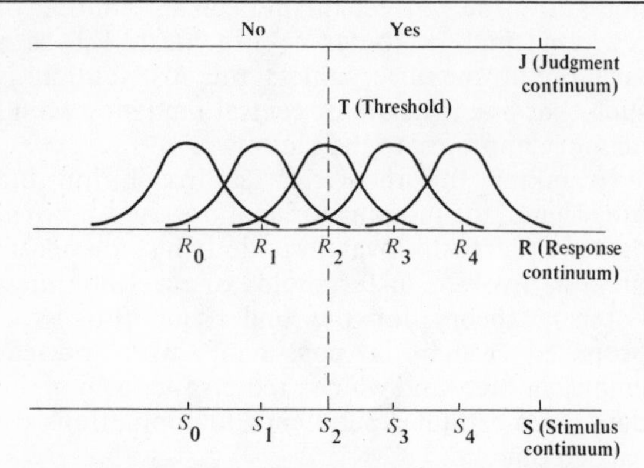


**Figure 2.5** The three continua—judgment ($J$), internal response ($R$), and stimulus ($S$)—proposed by the classical theory of thresholds. Stimulus $S_2$ is defined as the absolute threshold ($T$) since half the time that it is presented it elicits a yes response. (After Corso, 1967.)

not exceed his threshold. According to the classical definition of the threshold, stimulus $S_2$ is the value of this subject's absolute threshold. The threshold corresponds to the mean of the response distribution which $S_2$ produces because the distribution is normal. Since a normal distribution is symmetrical, half of the time stimulus $S_2$ is presented it exceeds threshold, and the other half of the time it does not. Stimulus $S_1$ sometimes exceeds threshold, stimulus $S_3$ usually does, and stimulus $S_4$ always does. Stimulus $S_0$ is the null stimulus, or the "stimulus" present when the to-be-detected stimulus is omitted, as on catch trials. In other contexts, it is called *noise alone*. The classical theory assumes that the null stimulus or noise alone never exceeds the threshold, and for this reason the classical theory is sometimes referred to as a high-threshold theory.

For stimuli spaced closely enough along the stimulus continuum, a plot of stimulus intensity against detection probability will produce a psychometric function corresponding to a normal ogive, which is the cumulative of the normal distribution. Thus the classical theory accounts for the variability in judgments of a constant stimulus, the ogival form of the psychometric function, and the statistical definition of the threshold.

The two relatively modern theories considered here—neural quantum and signal detection—are really theories of increment detection because they are tested with procedures in which an increment is added to a constant background such as a pure tone or noise.

*Neural quantum theory*

Neural quantum theory asserts that sensory discrimination is a discrete, all-or-none process rather than a continuous one. The theory maintains that a true sensory threshold exists and that sensation increases from that point in *discrete units,* or *quanta*. Thus, although stimulus intensity is continuous, its effects on the observing organism are discrete. It is like the classical theory in postulating a true sensory threshold, but unlike the classical theory it postulates discrete changes in sensation with increases in stimulation. Quanta are not identified with any specific neural units, although the quantal nature of sensation is assumed to be closely associated with neural events.

According to neural quantum theory, the observer in a detection experiment is aware of a stimulus change whenever such a change excites an integral number of additional neural quanta. However, the observer is assumed to fluctuate slowly in sensitivity over time, due to background events and neural noise. Together, these two factors excite a certain base number of quanta and, in addition, there will typically be a surplus, or *residue,* of excitation from these two sources over and above the exact amount necessary to excite an integral number of quanta. Picture, as a physical analogy to this process, a vessel filled with water whose level is slowly fluctuating and which contains rows of horizontally strung wires. Whenever the water level exceeds the $n$th wire from the bottom, we say that $n$ quanta are excited, and the excess water above that wire we call the residue. This residue is assumed to be available to sum with the effects of a stimulus. Hence, a constant stimulus increment does not always excite the same number of additional quanta because the amount of residue is not identical from trial to trial. Furthermore, it is assumed that the residue can lie anywhere between two quantal boundaries with equal probability. Stated in another way, the distribution of residues between any two quantal boundaries is assumed to be rectangular.

The careful observer in a quantum experiment adopts some criterion such that the background stimulus seldom if ever exceeds the criterion but many signals do. Although changes in sensitivity are large relative to the size of the quantum, they are assumed to be gradual so that within a short interval of time the background stimulation may excite an additional one quantum but rarely an additional two quanta. Thus, the observer is often assumed to set a two-quantum criterion. In this case, a signal having energy that excites exactly two quanta (or more) is always detected by the observer, a signal that excites one quantum (or less) is never detected, and signals of intermediate intensity are sometimes detected and sometimes not because their effects are added to the available residue from the background.

The preceding assumptions predict that an observer maintaining a two-quantum criterion will produce a psychometric function on which $p$ reaches 1.0 when the increment in stimulus energy above the background is twice the increment at which $p = 0$. In other words, the smallest stimulus increment for which the probability of detection is just 1.0 will be twice that of the largest stimulus increment for which the probability of detection is still 0. In general, an observer maintaining an $n$-quantum criterion will produce a psychometric function whose $p = 1.0$, $p = 0$ intercepts stand in the ratio of $n:n - 1$ in terms of stimulus energy. By assuming that residues are distributed rectangularly between any two quantal boundaries, the theory further predicts that the psychometric functions will be linear.

Experiments testing the theory in the recommended way have generally yielded linear psychometric functions with $n:n - 1$ (usually 2:1) intercepts (von Békésy, 1960; Larkin & Norman, 1964; Stevens, Morgan, & Volkmann, 1941). The recommended procedure is to make the task as simple as possible, let the observer know what to expect on every trial, and avoid large changes in stimulus intensity between trials (as in the method of constant stimuli). It is felt that unexpected changes in stimulus intensity will introduce large sensitivity changes in the observer.

Typically, well-practiced and highly motivated observers, often the investigators themselves, serve as subjects. It has been observed that presenting each stimulus increment in a block of about twenty-five trials produces better neural quantum functions than randomizing the stimulus increments, although Stevens (1972) has pointed out that some investigators have found neural quantum results with a randomized procedure. It is essential, however, to keep the interval between the background stimulus and the increment very short, for increasing the interval between the background or standard and the increment produces a classical ogival psychometric function (Stevens, 1972). Indeed, as pointed out earlier, most neural quantum experiments are run as increment detection experiments in which there is zero interval

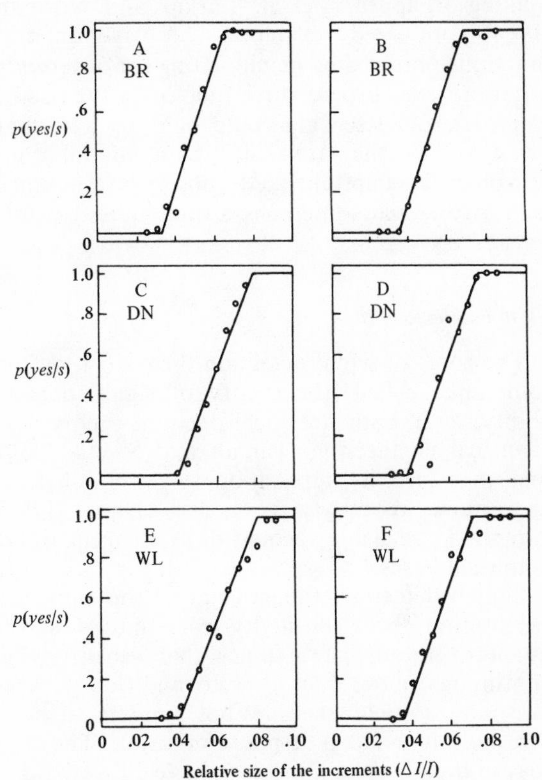


**Figure 2.6** Psychometric functions from neural quantum experiments. The lines were fitted to the data points by eye, with the restriction that the $p(yes/s) = 1.0$ and $p(yes/s) = 0$ points intersect at stimulus values having 2:1 ratios. (From Larkin & Norman, 1964.)

between the background and the increment. Although the theory has been tested primarily with increments in frequency or intensity of pure tones against a pure-tone background, Stevens (1972) has recently shown that a reanalysis of some classical studies in detection of brightness increments also yields linear psychometric functions with 2:1 intercepts.

Figure 2.6 shows some representative psychometric functions for three observers who detected an increment in the intensity of a 1000-Hertz tone. The data points are well fit by linear psychometric functions with 2:1 intercepts.

Some investigators (e.g., Corso, 1956) have failed to find either the linearity or the 2:1 intercepts. However, proponents of the neural quantum theory point out that any defects in the experiment, such as low motivation or failure of the observer to maintain a strict criterion, distort the function, making it appear ogival. Larkin and Norman (1964) presented examples of psychometric functions obtained by manipulating the observer's criterion from two to three quanta by the use of catch trials. These data could be fit by a normal ogive, and yet they are well fit by a quantal function on the assumption that the observer sometimes uses a two- and sometimes a three-quantum criterion.

### *Signal detection theory*

The roots of signal detection theory (or, as it is sometimes called, the theory of signal detectability) lie in both statistical decision theory and electrical engineering. Tanner and Swets (1954) first proposed its application to psychophysics, and more recently Green and Swets (1966) compiled a readable account of its theoretical and empirical bases.

Signal detection theory makes the opposite assumption about sensitivity from that of neural quantum theory; it assumes that sensitivity is continuous rather than discrete, and that no true sensory threshold exists. What appears to be a threshold is in fact a response criterion. The only reason the observer appears to have a threshold is that he is forced to distinguish between a signal and noise. The noise either is produced by internal events, such as random activity of neural units, or is introduced by the experimenter as background.

Since the observer's sensation is continuously variable rather than discrete, he must set some criterion for deciding whether a signal was presented or not. When a sensation exceeds the criterion, he responds as if a stimulus had been present, and when the sensation does not exceed the criterion, he responds as if no stimulus had been present. His task is like that of a statistical decision maker who, on the basis of noisy or variable data, must decide whether or not his experimental manipulation produced a true difference. The decision maker is well aware that even a large difference could have been produced by a combination of chance factors. He therefore sets some criterion, called the *significance level,* that defines the risk he is willing to take for accepting the difference as a true one (or rejecting the null hypothesis), when in fact there is no difference. The probability of this incorrect decision is set to some small fixed value such as .05 or .01.

Unlike the statistical decision maker, who maintains a fixed criterion, the signal detection observer is assumed to be more flexible. In particular, as is shown later, the location of his criterion is assumed to be affected by nonsensory aspects of the experiment, such as the probability that the signal is presented, or the rewards and costs of right and wrong decisions.

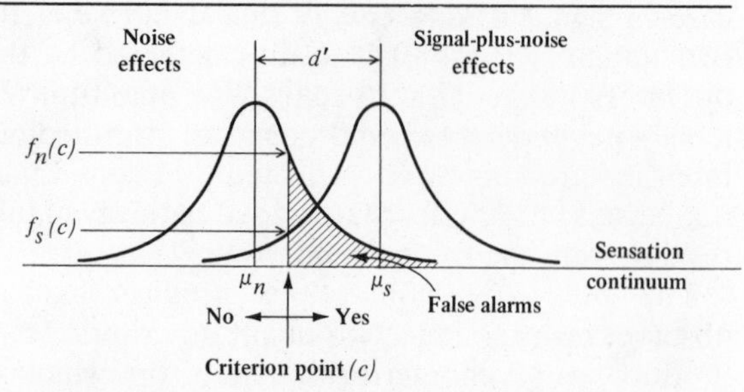


**Figure 2.7** Sensation continuum proposed by signal detection theory. If the observer's criterion is set at the criterion point, the shaded portion of the noise distribution represents the theoretical probability of a false alarm. (After Galanter, 1966.)

A necessary experimental condition to test signal detection theory is the inclusion of a substantial proportion of noise trials on which no signal is presented. In the classical methods, these are known as catch trials. Thus there are two types of trials: signal present, occurring on proportion $p$ of the trials, and signal absent, occurring on $1 - p$ proportion of the trials. Because the signals are generally presented in a noise background, the first type of stimulus is called *signal plus noise,* and the second type is called *noise alone*.

The effects of both noise alone and signal plus noise are assumed to be normally distributed. Since the two distributions overlap, a sensation of given magnitude could be produced either by noise alone or by signal plus noise. In the simplest situation, the standard deviations of the noise ($n$) and signal ($s$) distributions are assumed to be equal. The theoretical sensation continuum, with a criterion or decision point, is shown in Figure 2.7.

The measure of the observer's sensitivity is the distance between the means of the two distributions, $\mu_n$ and $\mu_s$. It is expressed in units of the common standard deviation, $\sigma$, and is called $d'$. The equation is: $d' = (\mu_s - \mu_n)/\sigma$. The criterion measure, called $\beta$, is defined as the ratio of the ordinate of the signal distribution to the ordinate of the noise distribution at the criterion point $c$. The equation is $\beta = f_s(c)/f_n(c)$, where $f$ stands for the frequency of occurrence.

The larger the value of $\beta$, the more conservative the observer; the smaller the value, the more liberal the observer. An observer who adopts a criterion at the mean of the noise distribution in Figure 2.7 would be considered to have a liberal criterion; that is, he requires a relatively small sensation to conclude that a signal was presented. He is like the radar operator for whom almost every small speck on the radar screen is seen as an enemy plane. An observer who adopts a criterion at the mean of the signal distribution would be considered to have a conservative criterion; he requires a relatively large sensation before he concludes that a signal was presented. He is like the aircraft pilot who requests fire-fighting equipment at his landing only when the probability of a crash is fairly high.

In the typical signal detection experiment, the location of the subject's criterion is manipulated experimentally by variations in either signal presentation probabilities or explicit payoffs for right and wrong decisions. However, the tendency of subjects to adopt conservative or liberal criteria in the absence of explicit payoffs or of knowledge about presentation probabilities has been studied in its own right, and provides an important basis for differentiating between different types of observers.

Both $d'$ and $\beta$ can be calculated from the *hit rate,* the proportion of trials on which the subject responds "signal" ($S$) to a signal presentation, or $Pr(S/s)$, and the *false alarm rate,* the proportion of trials on which he responds "signal" to a noise presentation, or $Pr(S/n)$. Two other events can occur. The subject can respond "noise" ($N$) to a signal presentation; this event is called a *miss,* and its probability, $Pr(N/s)$, is equal to $1 - Pr(S/s)$. Or the subject can respond "noise" to a noise presentation; this event is a *correct rejection,* and its probability, $Pr(N/n)$, equals $1 - Pr(S/n)$. Thus the subject can be right in two ways, by making a hit or a correct rejection, and wrong in two ways, by making a false alarm or a miss.

To estimate these probabilities, the proportion of noise or catch trials may be varied from 10 percent to 90 percent. This is in marked contrast to most quantal experiments in which the stimulus is present on every trial, and the subject knows it. It might appear as if the signal detection experimenter is trying to trick the subject, but in fact such a procedure is absolutely required by the theory.

For a given observer and a given signal intensity, $d'$ is assumed to remain constant; however, $\beta$ is assumed to be sensitive to nonsensory aspects of the experiment, such as presentation probabilities and payoffs. The results of a signal detection experiment are often summarized by plotting the probability of a hit against the probability of a false alarm in what is known as a *receiver operating characteristic (ROC) curve,* also sometimes referred to as an *isosensitivity curve.* For a fixed stimulus, an ROC curve can be traced out by systematically varying the probability of a signal presentation or by varying the relative payoffs for correct responses and errors.

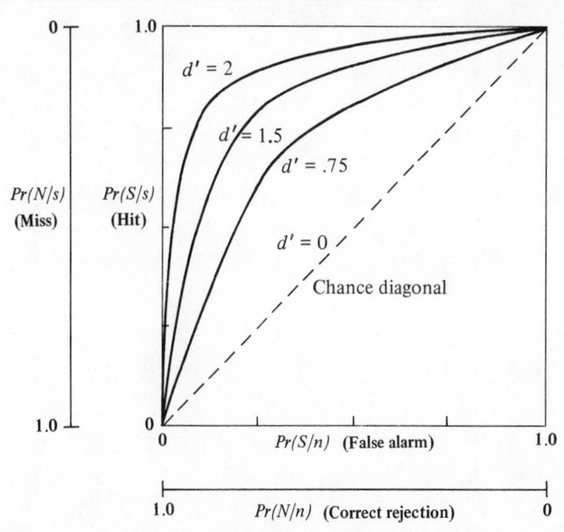


**Figure 2.8** Some theoretical ROC curves for various values of $d'$, under the equal-variance assumption for signal and noise distributions.

Figure 2.8 presents some examples of ROC curves for different values of $d'$ and different criteria. As indicated in the figure, the probability of a miss is the complement of the hit probability, that is, the two probabilities always sum to 1.0; similarly, the probability of a correct rejection is the complement of the false alarm probability. High-intensity signals (or a highly sensitive subject) generate a curve that lies in the upper left-hand corner and has a large $d'$, whereas low-intensity signals (or an insensitive subject) generate ROC curves that are closer to the main diagonal and have small $d'$s. The main diagonal, shown in the figure by the dotted line from 0,0 to 1.0,1.0, represents chance performance (and a $d'$ of 0) since the hit and false alarm rates are equal. Movement along any particular ROC curve indicates changes in the response criterion without changes in $d'$.

Figure 2.9 shows an ROC curve generated by varying the probability of signal presentation, that is, the proportion of signal-plus-noise trials. Each point on the graph was obtained with a different probability: 0.1, 0.3, 0.5, 0.7, or 0.9. The estimated $d'$ was constant at 0.85. The insert shows the

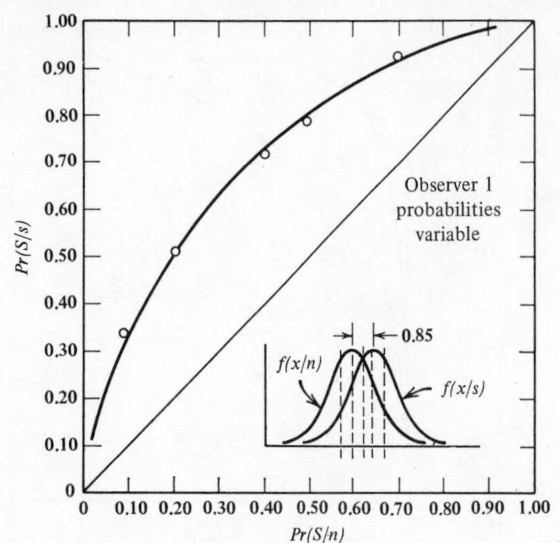


**Figure 2.9** ROC curve for detection of an auditory signal in noise. The empirical data points were obtained by varying the signal presentation probabilities, and the theoretical curve is for $d' = 0.85$ and equal-variance noise and signal distributions. (From Green & Swets, 1966.)

theoretical distributions of signal and noise distributions for the ROC curve drawn through the data points. Each dashed line in the insert represents one of the five criteria used by the observer under each of the presentation probabilities.

Figure 2.10 shows an ROC curve generated by varying only the payoff, in accordance with the five matrices shown in Table 2.2; signal intensity was constant and the signal presentation probability was fixed at 0.5. The payoff matrix shows the reward or cost, in points or money, for each of the four types of responses. Under payoff matrix A, the subject wins one point for correctly detecting the signal, loses nine points for making a false alarm, wins nine points for a correct rejection, and loses one point for a miss. This particular payoff matrix is designed to induce the subject to adopt a conservative criterion, that is, to report the signal as present only when he is quite sure it was. Although theoretically the various payoffs and presentation probabilities (Figures 2.9 and 2.10) should have produced the same criteria, extreme payoffs were much more effective than extreme presentation probabilities in inducing the observer to adopt extreme criteria.

Signal detection theory specifies explicitly what sort of decision rule a so-called *ideal observer* should adopt, depending on his goal. If the observer wishes to minimize the number of errors, he should adopt one type of decision rule; if he wishes to maximize expected value, he should use another. Because most signal detection experiments are run with payoff matrices and because it seems reasonable that subjects will want to win as much money as possible, it is usually assumed that the ideal observer will adopt a criterion to maximize expected value, that is, to maximize his average winnings in the experiment. In the latter case, he takes into account both the presentation probabilities and payoffs to compute the optimum value of $\beta$ as follows:

$$\beta_{opt} = \frac{Pr(n)}{Pr(s)} \times \frac{\text{Value (correct rejection)} + \text{Cost (false alarm)}}{\text{Value (hit)} + \text{Cost (miss)}} \quad [4]$$

When $Pr(n) = Pr(s) = 0.5$ and the payoff matrix is symmetrical in that values of both types of correct decisions and costs of both types of errors are the same (as in payoff matrix C in Table 2.2) $\beta_{opt} = 1$. This means that the ideal observer will set his criterion at the intersections of the $n$ and $s$ distributions. At their intersection points, $f_n(x) = f_s(x)$, and their ratio is 1. (Note that $x$ stands for a particular value along the abscissa of a response distribution such as that shown in Figure 2.7.)

For intermediate probability and payoff values,

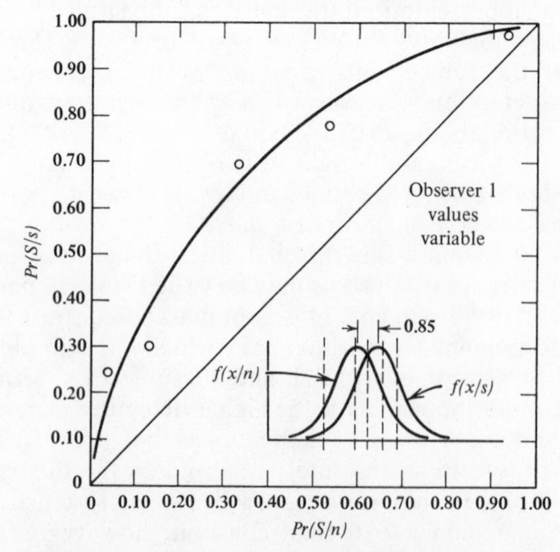


**Figure 2.10** ROC curve obtained by varying payoffs rather than presentation probabilities, for the same observer as in Figure 2.9. (From Green & Swets, 1966.)

criteria actually adopted by subjects in signal detection experiments agree fairly well with the optimum $\beta$ as defined here; for extreme probabilities or payoffs, however, subjects' criteria tend to be more moderate than predicted.

The method of signal detection has been applied in some fascinating contexts. For example, the flicker-fusion threshold has often been reported to be higher for psychiatric patients than for normal subjects (Granger, 1953, 1957). The flicker-fusion threshold is defined as the lowest frequency of interruption of a light source at which the observer reports the light to appear steady. Thus, psychiatric patients require a higher rate of flicker to report a steady stimulus. Because these thresholds are also altered by brain injury and by biochemical changes in the central nervous system, the higher thresholds in psychiatric patients might imply similar biochemical or structural changes in these patients. However, a series of experiments by Clark and his associates has provided convincing evidence that this difference in flicker threshold is a difference in criterion rather than in sensitivity.

Clark (1966) found that schizophrenic subjects could be induced to vary their criteria for reporting flicker depending on whether they were given facilitating or conservative instruction sets, even though $d'$ did not change. Clark, Brown, and Rutschmann (1967) found that under a method of forced choice, a technique that is much less affected by differences in response criterion than the yes-no procedure, thresholds were the same for psychiatric and normal subjects, whereas under the method of limits, psychiatric subjects had higher thresholds than normal subjects.

Psychiatric patients adopt more conservative criteria for reporting flicker than do normal subjects because, according to Clark et al., they are particularly anxious not to report anything they are not sure is there: They know the stimulus is intermittent and are reluctant to report it as steady until there can be no mistake about their perception.

Stunkard and Koch (1964) have applied signal detection methods to a novel stimulus. In an elaboration of the classic study by Cannon and Washburn (1912), Stunkard and Koch had obese and normal men and women swallow stomach balloons, and recorded their stomach contractions. Subjects were asked during the course of the four-hour experimental session whether or not they were hungry, experienced a feeling of emptiness, or had a desire to eat. Reports were taken when stomach contractions were actually present, as indicated by the recording, and when no contractions were recorded. The stomach contraction served as the signal, and the absence of a contraction served as the noise. Reports of hunger (or emptiness or desire to eat) when contractions were present were defined as hits, and when they were absent, as false alarms. Unlike usual signal detection experiments, the experimenter had no control over the signal presentation since it was a naturally occurring event.

**Table 2.2 Payoff Matrices, and Observed Response Probabilities, in a Yes-No Signal Detection Experiment, Where the Signal Is a Tone Burst in a Background of White Noise and $d' = 0.85$**

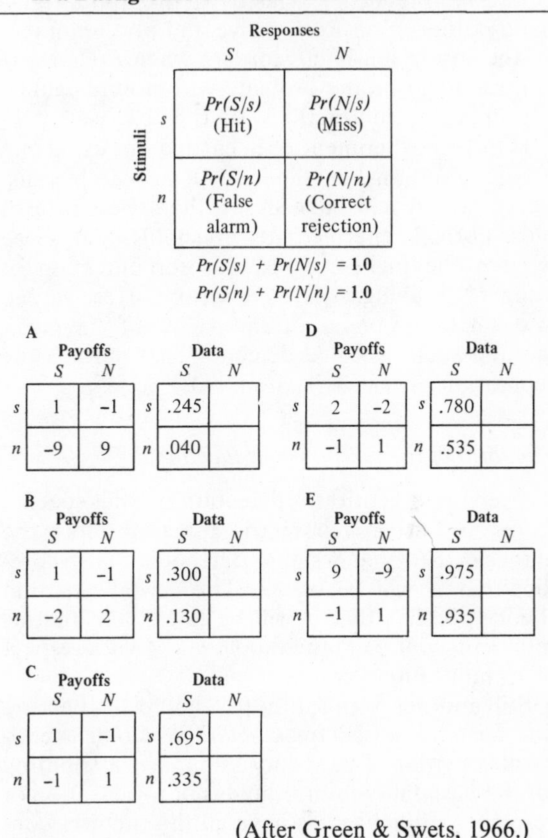

| Stimuli | Responses: *S* | Responses: *N* |
|---|---|---|
| *s* | *Pr(S/s)* (Hit) | *Pr(N/s)* (Miss) |
| *n* | *Pr(S/n)* (False alarm) | *Pr(N/n)* (Correct rejection) |

$Pr(S/s) + Pr(N/s) = 1.0$

$Pr(S/n) + Pr(N/n) = 1.0$

A

| | Payoffs *S* | Payoffs *N* | Data *S* | Data *N* |
|---|---|---|---|---|
| *s* | 1 | -1 | .245 | |
| *n* | -9 | 9 | .040 | |

B

| | Payoffs *S* | Payoffs *N* | Data *S* | Data *N* |
|---|---|---|---|---|
| *s* | 1 | -1 | .300 | |
| *n* | -2 | 2 | .130 | |

C

| | Payoffs *S* | Payoffs *N* | Data *S* | Data *N* |
|---|---|---|---|---|
| *s* | 1 | -1 | .695 | |
| *n* | -1 | 1 | .335 | |

D

| | Payoffs *S* | Payoffs *N* | Data *S* | Data *N* |
|---|---|---|---|---|
| *s* | 2 | -2 | .780 | |
| *n* | -1 | 1 | .535 | |

E

| | Payoffs *S* | Payoffs *N* | Data *S* | Data *N* |
|---|---|---|---|---|
| *s* | 9 | -9 | .975 | |
| *n* | -1 | 1 | .935 | |

(After Green & Swets, 1966.)

Stunkard and Koch found that normal men and women tended to report hunger when stomach contractions were present and no hunger when they were absent, with no obvious bias toward one or the other extreme. Obese men and women, on the other hand, showed extreme and opposite response biases. Obese women showed a marked *nay-saying bias* in that they denied hunger in general, even when contractions were objectively present; obese men, on the contrary, had a *yea-saying bias* and tended to report hunger all the time, even when no contractions were recorded. Obese men tended to cluster at the upper right-hand corner of an ROC curve and obese women, at the lower left-hand corner, when *Pr*(hunger/contractions) on the ordinate was plotted against *Pr*(hunger/no contractions) on the abscissa.

Had this experiment been carried out using one of the traditional methods, with no catch trials, obese men would have shown the lowest thresholds, normals intermediate thresholds, and obese women the highest thresholds for detection of hunger through gastric contractions. Here we see a dramatic example of the value of having a method such as signal detection that permits the separation of sensitivity from bias.

### *The form of the psychometric function*

The three theories of detection predict specific forms for the psychometric function. Both the classical theory and signal detection theory predict that it will be ogival. The neural quantum theory predicts that it will be linear and that its intercepts will be in the ratio $n{:}n - 1$ with respect to stimulus intensity.

Still another form for the psychometric function has been proposed for *absolute detection* experiments in vision. This theory is unique in attributing all the variability in thresholds not to sensation or response variability, as have all the theories considered thus far, but rather to variability within the stimulus itself.

Hecht, Shlaer, and Pirenne (1942), considering the light stimulus in terms of its particle rather than its wave nature, computed how many photons of light from a threshold stimulus were likely to be absorbed by the photosensitive substance in the rods (see Chapter 7). A threshold stimulus for their subjects, who were tested under optimum conditions for sensitivity, consisted of approximately 50 to 150 photons of light. However, some of these are lost through reflection from the cornea, some are lost from scattering in the media of the eyeball, and not all that reach the rods are absorbed by the photosensitive substance. Hecht et al. concluded that the average number of photons actually absorbed by the retina from this threshold stimulus is of the order of only 5 to 14. This means that different numbers of photons will be absorbed from the identical physical stimulus from one trial to the next. Thus, if the subject himself were absolutely constant, in the sense that he reported a stimulus as present anytime *n* or more photons were absorbed, he will exhibit variability in his responses in that the same stimulus will sometimes be detected by him and sometimes not. The frequency distribution for the number of photons delivered by a particular stimulus is described by the *Poisson distribution*.[1] The cumulative Poisson distribution is then the appropriate form for the psychometric function, which in this context is called a *frequency-of-seeing* curve. Hecht et al. obtained good fits to data by using the cumulative Poisson distribution. Their results suggest that for absolute detection of visual stimuli by well-trained observers, all response variability can be attributed to variability in the physical stimulus.

## The Weber fraction and Fechner's law

The relationship of the jnd to the size of the standard has been a topic of deep and lasting interest to psychologists. Intuitively, it would seem that a small change is more noticeable against a small-magnitude background than against a large-magnitude background: Lighting a candle in a completely dark room can have a blinding effect, but will make no noticeable difference in a brilliantly lighted room. A person's whisper is audible in silence, but is completely masked at a jet airfield. Similarly, a small difference between stimuli of small magnitude is more noticeable than that same difference between stimuli of large magnitude. It is easier to tell that two lemons are of unequal weight than that two melons are unequal even though the inequality is the same.

The German physiologist E. H. Weber (1795–1878) was the first to systematically explore the relation between the jnd and the size of the standard. In 1846 he published his researches on the jnd for lifted weights, reporting that the jnd was a constant proportion (1/30) of the standard weight. For a 300-gram weight, the jnd was approximately 10 grams, and for a 1000-gram weight, it was approximately 33 grams.

Weber's law is often expressed as $\Delta I/I = k$, where $\Delta I$ is the magnitude of the jnd, $I$ is the magnitude of the standard or background, and $k$ is a constant less than 1. The value of $k$ is often referred to as the *Weber fraction*.

The publication of Weber's results led other investigators to determine whether the law held for other stimuli and modalities, such as bright-

[1] The Poisson distribution is a continuous approximation to the binomial distribution when *p* is close to zero.

**Table 2.3 The Weber Fraction for Various Modalities in the Optimum Range of Sensitivity**

| Sense modality | Weber fraction |
|---|---|
| Deep pressure, from skin and subcutaneous tissue | 1/77 |
| Visual brightness | 1/60 |
| Lifted weights | 1/52 |
| Loudness of a 1000-Hz tone | 1/12 |
| Smell for rubber | 1/11 |
| Cutaneous pressure | 1/7 |
| Taste for saline solution | 1/5 |

(After Boring, Langfeld, & Weld, 1935.)

ness, loudness, taste, and pressure. In general, Weber's law is valid for the middle ranges of stimulus magnitude, but the fraction increases markedly toward threshold. A possible explanation for the breakdown of Weber's law near threshold is the existence of intrinsic noise within the observer which might interfere with discrimination between near-threshold stimuli. In weight-lifting experiments, the subject must discriminate the weight of his arm plus weight A from the weight of his arm plus weight B. If weights A and B are small, the weight of the subject's arm contributes heavily to the discrimination. Likewise, in visual discrimination of very dim lights, the intrinsic noise contributed by spontaneous nerve firings or spontaneous breakdown of the photosensitive substance in the eye interfere with this discrimination. One can obtain much better approximations to Weber's law at low intensities by adding to the standard intensity $I$ the absolute threshold intensity $I_t$, which is taken as an estimate of intrinsic noise. The correction to Weber's law, first introduced by Helmholtz, is

$$\Delta I/(I + I_t) = k \qquad [5]$$

and is more nearly approximated by experimental data.

Table 2.3 presents minimum Weber fractions for various modalities and stimuli. A large fraction means poor discrimination and a small one means good discrimination.

Fechner saw in Weber's law the possibility of constructing a function relating sensation to physical intensity. Because an earlier development in economic thought influenced his approach to the problem, we first turn to the work of the mathematician Daniel Bernoulli who, in 1738, proposed that the *utility* or subjective value of money increases more slowly than its objective value. He made this proposal in response to a gambling paradox presented to him by his cousin, Nicolas Bernoulli. Referred to as the *St. Petersburg* paradox because of the journal in which Daniel Bernoulli's solution to it was published, the problem can be stated in the following manner.

Peter offers Paul the chance to engage in the following gamble: Peter will throw a coin until it lands heads. If it lands heads on the first throw, Paul wins 1 ducat; if on the second, 2 ducats; if on the third, 4 ducats; and if on the fourth, 8 ducats. In general, the number of ducats won when the coin lands heads on the $n$th toss is $2^{n-1}$.

How much should Paul pay Peter to participate in this gamble? Most people would agree that although they might very well pay 2, 3, or possibly even 4 ducats for the chance, they would certainly never pay as much as, say, 20 ducats to participate. What is the fair price for the gamble? According to the earliest classical theory of utility and risk taking, the *expected value (EV)* of a gamble may be calculated by multiplying the probability of each outcome by the value, in ducats or dollars, of that outcome.

There are an infinite number of outcomes in this gamble, since the coin could land heads on any trial from $n = 1$ to $n =$ any positive digit. Hence, the EV of the bet is

$$\begin{aligned} EV &= 1/2 \cdot 1 + 1/4 \cdot 2 + 1/8 \cdot 4 + \ldots \\ &= 1/2(1 + 1 + 1 + 1 + \ldots \\ &= \overset{\infty}{\Sigma}(1/2). \end{aligned}$$

This sum has no limit, so the rational individual should be willing to pay any amount to participate in the gamble. Since supposedly rational people are not willing, there must be something wrong with the expected-value approach.

Bernoulli solved the paradox by introducing the concept of utility to replace objective value. He assumed that the marginal utility of an additional unit of money is inversely proportional to the number of units already possessed. For example, if a man with $1,000 in the bank were willing to pay $2 for a meal, a man with $100,000 should be willing to pay $200 for the same meal if the utilities of the meal were the same for both of them. Likewise, the utility of winning $10 at poker for the first man is equal to the utility of winning $1,000 at poker for the second. Bernoulli showed that if marginal utility is proportional to value of money already possessed, then the utility of money is a logarithmic function of the value of money, or

$$U(M) = C \log M. \qquad [6]$$

Applying this result to the St. Petersburg paradox, Bernoulli (1738) showed that if Paul owned nothing, he should rationally pay only 2 ducats for the gamble; if he owned 10 ducats, he should pay 3 ducats; and even if Paul had a fortune of 1000 ducats, he should still only pay 6 ducats for the gamble.

Fechner, like Bernoulli, wanted to find the function relating a subjective continuum to a physical continuum. Bernoulli was looking for the relationship of utility to amount of money; Fechner was looking for the relationship of sensation to stimulus magnitude. Fechner made three assumptions. First, he assumed that Weber's law was correct. As noted earlier, the law is true over an intermediate range of stimulus values, although it fails at the lower extreme. Second, he assumed that jnd's were subjectively equal, that is, that a difference which is detected 50 percent of the time is of the same subjective magnitude regardless whether it is a large difference between two large-magnitude stimuli or a small difference between two small-magnitude stimuli. Third, he assumed something which he called the *mathematical auxiliary principle,* which maintains that small sensation increments are proportional to stimulus increments; that is, if the physical difference between two stimuli is doubled, then so is the sensation difference.

These three assumptions led him to his *fundamental formula,* which is:

$$\Delta S = k\frac{\Delta I}{I}, \qquad [7]$$

where $\Delta S$ is the change in sensation, $k$ is a constant, and $\Delta I$ is a small change in physical intensity. When $\Delta I$ represents the jnd, this fundamental formula represents both Weber's law and the assumption of subjective equality of jnd's.

The use of the small changes in physical and subjective intensities, $\Delta I$ and $\Delta S$, suggest differentials, and indeed Fechner treated the fundamental formula as a differential equation, integrated it, and produced his version of the psychophysical function, which we now call *Fechner's law:*

$$S = k \log I, \qquad [8]$$

where $S$ is the amount of sensation produced by a stimulus of magnitude $I$, expressed in units of the absolute threshold, and $k$ is a constant. In his own words,

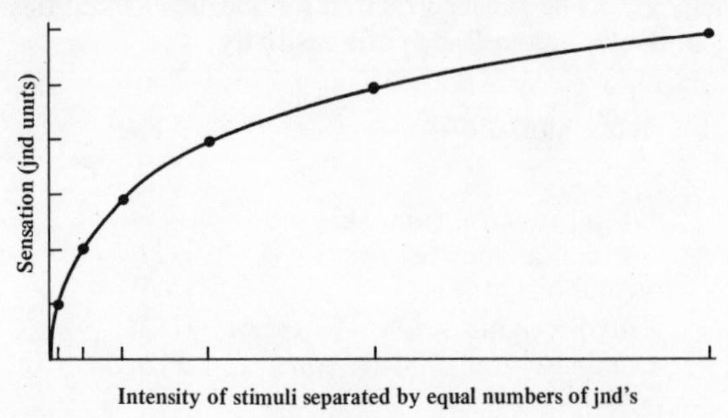


**Figure 2.11** Logarithmic relationship between sensation and stimulus intensity proposed by Fechner.

> The magnitude of the sensation ... is not proportional to the absolute value of the stimulus..., but rather to the logarithm of the magnitude of the stimulus, when this last is expressed in terms of its threshold value ..., i.e., that magnitude considered as unit at which the sensation begins and disappears. In short, it is proportional to the logarithm of the fundamental stimulus value [translated in Dennis, 1948, p. 211].

Some examples may clarify this relationship. Figure 2.11 shows a graph of stimuli along the abscissa separated by equal numbers of jnd's. If Weber's law is true, the physical magnitudes of the stimuli must be logarithmically spaced. For example, if the stimuli are separated by steps of one logarithmic unit so that $I_1 = 1, I_2 = 2, I_3 = 4, I_4 = 8$, and, in general, $I_n = 2^{n-1}$, then

$$\begin{aligned} \Delta I_1 &= I_2 - I_1 = 1 \\ \Delta I_2 &= I_3 - I_2 = 2 \\ \Delta I_3 &= I_4 - I_3 = 4 \\ \Delta I_n &= I_{n+1} - I_n = 2^n - 2^{n-1} \end{aligned}$$

and the ratio of $\Delta I_n$ to $I_n$ is

$$\frac{\Delta I_n}{I_n} = \frac{1}{1} = \frac{2}{2} = \frac{4}{4} = \frac{2^n - 2^{n-1}}{2^{n-1}} = 1 = k.$$

The logarithmic spacing of the stimuli is such that $\Delta I/I = k$, which satisfies Weber's law.

The consequences of assuming that jnd's are subjectively equal produces the function shown in Figure 2.11, in which a logarithmic unit on the abscissa representing physical magnitude corresponds to a linear unit on the ordinate corresponding to sensation. Thus sensation is a logarithmic function of stimulus intensity.

A consequence of the logarithmic law is that equal stimulus-magnitude ratios produce equal sensation differences. To illustrate, the sensation differences between $I_n$ and $I_{n-1}$ in the previous example are equal for all $n$, since jnd's are assumed to be subjectively equal. The stimulus magnitude ratios

$$\frac{I_{n+1}}{I_n} = \frac{2^n}{2^{n-1}} = 2$$

are also equal for all $n$. Thus equal stimulus ratios produce equal sensation differences.

Fechner's use of discrimination data to generate the psychophysical function was not accepted without resistance, however, particularly among psychologists of an introspectionist bent who on the basis of their own experience doubted that sensations could be analyzed into components. One of the most articulate of Fechner's critics was William James, who wrote:

> The fundamental objection to Fechner's whole attempt seems to be this, that although the outer *causes* of our sensations may have many parts, every distinguishable degree, as well as every distinguishable quality, of the *sensation itself* appears to be a unique fact of consciousness. Each sensation is a complete integer.... Surely our feeling of scarlet is not a feeling of pink with a lot more pink added; it is something quite other than pink. Similarly with our sensation of an electric arc-light: it does not contain that of many smoky tallow candles in itself. Every sensation presents itself as an indivisible unit; and it is quite impossible to read any clear meaning into the notion that they are masses of units combined [1892, p. 23].

Despite these sorts of attacks, Fechner's law was generally held to be correct. More recently, however, Stevens (1957, 1961, 1962a), using a direct method to measure sensation rather than Fechner's indirect one of adding jnd's, has amassed a great deal of evidence for a very different psychophysical function. These findings will be described in the section on scaling.

## Reaction time in detection and discrimination

### *Detection*

The data available to the experimenter from most detection experiments are generally confined to the conditional probabilities of yes and no responses in the presence and absence of the signal. However, the subject in such an experiment may be able to categorize his sensation into more than the two yes-no categories. In fact, when the same stimulus is repeatedly presented in a signal detection paradigm and subjects are asked to give confidence ratings, the ratings are positively related to the probability of detecting a stimulus (Green & Swets, 1966). The more likely that the subject detected the signal, the more confident he is about his judgment. Similarly, the time it takes the subject to indicate a yes or no response may also be used as an index of the magnitude of his sensation. In fact, reaction times, like confidence ratings, show certain lawful relationships to the probability of detection and also decrease with increases in stimulus intensity at suprathreshold levels, that is, when the probability of detection has reached 1.0.

Steinman (1944), using increments in the intensity of a patch of white light, and Flynn (1943), using increments in the frequency of a pure tone, measured simple RTs in response to increments of various sizes in a modified quantal method. Steinman's purpose was to determine the adequacy of simple RT as a psychophysical response to change. As such, she sought to relate changes in RT to the Weber fraction ($\Delta I/I$) at various luminance levels. The Weber fraction for the detection of light increments decreases rapidly as the background luminance rises above threshold, remains constant over a middle range of intensities, and then increases slightly at high intensities. Steinman found a similar U-shaped relationship between mean RT and background intensity for fixed suprathreshold values of $\Delta I/I$. She also found that when she increased the value of $\Delta I/I$, RT decreased rapidly at first, and then reached an asymptote.

Steinman used values of $\Delta I$ for which the probability of detection was 1.0. However, Flynn (1943) used increments in the frequency of pure tones for which the probability of detection was between 0 and 1.0. He found an inverse relationship between RT and detection probability for two of his three subjects. As the size of the increment increased, probability of detection increased and RT decreased.

In detection, then, RT is a sensitive and predictable measure that decreases as probability of detection increases. It is of particular value in indicating changes in sensation for perfectly detectable signals. This is also its advantage in discrimination experiments.

### *Discrimination*

Several studies are based on choice RT as a measure of the discriminability of two stimuli. It is assumed that less discriminable stimuli produce both longer choice RTs and more errors, while more discriminable stimuli produce shorter RTs and fewer errors.

Johnson (1939), presenting pairs of lines differing in length, asked subjects to indicate whether the variable line was longer or shorter than the standard by depressing one of two telegraph keys. Subjects also indicated how confident they felt about each judgment.

Figure 2.12 presents the three response measures—proportion of longer responses, mean confidence rating, and mean choice RT—obtained for each line length. Confidence and RT both continue to change well after the percent of correct responses exceeds 100. Thus, both response measures are sensitive to stimulus differences that are always detected and can be said to extend the subjective measure of stimulus differences beyond the jnd. Indeed, Cattell (1902) suggested that differences that require equal choice RTs for discrimination be considered subjectively equal. He proposed that sensation be measured in *equal time units,* instead of the *equal discriminability units* of the jnd.

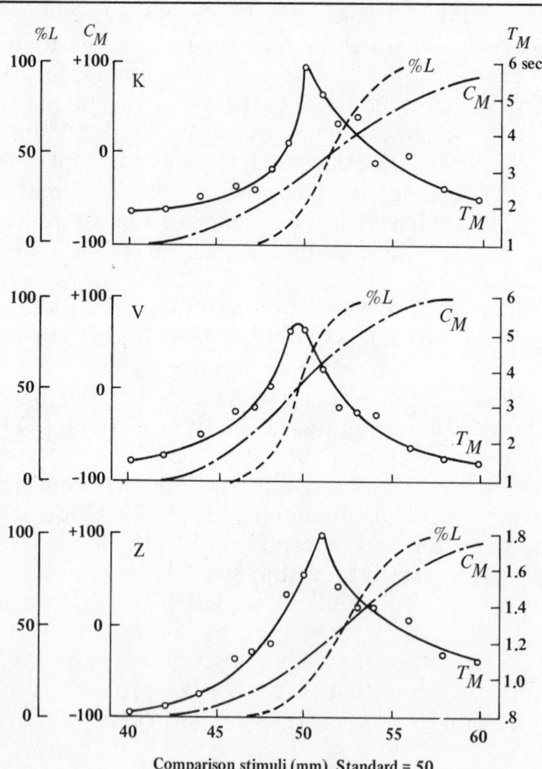


**Figure 2.12** The relationship between percent longer judgments (%$L$), mean confidence rating ($C_M$), and mean choice RT ($T_M$) as a function of the value of the variable, for a standard of 50 mm. Data are plotted separately for three subjects. (From Johnson, 1939.)

### Theories of reaction time

Just as detection theorists disagree about whether sensation is continuous or discrete, so among reaction time theorists there is a similar discrete vs. continuous controversy. The classical view holds that time is psychologically, as well as physically, continuous, so RT is a continuously varying function of stimulus, subject, and situational parameters. The quantal view holds that psychological time is quantized into discrete chunks. The two views differ primarily about the form of the theoretical distribution of RTs.

The form of the distribution of RTs is important for several reasons. First, it allows us to accept or reject certain hypotheses about the process underlying RT, and, second, it tells us which of the several possible measures of central tendency and variability are most suitable to calculate from the empirical RT distributions. We consider here only theories for simple RT situations.

In the simple RT experiment, the subject is instructed to make a motor response, such as pressing or releasing a telegraph key, to the onset of a brief stimulus, the *reaction signal.* The reaction signal is usually preceded by a *warning signal,* and the interval of time separating them is called the *foreperiod.* The reaction signal starts a timer, which is stopped by the subject's response, and the period between stimulus onset and response is the RT.

Simple RT is affected by many factors. It is different for different sensory modalities; for example, RT to sound and shock is faster than to light. Within a given modality, RT decreases as stimulus intensity is increased. RT is also sensitive to certain motivational and attentional factors. Payoffs for fast responses reduce RT; either lengthening the foreperiod beyond some optimum duration (usually 1 or 2 seconds) or making it more variable increases RT. Two-choice RT, in which one of two stimuli is presented and must be responded to with one of two responses, is slower by at least 100 milliseconds than simple RT. Generally, choice RT increases with the number of stimulus-response pairs.

A ubiquitous problem in simple RT experiments is the occurrence of near-zero or negative RTs, that is, responses that occur immediately after or even somewhat before the reaction signal. These are called *anticipations,* and some investigators (e.g., Snodgrass, Luce, & Galanter, 1967) believe them to be voluntary estimates of the foreperiod which are triggered by the warning signal. In this view, anticipations are produced by a different process than true RTs, which are triggered by the reaction signal, and so anticipations should be eliminated from the distribution of RTs either during the data analysis or by some experimental manipulation.

Any RTs which are faster than some minimum time, called the *irreducible minimum* RT (Woodworth, 1938), are presumed to be anticipations rather than true RTs. The irreducible minimum is typically held to be about 100 milliseconds and is often estimated as the mean RT to the most intense stimulus possible, exclusive of anticipations. To eliminate anticipations, then, some investigators simply discard RTs which are faster than the irreducible minimum prior to the data analysis. Two experimental procedures may be used to discourage anticipations during the experiment proper: First, variable rather than fixed foreperiods may be used so that subjects will be less able to estimate the foreperiod duration and hence to anticipate. Second, catch trials during which no reaction signal is presented may be introduced, and subjects who respond on catch trials may be warned.

Other investigators (e.g., John, 1967) view the simple RT experiment as analogous to a signal detection experiment. Anticipations are viewed as reflecting a reduced criterion for the presentation of a signal, in much the same way that a high false alarm rate in a detection experiment reflects a similar lowering of a response criterion. Accordingly, anticipation rates, like false alarm rates, should be carefully measured and manipulated by varying the payoffs for fast responses and the signal presentation probabilities, since anticipations are produced by the same process that produces true RTs.

Because so many psychological phenomena follow a normal distribution, it was originally thought that RTs might also be normally distributed. However, RT distributions, particularly simple ones, are almost invariably positively skewed, whereas the normal distribution is symmetric. Woodworth and Schlosberg (1954) proposed as a substitute the *log normal distribution,* in which RTs are converted to logarithms before being plotted. Taking logarithms expands the lower end of the RT scale and contracts the upper end, thereby pulling in the long tail of a positively skewed distribution.

More recently, distributions of RTs have been derived from a consideration of the possible mechanisms underlying the reaction process, by postulating a series of intervening, unobservable steps in a chain between the stimulus and the manifest response. Some modern theories have assumed three steps: neural input, decision, and motor response; the sum of the times of these three processes is supposedly reflected in the RT. Often, the neural input time is identified with the irreducible minimum, and so taken to be about 100 milliseconds for the auditory mode. A model of simple RT proposed by McGill (1963) will illustrate this approach. He assumes that stimulus and motivational effects have their locus in the decision process, which is of primary interest here. He proposes a *counting* model in which two counters accumulate information, one about the effects of noise in the neural channels and the other about the stimulus. When the difference between the noise and the stimulus counters exceeds the subject's criterion, the subject terminates the decision process and makes his motor response. Thus two factors affect decision time: the rate at which the two counters diverge, and the criterion. The first factor will be affected by the intensity of stimuli, and hence McGill's model predicts that RT will decrease as stimulus intensity increases, as indeed it does. The second factor, the criterion, will be affected by motivational and perhaps attentional factors. Payoffs for fast responses should decrease RT by lowering the criterion, and penalties for anticipations should increase RT by raising the criterion.

McGill made certain assumptions about the three RT components. He assumed that the neural input time has virtually no variability, that the decision process is normally distributed, and that the motor response is exponentially distributed. Thus McGill's model predicts that RTs will follow a distribution formed by the convolution of a normal and exponential distribution displaced by a constant equal to neural input time. The prediction was fulfilled by Hohle's (1965) measures of simple RT, but Snodgrass, Luce, and Galanter (1967) found that a different theoretical distribution fit their simple RT data better.

The name most closely associated with *quantal time* is that of Stroud (1955), who termed the unit of time the *psychological moment*. According to Stroud, psychological time is divided into discrete chunks, called moments, that vary in duration from 50 to 200 milliseconds. A moment defines the *psychological now* of subjective experience, and events that occur within a single moment are not perceived as ordered. Order is only possible when events occur in separate moments. Furthermore, moments are *modality specific*. Stimuli in different modalities occurring simultaneously in physical time can only be perceived in different moments. Similarly, a motor response to a stimulus cannot be initiated until the end of the moment in which the stimulus occurs. It is this latter assumption that is relevant to predictions about RT distributions.

Specifically, Stroud assumes some constant time lag, *K*, between stimulus and response in the simple RT situation. The value of *K* reflects the sum of stimulus-input and motor-output times, and corresponds to the irreducible minimum RT of other investigators. In addition to *K*, there is a variable time lag in RT which is determined by the instant at which the stimulus occurs in the psychological moment. Because the subject must wait until the end of the psychological moment to begin his response, the variable time lag can be as short as zero (if the stimulus occurs at the very end of the moment) or as long as the duration of the moment (if the stimulus occurs at its beginning). Stroud assumes that when the stimulus onset is unpredictable, as when foreperiods are long and/or variable, the reaction signal will occur anywhere within a moment with equal probability. These assumptions lead to the prediction that the distribution of RTs is rectangular, with a width equal to the duration of a moment, *Q*, and displaced along the time axis by a value equal to *K*.

To test the moment hypothesis, Stroud used Woodrow's (1914) data on simple RTs to auditory stimuli presented at various intervals after a warning signal. Stroud found that certain distributions of RTs, obtained after fairly long (16–24 seconds) foreperiods, exhibited the predicted rectangular shape, and he estimated *Q* from the width of the distributions to be between 56 and 62 milliseconds, and *K* to be between 40 and 60 milliseconds.

However, Woodrow's data are exceptional in that most RT distributions are not rectangular in shape; in fact, recently it has been shown that the more control that is established over RT, by means of feedback and payoffs that encourage true RTs and discourage anticipations, the more peaked the distribution of RTs becomes (Snodgrass, 1969; Snodgrass, Luce, & Galanter, 1967).

## SCALING

> The ape-man reached out through the darkness and found Jana's hand. Carefully he led her through the stygian darkness toward the mouth of the fissure. Feeling his way step by step, groping forward with his free hand, the ape-man finally discovered the entrance to the trail.
>
> Clambering upward over broken masses of jagged granite through utter darkness, it seemed to the two fugitives that they made no progress whatever. If time could be measured by muscular effort and physical discomfort, the two might have guessed that they passed an eternity in this black fissure, . . . [Burroughs, 1929, p. 166].

Thus the scaling problem is described for us by Burroughs as Tarzan and Jana judge the subjective passage of time by muscular effort and physical discomfort. Although their estimate of this time interval as an eternity might not be manageable in terms of usual psychophysical scaling techniques, it illustrates the aim of psychophysical scaling methods: to obtain numerical measures of subjective quantities and relate them to objective quantities.

Scaling is closely related to the problem of measurement, which is the assignment of numerals to properties of stimuli or events according to rules (see Stevens, 1951). In scaling we obtain responses to stimuli in such a way that we can assign numbers to the stimuli according to a nominal, ordinal, interval, or ratio scale of measurement.

In the simplest kind of measurement, *nominal* scaling, the numbers or other symbols assigned to the stimuli categorize them as different with respect to the measured response, but say nothing about how they are ordered, how different they are from each other, or how big they are. In *ordinal* scaling, the stimuli can be ordered with respect to a property, and the assigned numbers reflect that order, but nothing else. In *interval* scaling, the assigned numbers reflect differences between stimuli, as well as order. Finally, in *ratio* scaling, the assigned numbers reflect both differences and ratios between stimuli.

### Measurement

Measurement is the assignment of symbols, usually numbers, to properties of objects or events according to rules. Objects themselves are not measured, only their properties. A further distinction is made by Torgerson (1958) between *systems,* which include tangible objects such as books, telephones, and hands, as well as less tangible things such as spots of light and tones, and *properties,* which are observable dimensions such as weight, length, color, and loudness. In Torgerson's terminology, systems are never measured, only their properties. For our purposes, systems are

**Table 2.4 Examples of Measurement on Four Types of Scales**

| Team member | I Number on jersey (Nominal) | II Order at finish line (Ordinal) | III Time at finish line (Interval) | IV Running time in minutes (Ratio) |
|---|---|---|---|---|
| A | 52 | 1 | 2:01 | 1.0 |
| B | 6 | 2 | 2:02 | 2.0 |
| C | 74 | 3 | 2:04 | 4.0 |
| D | 106 | 4 | 2:05 | 5.0 |

stimuli and the sensations they evoke, and properties of stimuli refer to attributes such as hue, intensity, form, and size.

Depending on which rules are used, the numerals that are assigned to properties form one of four types of scales: nominal, ordinal, interval, or ratio. The scale type determines the operations that may be performed on the assigned numerals. Numbers themselves are on a ratio scale; that is, the number 10 is twice as large as the number 5; the number 50 is ten times as large as the number 5, and so on. We can take logarithms of numbers, raise them to powers, and perform any mathematical operation on them we wish. However, the numbers that are assigned to properties or events may or may not be treated as true numbers, depending on which rules were used in constructing the scale and, hence, on the scale type. To illustrate the different scales, imagine the following situation.

Four members of a track team run a race. Runner A has the number 52 on the back of his jersey, runner B has the number 6, C is number 74, and D is number 106. An observer at the finish line determines that A comes in first, B is second, C is third, and D is fourth. A timekeeper determines that A crosses the finish line at 2:01 P.M., B at 2:02 P.M., C at 2:04 P.M., and D at 2:05 P.M. An official of the track meet determines the actual running time of each man in minutes by subtracting from the clock time at finish the time the race was started—in this case, 2:00 P.M.—so that the running time for A is 1 minute, time for B is 2 minutes, time for C is 4 minutes, and time for D is 5 minutes. These four sets of measurements, representing measurement on each of the four scale types, are shown in Table 2.4.

The number of the runner (column I) is on a nominal scale of measurement; each runner's number only identifies or names him. The number indicates nothing about the relationship between team members on any attribute except that they are different. In nominal scale measurement, numerals are merely names that distinguish one object from another. None of the usual mathematical operations such as subtraction, division, or multiplication can be performed on them. Moreover, they can be changed in any way desired—to other numbers, to letters, to proper names, etc.—so long as no two objects or classes of objects are assigned the same symbol or number.

The numbers indicating the order in which runners crossed the finish line (column II) are on an ordinal scale. The order of the numbers is essential, but differences or ratios among them are not. They can be changed in any way that preserves the order among them. The type of transformation that preserves order, but does not necessarily preserve differences or ratios, is the *simple increasing monotonic transform*. Such a function increases without reversal. Thus, instead of order at the finish line, the amount of money won by each of the runners could be used to rank them. Suppose the first one across the line won $10; the second, $5; the third, $2; and the fourth, $1. The values of the prizes also form an ordinal scale in that they indicate only the order of arrival.

Time at finish line (column III) is measured on an interval scale. Here, time of arrival indicates differences between running times, but nothing about their ratios. We know from time of arrival that B was slower than A by the same amount of time that D was slower than C; the difference between B and A, 2:02 − 2:01, is equal to the difference between D and C, 2:05 − 2:04. However, not knowing the starting time, we have no idea whether B was twice as fast or ten times as fast as A. With no knowledge of starting time, the ratios between the running speeds are not known. Interval-scale numbers may be transformed by the formula $X' = aX + b$ (where $a$ is positive). The constant $a$ changes the unit of measurement, and the constant $b$ changes the zero point. Such a transformation preserves the ratio of *differences* among the times and the order, but not the direct ratios among the times themselves.

Running time in minutes (column IV) illustrates ratio-scale measurements; ratios between running times of the different players are now meaningful. Now it can be said that A ran twice as fast as B, and B ran twice as fast as C. The only permissible transformation for ratio-scale measurements is by the rule $X' = aX$ (where, again, $a$ must be positive). The unit of measurement, $a$, can change but the zero point is fixed. Thus, running times could be multiplied by 60 to transform minutes into

**Table 2.5 Comparisons Among the Four Scales of Measurement**

| Scale | Necessary operation for creating scale | Permissible transformations | Permissible statistics |
|---|---|---|---|
| Nominal | Determination of equality | $X' = f(X)$, where $f(X)$ is any one-to-one substitution | Number of cases<br>Mode<br>Contingency correlation |
| Ordinal | Determination of greater or less | $X' = f(X)$, where $f(X)$ is any increasing monotonic function | Median<br>Percentiles<br>Rank order correlation |
| Interval | Determination of equality of intervals or differences | $X' = aX + b$<br>$(a > 0)$ | Mean<br>Standard deviation<br>Product-moment correlation |
| Ratio | Determination of equality of ratios | $X' = aX$<br>$(a > 0)$ | Geometric mean<br>Coefficient of variation<br>Decibel transformations |

(After Stevens, 1951.)

seconds. Such a transformation keeps both the ratios and the ratios of differences constant.

Knowing the scale of measurement has great practical importance because the statistics that may be used on the data depend on the permissible transformations of the data, which in turn depend on the scale on which the responses have been measured. Table 2.5 lists the scales of measurement, the necessary operations for creating the scale, the permissible transformations of the numerals so assigned, and the permissible statistics (Stevens, 1951). Note that use of the mean and the standard deviation requires measurement on at least an interval scale, whereas use of the coefficient of variation requires ratio-scale measurement.

Table 2.6 illustrates the effect that transformations of three sets of scores measured on interval and ratio scales have on the means, standard deviations, and coefficients of variation. Interval measurement requires a method of determining equality of intervals or differences, and thus under interval transformation equal differences among means and standard deviations must be preserved. In the original set of data, $\mu_{B_0} - \mu_{A_0} = \mu_{C_0} - \mu_{B_0} = 1.0$, and $\sigma_{B_0} - \sigma_{A_0} = \sigma_{C_0} - \sigma_{B_0} = 0.5$. In the transformed data $\mu_{B_1} - \mu_{A_1} = \mu_{C_1} - \mu_{B_1} = 2.0$, and $\sigma_{B_1} - \sigma_{A_1} = \sigma_{C_1} - \sigma_{B_1} = 1.0$. However, the coefficient of variation, which was the same for all three sets of measurements in the original data, does not remain invariant across sets under the interval transformation, illustrating that the coefficient of variation is not a permissible statistic to use with interval measurement.

Ratio measurement requires a method of determining equality of ratios; this equality is preserved under the ratio transformation; i.e., $\mu_{A_0}/\mu_{B_0} = \mu_{A_2}/\mu_{B_2}$, $\mu_{B_0}/\mu_{C_0} = \mu_{B_2}/\mu_{C_2}$ and $\sigma_{A_0}/\sigma_{B_0} = \sigma_{A_2}/\sigma_{B_2}$, $\sigma_{B_0}/\sigma_{C_0} = \sigma_{B_2}/\sigma_{C_2}$. Furthermore, the coefficient of variation remains invariant across sets under the ratio transformation, illustrating that the coefficient of variation is a permissible statistic under ratio-scale measurement.

### Nominal scaling: Recognition

In the recognition experiment, also referred to as the *identification* or *absolute-judgment situation,* one of $n$ stimuli is presented to the subject who tries to identify or recognize it. His response may be a number, a name, or even a key-press. We classify recognition as nominal scaling because even when numbers are used as responses, the numbers themselves serve only to identify the stimuli and do not necessarily reflect ordinal, interval, or ratio characteristics among the stimuli with respect to some property.

Unlike stimuli in discrimination experiments, those in recognition experiments are usually perfectly discriminable from one another when presented simultaneously in pairs. However, because recognition stimuli are presented successively, the subject must compare each stimulus to some internal standard developed through experience with the stimuli. His ability to do this is the subject of study in recognition experiments.

The stimuli in recognition experiments may vary along a single dimension, such as intensity,

**Table 2.6 Comparison of the Effect of Two Types of Scale Transformation on the Mean ($\mu$), Standard Deviation ($\sigma$), and Coefficient of Variation ($V$)**

| | Original data | | | Interval transformation* | | | Ratio transformation** | | |
|---|---|---|---|---|---|---|---|---|---|
| | $A_0$ | $B_0$ | $C_0$ | $A_1$ | $B_1$ | $C_1$ | $A_2$ | $B_2$ | $C_2$ |
| $\mu$ | 5.0 | 6.0 | 7.0 | 20.0 | 22.0 | 24.0 | 20.0 | 24.0 | 28.0 |
| $\sigma$ | 2.5 | 3.0 | 3.5 | 5.0 | 6.0 | 7.0 | 10.0 | 12.0 | 14.0 |
| $V = 100\,\sigma/\mu$ | 50.0 | 50.0 | 50.0 | 25.0 | 27.2727 | 29.1666 | 50.0 | 50.0 | 50.0 |

$*X_1 = 2X_0 + 10$ $**X_2 = 4X_0$

wavelength, or frequency, or simultaneously along a combination of dimensions. A question of major interest is the number of different stimuli that can be correctly identified as a function of the number of dimensions along which they vary and their relative spacing along those dimensions.

A common and persistent finding has been that the number of *unidimensional* stimuli that can be identified without error is of the order of seven, plus or minus two, regardless of the dimension involved (Miller, 1956). That is, if stimuli vary with respect to only one attribute, such as pitch, loudness, degree of saltiness, or position on a line, subjects can identify only about seven different stimuli without error. Sometimes the number is larger, as for points on a line, and sometimes it is smaller, as for saltiness. It is surprising that this number is so small since in our daily life we recognize a much larger number of faces, spoken and written words, paintings, and so on. However, the objects we encounter in our daily life are not unidimensional; faces vary on some undetermined but large number of dimensions, and we probably use quite a few of them to make our identifications. Therefore, an obvious question in recognition experiments is what happens to the number of stimuli that can be recognized when they vary on more than one dimension.

Subjects can recognize perfectly about six tones differing only in pitch, and about five tones differing only in loudness. Suppose subjects are presented tones differing both in pitch and in loudness in all possible combinations; it might be expected that in combination the subject could recognize thirty tones (5 × 6) differing in both. However, when pitch and loudness are combined the subject can recognize only about nine tones without error (Pollack, 1952, 1953). Recognition of stimuli which vary on two dimensions simultaneously is better than recognition of stimuli varying on any single dimension, but the improvement is not as great as might be expected from performance on each dimension separately. Furthermore, the spacing of stimuli along a single dimension does not affect recognition performance as much as might be expected. The limit in recognition appears to be set by the subject's internal standard and not by the physical characteristics of the stimuli to be recognized.

### *Information theory in the recognition experiment*

It would be desirable to have a statistic that would summarize the subject's performance in a recognition experiment, so that the experimenter could take into account the number of stimuli presented, their relative frequencies of presentation, the frequency of errors, and the degree of dispersion of the errors. The field of communication engineering has provided a concept—information—and a method of measuring it that psychologists have found useful in the recognition context, as well as in a number of other areas (Miller, 1953).

There are four information statistics: the information in any particular message, denoted $h_i$; the average information in a set of messages, denoted $H$; the uncertainty prior to the delivery of a message, denoted $U$; and the amount of information actually transmitted from a source to a receiver, denoted $T$.

The information in a particular message is inversely related to its probability of occurrence. This accords well with common-sense notions about information, since the less likely a message is, the more information it conveys. For example, in response to your query "How are you?" your friend is more informative when he replies "Terrible, I have the flu" than when he replies "Fine, thank you," because the former reply is less probable than the latter. Specifically, the amount of information, $h_i$, in the $i$th message is

$$h_i = \log \frac{1}{p_i} = -\log p_i, \quad [9]$$

where $p_i$ is the probability of the $i$th message and the logarithms are to the base two.

The average information in a set of messages is calculated by multiplying the information in each message by its probability of occurrence and summing over the set of messages, so

$$H = -\Sigma p_i \log p_i. \qquad [10]$$

Uncertainty $U$ is numerically identical to average information $H$, but refers to the state of affairs prior to delivery of the message, whereas $H$ is often used to refer to the state of affairs after delivery. To illustrate, before you turn on the radio for the evening news you have a certain amount of uncertainty about what will be said with respect to each of several categories of news. This uncertainty is the same as the average amount of information that has been conveyed or can be conveyed about each category. The news commentator delivers a single message in each of the categories, and the $h$ value for these individual messages is inversely related to their a priori probabilities of occurrence. Noteworthy news is surprising, and to the degree it is surprising, it is informative. The extent to which you correctly receive the set of messages is the amount of information transmitted $T$: you can never receive more information than was sent, but if you miss or mishear some details, you will receive less.

As originally proposed by Shannon (1948), information measurement was used to measure *channel capacity* of a communication line. Channel capacity is determined by comparing the amount of information received at the end of the channel with the amount of information present at the source. In order to translate the concepts of the communication engineer to those relevant to psychology, we will consider a *source* as a set of stimuli in the recognition experiment, the *channel* as the human subject, and the *receiver* as the subject's responses as measured by the experimenter. Our problem is to evaluate the capacity of the subject as a channel or information transmitter. To do this, we must first compute $H(s)$, the amount of information in the stimulus set.

Basically, $H(s)$ is a nonmetric measure of *variance* for a set of stimuli on a nominal scale of measurement. It takes into account only the number and relative frequencies of occurrence of a set of stimuli. It does not take into account actual values of stimuli or their spacing, as would the traditional variance measure for stimuli measured on interval or ratio scales. Because it is the number and presentation probabilities of stimuli rather than their absolute values and spacings which are of paramount importance in recognition experiments, the information statistic seems ideally suited for application to this area.

The amount of information in a set of $n$ stimuli, each having the same probability of presentation, can be defined as the number of yes-no questions that must be asked in order to identify the stimulus. For example, in order to find out which of the digits 1 through 8 is written on a slip of paper your friend is holding, you need to ask him only three yes-no questions, as outlined below.

Note that for optimum efficiency the questions are so phrased that each answer halves the number of alternatives, provided they are all equally likely. Although on a single trial one might find the answer

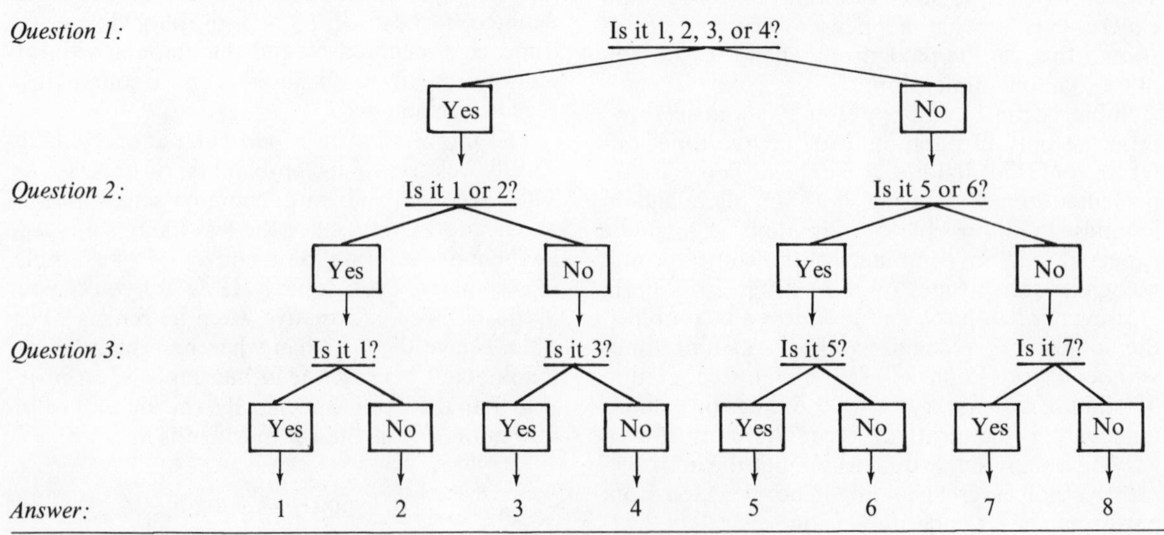

in fewer questions by eliminating them one by one, e.g., Is it 1? Is it 2? etc., the average number of questions that would have to be asked with this inefficient strategy is 4.5. In guessing games, people tend to adopt the more efficient strategy. In the game Twenty Questions, good players try to ask questions so as to eliminate half of the remaining possibilities, such as "Is the person a man?" "Is he living?" etc.

The number of yes-no questions, or *binary decisions,* necessary to decide among $n$ equally probable alternatives is $\log_2 n$, and hence the average amount of information, $H(s)$, in a set of $n$ equally probable messages is $\log_2 n$. This equation can be derived from our original formula for $H$:

$$H = -\Sigma p_i \log_2 p_i.$$

$p_i = 1/n$ for equally likely alternatives, so

$$\begin{aligned} -\Sigma\, p_i \log_2 p_i &= -\Sigma \frac{1}{n} \log_2 \frac{1}{n} \\ &= -n\left(\frac{1}{n} \log_2 \frac{1}{n}\right) \\ &= -\log_2 \frac{1}{n} \\ &= \log_2 n. \end{aligned} \qquad [11]$$

Information is measured in *bits*, which is the contraction for *binary digits*. The number of binary digits required to code messages optimally is equal to their $h$ value in bits. For example, a stimulus set containing four equally likely alternatives has an average information value of two bits, each of the individual messages has an $h$ value of two bits, and two binary digits are required to code the messages.

The average amount of information in a stimulus set is maximum for equally probable alternatives and decreases monotonically as the probabilities become less equal. Table 2.7 illustrates this rule by showing how information $h_i$ in single alternatives and average information $H$ in two-alternative sets vary with the probability values. Although the information in a single alternative is greatest when $p_i$ is smallest, the average information in a two-alternative set is greatest when the two component $p_i$s are the same and equal to 0.5.

In order to calculate transmission or channel capacity from a recognition experiment, two quantities are necessary: the amount of information in the stimulus set, $H(s)$, and the amount of information remaining in the stimulus set when the subject's responses are known, $H_r(s)$. Information transmitted, $T$, is defined as $H(s)$ minus $H_r(s)$. If the subject never makes an error, no information is left in the stimulus once his responses are known,

**Table 2.7 Information ($h_i$) in Individual Alternatives Whose Probability Is $p_i$, and Average Information ($H$) in Two-Alternative Sets, One of Whose Components Has a Probability of $p_i$ and the Other 1.0 − $p_i$**

| Single alternatives | | Double alternatives | |
|---|---|---|---|
| $p_i$ | $h_i = \log_2 p_i$ | $p_i, 1.0 - p_i$ | $H = -\sum^2 p_i \log_2 p_i$ |
| .10 | 3.322 | .01, .99 | 0.0788 |
| .20 | 2.322 | .05, .95 | 0.2864 |
| .30 | 1.737 | .10, .90 | 0.4690 |
| .40 | 1.322 | .20, .80 | 0.7220 |
| .50 | 1.000 | .25, .75 | 0.8113 |
| .60 | 0.737 | .30, .70 | 0.8813 |
| .70 | 0.515 | .40, .60 | 0.9710 |
| .80 | 0.322 | .45, .55 | 0.9928 |
| .90 | 0.152 | .50, .50 | 1.0000 |

so $H_r(s) = 0$ and $T = H(s)$. The subject has transmitted all the information in the stimulus set.

Table 2.8 contains the results of a recognition experiment carried out as part of an undergraduate laboratory course. These data are used to illustrate the calculation of $T$. Ten subjects identified ten tones by their letter names when the tones, which were played on the piano, were closely spaced, moderately spaced, and spaced far apart. The number in each cell is the number of subjects who gave the indicated response to each stimulus.

The 10 stimuli were presented equally often, so $H(s) = \log_2 10 = 3.322$ bits. $H_r(s)$ is calculated by treating each column (i.e., response) as a unit, calculating the average amount of information in each column, weighting that average by the proportion of all 100 responses which that column represents, and summing across columns. Note that if all 10 subjects had responded correctly to each stimulus, the average information in each column would be 0, $H_r(s)$ would be 0, and the subjects would have transmitted all the information in the stimulus set, that is, 3.322 bits.

In fact, the subjects made errors, and $T$ for Array 1, small range, is 1.750 bits; for Array 2, moderate range, $T$ is 1.668 bits; and for Array 3, large range, it is 1.829 bits. Theoretically, $T$ is the log to the base two of the number of stimuli that could be identified without error, so fewer than four stimuli ought to be absolutely identified by these subjects in a similar situation. This number is somewhat less than the six tones differing in pitch that were correctly identified in the experiment referred to earlier (Pollack, 1952). These data illustrate the point that the range of stimulus values does not have a large effect on the number of stimuli that can be recognized without error.

**Table 2.8 Confusion Matrices for Three Ranges of Frequencies of Tones. The Entry in Each Cell Is the Number of Subjects Who Gave the Indicated Response to Each Stimulus**

Array 1 (small range)

| | | Response | | | | | | | | | | |
|---|---|---|---|---|---|---|---|---|---|---|---|---|
| | | 1 | 2 | 3 | 4 | 5 | 6 | 7 | 8 | 9 | 10 | Total |
| | 1 | 7 | 2 | 1 | | | | | | | | 10 |
| | 2 | | 5 | 3 | | 2 | | | | | | 10 |
| | 3 | 1 | 3 | 5 | 1 | | | | | | | 10 |
| | 4 | | | 1 | 7 | 2 | | | | | | 10 |
| Stimulus | 5 | | | 1 | 2 | 4 | 1 | 1 | 1 | | | 10 |
| | 6 | | | | 2 | 4 | 3 | 1 | | | | 10 |
| | 7 | 1 | | | | | 5 | 3 | | 1 | | 10 |
| | 8 | | | | | 1 | 1 | 2 | 4 | 2 | | 10 |
| | 9 | | | | | | | 2 | 1 | 7 | | 10 |
| | 10 | | | | | | | 1 | 1 | | 8 | 10 |
| *Total* | | 9 | 10 | 11 | 12 | 13 | 10 | 10 | 7 | 10 | 8 | 100 |

Array 2 (moderate range)

| | | Response | | | | | | | | | | |
|---|---|---|---|---|---|---|---|---|---|---|---|---|
| | | 1 | 2 | 3 | 4 | 5 | 6 | 7 | 8 | 9 | 10 | Total |
| | 1 | 8 | 1 | | 1 | | | | | | | 10 |
| | 2 | 1 | 2 | 3 | 4 | | | | | | | 10 |
| | 3 | 1 | 3 | 4 | 1 | 1 | | | | | | 10 |
| | 4 | | | 5 | 3 | 1 | | 1 | | | | 10 |
| Stimulus | 5 | | 1 | 2 | 2 | 3 | 2 | | | | | 10 |
| | 6 | | | 1 | | 2 | 3 | 4 | | | | 10 |
| | 7 | | | | 1 | 1 | 3 | 3 | 2 | | | 10 |
| | 8 | | | | | | 1 | 2 | 4 | 3 | | 10 |
| | 9 | | | | | | | | 2 | 7 | 1 | 10 |
| | 10 | | | | | | | | | 1 | 9 | 10 |
| *Total* | | 10 | 7 | 15 | 12 | 8 | 9 | 10 | 8 | 11 | 10 | 100 |

Array 3 (large range)

| | | Response | | | | | | | | | | |
|---|---|---|---|---|---|---|---|---|---|---|---|---|
| | | 1 | 2 | 3 | 4 | 5 | 6 | 7 | 8 | 9 | 10 | Total |
| | 1 | 6 | 2 | 1 | 1 | | | | | | | 10 |
| | 2 | | 7 | 1 | | 2 | | | | | | 10 |
| | 3 | 2 | 1 | 4 | 2 | | 1 | | | | | 10 |
| | 4 | | 1 | | 5 | 1 | 2 | 1 | | | | 10 |
| Stimulus | 5 | | | 2 | 3 | 4 | | 1 | | | | 10 |
| | 6 | | | | | 2 | 5 | 3 | | | | 10 |
| | 7 | | | | | | 2 | 4 | 2 | 2 | | 10 |
| | 8 | | | | | | | 2 | 5 | 2 | 1 | 10 |
| | 9 | | | | | 1 | | 1 | | 8 | | 10 |
| | 10 | | | | | | | | | | 10 | 10 |
| *Total* | | 8 | 11 | 8 | 11 | 10 | 10 | 12 | 7 | 12 | 11 | 100 |

(Data were collected by H. B. Barsky.)

*Choice reaction time and information*

An experiment by Hyman (1953) illustrates how information theory has been used in choice RT experiments. Hyman varied the amount of information in a set of stimuli in three ways: (a) by varying the number of equally probable alternatives from one to eight, (b) by varying both the probability of occurrence and the number of alternatives, and (c) by introducing *sequential dependencies* into the presentation schedule of stimuli. For example, in a two-alternative situation where both alternatives were equally probable across trials, the probability of a change from one alternative to the other from trial $n$ to $n + 1$ was 0.80, and thus the probability of repeating the same stimulus was 0.20. Less information is conveyed by a stimulus in this situation than in one without sequential dependencies because the presentation of a specific stimulus on trial $n$ changes the presentation probabilities on trial $n + 1$ from .50/.50 to .80/.20.

Although the several conditions resulting from these three types of manipulations are qualitatively different, they yield equivalent values for $H(s)$, the average information in the stimulus set. The amount of information varied from 0 bits (simple RT) to 3 bits. Hyman found that mean RT was a linear function of average information in the stimulus set regardless how the information was produced and that, except for one of the four subjects, the slopes and intercepts of the regression line relating information to RT were the same across the three sets of conditions. In this case, then, RT behaves analogously to *error rate*. Subjects take longer to process a stimulus that conveys more information, as in Hyman's study, or they make more errors when required to identify a high-information stimulus, as in the recognition studies previously discussed.

### Ordinal scaling: The method of paired comparisons and ranking

Stimuli can be placed on an ordinal scale if subjects can rank-order them with respect to some attribute. Suppose the subject is to rank $n$ stimuli with respect to property $X$, where $X$ could be intensity, esthetic value, utility, degree of preference, and so on. He can be given subsets of $k$ stimuli from the set of $n$ and asked to rank within that subset, giving the rank of 1 to the stimulus with the most $X$ and the rank of $k$ to the stimulus with the least. When $k = 2$, the method is called *paired compari-*

*sons;* when $k = n$, all the stimuli are ranked at once, and the method is called *ranking;* when $k = 3$, it is the method of *triads*. Coombs (1964, Ch. 2) analyzes the efficiency of various methods for various values of $n$ and $k$.

When $k < n$, the rank of stimulus A is obtained by ranking the frequency with which it is chosen over all other stimuli. Typically, each stimulus is compared at least once with every other stimulus. To determine how many sets of $k$ must be presented so that each stimulus is compared once with every other stimulus, we use the formula for combinations, which tells us the total number of ways to take $n$ things $k$ at a time, or

$$\binom{n}{k} = \frac{n!}{k!\,(n-k)!}. \qquad [12]$$

This formula will be familiar to many readers as that for a binomial coefficient.

Suppose, for example, we want to compare sixteen foods by the method of paired comparisons. According to the formula for combinations,

$$\binom{16}{2} = \frac{16!}{2!\,14!} = \frac{16 \times 15}{2} = 120,$$

that is, there are 120 pairs for $n = 16$.

Obviously the method of ranking is much faster than the method of paired comparisons. However, the latter method has two advantages: First, the subject's task is simpler, and second, *transitivity of judgments* can be tested. One of the characteristics of an ordinal scale is transitivity; that is, if A is preferred to B, and B is preferred to C, then A must be preferred to C (where *preferred* may be replaced by any statement of the form "is judged to have more of attribute $X$"). In fact, judgments of this sort rarely show perfect transitivity, especially if the number of objects being compared is large. However, the following section shows how one model of scaling turns the lack of transitivity to advantage in deriving scale values for stimuli.

### *Thurstonian scaling*

Thurstone (1927) was one of the first to adapt the methods of psychophysical scaling to psychological continua. He saw that one could make use of *confusability* among stimuli differing along a psychological continuum to obtain scale values for them in much the same way Fechner used confusability among psychophysical stimuli to scale them by adding up jnd's. Thurstonian scaling uses the method of paired comparisons, whereas jnd's are generally measured with the two-category method of constant stimuli. The two methods differ in two ways: First, in paired comparisons all stimuli are compared with one another, rather than each with a standard stimulus of constant value. The reason for this is that the standard in psychophysics is generally chosen from the middle of the range of variables, whereas in psychological scaling the experimenter often does not know the underlying order of the stimuli before the experiment. Second, in paired comparisons the same stimulus is usually not compared with itself, since the stimuli used in psychological scaling experiments are highly discriminable with regard to certain physical attributes, even though they may not be with regard to the psychological attribute under study. For example, a subject may find it difficult to discriminate between roast beef and steak on the basis of his preference, yet he has no trouble discriminating between them on other grounds. Thus in psychological scaling it usually does not make sense to ask a subject which he prefers, roast beef or roast beef, although it does make sense in psychophysical procedures, as when studying the time-order error, to ask a subject which of two identical tones is louder.

Just as intransitivities occur within a given subject's data in discrimination experiments, intransitivities occur within psychological judgments. Thurstone's *law of comparative judgment* assumes that the underlying basis for these intransitivities is the same as that which the classical theory of thresholds assumes for intransitivities within threshold judgments.

Thurstone assumes that each presentation of a stimulus object generates a *discriminal* process in the subject that differs somewhat from moment to moment or from trial to trial. Thus a frequency distribution of discriminal processes is associated with each stimulus, which is assumed to be normally distributed, whose mean is taken as its scale value, and whose standard deviation is known as its *discriminal dispersion*. Let us call $s_j$ and $s_k$ the scale values of stimuli $j$ and $k$, $\sigma_j$ and $\sigma_k$ their discriminal dispersions, and $d_j$ and $d_k$ the particular value of discriminal process excited by stimuli $j$ and $k$ on a particular trial. In the simplest case, known as Case V, Thurstone assumes that $\sigma_j$ and $\sigma_k$ are equal for all $j$ and $k$, and the correlation, $r$, between $d_j$ and $d_k$ is zero.

To make his judgment, the subject compares the individual discriminal processes $d_j$ and $d_k$. For example, assume that the subject's task is to indicate his preference for soft drinks; $d_j$ is his momentary preference for cola and $d_k$ is his momentary preference for root beer. When this pair is presented, he looks at the difference $d_j - d_k$; if it is positive, he chooses cola, and if negative, root beer. The distribution of differences between $d_j$ and $d_k$ will be normal with a mean $= s_j - s_k$ and a standard deviation $= \sqrt{\sigma_j^2 + \sigma_k^2 - 2r\sigma_j\sigma_k}$. Because it is assumed that $r = 0$, and $\sigma_j = \sigma_k = \sigma$, the standard deviation of the difference distribution $= \sqrt{2}\sigma$. Since this procedure yields interval-scale values, the unit and the zero point are not fixed so we can take $\sqrt{2}\sigma$ as our unit.

Experimentally, stimuli are presented repeatedly in the method of paired comparisons either to the same subject, to different subjects, or both, and the proportion of choices of stimulus $j$ over stimulus $k$ are tabulated. When stimuli are presented by name, as in a preference experiment for soft drinks, the names are quite discriminable, and presenting the same pair repeatedly to the same subject might bias his subsequent responses toward his previous judgments; in this case, the judgments are often collected across subjects rather than within subjects. On the other hand, if the subject were presented with tastes of the actual drink and asked to choose between unmarked glasses of cola and root beer, it would be feasible to present the same pair of liquids to him over and over again.

To illustrate how scale values are derived, let us take a simple example. A candy manufacturer wants to scale goodness of three of his candy bars, A, B, and C. All possible pairings of the three have been presented to a large number of children, and the proportion of children who prefer A to B, B to C, and A to C are as follows:

$$Pr(\text{A P B}) = 0.80$$
$$Pr(\text{B P C}) = 0.65$$
$$Pr(\text{A P C}) = 0.89$$

The theoretical distribution of differences between stimuli $j$ and $k$ is shown in Figure 2.13. The mean of the distribution, $x_{jk}$, is the difference in scale values $s_j - s_k$ expressed in $\sqrt{2}\sigma$ units. The shaded portion to the right of the zero point is the probability that the difference $d_j - d_k$ is positive, and corresponds to the proportion of times $j$ was preferred to $k$. To find the value of $x_{jk}$, we find the number of $z$ scores (from the unit normal curve) that the zero point lies away from the mean. The negative of the $z$ score is the value of $s_j - s_k$ in units of $\sqrt{2}\sigma$.

For our example, the area in the theoretical distribution of differences between candy bar A and candy bar B to the right of the zero point is esti-

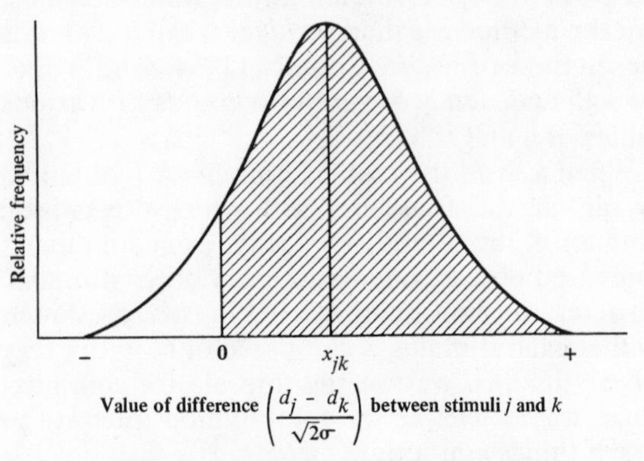


**Figure 2.13** The distribution of discriminal differences between stimuli $j$ and $k$. The shaded area to the right of the zero point is the proportion of times stimulus $j$ was preferred to stimulus $k$. The mean difference $x_{jk}$ is measured in $\sqrt{2}\sigma$ units. (From Torgerson, 1958.)

mated from the proportion of preferences for A over B as 0.80. A table of the normal distribution yields a $z$ score of $-0.84$ for the zero point, so the mean, $x_{AB}$, of the distribution is $+0.84$, or $s_A - s_B = +0.84$. Similarly, the area for the distribution of differences between B and C is 0.65, yielding a $z$ score of $-0.39$ and a mean difference, $x_{BC}$, of $+0.39$. Finally, for A and C the area is 0.89, the $z$ score is $-1.23$, and the mean difference, $x_{AC}$, is $+1.23$. In summary,

$$s_A - s_B = +0.84,$$
$$s_B - s_C = +0.39, \text{ and}$$
$$s_A - s_C = +1.23.$$

Error-free data produce additive distances, that is, $(s_A - s_B) + (s_B - s_C) = s_A - s_C$, as shown in the preceding example. In practice, however, distances computed from empirical data rarely show perfect additivity, so that certain statistical techniques have been developed to combine the various distance estimates in optimum ways (Torgerson, 1958, Ch. 9). Once the distances have been obtained, it is a simple matter to compute the scale values themselves. Because the zero point is arbitrary, the value of 0 is often assigned to the least-preferred alternative, and the other scale values are found by accumulating intervening distances. In the illustration, $s_C = 0$, $s_B = +0.39$, and $s_A = +1.23$.

### *The unfolding technique*

Another approach to ordinal scaling is to assume that subjects differ with respect to stimuli. Consider as an example of stimuli candidates for political office. On the one hand, we might be interested in obtaining scale values for the candidates along a dimension of conservatism-liberalism. In this case, we would expect subjects to show a certain degree of agreement in their judgments, and so the Thurstonian scaling method might very well be appropriate. On the other hand, if we were interested in obtaining people's preferences for candidates, we would expect certain idiosyncratic preference patterns to emerge depending on the subject's view of the ideal degree of conservatism-liberalism. We might assume that each subject views the candidates in a similar way along the conservatism-liberalism dimension, but that his preferences will be determined jointly by the position of the candidates along this dimension and the subject's own *ideal point* with respect to the dimension. The concept of the individual ideal point is central to the unfolding technique. It is assumed that each subject most prefers the candidate with the amount of liberalism (or conservatism) closest to his ideal point and prefers candidates less and less the farther from his ideal point they are perceived to lie. The location of the ideal point would be expected to vary from person to person or from group to group; in this example, members of the Communist party would have ideals rather distant from those of John Birch Society members.

Coombs (1950, 1964) has presented a theory which takes account of idiosyncratic preference patterns of the sort we have described. Unfolding theory assumes that the stimuli have an underlying order with respect to some attribute and a unique spacing, and that these are the same for all subjects. The stimulus scale is called the *joint* or *J scale,* referring to the fact that both stimuli and the individual's ideals are jointly located along the scale. However, each individual is assumed to have one ideal point along this continuum, and his preferences among the stimuli are determined by their distances from his ideal point. The subject makes his preference judgments by *folding over* the *J* scale at his ideal point and ranking the stimuli according to the rank of the distance of each stimulus from the ideal. The *individual* or *I scale* is the subject's ranking and will differ from subject to subject depending on the location of the ideal point.

If the data for each subject are transitive and if enough subjects are sampled to obtain a range of ideal points, stimuli can be placed on a scale somewhat between an interval and an ordinal scale, since both the order of stimuli and the order of differences between the stimuli on the *J* scale may be determined.

We illustrate the precise analytic technique that is followed in unfolding theory by a simple example. Suppose we give samples of four colors—yellow, chartreuse, green, and blue green—to a large group of observers and ask for preference rankings. The questions that we ask of our data through unfolding theory are: (1) whether the colors lie along a single dimension; (2) if so, what is their ordering; and (3) do the data permit an ordering of the intervals between stimuli, as well as the ordering of the stimuli themselves. The scale in (2) is called a *qualitative J scale,* and the scale in (3) is a *quantitative J scale.*

It is theoretically possible to obtain 24 different *I* scales, given by all the permutations of 4 stimuli (4! = 24). However, unfolding theory requires that only 7 distinct *I* scales, having a very restricted pattern, be obtained. A possible set of 7 *I* scales, corresponding to a unique qualitative and quantitative ordering, is given here. For convenience in later discussions, we give the ordering in terms of first letters of the colors, and then relabel the colors A, B, C, and D according to their order on the qualitative *J* scale.

| | Color name ordering | Relabeling |
|---|---|---|
| $I_1$ | Y C G B | A B C D |
| $I_2$ | C Y G B | B A C D |
| $I_3$ | C G Y B | B C A D |
| $I_4$ | C G B Y | B C D A |
| $I_5$ | G C B Y | C B D A |
| $I_6$ | G B C Y | C D B A |
| $I_7$ | B G C Y | D C B A |

A set of *I* scales consistent with unfolding theory has several characteristics. First, the end or least-preferred color is always yellow or blue green. A physical model for unfolding theory will make this requirement obvious. Imagine that the single dimension along which the stimuli lie is represented by a string, and the location of the stimuli by knots. The subject picks up the string at his ideal point and orders the stimuli from highest to lowest by the distance of the knots from the folding point. The last knot he comes to—the lowest hanging one—will always be one of the end knots along the *J* scale.

Having identified the end stimuli, we can identify the qualitative *J* scale by finding the two *I* scales beginning and ending with those stimuli. In our example, $I_1$ and $I_7$ represent the *J* scale and its mirror image.

The task of identifying the order of intervals between stimuli is somewhat more complicated.

The first step is to order the $I$ scales as they are in the example, so that they begin with the qualitative $J$ scale and end with its mirror image, and that successive $I$ scales differ from one another only in that a pair of adjacent stimuli have their positions reversed. For example, the only difference between $I_3$ and $I_4$ is that AD is reversed to DA. This list of $I$ scales can be generated by moving the ideal point along the $J$ scale from the left to the right. Each time the ideal point crosses one of the six possible midpoints between stimuli, the $I$ scale changes. The order of the midpoints determines the order in which the adjacent $I$ scales are reversed, and in turn the distances between stimuli depend on the order of the midpoints. In going from left to right along the $J$ scale, the first midpoint which is crossed is always the one between the first and second stimuli, and the second is always that between the first and third. Thus the first three $I$ scales are fixed. It is the fourth $I$ scale, and in this example, only the fourth, which gives us information about interval order. In the case of four stimuli, only the order of two of the three interstimulus distances, those between the first and second and the third and fourth, are obtainable. For larger numbers of stimuli, all of the intervals may be ordered if a sufficient variety of $I$ scales has been collected.

Figure 2.14 presents the two possible quantitative $J$ scales for four stimuli, one in which the distance between C and D is less than that between A and B ($J$-1) and the reverse situation ($J$-2). Four of the six midpoints are shown. We refer to midpoints as AB, and to distances between stimuli as $\overline{AB}$. The only two of interest are the midpoints AD and BC. If AD comes before BC, then $\overline{CD} < \overline{AB}$. If BC comes before AD, then $\overline{CD} > \overline{AB}$. This can be shown algebraically, as follows.

The midpoint AB $= (A + B)/2$ and the distance $\overline{AB} = B - A$, where A and B stand for scale values associated with stimuli A and B. If AD < BC, then

$$\frac{A + D}{2} < \frac{B + C}{2},$$

$$A + D < B + C,$$

$$D - C < B - A, \text{ and}$$

$$\overline{CD} < \overline{AB}.$$

Just the converse can be shown if BC < AD.

In Figure 2.14, the critical $I$ scale is generated for each $J$ scale. An $I$ scale BCDA implies that the first $J$ scale is the correct one, and an $I$ scale CBAD implies that the second is correct.

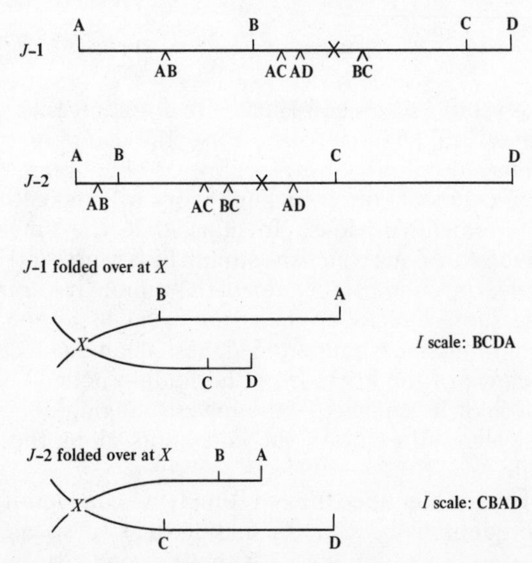


**Figure 2.14** Two hypothetical $J$ scales for four stimuli on one dimension, and their resulting $I$ scales when folded over at the ideal point indicated by $X$.

*Reaction time in paired-comparison studies*

Preference studies employing the paired-comparison methods and also measuring choice RTs have consistently found that (a) decision time lengthens as distance (defined as number of ranks separating two stimuli) decreases; and (b) for a given distance, decision time is longer between lower-ranked or less-preferred pairs.

Shipley, Coffin, and Hadsell (1945) showed pairs of colors to 40 female undergraduates who indicated their preference by pressing the key associated with the preferred color. Six hues were presented in all possible pairs. The relation between RT (expressed as percent of each subject's mean RT) and affective distance was linear and negative. In addition, higher RTs tended to be associated with low-ranking pairs.

Barker (1942) asked 19 boys to indicate their preferences among 7 liquids by moving a lever from a center position completely to the right or left. The names of the liquids were exposed in pairs until the subject had made his choice. Two payoff structures were used: a hypothetical one, in which the subject's choice had no effect on which liquid he subsequently drank, and a real one, in which the subject's choice determined which liquid he was to drink. Barker measured two responses in addition to choice frequency: time required to move the lever to its final position, and number of *vicarious trial and errors,* operationally defined as a movement of the lever in one direction less than the required distance followed by a movement back to center position. He found, in agreement with previous studies, that decision time and number of vicarious trial and errors were negatively and linearly related to *preference distance,* defined as difference in ranks computed from the choice frequencies. Both measures were higher for undesirable beverages. The payoff structure had a differential effect only for the subjects who received the real payoff first; for them overall decision time was longer but number of vicarious trial and errors was unaffected.

**Interval scaling: Category scales**

In category scaling, subjects are given some number of categories prior to the experiment and instructed to assign stimuli, presented one at a time, to one of the $n$ categories. Subjects are instructed to make the subjective widths or intervals of the categories equal and, for this reason, the method is sometimes called the method of *equal-appearing intervals.* These instructions imply that responses are on an interval rather than an ordinal scale. Thus, in analyzing the data, the experimenter assigns numbers to these categories so that the difference between adjacent numbers is equal, and each stimulus' scale value is the mean of its category values.

Typically, the number of categories is odd, and the subject is presented with the extremes of the stimulus range at the beginning of the experiment in order to *anchor* his judgments. For example, if loudness of tones is being judged, he is presented with the loudest and softest tones that will appear in the series and told that these should be assigned to the extreme categories. These anchoring stimuli provide extreme standards against which other tones may be judged. The categories may be numbers such as 1 through 5, or adjectives such as *very soft, soft, medium, loud,* and *very loud.* Whether labels or numbers are used does not change the form of the category scale very much (Stevens & Galanter, 1957).

Category scaling was used in early attempts to verify Fechner's law. Generally, when quantitative continua such as loudness, brightness, and weight are scaled by the category method, the psychophysical function is nearly logarithmic, thereby offering support for Fechner's law. However, when qualitative continua such as hue, pitch, and position are scaled, the function is not logarithmic but rather is close to the form of the psychophysical function obtained by the method of *magnitude estimation.*

Stevens and Galanter (1957) have termed quantitative continua *prothetic* and qualitative continua *metathetic.* Prothetic continua are defined as attributes "for which discrimination appears to be based on an additive mechanism by which excitation is added to excitation at the physiological level," and are exemplified by loudness, weight, brightness, and saturation. Metathetic continua are defined as attributes "for which discrimination behaves as though based on a substitutive mechanism at the physiological level," and are exemplified by hue, pointer position, and pitch [p. 377].

Stevens and Galanter make two specific distinctions between the two types of continua. First, for prothetic continua the *subjective* size, as well as the physical size, of the jnd increases with absolute stimulus magnitude, but for metathetic continua the subjective size is nearly constant over the whole stimulus range. In other words, Fechner, in assuming that the subjective jnd is constant, was right only about metathetic continua. For some metathetic continua, the physical size of the jnd is also constant over the stimulus range; that is, Weber's law does not hold, but rather $\Delta I = k$ for all values of $I$. Second, according to Stevens and Galanter, the time-order error is typically observed only for prothetic continua.

Table 2.9 presents some examples of prothetic and metathetic continua; both the stimulus attribute giving rise to the sensation and the sensation attribute are listed. Thus sound intensity is a physical stimulus attribute, and loudness is a psychological attribute of the resulting sensation. One metathetic-prothetic distinction which may need clarification is that between numerousness and proportion. Numerousness of dots (or of any other elements) is a prothetic continuum because the absolute size of the difference threshold increases with number: It is harder to tell the difference between 100 and 101 dots than it is between 10 and 11 dots. However, if the total number of dots of two colors is kept constant, and the proportion of one color of dots is varied, the difference threshold does not increase as the proportion of one color is increased. Indeed, discrimination is better at the extreme proportions and also in the middle around 50 percent. Therefore, proportion is a metathetic continuum, but numerousness is a prothetic continuum.

Because of these differences between the two types of continua, Stevens and Galanter have argued that category scaling is not a valid method

**Table 2.9 Examples of Some Prothetic and Metathetic Continua**

| | Prothetic | | Metathetic | |
|---|---|---|---|---|
| Sense modality | Stimulus attribute | Sensation attribute | Stimulus attribute | Sensation attribute |
| Audition | intensity of sound | loudness | frequency of pure tones | pitch |
| | duration of sound | apparent duration | | |
| Vision | intensity of light | brightness | wavelength of light | hue |
| | visual length | apparent length | position on a line | apparent position |
| | visual area | apparent area | | |
| | saturation | apparent saturation | visual inclination | apparent inclination |
| | number (of dots) | numerousness | proportion (of dots) | apparent proportion |
| Touch | shock intensity | touch or pain intensity | position of shock | position of touch or pain |
| | temperature | warmth; cold | | |
| | weight | heaviness | | |

of obtaining the psychophysical function for prothetic continua, although it may be for metathetic continua. The reasons for this are twofold. First, since on prothetic continua the subjective jnd is smaller at the low end of the scale than at the high end, the subject tends to make the subjective size of his category intervals narrow at the low end and wide at the high end, despite instructions to keep the intervals the same size.

Of course, Fechner would say that if the size of the category intervals were proportional to discriminability or to the size of the jnd, then category intervals would be subjectively equal. Stevens and Galanter's argument rests on the assumption that Fechner's logarithmic law is not valid, but rather that the form of the psychophysical function is a power function. (This assumption will be examined in detail in the section on ratio scaling.) For the moment, we simply assert that a power function implies that jnd's are not subjectively equal; rather, it is the ratio of the jnd to the standard that is subjectively equal. If the width of the category intervals were strictly proportional to the discriminability of the stimuli, then the graph plotting mean category scale against physical stimulus magnitude would be logarithmic in form. However, such a graph is usually some compromise between a logarithmic function and a power function, indicating to Stevens and Galanter that the subject makes some compromise between instructions and discriminability.

The second biasing factor in category scaling is that subjects usually try to use all categories equally often. If the spacing of stimuli along the physical continuum changes, the form of the category scale function changes. If stimuli are more closely spaced at one end or the other, the curve steepens in that region because the subject tends to avoid using that category as much as he ought to and spreads out the stimuli across categories in that part of the scale.

Stevens and Galanter propose an interesting method for determining the true category scale. If the stimuli were equally spaced along the sensation continuum, then the subject would use each category equally often. In order to find the physical spacing that corresponds to equal spacing along the sensation continuum, one could continue respacing stimuli along the physical continuum in accordance with the subject's previous usage of the categories until he uses the categories equally often. This method should then produce the true psychophysical function for category scales.

The results of category scaling are valid only

if the stimuli are not perfectly discriminable, there are more stimuli than categories, or both. For example, if in a five-category scaling experiment, only five stimuli were presented and they could be recognized perfectly, the subject would probably assign each to a different category. Then the form of the psychophysical function would be completely determined by the physical spacing of the five stimuli.

## Ratio scaling: The magnitude methods

We have seen how Fechner, using the data from discrimination, indirectly constructed the psychophysical function by assuming that jnd's are subjectively equal. Fechner used this approach because he firmly believed that sensation could never be measured directly, but only inferred by measuring discrimination ability. However, Stevens (1957, 1961, 1962a), using a direct method of measuring sensation, has accumulated an impressive amount of evidence that the psychophysical function is a power function rather than a logarithmic function. These direct methods are known as *magnitude methods*.

### *Magnitude estimation*

Stevens' solution to the problem of measuring sensation was simple: He merely asked subjects to report directly, with numbers, how intense various stimuli appeared. In magnitude estimation the subject is presented with a standard stimulus to which the experimenter assigns an easily remembered, simply manipulated number, such as 10. To subsequent stimuli of differing intensities the subject is asked to assign numbers such that the ratio between the assigned numbers and the number 10 reflects the ratios between the sensation produced by the variable and the sensation produced by the standard. For example, he is told to assign the number 20 to a stimulus that appears twice as loud as the standard, the number 5 to a stimulus that appears half as loud, the number 100 to the stimulus that appears 10 times as loud, and so on. (In a more recent version of the method, which yields more consistent data, no standard is given. The subject assigns whatever numbers seem to correspond to his sensation magnitude.) Typically, each variable stimulus is presented only two or three times to a single subject, and data are pooled across about a dozen subjects. The method is a form of ratio scaling because the subject judges subjective ratios rather than subjective differences, as in the method of category scaling, or subjective order, as in ordinal scaling.

Using the method of magnitude estimation, or one of several related methods, Stevens finds that on prothetic continua the psychophysical function is a power function, rather than a logarithmic function, of the form:

$$S = aI^b, \quad [13]$$

where $a$ and $b$ are constants, $S$ is psychological magnitude, and $I$ is the physical magnitude of the stimulus.

One of the properties of power functions is that on log-log coordinates the functions plot as straight lines with an intercept of $\log a$ and a slope of $b$. That a power function is linear on log-log coordinates can be shown by taking logarithms of both sides of Equation 13:

$$\log S = \log a + b \log I. \quad [14]$$

Thus a convenient way of determining whether a set of magnitude estimations follows a power function is to plot the data on log-log coordinates.

Power functions plotted in linear coordinates may be concave upward, concave downward, or straight, depending on the value of the exponent. Figures 2.15 and 2.16 show three psychophysical functions obtained by the method of magnitude estimation for three modalities: apparent intensity of electric shock, apparent length of lines, and

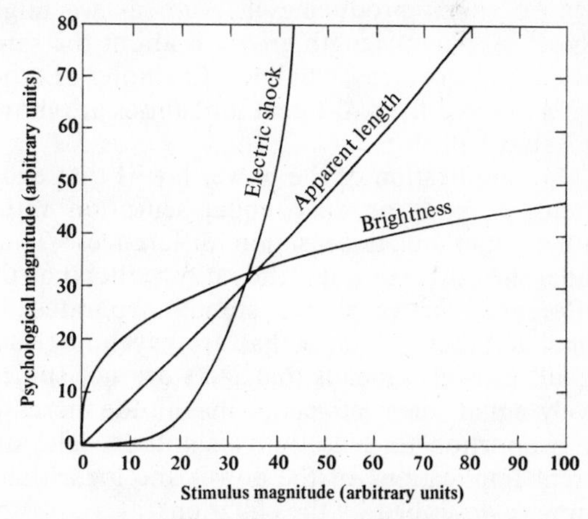


**Figure 2.15** Three psychophysical functions obtained by the method of magnitude estimation. The functions plotted are power functions with exponents of 3.5 for electric shock, 1.1 for apparent length, and 0.33 for brightness. (From Stevens, 1961.)

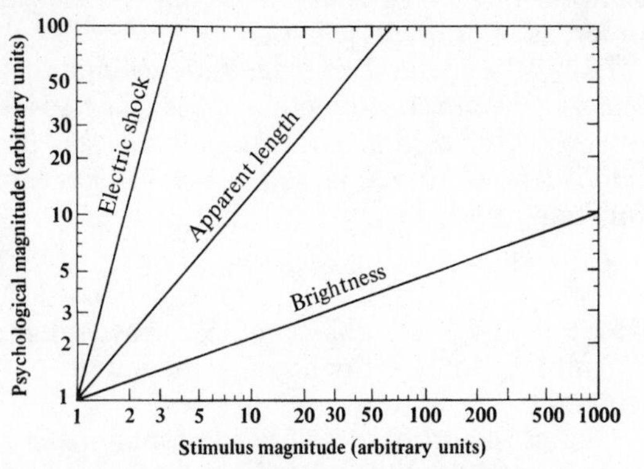


**Figure 2.16** The same psychophysical functions as in Figure 2.15 are plotted on log-log coordinates. The slopes of the functions correspond to the exponents of the power functions. (From Stevens, 1961.)

brightness of lights. The data are plotted in linear coordinates in Figure 2.15 and in log-log coordinates in Figure 2.16.

It is clear that a power function describes the psychophysical function very well. It is also clear that the sensation continua for different sensory modalities grow at different rates, that is, they exhibit different exponents. For example, brightness grows as a cube root of light energy. Perceived intensity from shock, on the other hand, grows at a much greater rate than does the intensity of the electric shock producing it. And, as we might expect, apparent length grows at about the same rate as physical length of lines. Examples of exponents derived from different modalities are shown in Table 2.10.

One implication of the power law is that equal intensity ratios produce equal sensation ratios rather than equal sensation differences. Thus, under the power law, it is the ratios rather than the differences between two stimuli separated by equal numbers of jnd's that are psychologically equal. This also means that jnd's are not subjectively equal; their subjective magnitude increases in proportion to sensation magnitude. The different implications of the power and logarithmic laws are described by the equations

Power law: $$\frac{I + n(\Delta I)}{I} = \text{constant sensation} \quad [15]$$

and

Logarithmic law: $$I + n(\Delta I) - I = \text{constant sensation}, \quad [16]$$

where $\Delta I$ is the size of the jnd and $n$ is the number of jnd's by which the two stimuli are separated.

In treating the data, Stevens assumes that the numbers the subject emits are directly proportional to his perceived sensations. This assumption has been criticized on the ground that the numbers may tell us more about the subject's number habits than about his sensation. To counter this criticism, Stevens has used other methods such as cross-modality matching, inverse scaling, and magnitude production to validate the results of magnitude-estimation experiments.

*Cross-modality matching*

In cross-modality matching the subject matches the perceived intensity from one modality with the perceived intensity from another, usually by the method of adjustment. For example, the subject might adjust the intensity of a sound so that it matches the intensity of a light, or he might vary the strength with which he squeezes a device called a *dynamometer* so that the perceived tension matches the perceived intensity of an electric shock.

If the psychophysical function is a power function and Stevens' method is valid, the relationship between the intensities of the two matched stimuli should also be a power function with an exponent predicted from the magnitude-estimation data for those two modalities. To illustrate, let us assume that magnitude estimations have been obtained for the intensities of sound ($S$) and light ($L$), the power law was verified, and the exponents for the two modalities are $b$ and $b'$ respectively, so

$$S_S = a\,I_S{}^b \quad [17]$$

and

$$S_L = a'\,I_L{}^{b'}, \quad [18]$$

where $I_S$ and $I_L$ refer to the physical intensities of sound and light and $S_S$ and $S_L$ refer to the magnitudes of sensation of sound and light.

When, in the cross-modality matching experiment, $I_S$ is matched to $I_L$ this implies that $S_S = S_L$. Therefore,

$$a\,I_S{}^b = a'\,I_L{}^{b'} \quad [19]$$

$$I_S = \frac{a'}{a}^{1/b} I_L{}^{b'/b} \quad [20]$$

This equation can be simplified by substituting for

**Table 2.10 Representative Exponents of the Power Functions Relating Psychological Magnitude to Stimulus Magnitude on Prothetic Continua**

| Continuum | Exponent | Stimulus condition | Continuum | Exponent | Stimulus condition |
|---|---|---|---|---|---|
| Loudness | 0.6 | 1000-Hz tone | Finger span | 1.3 | thickness of wood blocks |
| Brightness | 0.33 | 5° target—dark-adapted eye | Pressure on palm | 1.1 | static force on skin |
| Brightness | 0.5 | point source—dark-adapted eye | Heaviness | 1.45 | lifted weights |
| Lightness | 1.2 | reflectance of gray papers | Force of handgrip | 1.7 | precision hand dynamometer |
| Smell | 0.55 | coffee odor | Vocal effort | 1.1 | sound pressure of vocalization |
| Smell | 0.6 | heptane | Electric shock | 3.5 | 60 Hz—through fingers |
| Taste | 0.8 | saccharine | Tactual roughness | 1.5 | felt diameter of emery grits |
| Taste | 1.3 | sucrose | Tactual hardness | 0.8 | rubber squeezed between fingers |
| Taste | 1.3 | salt | Visual velocity | 1.2 | moving spot of light |
| Temperature | 1.0 | cold–on arm | Visual length | 1.0 | projected line of light |
| Temperature | 1.5 | warmth—on arm | Visual area | 0.7 | projected square of light |
| Vibration | 0.95 | 60 Hz—on finger | | | |
| Vibration | 0.6 | 250 Hz—on finger | | | |
| Duration | 1.1 | white-noise stimulus | | | |
| Repetition rate | 1.0 | light, sound, touch, and shocks | | | |

(After Stevens, 1962b.)

the constant term, $\left[\frac{a'}{a}\right]^{1/b}$, the symbol $c$. Then we have

$$I_S = c\, I_L{}^{b'/b}. \qquad [21]$$

The last equation means that when the intensity of the adjusted sound is plotted against the intensity of the light, the form of the function should be a power function with an exponent equal to $b'/b$.

Stevens has found, across a wide variety of different modalities, that cross-modality matches produce power functions with the predicted exponents, thus providing strong support for the power law.

*Inverse scaling*

Instead of estimating the magnitude of an increasing sensation, such as loudness or heaviness, subjects may be instructed to estimate the magnitude of the inverse sensation, such as softness or lightness. The magnitude estimates for the inverse function should result in a power function with an exponent equal to the negative of the exponent for the positive function. Such a relationship has been verified for longness and shortness of lines, largeness and smallness of circles, loudness and softness of tones, and brightness and dimness of lights (Stevens & Guirao, 1962, 1963).

*Magnitude production*

In magnitude production the subject is required to produce a stimulus whose subjective magnitude matches the magnitude of a number presented to him by the experimenter. This procedure is the opposite of magnitude estimation, in which the experimenter produces the stimulus and the subject produces the number. Although magnitude production normally yields a power function relating the adjusted stimulus magnitude to the experimenter's number, thus confirming the power law, the exponent is usually slightly larger than is measured with magnitude estimation. This difference between production and estimation has been attributed to the subject's tendency to constrict the range of his responses, whether the responses be numbers or adjusted magnitudes.

*Magnitude estimation by individual subjects*

There is some question whether magnitude estimations collected from individual subjects are well characterized by a power function, or whether the power function for group data arises from averaging across individual functions that have assorted shapes. Pradhan and Hoffman (1963) concluded from an analysis of individual functions for apparent weight that the power function is an artifact of averaging; none of their subjects actually exhibited the power function individually, although the group did. Similarly, Luce and Mo (1965) found that for apparent weight and loudness, the psychophysical functions of individual subjects showed characteristic and idiosyncratic curvature on log-log plots. Stevens and Guirao (1964), on the other hand, found that their individual subjects showed excellent power functions for loudness estimations, although the slopes of the functions on log-log plots differed from subject to subject.

*Simple reaction time as magnitude estimation*

Like magnitude estimation, simple reaction time is a response that may provide information about the perceived intensity of a stimulus. Chocholle (1940), in a classic study, measured simple RTs of three subjects to pure tones of several frequencies which were varied in intensity from threshold to 100 dB above threshold. The RTs he obtained showed consistent and regular decreases with increased stimulus intensity at each frequency. Furthermore, tones of different frequencies that were judged to be equally loud by his subjects produced equal mean RTs.

### The psychophysical function: Power law or logarithmic law?

Evidence from magnitude-estimation experiments supports Stevens' power law, whereas evidence from category-scaling experiments supports Fechner's logarithmic law. Which is correct? According to one investigator (Torgerson, 1961), the question cannot be decided on empirical grounds, so that the form of the psychophysical function is a matter of choice, not of discovery.

Torgerson conducted an experiment in which subjects were required to scale the degree of lightness or darkness of *Munsell* gray color chips. He found that the subjects judged either ratios or differences, depending on instructions. When they judged ratios, they produced power functions; when they judged differences, they produced logarithmic functions.

To use a concrete example, suppose a subject in the method of magnitude estimation judged stimulus A to be twice as great as stimulus B, and stimulus B to be twice as great as stimulus C. When he judged these same three stimuli in the method of category scaling or *bisection,* he judged B to be halfway between A and C. If subjects have an internal numerical representation of these stimuli, these two sets of judgments are obviously in conflict. For example, a numerical representation of stimuli A, B, and C that would be congruent with the magnitude-estimation data might be A = 10, B = 20, and C = 40. On the other hand, this numerical representation is not congruent with the category-scaling data: B is not halfway between A and C in its numerical representation. Torgerson's view is that subjects do not perceive ratios or differences in numerical terms; rather, they perceive the stimuli to be different, and they express this difference either in terms of ratios or in terms of differences, depending on the instructions of the experiment.

Some scientists feel that the ultimate validity of either law can be determined on the basis of physiological evidence. For example, if the nervous system were found to convert physical intensity into some physiological response, such as rate of nerve firing, by a logarithmic transformation, this would be evidence for Fechner's law. On the other hand, if the transformation between physical intensity and physiological response were found to be a power function, Stevens' law would be supported. Indeed, both types of physiological transformations have been observed (Teitelbaum, 1967), although Stevens (1970) has argued that many transformations originally thought to be logarithmic are, in fact, better described by a power function. He has marshaled considerable evidence—in experiments on vision, hearing, touch, and taste—that stimulus input is converted to neural response according to a power law.

Galanter (1966), however, has disagreed with this approach, arguing that even if the evidence for one or the other physiological transformation were unequivocal, that would still not tell us which psychological transformation between physical intensity and sensation is correct. In his words,

> There is a sense . . . in which no physiological representation really supports a psychophysical representation. Suppose, for example, that we found that the rate of firing of the nerves in the ear increases as a power function of the physical intensity. Would this support Stevens' view? The answer is no, for how do we know that later in the nervous system, or somewhere in the muscles, this particular power function of the physical energy is not subsequently transformed by the logarithm into what Fechner would have expected and that these transformed impulses are the physiological "causes" of the loudness. There is, of course, no way to know, and so physiological evidence cannot constitute the basis for acceptance or rejection of psychophysical theories. Rather, it is the other way around. Only when we understand something about the psychophysical processes are we able to know what to look for in the physiological system itself [p. 215].

## THE OUTCOME STRUCTURE IN PSYCHOPHYSICAL EXPERIMENTS

Most psychophysical experiments can be characterized as choice experiments. As defined by Bush, Galanter, and Luce (1963), a choice experiment is

> one in which there is a set of two or more empirically defined alternative responses from which the subject chooses just one whenever he is given an opportunity to do so. We call these opportunities "trials." The set of response alternatives is usually finite, often having only two or three elements, but occasionally infinite sets are employed [p. 79].

Each trial of a choice experiment consists of three events: a stimulus, a response, and an outcome. Often, particularly in older psychophysical experiments, the outcomes are implicit rather than explicit. However, modern psychophysicists see the lack of explicit outcomes as a flaw in the traditional methodology and some current psychophysical techniques include explicit payoffs or outcomes as an intrinsic part of the experiment.

In certain cases, the choice set from which the subject makes his response is very large indeed. For example, in the method of magnitude estimation, the subject theoretically has available to him an infinite set of responses (all the positive numbers), although in practice he undoubtedly chooses from a much smaller finite set of responses.

An important aspect of the analysis of choice experiments by Bush et al. is the concept of an *identification function,* which informs the subject which response is correct for which stimulus. For example, the identification function for a detection experiment identifies the verbal response "yes" (or the press of a "yes" button) as correct for the stimulus *signal present,* and the verbal response "no" (or the press of a "no" button) as correct for the stimulus *signal absent*. In recognition experiments, the experimenter gives the subject the identification function at the beginning of the experiment by instructing him which response is correct for which stimulus. On the other hand, in scaling experiments, the identification function is what the experimenter hopes to discover from his subject.

Perhaps the most important characteristic that differentiates the psychophysical methods we have reviewed is whether or not there is a criterion for correct responses. In detection, discrimination, and recognition studies, the experimenter can score the subject's response as right or wrong by reference to an external criterion. In detection, the experimenter can record whether or not a stimulus was presented on a trial when the subject reported it was there. In discrimination, the experimenter can determine whether one of two stimuli was actually of greater magnitude when the subject reported it as louder, brighter, or heavier. In recognition, the experimenter can score the response as correct when the subject's identification of a stimulus corresponds to that of the experimenter.

In scaling, on the other hand, the experimenter may question the subject about what magnitude of sensation is produced by a particular stimulus, which painting is most pleasing, or which statement of opinion the subject agrees with most. Since the experimenter does not have access to the subject's internal states, the experimenter has no criterion for scoring the subject's responses as correct or incorrect.

In simple reaction-time experiments, there is an identification function over a range of times, rather than over discrete responses. For example, instructions to the subject in the simple RT experiment may be of the form: "Do not respond until the red light flashes, but when it does flash, respond as quickly as you can." These instructions define a payoff function that is negatively valued in the foreperiod, highly valued immediately after the reaction signal, and decreasingly valued thereafter.

In choice RT experiments, the identification function is over discrete responses as well as time. The subject is instructed to be both correct and fast. Thus fast correct responses are highly valued, slow correct responses are less valued, and errors are negatively valued.

Typically, the outcome or payoff structure is consonant with the identification function, so that the subject is rewarded for correct responses and penalized for incorrect ones. An implied assumption in the use of payoffs is that the subject prefers winning money to losing money, or, if only information feedback is given, that the subject prefers being correct to being incorrect.

Experimentally, the identification function is often conveyed to the subject both prior to the experiment and after every response in the form of *information feedback.* Feedback informs the subject whether his response was right or wrong, and it may also inform him how much money he has won for that trial. The use of information feedback and payoffs permits greater control and manipulation of the subject's attitudes and motivation. Although the criterion of *accuracy* is most commonly used as the basis for feedback and payoffs, another criterion, *consistency,* may also be used as that basis.

**Accuracy criteria**

Usually accuracy criteria exist only for truly psychophysical situations, including all recognition experiments and certain detection and discrimination experiments. Truly psychophysical experiments are those employing stimuli which are measurable on a physical scale. Outcomes based on accuracy do not appear feasible for scaling experiments.

In detection experiments, there is an accuracy criterion whenever catch trials are employed. In the method of signal detection, in which catch trials play a major role, both feedback and payoffs are an intrinsic part of the experiment. The subject is rewarded for hits and correct rejections, and is penalized for false alarms and misses.

Experiments testing neural quantum theory, on the other hand, which do not usually employ catch trials, provide no basis for an outcome structure. The signal is always present, but the subject is not expected to detect it on every trial. In classical detection or absolute-threshold experiments, unless catch trials are employed, no accuracy criterion exists. When catch trials are used, however, an accuracy criterion does exist, but in a different sense from that in signal-detection experiments. Classical theory assumes that while a signal presentation may or may not exceed the subject's threshold, a noise presentation never will. This view is referred to as *high threshold theory,* because the subject's threshold is assumed high enough never to be exceeded by noise alone. Thus, when a subject makes a false alarm on a catch trial, according to high threshold theory he is not reporting his sensation correctly. The usual experimental procedure in this case is to warn the subject when he makes a substantial proportion of false alarms and to discard his data if necessary. Thus, in classical theory, the subject is incorrect when he makes a false alarm but not when he makes a miss.

Signal detection theory, on the other hand, assumes that sometimes a noise presentation will exceed the subject's criterion and that the resulting internal observation will be indistinguishable from the same observation resulting from a signal presentation. Thus, the subject is penalized not on the basis of his internal observation, but on the basis of the state of the external world, that is, the world controlled by the experimenter. In short, accuracy criteria in detection experiments exist whenever there are catch trials, but the definition of an error varies with the particular theory of thresholds.

In discrimination experiments, there would appear to be a clear accuracy criterion. The subject is correct whenever his judgment of differences in apparent magnitude coincides with differences in physical magnitude. There are, however, two problems with this view, one involving the constant errors and the other regarding comparisons between heterogeneous stimuli.

As we have seen, certain constant errors, especially for temporally distinct stimuli, are often observed in discrimination experiments. Let us assume for the moment that when a negative time-order error in auditory intensity discrimination occurs, it is the result of a true sensation difference between two temporally distinct stimuli, rather than the result of response biases of one sort or another. Were we to use feedback and payoffs for correct discrimination responses in such an experiment, the subject could probably compensate for the phenomenological difference in the two stimuli and eliminate his time-order error. If the value of the constant error were $k$, the subject could simply require that a second stimulus appear louder by the amount $k$ in order to judge them equal; if the subjective difference were less than *k*, he would respond "less than," and if greater than *k*, "greater than." Ironically, however, we have, by introducing feedback and payoffs into this situation, increased response bias to a degree proportional to the size of the constant error, whereas the purpose of feedback and payoffs is to decrease, or at least more closely control, response biases.

The second problem has to do with comparisons between heterogeneous stimuli. Most discrimination experiments deal with unidimensional stimuli; that is, if we study discrimination of pure tones on the basis of intensity, the tones are kept identical in frequency, duration, and phase, and differ only in intensity. However, suppose we wish to compare tones of different frequencies and intensities. Because frequency and intensity interact in that tones of different frequencies and the same intensity are not necessarily equally loud, it is difficult to use an accuracy criterion until it is known which intensity-frequency combinations are subjectively equal. This information must come from experiments in which no outcome structure exists.

The clearest argument for an accuracy criterion can be made for experiments in recognition. The experimenter conveys the identification function to the subject at the beginning of the experiment by pairing labels with the stimuli to be used. The label may be arbitrary, as numerals for random shapes, or the label may be well learned, as common color names for colors. In still other cases, the ordering of the labels may match the ordering of the stimuli: If tones of different frequencies are used as stimuli and numerals are used as responses, typically the order of the *n* frequencies from low to high will match the ordering of the numerals from 1 to *n*.

In scaling experiments, feedback and payoffs are almost never used. Even when a physical scale exists for the stimulus, the subject is virtually never rewarded for reproducing the physical scale in his responses. The reasons for this are twofold. First, for many modalities there is more than one physical scale available. For example, the intensity of acoustic stimuli may be measured in *absolute power units, absolute pressure units, log relative power units,* or *log relative pressure units*. (The latter two are decibel scales; see Chapter 4.) The ratios are not the same for the various units, so which of these physical scales should the experimenter take as the basis for an accuracy criterion in ratio scaling?

The second, more fundamental problem is that of interpretation. As in discrimination experiments, the subject could probably learn to respond to acoustic stimuli so as to reproduce the physical scale in decibels or in absolute power or pressure units, or he could learn to estimate area in square centimeters or inches. However, the experimenter is interested in how magnitude of subjective sensation varies with physical magnitude, not how well a subject can learn to reproduce an arbitrary scale. We shall consider one possibility for interpretation of scaling experiments with outcome structures when we discuss consistency criteria.

Table 2.11 presents some examples of psychophysical and psychological experiments for which accuracy criteria do exist (Type I tasks) and for which they do not exist (Type II tasks). Psychophysical tasks are indicated by an asterisk. With the exception of recognition tasks, no psychological tasks are Type I, but there are many psychophysical tasks that are Type II.

### *Absolute thresholds*

Determining the absolute threshold for heat, a psychophysical task, has a clear criterion for accuracy. When the heat stimulus is present and the subject detects it, he is correct, and when it is absent and he responds appropriately, he is again correct. Otherwise, he is incorrect. The absolute threshold for pain produced by heat, on the other hand, does not have a clear accuracy criterion. Some heat stimuli produce a sensation of heat but not pain, some may produce pain but not heat sensation, some produce both sensations, and some produce neither (see Chapter 5). If the subject were rewarded for reporting pain every time a heat stimulus was present, he could adopt the strategy of reporting pain whenever he experienced heat, and little if anything would be learned about the detection of pain itself. Although there have been attempts to apply signal detection methodology to heat and pain thresholds (e.g., Clark, 1969), these experiments have been conducted without feedback and payoffs for accuracy because of the lack of accuracy criteria.

### *Difference thresholds*

For difference thresholds for line lengths, where the variable and standard are presented simultaneously but in different spatial positions, it seems reasonable to use feedback and payoffs for correct responses; hence, this is a Type I task. We classify it as such primarily because there is little

**Table 2.11 Classification of Experimental Tasks by Applicability of Accuracy Criteria**

| | | Type I tasks (Accuracy criteria exist) | Type II tasks (Accuracy criteria do not exist) |
|---|---|---|---|
| THRESHOLDS | | | |
| | Absolute | Absolute threshold for heat* | Absolute threshold for pain from heat* |
| | | | Absolute threshold for complexity |
| | Difference | Difference threshold for line length* | Difference threshold for horizon and zenith moons* |
| SCALING | | | |
| | Nominal | Recognition of tones of different frequencies* | Sorting photographs of faces by similarity |
| | | Recognition of photographs | Sorting words by similarity and meaning |
| | Ordinal | Ranking degree of sourness of solutions of different vinegar concentrations* | Ranking degree of pleasantness of solutions varying in several taste dimensions* |
| | Interval | Category rating of durations of tones with feedback and payoff for equal differences in judged duration* | Category rating of durations of tones by usual methods* |
| | | | Category rating of severity of crimes |
| | Ratio | Bisecting straight line* | Bisecting Müller-Lyer illusion* |
| | | Magnitude estimation of areas of figures with feedback and payoff for judging ratios of areas* | Magnitude estimation of areas of figures with usual procedures* |
| | | | Magnitude estimation of esthetic value of handwriting |

*Psychophysical task

evidence of a constant error when this experiment is conducted without feedback and payoffs.

Illustrations of Type II tasks can be taken from any of those errors in perception called *illusions*. A well-known example is the moon illusion, in which the moon over the horizon appears larger than the moon at its zenith, even though its retinal size is constant. This illusion has been related to the fact that the horizon sky is perceived farther away than the zenith or overhead sky (Rock & Kaufman, 1962). Generally, the same object at different distances produces different retinal sizes and yet we see the object as the same size at different distances. This is known as size constancy. Since the moon has the same retinal size on the horizon and zenith but different apparent distances, the horizon moon looks larger.

The moon illusion can be demonstrated with an artificial moon projected on a viewing glass through which the observer looks at the horizon or zenith sky. Suppose we were to conduct a discrimination experiment with moons projected at the horizon and zenith, using feedback and payoffs for correct discriminations. Because there is an illusion, the subject will have to correct his phenomenal judgments for this space error, and our data will be relatively meaningless. Hence, this is a Type II task.

### *Nominal scaling*

Recognition of tones of different frequencies and recognition of photographs of faces are both Type I tasks, although there is a relevant physical measure for the tones but not for the photographs. A Type II nominal-scaling task might be one in which subjects are instructed to sort photographs in some specified number of piles on the basis of their similarities. The sorting task would differ from the recognition task in that the number of categories would have to be smaller than the number of stimuli to be sorted. The sorting task entails nominal scaling because the categories are not ordered on any dimension.

Such a sorting task has been used by Miller (1967) to study the similarity and meaning of words. A sample of words typed singly on index cards was given to subjects, who were instructed to sort the words into as many piles as they wished on the basis of meaning and similarity. In contrast to recognition experiments, the number of categories was left up to the subject and there were no correct sorting strategies.

Miller has found significant differences among various groups of subjects in the criteria used to classify words, or in the clusters of words produced. If different parts of speech make up the sample of words, one basis for classification is syntax; verbs are grouped with verbs, nouns with nouns, and so forth. Another basis for classification is semantics or meaning. Miller found that adults tend to sort by syntactic categories, whereas children tend to sort by semantic categories. For example, a major cluster produced by the children in Miller's study included *sadly, suffer, weep, doctor,* and *needle,* whereas a major adult cluster for the same sample of words was *doctor, foot, needle, house,* and *table* and a second cluster was *sadly, suffer,* and *weep*. The children's cluster is syntactically heterogeneous but semantically homogeneous (and one must conclude that these children have had unfortunate experiences with doctors), whereas the adult clusters are syntactically homogeneous, except that the second cluster mixes two verbs with an adverb.

*Ordinal scaling*

An example of a Type I task is the ranking of degree of sourness of solutions differing in concentration of vinegar. When this experiment utilizes feedback and payoffs, it becomes a recognition experiment of the type referred to earlier, one in which the order of the numerical labels corresponds to the ordering of the stimuli on the dimension being judged. The same would be true of recognition experiments involving any set of stimuli varying on a unidimensional continuum, such as pitch or intensity of tones or position of a pointer on a line, in which numbers are used as labels and their order matches the ordering of the stimuli.

An example of a Type II task is the ranking of pleasantness of solutions varying in several taste dimensions, such as sourness, sweetness, and bitterness. This task is of Type II because the judgments may not show any simple functional relationship to taste dimensions.

*Interval scaling*

An example of a Type I category-scaling task is one in which a subject is given feedback and payoffs for categorizing pure-tone stimuli into equally spaced intervals in terms of duration. For stimuli ranging from 1 to 6 seconds and a five-interval category scale for duration, the following would be an appropriate identification function:

| *Stimuli falling in interval* | *Correct category* |
|---|---|
| 1–2 sec | 1 |
| 2–3 sec | 2 |
| 3–4 sec | 3 |
| 4–5 sec | 4 |
| 5–6 sec | 5 |

The typical category-rating experiment is a Type II task and may be psychophysical, as category rating of durations of tones, or psychological, as category rating of severity of crimes.

*Ratio scaling*

Bisection experiments are those in which the subject adjusts a middle stimulus until it appears to bisect the interval between two extreme stimuli. An example of a Type I bisection task is one in which the subject adjusts a vertical line until it appears to bisect a horizontal line. Here feedback and payoffs may be used for bisections that lie within some error interval of the true bisection point. It makes sense to treat this as a Type I task because in the absence of feedback and payoffs subjects perform this task rather accurately, with little or no *space-order error,* in which the spatial location of the stimulus affects its perceived magnitude. We referred to one type of space-order error, the moon illusion, previously.

Another space-order error can be demonstrated for the Müller-Lyer illusion (see Figure 2.17) by having a subject adjust the middle arrow until both horizontal segments of the line appear equal. Subjects will adjust the middle arrow so that the left segment is shorter than the right segment, as shown in Figure 2.17B, and the measure of the magnitude of the illusion (the constant error) is the difference in length between the two line segments.

When subjects are given feedback and payoffs for adjusting two halves to objective equality, the

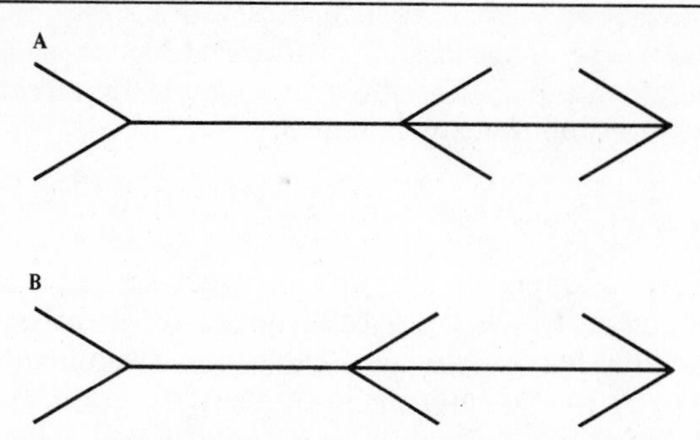


**Figure 2.17** The Müller-Lyer illusion: Panel A shows a Müller-Lyer adjusted so that the two horizontal line segments are physically equal, and panel B shows the two halves adjusted so that they are approximately psychologically equal.

constant error quickly approaches zero. Nonetheless, subjects often report that the illusion is still present but that they have learned to make the appropriate correction to compensate for it. However, our interest is in the magnitude of the illusion itself, not the subject's ability to compensate for it. We shall consider how feedback and payoffs based on a consistency criterion may be used to measure the magnitude of the illusion.

Another Type I task is magnitude estimation of areas of figures with feedback and payoffs for producing numbers whose ratio to the number of the standard reflects the ratio of the physical area of the variable figure to the physical area of the standard figure. Typically, however, magnitude-estimation experiments are conducted as Type II tasks. Magnitude-estimation methodology has been used for such psychological continua as esthetic value of handwriting and drawings, and severity of crimes (Stevens, 1966), and these cases are of necessity Type II tasks since there is no physical stimulus measure.

It should be clear from the foregoing discussion that the classification of tasks as Type I or Type II is somewhat arbitrary; only signal detection and recognition tasks are unequivocally Type I, and for the others, the decision as to whether feedback and payoffs for accuracy are appropriate depends on considerations about how likely the subject is to have sensations that are highly correlated with stimulus magnitude.

### Consistency criteria

Two consistency criteria can be employed: *intrasubject* consistency, or the degree to which a subject gives the same responses to the same stimuli within an experimental session or between two sessions; and *intersubject* consistency, or the degree to which a subject gives the same responses as other subjects to the same stimuli. Both these criteria are used informally in psychological research, not as a basis for feedback and payoffs, but as a basis for discarding subjects. If a subject either is not self-consistent or responds differently from other subjects, his data are often eliminated from the analysis or at least reported separately from the data of other subjects. Here we consider criteria based only on intrasubject consistency.

We first examine the use of an intrasubject consistency criterion in the measurement of the Müller-Lyer illusion. Suppose the magnitude of the illusion is $+k$ centimeters; that is, the right-hand portion of the horizontal line segment of Figure 2.17 must be $k$ centimeters longer than the left-hand segment in order for the two lines to appear equal. Consider two feedback and payoff functions: one that rewards the subject for setting the middle arrow at $+k$, i.e., at his true PSE (point of subjective equality) and one that rewards the subject for setting the middle arrow at zero, i.e., at the PE (point of physical equality). In the first case, the subject merely has to set the arrow so that both line segments appear equal, or at his PSE; in the other, he must set the arrow at the PSE $- k$. It seems apparent that the first task will be easier than the second. Furthermore, since the second adjustment involves subtracting a subjective constant, $k$, from a subjective value, the PSE, and both these values presumably include intrinsic variability, the second type of adjustment should be more variable than the first type.

To test this prediction an independent research project was carried out as part of an undergraduate experimental psychology course.[2] (As such, the obtained data should be considered illustrative rather than definitive.) A single subject was tested on an adjustable Müller-Lyer illusion board. First, he adjusted one line segment until it appeared equal to the second for several trials, and the constant error was found to be −3.0 centimeters. The subject was subsequently given feedback for adjusting the illusion to a constant error of 0 (i.e., to physical equality), to a constant error of −3.0 centimeters (i.e., to psychological equality), and to a constant error of −6.0 centimeters. After each trial, he was told whether his adjustment was longer or shorter than the constant error in force.

[2] These data were collected by Marilyn L. Goldstein.

The variance of his adjustments was lowest (less than 0.5 centimeters) when the correct adjustment was to the PSE, and about equally high (over 2.0 centimeters) when the correct adjustment was to the PE or to a CE of −6.0 centimeters. Thus, the subject was more consistent in his adjustments when feedback was given for adjusting the illusion to apparent equality than to either of the other two points.

Although in this experiment the subject's PSE was obtained during trials conducted without feedback, we could define the PSE on the basis of the subject's responses under feedback and payoffs for various adjustment positions. Suppose we give feedback and payoffs for responses that are within a small interval of a target setting, *A*, and vary the value of *A* over a range which probably includes the PSE. The PSE is then defined as that value of *A* for which the subject's adjustments exhibit minimum variability. Based on the reasoning given previously, the subject should be most consistent when he adjusts the two halves of the illusion to subjective equality.

A similar approach has been taken in rewarding and identifying the true RT distribution. Snodgrass, Luce, and Galanter (1967) used feedback and payoffs for RTs falling within a small time interval and varied the position of this time interval over a range that bracketed the probable location of the true RT distribution. The true RT distribution was defined as the one showing minimum variability, obtained under an optimum payoff interval.

In these examples, both consistency and accuracy are used as criteria in the sense that in the RT and Müller-Lyer experiments, arbitrarily correct target intervals—spatial in the Müller-Lyer case and temporal in the RT case—are established and the subject is given feedback and payoffs for consistent responses and for responses within that interval. Subsequently, a consistency criterion is used to identify the true PSE or the true RT distribution.

A similar procedure might be used for ordinal, interval, or ratio scaling. For ordinal scaling, an arbitrarily correct order over stimuli on the basis of values on some dimension, or combination of dimensions, could be defined as the correct ordering; subjects would then be given feedback and payoffs for adhering to this arbitrary ordering, and the ordering to which they could most consistently adhere might be taken as the true underlying order. Similarly, in interval or ratio scaling of unidimensional stimuli, subjects could be given feedback and payoffs for giving category responses or magnitude estimations that follow a power, logarithmic, or linear function. The payoff function that most closely represents the subject's true psychophysical function should be the simplest for the subject to follow, and hence the variability of his responses under that payoff function should be minimal.

A disadvantage of this procedure for scaling, however, is the large number of possible functions one might reward. The task of identifying the true psychophysical function by such a procedure seems much more monumental than identifying the true RT distribution by rewarding different latency intervals. In scaling situations, perhaps a somewhat different consistency criterion should apply—one that rewards the subject not on the basis of some arbitrarily defined function but on the basis of his previous performance.

Suppose we want to obtain rank preference data from subjects for various simple patterns so that we can determine which objectively measurable characteristics of these patterns affect degree of preference. How shall we reward the subject for producing his true preference ranking, as uncontaminated as possible by error and carelessness? We could use a consistency criterion based on that subject's past performance by having him carry out this task at least twice. The subject could be rewarded at the end of two sessions on the basis of the degree of correlation between his preference ranking in session 1 and his ranking in session 2. If the stimuli are sufficiently numerous or sufficiently similar so that their original ordering cannot be memorized, it would seem that the subject's best strategy under these payoff conditions is to give his true preference ranking in both sessions, since this ranking ought to be the easiest for him to reproduce.

Similar procedures might be used for interval and ratio scaling. Subjects could be tested twice, preferably on different samples of stimuli, and instructed that their payoff will be based on the degree of consistency between the psychophysical functions obtained from the two scaling sessions. It would seem that the subject would be wise to try to duplicate, insofar as he can, the magnitude of his true sensation as expressed in category ratings or magnitude estimations.

We have seen that the areas of motivation and control in psychophysical experiments have been overlooked for far too long. We would look to the new generation of psychophysicists, to which some of the present readers may belong, to devise new and ingenious outcome structures in order to shed new light on these very old problems in psychophysics.

## SUMMARY AND CONCLUSIONS

The main purpose of psychophysics is to describe the function that relates the physical world to the mental world, that is, the function that relates physical intensity to psychological intensity. Two aspects of the psychophysical function are of primary interest: the point at which the function begins, and the rate at which the function grows with physical stimulus magnitude.

Determination of the absolute threshold gives the starting point—that is, how much physical intensity is required before the subject becomes aware of any sensation whatever. The subject's task is to discriminate the presence of a stimulus from its absence, or to discriminate the effects of a stimulus from the effects of a silent background. In absolute detection, the subject must detect the difference between some threshold amount of stimulation and no stimulation.

It is natural to extend absolute detection to the discrimination of an increment in some standard level of background intensity, where the particular background level can be set at any value. This increment is the difference threshold.

Classical theories of threshold assume that a barrier within the nervous system must be overcome in order for the subject to detect either the difference between a stimulus and its absence, for the absolute threshold, or the difference between a stimulus increment and a background intensity, for the difference threshold. That is, the classical theories propose that the threshold is real, and can be found within the subject's nervous system. A modern version of classical threshold theory is neural quantum theory, which maintains that discontinuities in discrimination can be observed under proper experimental conditions. Neural quantum theory holds that a continuously increasing stimulus produces a series of discrete steplike changes in sensation, mediated by successive triggering of neural quanta. Such discontinuities are experimentally manifest in a psychometric function that is linear. The theory also predicts that the minimum intensity increment always detected by a subject is an integral multiple of the maximum increment never detected.

In contrast to both classical and neural quantum theories, signal detection theory maintains that no true threshold exists as a barrier within the nervous system, but rather humans are sensitive to continuous changes in intensity, whether those changes occur against a silent background or against a noise background. According to signal detection theory, the subject does not show perfect discrimination because there is noise in the system—generated both from within by the nervous system and from without by the experimenter himself. Such noise forces the subject to adopt a response criterion for deciding whether or not a particular effect was more likely the result of signal or of noise; however, such a response criterion is not a threshold in the classical or neural quantum sense, because its location is easily manipulated by nonsensory aspects of the experimental situation, such as payoffs.

The controversy over whether a sensory (as opposed to a response) threshold exists is important for both theoretical and practical purposes. Each theory prescribes its own methods for measuring discrimination, and so the methods used to measure thresholds are directly tied to theories about whether they exist or not.

Controversies also rage over how to measure the form of the psychophysical function—that is, how to determine the manner in which sensation grows with physical stimulus intensity. Fechner, the father of psychophysics, used the difference threshold, or jnd, as the unit of measurement along the sensation scale. He made the reasonable suggestion that the *subjective* difference between any two just noticeably different stimuli must always be equal, even though their *physical* difference varies widely with the absolute physical intensity of those stimuli. Thus Fechner proposed that while the physical jnd, $\Delta I$, increases with the intensity of the standard, the subjective jnd, $\Delta S$, remains constant, and so can be used as the unit of measurement for the psychophysical function. Weber had previously shown that the size of the physical jnd is a constant fraction of the size of the standard, at least over the middle range of intensities, a generalization known as Weber's law. By assuming that Weber's law was true, and that the subjective jnd was constant, Fechner derived the law bearing his name: Sensation grows as the logarithm of physical intensity, or $S = a \log I$.

Fechner derived the psychophysical function indirectly by measuring difference thresholds. However, since Fechner's time, direct methods of scaling sensory magnitude have been developed, including category scaling and the magnitude methods of S. S. Stevens. When subjects directly estimate the magnitude of their sensations by assigning numbers to them, as in magnitude estimation, the resulting psychophysical function is not at all like Fechner's logarithmic function. Instead, it is a power function, expressed as $S = aI^b$, where the exponent $b$ describes the rate at which sensation magnitude grows with stimulus magnitude. The power function is more versatile than the logarithmic function: The logarithmic function says that sensation always grows more slowly than physical magnitude. Power functions with exponents less than 1.0 also indicate that sensation lags behind physical intensity; however, with an exponent equal to 1.0, such as for line length and duration, sensation (i.e., perceived length or perceived duration) grows at the same rate as physical magnitude, and an exponent greater than 1.0 indicates that sensation races ahead of physical intensity, as for sweetness or perceived shock intensity.

Between the two extremes of Fechner's indirect scaling methods and Stevens' direct methods lie a variety of other techniques for scaling psychological continua. Psychological continua, such as liberalism-conservatism, esthetic value, and severity of crimes, have no corresponding, well-defined physical measure. Hence, it is impossible to obtain a psychophysical function for them. A psychological scale can say how different in severity two crimes seem to be, but that psychological difference cannot be related to any objectively measurable difference.

Thurstonian scaling is one example of a technique used to derive a psychological scale. Thurstonian scaling, like Fechnerian scaling, uses the degree of confusion among items to construct a scale. The unfolding technique is another procedure, one that introduces individual differences to scaling. Different subjects may have different "ideal points" along a particular psychological dimension, even though all the subjects have the identical underlying scale. Unfolding analysis produces a scale between an ordinal and an interval scale; both the order of stimuli and the order of their differences are measured.

Recognition does not yield a scale of the stimuli presented. Rather, the results of a recognition experiment tell how accurately subjects can absolutely identify a set of stimuli as a function of their spacing along the physical stimulus dimension and their dimensionality. An often-quoted result from recognition experiments is that only about seven (plus or minus two) unidimensional stimuli can be identified without error, regardless of what the dimension is or how the stimuli are spaced. The subject appears to have a flexible internal "yardstick" which he can stretch here and compress there, but which has only about seven compartments along it into which he can place, without error, each of seven stimuli.

An interesting development in modern psychophysics has been explicit payoffs for desired performance, in lieu of vague instructions either to be as accurate as possible in a detection experiment, or as fast as possible in a reaction-time experiment. Payoffs for correct responses occur naturally within the signal detection experiment and within the recognition experiment. However, payoffs for correct responses in scaling experiments are difficult to envisage. Without access to the subject's internal states, the experimenter cannot know when the subject is reporting the magnitude of his sensation correctly, and so cannot know when to reward him. Perhaps, payoffs could be based on consistency instead of accuracy, since those subjects who do correctly report their internal states ought to be more consistent than those who do not.

# REFERENCES


**Barker, R. G.** An experimental study of the resolution of conflict by children: Time elapsing and amount of vicarious trial-and-error behavior occurring. In Q. McNemar & M. A. Merrill (Eds.), *Studies in personality.* New York: McGraw-Hill, 1942. Pp. 13–34.

**Bartlett, R. J.** Measurement in psychology. *Advancement of Science,* 1939, **1**, 1–20.

**Békésy, G. von.** *Experiments in hearing.* New York: McGraw-Hill, 1960.

**Bernoulli, D.** Specimen Theoriae Novae de Mensura Sortis, *Commentarii Academiae Scientiarum Imperialis Petropolitanae,* Tomus V (*Papers of the Imperial Academy of Sciences in Petersburg,* Vol. V), 1738. Pp. 175–92. (Reprinted as Exposition of a new theory on the measurement of risk, translated by L. Sommer, *Econometrica,* 1954, **22**, 23–36.)

**Blough, D. S.** Dark adaptation in the pigeon. *Journal of Comparative and physiological psychology,* 1956, **49**, 425–30.

**Boring, E. G.** *A history of experimental psychology.* (2nd ed.) New York: Appleton-Century-Crofts, 1950.

**Boring, E. G., Langfeld, H. S., & Weld, H. P.** *Psychology: A factual textbook.* New York: Wiley, 1935.

**Burroughs, E. R.** *Tarzan at the earth's core.* New York: Ace Books, 1929.

**Bush, R. R., Galanter, E., & Luce, R. D.** Characterization and classification of choice experiments. In R. D. Luce, R. R. Bush, & E. Galanter (Eds.), *Handbook of mathematical psychology.* Vol. 1. New York: Wiley, 1963. Pp. 77–102.

**Cannon, W. B., & Washburn, A. L.** An explanation of hunger. *American Journal of Physiology,* 1912, **29**, 441–54.

**Catania, A. C.** Reinforcement schedules and psychophysical judgments: A study of some temporal properties of behavior. In W. N. Schoenfeld (Ed.), *The theory of reinforcement schedules*. New York: Appleton-Century-Crofts, 1970. Pp. 1–42.

**Cattell, J. McK.** On errors of observation. *American Journal of Psychology,* 1893, **5,** 285–93.

**Cattell, J. McK.** The time of perception as a measure of differences in intensity. *Philosophical Studies,* 1902, **19,** 63–68.

**Chocholle, R.** Variation des temps de réaction auditifs en fonction de l'intensité à diverses fréquences. *Année psychologique,* 1940–41, **41–42,** 5–124.

**Clark, W. C.** The *Psyche* in psychophysics: A sensory-decision theory analysis of the effect of instruction on flicker sensitivity and response bias. *Psychological Bulletin,* 1966, **65,** 358–66.

**Clark, W. C.** Sensory-decision theory analysis of the placebo effect on the criterion for pain and thermal sensitivity ($d'$). *Journal of Abnormal Psychology,* 1969, **74,** 363–71.

**Clark, W. C., Brown, J. C., & Rutschmann, J.** Flicker sensitivity and response bias in psychiatric patients and normal subjects. *Journal of Abnormal Psychology,* 1967, **72,** 35–42.

**Coombs, C. H.** Psychological scaling without a unit of measurement. *Psychological Review,* 1950, **57,** 145–58.

**Coombs, C. H.** *A theory of data*. New York: Wiley, 1964.

**Corso, J. F.** The neural quantum theory of sensory discrimination. *Psychological Bulletin,* 1956, **53,** 371–93.

**Corso, J. F.** *The experimental psychology of sensory behavior.* New York: Holt, Rinehart & Winston, 1967. Figure 7–1, page 22, Copyright © 1967 by Holt, Rinehart and Winston, Inc. Adapted and reprinted by permission of Holt, Rinehart and Winston, Inc.

**Dennis, W. (Ed.)** *Readings in the history of psychology*. New York: Appleton-Century-Crofts, 1948.

**Fechner, G. T.** *Elemente der Psychophysik*. Leipzig: Breitkopf und Härtel, 1860.

**Flynn, B. M.** Pitch discrimination: The form of the psychometric function and simple reaction time to liminal differences. *Archives of Psychology, New York,* 1943, **39,** No. 280.

**Galanter, E.** *Textbook of elementary psychology.* San Francisco: Holden-Day, 1966. Figure VI-15, p. 175, reproduced by permission.

**Granger, G. W.** Personality and visual perception: A review. *Journal of Mental Science,* 1953, **99,** 8–43.

**Granger, G. W.** Night vision and psychiatric disorders: A review of experimental studies. *Journal of Mental Science,* 1957, **103,** 48–79.

**Green, D. M., & Swets, J. A.** *Signal detection theory and psychophysics*. New York: Wiley, 1966.

**Guilford, J. P.** *Psychometric methods*. (2nd ed.) New York: McGraw-Hill, 1954.

**Hecht, S., Shlaer, S., & Pirenne, M. H.** Energy, quanta, and vision. *Journal of General Physiology,* 1942, **25,** 819–40.

**Helson, H.** *Adaptation-level theory*. New York: Harper & Row, 1964.

**Herrnstein, R. J., & van Sommers, P.** Method of sensory scaling with animals. *Science,* 1962, **135,** 40–41.

**Hohle, R. H.** Inferred components of reaction times as functions of foreperiod duration. *Journal of Experimental Psychology,* 1965, **69,** 382–86.

**Hyman, R.** Stimulus information as a determinant of reaction time. *Journal of Experimental Psychology,* 1953, **45,** 188–96.

**James, W.** *Textbook of psychology: Briefer course*. New York: Holt, Rinehart & Winston, 1892.

**Jastrow, J. A.** A critique of psychophysic methods. *American Journal of Psychology,* 1888, **1,** 271–309.

**John, I. D.** A statistical decision theory of simple reaction time. *Australian Journal of Psychology,* 1967, **19,** 27–34.

**Johnson, D. M.** Confidence and speed in the two-category judgment. *Archives of Psychology, New York,* 1939, **34,** No. 241.

**Kellogg, W. N.** An experimental comparison of psychophysical methods. *Archives of Psychology,* 1929, **17,** No. 106.

**Larkin, W. D., & Norman, D. A.** An extension and experimental analysis of the neural quantum theory. In R. C. Atkinson (Ed.), *Studies in mathematical psychology*. Stanford, Calif.: Stanford University Press, 1964. Pp. 188–200. Figure 1, p. 192, reproduced by permission.

**Luce, R. D., & Mo, S. S.** Magnitude estimation of heaviness and loudness by individual subjects: A test of a probabilistic response theory. *British Journal of Mathematical and Statistical Psychology,* 1965, **18,** 159–74.

**McGill, W. J.** Stochastic latency mechanisms. In R. D. Luce, R. R. Bush, & E. Galanter (Eds.), *Handbook of mathematical psychology*. Vol. 1. New York: Wiley, 1963. Pp. 309–60.

**Miller, G. A.** What is information measurement? *American Psychologist,* 1953, **8,** 3–11.

**Miller, G. A.** The magical number seven, plus or minus two: Some limits on our capacity for processing information. *Psychological Review,* 1956, **63,** 81–97.

**Miller, G. A.** Psycholinguistic approaches to the study of communication. In D. L. Arm (Ed.), *Journeys in science: Small steps—great strides*. Albuquerque: The University of New Mexico Press, 1967. Pp. 22–73.

**Needham, J. G.** The effect of the time interval upon the time-error at different intensive levels. *Journal of Experimental Psychology,* 1935, **18,** 530–43. Figure 2, p. 535, Copyright 1935 by the American Psychological Association, and reproduced by permission.

**Pollack, I.** The information of elementary auditory displays. *Journal of the Acoustical Society of America,* 1952, **24,** 745–49.

**Pollack, I.** The information of elementary auditory displays: II. *Journal of the Acoustical Society of America,* 1953, **25,** 765–69.

**Pradhan, P. L., & Hoffman, P. J.** Effect of spacing and range of stimuli on magnitude estimation judgments. *Journal of Experimental Psychology,* 1963, **66,** 533–41.

**Rock, I., & Kaufman, L.** The moon illusion: II. *Science,* 1962, **136,** 1023–31.

**Shannon, C. E.** A mathematical theory of communication. *Bell System Technical Journal,* 1948, **27,** 379–423, 623–56.

**Shipley, W. C., Coffin, J. I., & Hadsell, K. C.** Affective distance and other factors determining reaction time in judgments of color preference. *Journal of Experimental Psychology,* 1945, **35,** 206–15.

**Snodgrass, J. G.** Foreperiod effects in simple reaction time: Anticipation or expectancy? *Journal of Experimental Psychology Monograph,* 1969, **79** (No. 3, Part 2).

**Snodgrass, J. G., Luce, R. D., & Galanter, E.** Some experiments on simple and choice reaction time. *Journal of Experimental Psychology,* 1967, **75,** 1–17.

**Steinman, A. R.** Reaction time to change compared with other psychophysical methods. *Archives of Psychology, New York,* 1944, No. 292.

**Stevens, J. C., & Guirao, M.** Individual loudness functions. *Journal of the Acoustical Society of America,* 1964, **36,** 2210–13.

**Stevens, S. S.** Mathematics, measurement, and psychophysics. In S. S. Stevens (Ed.), *Handbook of experimental psychology.* New York: Wiley, 1951. Pp. 1–49.

**Stevens, S. S.** On the psychophysical law. *Psychological Review,* 1957, **64,** 153–81.

**Stevens, S. S.** The psychophysics of sensory function. In W. A. Rosenblith (Ed.), *Sensory communication.* Cambridge, Mass.: M.I.T. Press, 1961. Pp. 1–33. Figures 3 and 4, p. 11, reprinted by permission of The M.I.T. Press, Cambridge, Massachusetts. Copyright © 1961 by The Massachusetts Institute of Technology.

**Stevens, S. S.** The surprising simplicity of sensory metrics. *American Psychologist,* 1962, **17,** 29–39. (a)

**Stevens, S. S.** In pursuit of the sensory law. Second Klopsteg Lecture. Evanston, Ill.: Technological Institute, Northwestern University, November 7, 1962. (b) Table 1, p. 7, reprinted by permission.

**Stevens, S. S.** A metric for the social consensus. *Science,* 1966, **151,** 530–41.

**Stevens, S. S.** Neural events and the psychophysical law. *Science,* 1970, **170,** 1043–50.

**Stevens, S. S.** A neural quantum in sensory discrimination. *Science,* 1972, **177,** 749–62.

**Stevens, S. S., & Galanter, E.** Ratio scales and category scales for a dozen perceptual continua. *Journal of Experimental Psychology,* 1957, **54,** 377–411.

**Stevens, S. S., & Guirao, M.** Loudness, reciprocality, and partition scales. *Journal of the Acoustical Society of America,* 1962, **34,** 1466–71.

**Stevens, S. S., & Guirao, M.** Subjective scaling of length and area and the matching of length to loudness and brightness. *Journal of Experimental Psychology,* 1963, **66,** 177–86.

**Stevens, S. S., Morgan, C. T., & Volkmann, J.** Theory of the neural quantum in the discrimination of loudness and pitch. *American Journal of Psychology,* 1941, **54,** 315–35.

**Stroud, J. M.** The fine structure of psychological time. In H. Quastler (Ed.), *Information theory in psychology.* New York: The Free Press, 1955. Pp. 174–207.

**Stunkard, A., & Koch, C.** The interpretation of gastric motility: I. Apparent bias in the reports of hunger of obese persons. *Archives of General Psychiatry,* 1964, **11,** 74–82.

**Tanner, W. P., Jr., & Swets, J. A.** A decision-making theory of visual detection. *Psychological Review,* 1954, **61,** 401–409.

**Teitelbaum, P.** *Physiological psychology.* Englewood Cliffs, N.J.: Prentice-Hall, 1967.

**Thurstone, L. L.** A law of comparative judgment. *Psychological Review,* 1927, **34,** 273–86.

**Torgerson, W. S.** *Theory and methods of scaling.* New York: Wiley, 1958.

**Torgerson, W. S.** Distances and ratios in psychophysical scaling. *Acta Psychologica* (Amsterdam), 1961, **19,** 201–205.

**Underwood, B. J.** *Experimental psychology.* (2nd ed.) New York: Appleton-Century-Crofts, 1966. Figures 5–1, p. 136, and 5–10, p. 170, Copyright © 1966 by Meredith Publishing Company, and reproduced by permission of Prentice-Hall, Inc., Englewood Cliffs, New Jersey.

**Urban, F. M.** The method of constant stimuli and its generalizations. *Psychological Review,* 1910, **17,** 229–59.

**Woodrow, H.** The measurement of attention. *Psychological Monographs,* 1914, **17** (5, Whole No. 76).

**Woodworth, R. S.** *Experimental psychology.* New York: Holt, Rinehart & Winston, 1938.

**Woodworth, R. S., & Schlosberg, H.** *Experimental psychology.* (Rev. ed.) New York: Holt, Rinehart & Winston, 1954.

NEURAL ACTIVITY AND FUNCTION
- Physiology of the Neuron
- Synaptic Transmission
- Sensory Receptor Action

THE VISUAL SYSTEM
- Structure of the Eye
- Visual Receptors
- Visual Transduction
- The Visual Pathway
- Physiology of Visual Neurons

THE AUDITORY SYSTEM
- The Structure of the Ear
- Auditory Receptors
- The Auditory Pathway
- Physiology of Auditory Neurons
- The Vestibular System

THE OLFACTORY SYSTEM
- Olfactory Receptors
- The Olfactory Pathway
- Physiology of Olfactory Neurons

THE TASTE SYSTEM
- Taste Receptors
- The Taste Pathway
- Physiology of Taste Neurons

THE SOMATOSENSORY SYSTEM
- Anatomy of the Skin
- Cutaneous Receptors
- The Anatomical Pathway

SUMMARY AND CONCLUSIONS

# GENERAL BIOLOGY OF SENSORY SYSTEMS

# 3

**Thomas S. Brown**
**DePaul University**

*with the collaboration of*
*Ronald T. Verrillo*   Syracuse University*

The scent of the scarlet roses aroused me. The petals felt like velvet as I hurled them heavenward. I waited and listened to their cascading shower as they adorned me with royal garb and crowned me king of my world.

What these sentences describe is but a moment when an individual was being stimulated by a variety of physical energies and was reacting to those stimuli. In essence, these sentences describe the main emphasis of this chapter—the neural substrate of sensation and perception. Reread the first three sentences and embellish them with your experience as you scan Figure 3.1. This schema represents the series of events that occurs when an external stimulus excites some or all of our specialized receptor cells. Figure 3.1 illustrates the flow of afferent information from the receptors to the various sensory areas in the cerebral cortex. The flow is not continuous but proceeds from one neuron to the next, with critical transformations of the neural code taking place at the junctures between neurons, called *synapses,* which are discussed in a later section.

For humans the integrity of the sensory and association areas of the cerebral cortex is essential if complex stimuli are to be perceived. And, of course, how one perceives and responds to a stimulus is largely determined by its meaningfulness. Figure 3.1 omits a large number of perceptual variables, such as wants, needs, expectancies, interests, and values. These variables may also influence the neural transformations that occur throughout the system from receptor cell to cortical cell. However, the anatomical and physiological substrates for these influences are not understood.

In a sense, Figure 3.1 also presents an outline of this chapter, which reviews the anatomy and physiology of the sensory systems, emphasizing receptor-cell mechanisms and response characteristics of neurons in the various afferent pathways. Prior to the examination of the senses, the chapter reviews general neuron physiology and synaptic transmission.

## NEURAL ACTIVITY AND FUNCTION

The nerve cell, or neuron, is the functional unit of the nervous system. All neurons consist of three parts: a *cell body,* or *soma* (sometimes re-

*R. T. Verrillo wrote the section on The Somatosensory System and did the original drawings for Figures 3.36 and 3.37.

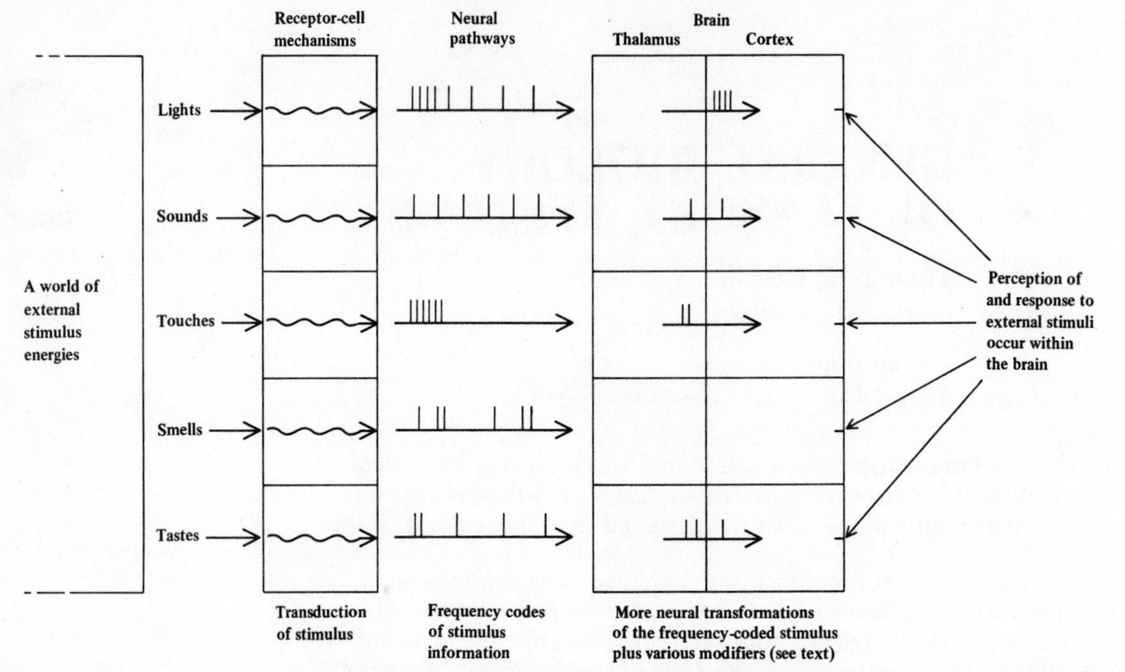


**Figure 3.1** Schema representing the flow of sensory information from the receptors to the brain.

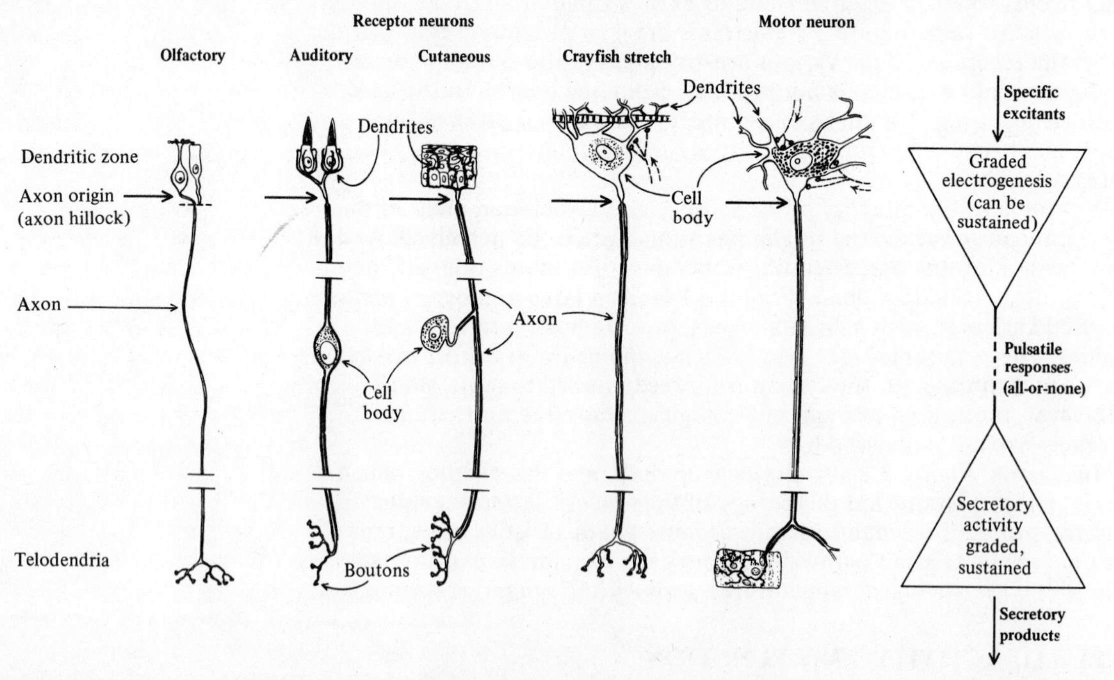


**Figure 3.2** Diagram of various types of neurons. On the far right is a schematic figure of the functional components of a generalized neuron as proposed by Grundfest (1957). The other diagrams are of various receptor neurons and a motor neuron indicating how their parts correspond to those of the generalized schema. (From Bodian, 1962.)

ferred to as the *perikaryon*), an *axon*, and *dendrites*. The axon is one of the many fine protoplasmic extensions of the soma; the rest are the dendrites. The dendrites branch out in complex patterns that vary greatly from neuron to neuron, so that neurons differ widely in appearance. Being a true living cell of the body, the neuron has many features common to all cells, for example, the various organelles within the soma and the difference in electrical potential that exists across the cell membrane. The dendrites and the axon are highly specialized portions of the neuron whose main functions are to initiate and propagate excitation along their length. Traditional definitions found in many textbooks of anatomy and physiology state that dendrites are the extensions that conduct impulses toward the cell body of the neuron, and the axon is the extension that conducts impulses away from the cell body. Such definitions may fit the structural features of many neurons, but the conduction of impulses is a physiological process and should not be specified by anatomical criteria.

Figure 3.2 compares a functional diagram of the generalized neuron as proposed by Grundfest (1957) with anatomical examples of various types of neurons. This diagram suggests that the position of the neuron's cell body is irrelevant to the functioning of the cell. Following Bodian (1962), then, the dendrites and axon can best be defined in functional terms. Thus, the dendritic zone of a neuron consists of a number of usually tapering cytoplasmic extensions that have synaptic connections with other neurons or are specialized to convert environmental stimuli into local-response-generating activity. The axon is the single, often branched cytoplasmic extension that conducts nervous impulses away from the dendritic zone. The *axon telodendria* (see Figure 3.2) is that portion of the membrane which is involved in synaptic transmission, or neurosecretory activity. The bulblike terminals of the telodendria, called *boutons*, generally contain a concentration of *mitochondria, synaptic vesicles*, or *secretory granules*. The cell body, which is the focal point of embryonic outgrowth of the dendrites and axon, is the metabolic center of the neuron. It contains the *Nissl bodies*, which are masses of granular endoplasmic reticulum that synthesize protein. From the cell body the protein moves out into the axon and dendrites. Devoid of Nissl bodies, the axon cannot synthesize protein. It is dependent on the cell body for its metabolic needs and dies once it is severed from the cell body. The fate of the protein is unknown, but it may be related to learning and memory.

## Physiology of the neuron

The human brain contains 10 to 12 billion neurons. Each one is a separate entity which makes functional connection via its axon terminals with many other neurons. Each neuron in turn receives synaptic influences from many (sometimes as many as 200 to 300) other neurons. Accordingly, the number of connections between neurons far surpasses the number of neurons. Yet each neuron can have only one of two effects on each neuron with which it makes contact; it either excites or inhibits, and it may excite some neurons at the same time that it inhibits others.

Despite the enormous complexity of the human nervous system, or perhaps owing to it, investigators have focused on the response of the axon. This response is the *all-or-none spike potential* that is propagated along the entire length of the axon without decrement. The usual and most informative way to examine the behavior of nerve axons is to measure electrical activity by placing a fine microelectrode into an axon. These measurements became possible with the development of the microelectrode in 1949 by Ling and Gerard.

When two electrodes are both placed either on the outside surface of the membrane or on the inside surface, no voltage difference can be recorded between them. The external and internal mediums are isoelectric; that is, they are of equal electrical potential or charge. However, if one electrode is placed inside the axon and the other outside, a potential difference of 70 millivolts (mV) is measured. Generally, the interior of the neuron is electrically negative with respect to the outside. A potential of $-70$ mV is measured when the neuron is not generating a nerve action potential, that is, when the cell is at rest. Hence, it is called the *resting membrane potential*. A resting neuron is considered to be *polarized*. Whenever the neuron is stimulated, the potential difference either decreases (moves toward the zero value) or increases (moves away from the zero value). Movement of the potential level toward zero is referred to as *depolarization*, and movement away from zero (so that the level becomes more negative, falling below the resting level, say to $-73$ mV) is referred to as *hyperpolarization*. Effective stimuli, then, either depolarize a neuron or hyperpolarize it.

A stimulus of moderate intensity applied to a neuron produces the complex and very rapid series of potential changes shown in Figure 3.3. Initially, a small depolarizing potential (A) moves the membrane potential to a level of $-60$ mV. Then there

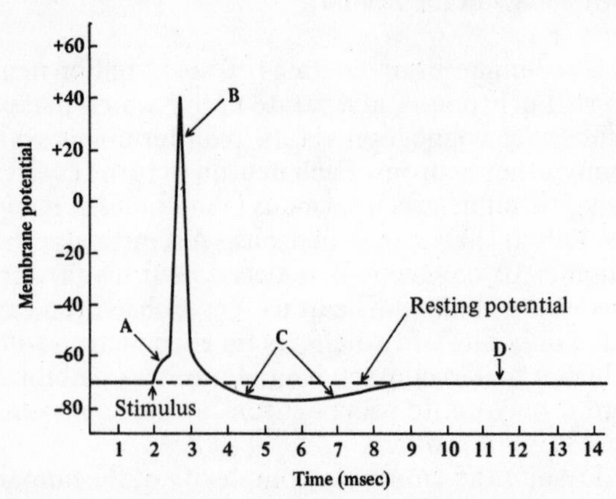


**Figure 3.3** The sequence of changes in the voltage of a neuron's membrane potential following effective stimulation. When a stimulus is applied to the cell at 2 msec, a nerve impulse is produced at B. See text for explanation.

suddenly occurs a large and rapid peak (B) as the membrane potential goes from −60 mV (inside negative) to a level of +40 mV (inside now positive with respect to outside) and quickly back to −60 mV (inside again negative). These changes all take place in about 1 msec. Then comes a period of hyperpolarization (C) which, in this example, lasts about 5.5 msec. Finally, the potential returns to its resting level (D) of −70 mV. These changes in the membrane potential flow along the entire length of the axon and constitute the *nerve action potential,* often also referred to as the *nerve impulse* or *spike potential*. It is the output of a neuron. Transmission of information throughout the nervous system is brought about by frequency coding of nerve impulses along fiber tracts, as well as by the identity of the fibers activated (see Chapter 1).

An interesting phenomenon shown in Figure 3.3 is the sudden development of the spike potential when the level of depolarization reaches −60 mV. This represents the threshold level for the neuron. Each neuron has its own threshold of depolarization which must be attained if a nerve impulse is to be triggered and propagated along the axon. A stimulus that is too weak to depolarize the neuron to its threshold level is below threshold. The wave of depolarization triggered by a subthreshold stimulus will passively spread along the cell membrane, subsiding as it flows away from the point of stimulation. In contrast, the amplitude of the nerve impulse does not undergo any change as it spreads along the membrane of the axon. All stimuli strong enough to depolarize to the threshold level will elicit the same maximal spike potential from that neuron. Subthreshold stimuli will produce only the small, subsiding potential.

Since all suprathreshold stimuli elicit the same full-sized potential from a given neuron, are all such stimuli essentially equivalent as far as that neuron is concerned? If so, can a neuron discriminate only between stimulation and no stimulation? In fact, neurons do not respond the same way to all suprathreshold stimuli. Within limits that depend on the sensory modality, the stronger the stimulus, the more rapidly a neuron responds. Stronger stimuli elicit more nerve impulses per second than weaker stimuli. This faster firing rate is achieved by a reduction in response *latency,* which is the time interval between the onset of a stimulus and the peak of the action potential. Suprathreshold stimuli of increasing strength trigger nerve impulses with shorter and shorter latencies. However, the speed at which a nerve impulse can be elicited from a cell is limited by the refractoriness of the neuron.

### *Refractory periods*

Immediately after propagating a nerve impulse, a neuron is unable to respond to a stimulus, no matter how strong it is. This *absolute refractory period* roughly corresponds to the duration of the spike potential. The second impulse cannot be elicited until the descending limb of the action potential has almost reached the foot (at about 3.5 msec in Figure 3.3). At the end of the absolute refractory period, the neuron is normally hyperpolarized and, although it can now respond to a stimulus, it is less sensitive than normal; that is, its threshold is raised and a stronger stimulus than usual is required to fire it. This *relative refractory period* is longer in duration than the absolute period and generally corresponds to the period of hyperpolarization that would normally follow a nerve action potential. The activity of a neuron is therefore characterized by a series of pulses rather than by a continuous steady stream. Consequently, the frequency of neural firing can provide information about the stimulus, and especially about stimulus strength.

### *Resting membrane potential*

The resting membrane potential is the result of ionic concentrations on either side of the membrane, and the nerve action potential reflects the

**Table 3.1 Concentrations of Small Ions in the Intra- and Extracellular Fluids, Expressed as Millimoles (mM) per Kilogram (kg). The Intracellular Fluid Is Also Characterized By a Relatively Large Amount of Negative Ions**

| Ions | Inside of cell | Outside of cell |
|---|---|---|
| $K^+$ | 400 | 20 |
| $Na^+$ | 50 | 440 |
| $Cl^-$ | 40 | 560 |
| $Ca^{++}$ | 0.4 | 10 |

(After Hodgkin, 1958.)

rapid flow of some of these ions through the neuron membrane. The internal and external ionic concentrations are shown in Table 3.1. The external fluids that bathe the neuron have relatively high concentrations of sodium ($Na^+$) and chlorine ($Cl^-$) ions and low concentrations of potassium ($K^+$), calcium ($Ca^{++}$), and magnesium ($Mg^{++}$) ions. The inside of the cell has a high concentration of $K^+$ and relatively low concentrations of $Na^+$ and $Cl^-$. Also in the cell is a number of organic anions which have a net negative charge. The neuron membrane is semipermeable; that is, some ions pass through the membrane rather freely, others only slowly and with difficulty, and still other large ions, such as the protein ions, do not pass through at all.

The resting level of the membrane potential is primarily due to the internal and external concentrations of potassium ions, as demonstrated by the work of A. L. Hodgkin and his colleagues (Baker, Hodgkin, & Shaw, 1961; Hodgkin & Katz, 1949). An increase in the external concentration of potassium ions (which normally is very low) reduces the resting membrane potential. A reduction in the resting membrane potential can also occur as a result of a decrease in the internal concentration of potassium ions. Although other ions may play some role in determining the value of the resting potential, they appear to be of minor consequence. For example, Hodgkin and Katz (1949) demonstrated that variations in the external sodium ion concentration did not alter the resting potential.

### *Nerve action potential*

At rest the cell is relatively impermeable to sodium ions, but not completely so. Sodium ions do leak into the cell, and they are extruded by *active transport;* that is, ions are moved against their concentration gradients. This movement requires the expenditure of metabolic energy. However, when a neuron is at rest the cell membrane is about 50 times more impermeable to sodium than it is to potassium, partly because the sodium ion is slightly larger.

The work of Hodgkin, Huxley, and Katz (1949) led to the formulation of the sodium hypothesis for the nerve action potential. They postulated that when a cell is stimulated the neuron becomes selectively permeable to sodium ions. Because of the large external concentration of sodium, these ions move down their concentration gradient and flow into the cell. This flow occurs during the rising phase of the nerve action potential, as the membrane potential rapidly shifts from −70 mV to +40 mV. Hodgkin and Katz (1949) demonstrated that the amplitude of the nerve action potential varies directly with the external sodium concentration: Lowering the external concentration of sodium ions reduces the size of the nerve impulse, and raising the concentration above its normal value increases the size of the nerve impulse. The size of the impulse is also altered if the internal concentration of sodium ions is changed (Baker, Hodgkin, & Shaw, 1961). Variations in the external potassium concentration do not affect the size of the impulse.

Perhaps the most significant evidence for the sodium hypothesis comes from the *voltage clamp technique,* used by Hodgkin, Huxley, and Katz (1949) to measure the current flows during a nerve action potential. Normally, as a neuron is conducting a nerve impulse, the membrane permeability, the membrane potential, and the current flow, or ionic movement, are all simultaneously changing. With the voltage clamp technique, the membrane potential can be held fixed at a chosen value and the membrane permeability can be measured. This is usually done in terms of membrane conductance as shown in Figure 3.4. The relationship between membrane conductance and membrane permeability is not a simple one. *Conductance* is a measure of the ease with which an ion passes through the membrane when driven by an electrical force. *Permeability,* on the other hand, is the ease of passage for a given ion when driven by a concentration force. For our purposes, we will consider membrane conductance as a measure of membrane permeability. Figure 3.4 presents the time course of changes in the membrane potential ($V$), and the time course of membrane conductance for sodium ($g_{Na}$) and potassium ($g_K$) ions. The

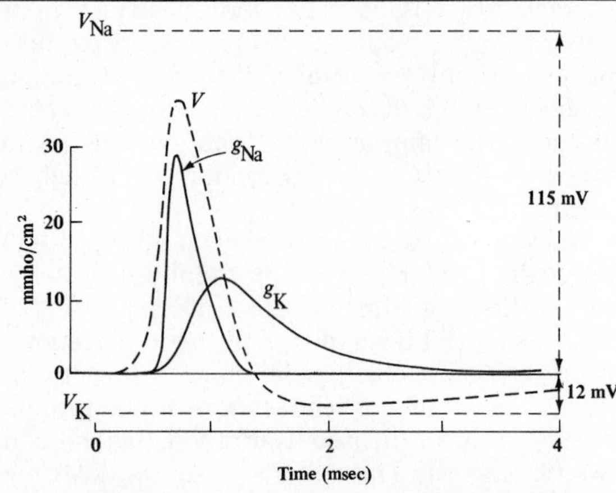


**Figure 3.4** Time course of theoretical changes in membrane potential and membrane conductances for sodium and potassium ions, based on the work of Hodgkin and Huxley (1952). $V_{Na}$ and $V_K$ represent the equilibrium potentials for sodium and potassium, respectively. Conductance is measured in millimhos (mmho). (From Hodgkin, 1958; after Hodgkin & Huxley, 1952.)

changes shown in Figure 3.4 are actually predicted values based on the results of the voltage clamp experiments of Hodgkin and Huxley (1952). The change in $g_{Na}$ lasts for about 1 msec. Its peak occurs with the rising face of the nerve action potential and then, almost as quickly, the membrane conductance for the sodium ions decreases to zero. The period of sodium conductance is accompanied by a movement of sodium ions into the cell. The time course of the potassium conductance is much slower than that of sodium. Its peak occurs with the falling face of the nerve action potential and its duration is about 3 msec. During this period, the potassium ions are moving out of the cell, thus aiding in the repolarization of the cell membrane. During each action potential, therefore, the cell accumulates a small amount of sodium and loses an equally small amount of potassium.

The movements of ions during the action potential are an inward flux of sodium, which is down its concentration gradient, and an outward flow of potassium, which is also down its concentration gradient. These ionic movements do not require the expenditure of energy. The amount of sodium that is accumulated in the cell and the amount of potassium that is lost during a single action potential is insignificant. Of course, after sustained periods of high activity the sodium-potassium balances would be less than optimal. However, in the long run the cell does not accumulate sodium, since a so-called *sodium pump* continually operates to extrude sodium from the cell. The existence of the pump has been demonstrated, but how it works is not yet understood (Caldwell & Keynes, 1957; Hodgkin & Keynes, 1955).

### *Propagation of the nerve impulse*

A brief electrical pulse applied to a nerve axon triggers two distinct events. First, electrons flow between the two electrodes; this is the current flow. Second, ions flow through the membrane. The direction of the electron flow is shown in Figure 3.5. Electrons move into the axon at the anode and out of the axon at the cathode. This current flow, called *electrotonus,* precedes the development of the nerve action potential. The movement of electrons out of the membrane at the cathode depolarizes the cell. If depolarization reaches the threshold level of the cell, a nerve action potential will develop at that point. The membrane becomes permeable to sodium ions which then move into the cell and initiate the action potential. Simultaneously, an outward flow of current at a more distant region of the axon acts to depolarize the cell there, and the nerve action potential will begin to develop at that point. Current flows in at that point and out at an adjacent region. This continuous process travels down the entire length of the axon. By this means the nerve impulse is conducted down the axon without any reduction in size. In the normal excitation of a neuron, the action potential is initiated at the region of axon origin (see Figure 3.2), also known as the *axon hillock,* which is the part of the neuron with the lowest threshold.

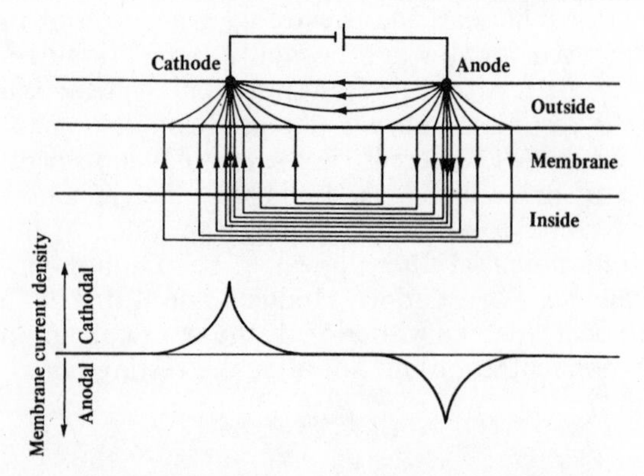


**Figure 3.5** The distribution and flow of current that develops in a nerve fiber when an external source of current is applied to it. The direction of the current flow is indicated by the arrows. (From Woodbury & Patton, 1960.)

## Synaptic transmission

Neurons are not in direct physical contact with each other, but are separated by a small space called the *synaptic space,* or *cleft.* This cleft generally measures about 200 Ångstroms (Å).[1] Some synapses, generally referred to as tight junctions, may have a synaptic cleft as small as 20 Å. The terminal arborizations of the axon are the axon *telodendria.* The telodendria are usually finely branched and exhibit a number of small swellings known as *synaptic boutons* or *synaptic knobs* or, more simply, *synaptic terminals.* A schematic illustration of a synapse is shown in Figure 3.6. The synaptic bouton is characterized by a large number of generally spherical objects called *synaptic vesicles.* These vesicles range in diameter from 300 to 600 Å and may appear empty or filled with a slightly dense, homogeneous material (De Robertis & Bennett, 1955). Two other types of synaptic vesicles range up to 1200 Å in diameter and appear as granulated objects (Grillo & Palay, 1962). Synaptic vesicles are clustered only in the boutons of the axon telodendria.

The synaptic junction is characterized in the electron micrograph by an increased opaqueness of the cell membrane opposite the synaptic bouton. Just behind the membrane, a subsynaptic web is often seen as in Figure 3.6. The synaptic cleft itself is frequently filled with intersynaptic filaments, which are also indicated in Figure 3.6. The function of the synaptic vesicles will become apparent in the section on the theory of synaptic transmission, but first it is necessary to discuss the transmission of excitation from one neuron to another.

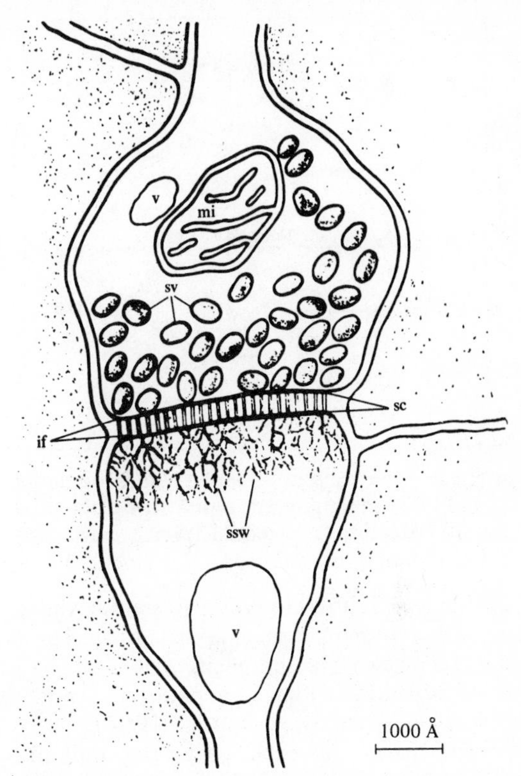


**Figure 3.6** Diagram of a synapse. The synaptic bouton in the upper half of the figure contains one mitochondrion (mi), one vacuole (v), and numerous synaptic vesicles (sv). The synaptic cleft (sc) contains a number of intersynaptic filaments (if). The membrane of the postsynaptic cell at the bottom is characterized by a well-developed subsynaptic web (ssw). (From De Robertis, 1964.)

### *Nature of interneuronal transmission*

Hypotheses concerned with the transmission of impulses from one neuron to another are classified as either chemical or electrical, depending on the nature of the proposed mechanism. Over the years, one or the other of these two hypotheses has been considered to be correct. Evidence at this time indicates that both modes of transmission exist. Chemical transmission occurs when a chemical, a neurotransmitter, is released from the presynaptic bouton as a result of nerve activity. The released chemical then acts on the postsynaptic neuron to either depolarize or hyperpolarize it. Electrical transmission, usually referred to as *ephaptic transmission,* occurs when the electrical fields resulting from nerve activity in one neuron affect the excitability in adjacent neurons. Chemical synapses are believed to be those whose synaptic cleft measures 200 Å or more, whereas electrical synapses are usually associated with tight junctions. While electrical synapses are found frequently in invertebrates and lower vertebrates (Bennett, 1965; Faber & Korn, 1973; Pappas & Bennett, 1966), they seem to be rare in the mammalian nervous system (Gray, 1969). In view of these findings, only chemical synaptic transmission will be treated in detail in this chapter.

### *Postsynaptic potentials*

When one neuron does affect another neuron across a synapse, the postsynaptic neuron will be either slightly depolarized or slightly hyperpolar-

[1] An Ångstrom is equal to $10^{-8}$ cm, or less than 200 millionths of an inch. The synaptic cleft spans less than 1 millionth of an inch.

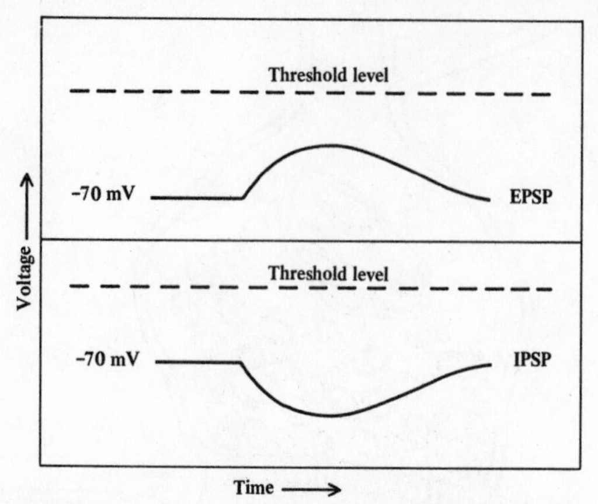


**Figure 3.7** The excitatory postsynaptic potential (EPSP) and the inhibitory postsynaptic potential (IPSP). Membrane potential level is plotted as a function of time.

ized. Figure 3.7 shows the small potentials that can be recorded from the postsynaptic neuron. The two potentials shown are the excitatory postsynaptic potential (EPSP), which is depolarizing, and the inhibitory postsynaptic potential (IPSP), which is hyperpolarizing. In each case, the membrane potential moves away from its resting level of −70 mV. The membrane potential moves toward threshold during an EPSP and away from threshold during an IPSP. Hence, the adjectives *excitatory* and *inhibitory* are used to describe the two potentials.

Postsynaptic potentials are not nerve impulses and have properties quite different from them. Postsynaptic potentials are graded responses with no refractory period, in contrast to the all-or-none behavior of a nerve impulse with its following refractory period. The EPSPs and IPSPs are additive, summing algebraically both spatially, over the membrane surface, and temporally. Spatial and temporal summation can occur simultaneously, although excitatory and inhibitory synapses tend to be located at different places on the surface of the neuron.

### *The chemical theory of synaptic transmission*

The chemical theory of synaptic transmission proposes that a nerve impulse results in the release of the transmitter substance, or neurotransmitter, which is stored in the vesicles of the synaptic boutons. The exact mechanism of the release is not known, but calcium ions are thought to be involved. It is postulated that the neurotransmitter, once released, diffuses across the synaptic cleft and alters the permeability of the postsynaptic membrane, either depolarizing or hyperpolarizing it, depending on the type of transmitter substance.

Several converging lines of evidence relate to the chemical theory in general and to the role of the synaptic vesicles as the storage site for the neurotransmitter in particular. Fatt and Katz (1952) demonstrated that transmitter substances are released in quanta of uniform size. One quantum probably contains several thousand molecules. DelCastillo and Katz (1956) reported a correlation between the presence of synaptic vesicles and the quantal release in synaptic transmission. Moreover, De Robertis and Vaz Ferreira (1957) have shown that a change in the number of vesicles is related to the frequency of stimulation.

The homogeneous vesicles mentioned earlier were first described by De Robertis and Bennett (1955) and are most likely cholinergic vesicles (i.e., they contain acetylcholine). The large granulated vesicles are apparently adrenergic vesicles (i.e., they contain an adrenaline-type neurotransmitter). Whether or not there exists a different vesicle for each separate synaptic transmitter substance is not known. But the effect on the postsynaptic cell, be it excitation or inhibition, is probably due to the nature of the transmitter released. Nevertheless, some instances have been reported which show that a single neuron releasing only one transmitter substance, acetylcholine, can excite some cells and inhibit other cells in invertebrates (Kandel, Frazier, Waziri, & Coggleshall, 1967; Tauc & Gerschenfeld, 1961). It would appear, therefore, that the effect of the neurotransmitter may sometimes be determined by the nature of the membrane of the postsynaptic cell (Tauc, 1969). It is not known whether such dual effects are common in the mammalian nervous system.

Anatomists have searched for structural features that distinguish inhibitory and excitatory synapses. Gray (1959) proposed a division into Type 1 (excitatory) and Type 2 (inhibitory) synapses based mainly on the thickenings present along the membrane at the synaptic cleft. That division, though still in use, is not without exceptions. A more promising division has been proposed by Uchizono (1965) based on his work with the cat cerebellum. Properly prepared, vesicles from known excitatory synapses look spherical or rounded under the electron microscope, whereas vesicles from inhibitory synapses look flat, ellipsoid, or oval. This difference, which has now been reported a number of times (e.g., Bodian, 1966; Gray, 1969; Westrum, 1966), may lead to important insights into the organization of the nervous system. For example, Westrum (1966) and Gray (1969) found that most of the synaptic boutons on the axon hillock contain flat vesicles. If these boutons are in fact inhibitory, then they would be maximally effective in preventing the neuron from firing since, as pointed out earlier, the hillock is that part of the neuron where a nerve impulse normally originates.

*Criteria for a chemical transmitter*

Although the chemical hypothesis assumes a chemical transmitter, so far it has not been possible to specify the chemical composition of transmitter substances. Researchers in the physiology and pharmacology of synapses have proposed a number of criteria that a chemical should satisfy in order to be classified as a transmitter substance (cf. McLennan, 1970). Although some chemicals, such as acetylcholine, are generally considered to act as neurotransmitters, no chemical has yet met all the criteria (Thompson, 1967). Despite this uncertainty, it is reasonable to assume that the chemical transmitters act on the postsynaptic membrane in the manner proposed by Eccles (1965), which is shown in Figure 3.8. Excitatory and inhibitory neurotransmitters are assumed to alter the membrane permeability in different ways. The excitatory transmitters affect the postsynaptic membrane so that sodium ($Na^+$) ions are allowed to flow into the cell which then becomes depolarized. Inhibitory transmitters presumably open channels that are too small for sodium ions, but are large enough to permit potassium ($K^+$) ions to flow out of and chloride ($Cl^-$) ions to flow into the neuron, thereby increasing the internal negativity of the cell and hyperpolarizing it.

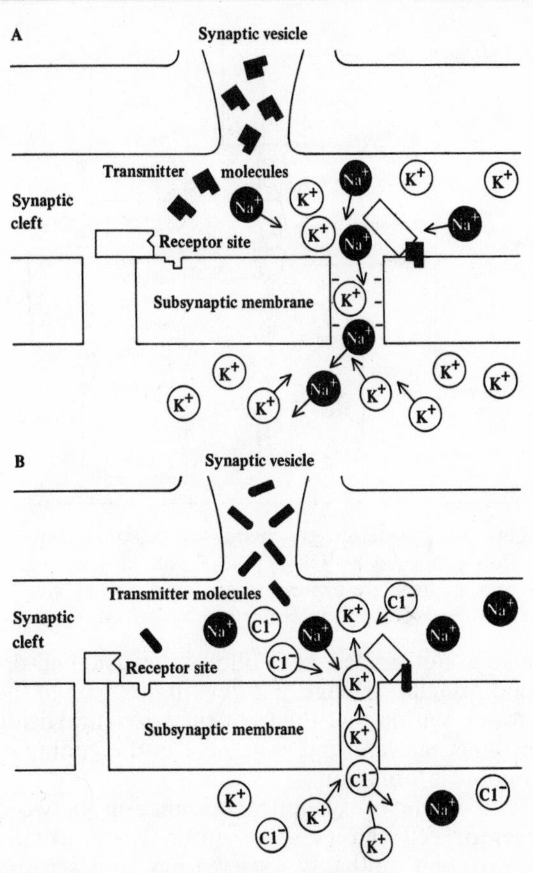


**Figure 3.8** Action of neurotransmitters at excitatory and inhibitory synapses as proposed by Eccles (1965). Panel A: The excitatory transmitter molecule would open large channels in the nerve cell membrane which would permit sodium ($Na^+$) ions to pour through freely, resulting in depolarization. Panel B: The inhibitory transmitter molecule would open channels too small for sodium, but an outflow of potassium ($K^+$) and/or inflow of chloride ($Cl^-$) ions would result in hyperpolarization. (From Eccles, 1965.)

**Sensory receptor action**

Figure 3.9 presents a general schema proposed by Davis (1961) for the action of sensory receptors. Functioning like a dendrite, the receptor cell receives the stimulus energies. The cell may or may not, depending on the particular sensory system, possess an axon that transmits a nerve impulse. The important feature of a receptor cell is its ability to respond in a graded manner to the amount of impinging stimulus energy. Davis (1961) calls this response the *receptor potential.* Those receptors which have no axon, as in the visual, auditory, and gustatory systems, elicit a response in the dendrites of a sensory neuron with which they have synaptic contact. Davis calls this response the *generator potential.* If the receptor cell does possess its own axon, as in the olfactory system, then the receptor and generator potentials are one and the same. Given the right conditions and a strong enough generator potential, the sensory neuron will then produce a nerve impulse. This impulse is the third step in the coding of the external stimulus. Thus, in the sequence (1) receptor potential, (2) generator potential, (3) nerve impulse, the first two potentials are graded, whereas the nerve im-

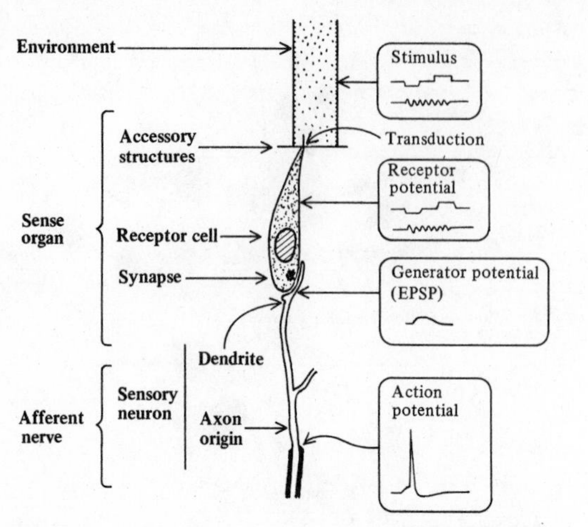


**Figure 3.9** Generalized schema for sensory reception proposed by Davis (1961). Not all features present here are present in all sense organs. See text for explanation. (From Flock, 1970.)

pulse is not graded and follows the usual all-or-none principle. Hence, it is here in the axon of the sensory neuron that the frequency of neural firing becomes relevant and can serve in the coding of stimulus information.

The mode of synaptic transmission between receptor cell and sensory neuron is not usually known and probably varies from one sensory system to another. A chemical transmitter may be involved, as seems to be true of most other types of synapses. Or, the receptor cell's receptor potential may activate the sensory neuron by means of an electrical field, as in the lateral line organ of fish and in the taste bud. A third possibility is that the receptor potential is completely absent, and the stimulus directly activates a chemical mechanism in the receptor cell that excites the sensory neuron.

### *Receptor and generator potentials*

Receptor cells are transducers—they transform one kind of energy into another. They are also analogous to specialized dendrites. Dendrites are the receptive pole of a neuron, and receptor cells are the receptive pole of the sensory system. The receptor potential is comparable to the postsynaptic potential. It is a sustained, graded response that varies with the intensity and duration of the external stimulus. Its amplitude varies as a direct function of stimulus intensity over a large range.

Although physiologists have recorded and described receptor potentials for numerous systems, the transduction mechanism itself is vaguely understood. It is not even known whether transduction is the same in different sensory systems. Presumably the external stimulus alters the receptor cell's permeability, thereby decreasing its membrane potential and depolarizing the cell. This alteration would allow a current flow as long as the stimulus is present. The amount of current flow would reflect the degree of permeability change, which in turn would depend on the intensity of the stimulus. *Adaptation,* however, complicates matters. Adaptation, which is found in all sensory systems, is the decrease in the amplitude of the receptor potential that results from prolonged stimulation. Figure 3.10 gives an example from the olfactory epithelium of the frog. In this particular instance, the recorded potential is both a receptor and a generator potential according to the schema presented in Figure 3.9. During 15 seconds of stimulation, the amplitude of the potential decreased gradually from its peak and then leveled off until the stimulus was discontinued at the arrow. The term *adaptation* also often refers to the decline in nerve impulse frequency in afferent pathways during sustained stimulation. This response decrement could result from adaptation of the receptor potential, the generator potential (where there is one), or even the axon's ability to generate nerve impulses. In view of this uncertainty, it is imperative to indicate the reference point when discussing adaptation. Moreover, the precise mechanism of adaptation is not clearly known.

## THE VISUAL SYSTEM

### The structure of the eye

Optically, the eye is designed to focus the rays of light from external objects upon the retina. A cross section of the human eye is shown in Figure 3.11.

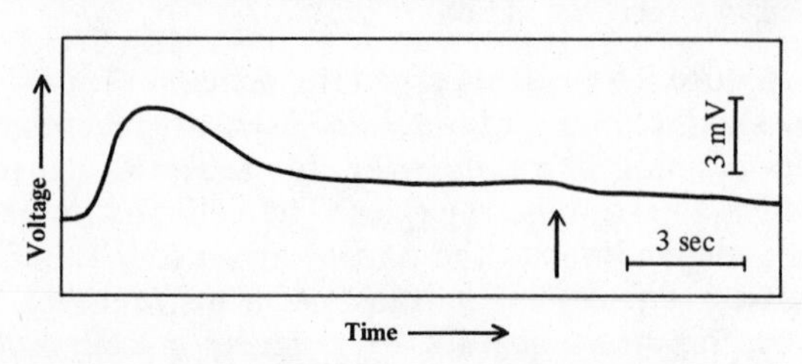


**Figure 3.10** Adaptation of the receptor potential of the olfactory epithelium under prolonged stimulation. Stimulus duration is 15 sec. Velocity of the stimulating air stream is 1 cc per sec. (From Ottoson, 1956.)

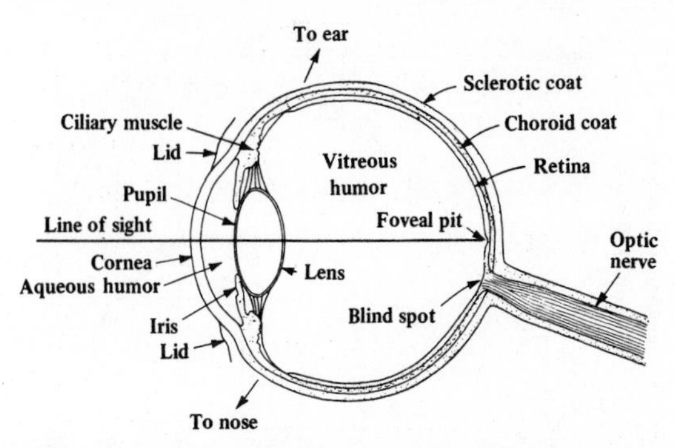


**Figure 3.11** Cross section of the human eye as seen in the horizontal plane. (From Judd & Wyszecki, 1963.)

The outer shell of the eyeball consists of three concentric layers. The outermost layer is the *sclerotic coat,* a tough protective membrane. Its transparent frontal portion is the *cornea.* The middle layer is the darkly pigmented *choroid coat* which serves to darken the inside of the eye. The anterior portion of the choroid layer is the *iris,* which forms the colored part of the eye. The innermost layer, the *retina,* houses the photosensitive receptor cells. The interior of the eye is filled with transparent substances, such as the *vitreous* and *aqueous humors,* and an elastic crystalline *lens* which is stretched across the anterior portion of the eyeball. The lens is attached on each side to the *ciliary muscles* whose contraction changes the thickness of the lens. The *pupil* is the opening or dark spot in the center of the eye. Its size is controlled reflexively by the muscles in the iris so that it becomes smaller in bright light and larger in darkness.

*Formation of the retinal image*

In forming an image on the retina, the eye acts essentially like an intricate convex lens composed of three refractive surfaces. At each refractive surface the entering light rays are bent or refracted, owing to a difference in the density of the medium on one side of the surface relative to the density on the other side. The eye's three refractive surfaces are: (1) the anterior surface of the cornea where the rays enter from the air into the denser material of the cornea; (2) the anterior surface of the lens where the rays enter a still denser medium; and (3) the posterior surface of the lens where the rays pass from the lens into the less dense medium of the vitreous humor. The refractive effects at these surfaces depend on the curvatures and the indices of refraction of the media. The *index of refraction* is the ratio of the speed of light in a vacuum to that in a given medium. In the eye, refraction is greatest at the cornea because the difference between the index of refraction of air and that of the cornea is greater than the difference at the lens and its surroundings.

Tracing the exact path of light through the eye becomes a complex and laborious task if all the refractive effects are individually considered. However, these complex effects can be simplified, without undue loss of accuracy, by using a *reduced eye* in which all refraction is assumed to occur at only one surface, the interface between air and the cornea. The eye is assumed to be composed of a homogeneous medium with the same refractive index as water, which is 1.333.

A diagram of the reduced eye appears in Figure 3.12. The refractive surface at the cornea of the reduced eye has a radius of 5 mm. Its center of curvature is the optical center, or *nodal point,* of the system. The retina lies 15 mm posterior to the nodal point and 20 mm from the surface of the cornea. Because these are the *interior* and *principal focal distances* of the system, images of distant objects are focused on the retina. The *anterior principal focus* is located 15 mm in front of the cornea and is the point at which rays parallel within the eye would converge upon emerging. The anterior focal distance differs from the interior focal distance because light travels through two mediums, air and the eye. It is determined by dividing the interior focal distance by the refractive index for the reduced eye. Thus,

$$\frac{20 \text{ mm}}{1.333} = 15 \text{ mm}.$$

As shown in the construction of the retinal image in Figure 3.12, all the rays of light from point $A$ that penetrate the eye will be focused at $a$, and all those from point $B$ will be focused at $b$. The image on the retina will thus be inverted and smaller than

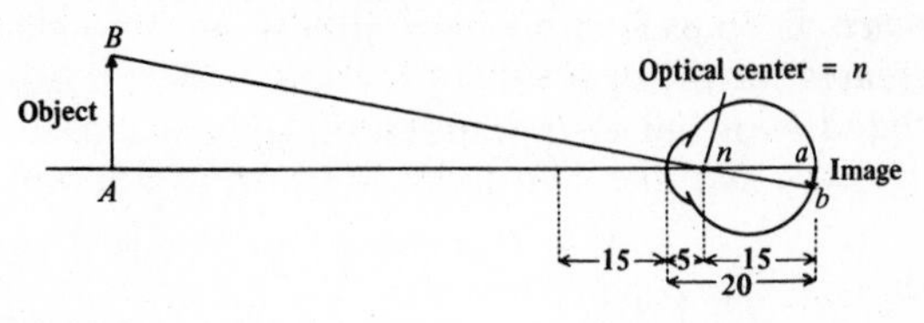


**Figure 3.12** Formation of the retinal image in the reduced eye. Distances are in millimeters. (From Houssay et al., 1955.)

the object. The angle formed at the nodal point by line segments *An* and *Bn* is known as the *visual angle*. It varies inversely with the distance of the object from the eye.

The size of the retinal image can easily be determined by trigonometry from the size of the object and its distance from the nodal point. The ratio of the object size to the image size equals the ratio of the distance between object and nodal point to the distance between image and nodal point, which is 15 mm in the reduced eye.

### *Accommodation*

As an object approaches the eye, the light rays coming from it become more and more divergent at the eye. Consequently, they would be focused at a point behind the retina if the eye remained unchanged, and the image would be unclear. However, the lens of the eye changes shape in response to changes in the distance of fixated objects, so that the image on the retina remains clear. Known as *accommodation,* this response of the eye involves changes primarily in the curvature of the anterior surface of the lens.

The *near point* in vision is that point at which an object can be directly seen with full accommodation, that is, maximal adjustment of the lens. The distance between the near point and the eye increases progressively throughout our lives owing to an ever increasing loss of plasticity in the lens. The gradual decline in our ability to accommodate has little impact until, between the ages of forty and fifty, it begins to interfere with reading or other close work and is then called *presbyopia*, or oldsightedness.

### *Convergence*

When an object is viewed at a distance of 20 ft. or more, the visual axes of both eyes are parallel. However, in viewing nearer objects, the eyes turn in and the visual axes converge to a point. Such convergent movements, or more simply *convergence,* keep us from seeing double. Convergence is greatest at the near point of vision, and so is associated with full accommodation. Objects closer to the eyes than the near point are seen as double.

### *Stereoscopic vision*

The retinal image formed in the right eye is slightly different from the retinal image in the left eye. This difference, known as *binocular parallax,*

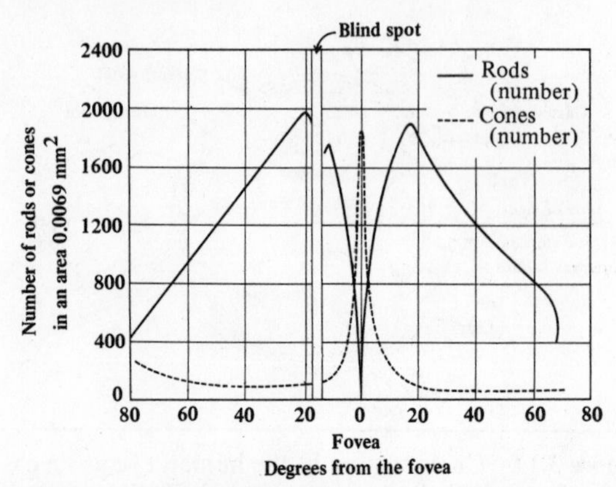


**Figure 3.13** The number of rods and cones per unit area across the horizontal meridian of the retina. The position of the blind spot is marked by the parallel vertical lines. (From Woodson, 1954; data from Østerberg, 1935, and Wertheim, 1894.)

provides cues for spatial discriminations, particularly depth or distance perception. The binocular parallax of any point in space is given by the angle formed at that point by two imaginary lines converging on it from the nodal points of the two eyes. Thus, objects at different distances up to about 20 ft. would subtend different angles.

## **Visual receptors**

The retina is an extremely complex tissue which contains two types of visual receptor cells, *rods* and *cones.* Besides these photoreceptors, there are *horizontal, amacrine, bipolar,* and *ganglion* cells. The horizontal and amacrine cells apparently collect and relay information within the retina, while the bipolar and ganglion cells relay information from the retina to the brain.

The spatial distribution of rods and cones across the human retina is shown in Figure 3.13. The central region of the retina, called the *fovea,* has almost no rods, only cones. The fovea is a shallow depression in the retina; from edge to edge it is about 1500 microns across and subtends a visual angle of about 5 degrees. Within the fovea, the center, or *fovea centralis,* is entirely devoid of rods. It corresponds to the floor of the foveal depression and is about 400 microns across, subtending a visual angle of 1 degree. The fovea centralis contains about 34,000 cones. Over the whole fovea, the density of cones is around 147,000 per mm$^2$. The cone density rapidly falls to about 5000 per mm$^2$ across the remainder of the retina. Concomitantly, the

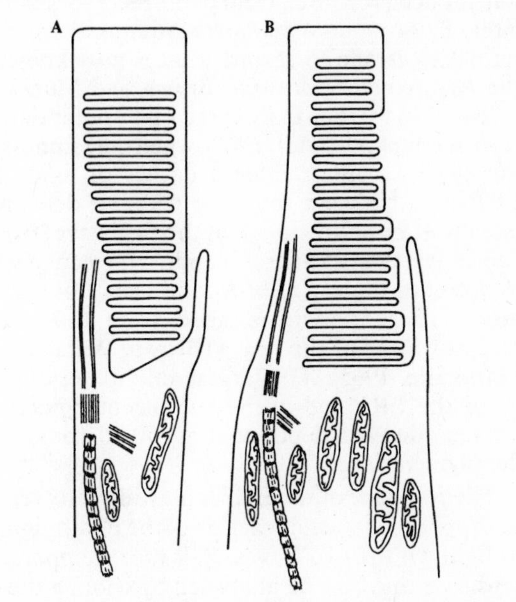


**Figure 3.14** Diagram of the discs in the outer segments of a typical rod (A) and cone (B). (From Cohen, 1963.)

number of rods greatly increases with increasing distance from the fovea centralis, as shown in Figure 3.13. The density of the rods is greatest (160,000 per mm$^2$) at an eccentricity of 20 degrees. The entire retina contains about 125 million rods and 6 million cones.

The use of the electron microscope has greatly advanced our knowledge of the fine structure, or *ultrastructure*, of the rods and cones, as well as other elements of the retina. Sjöstrand (1953) demonstrated that the outer segments of the photoreceptors consist of a pile of membranous discs enclosed within the cell membrane. Dowling (1965) has shown that the foveal cone's outer segment, which is about 40 microns long, contains about 1200 discs. Figure 3.14 is a schematized drawing of the outer segment of a typical cone and rod, each of which also contains stacks of discs. The membrane of a rod disc is 35 Å thick, whereas the membrane of a cone disc is as thick as the plasma membrane, 50 Å. In both rods and cones the discs are formed by invaginations or foldings of the plasma membrane at the base of the outer segment. The discs pinch off from the plasma membrane and appear to be free floating, especially in the rods. In the cones, the disc membrane tends to remain in continuity with the plasma membrane, as shown in Figure 3.14.

Young and Droz (1968) have shown that the discs are being renewed continually, at least in the rod where 25 to 36 new discs are formed each day. The protein necessary for new disc formation is synthesized in the organelles of the *myoid* region which lies in the photoreceptor's inner segment. The newly formed protein flows through the connecting cilium into the outer segment, where it is assembled into the membranous discs at the base. In the rods, the discs contain the photochemical rhodopsin which is incorporated as the discs are formed (Bargoot, Williams, & Beidler, 1969). The effect of light on rhodopsin could alter the disc membrane. As each new disc is formed, it is pushed up toward the apex of the outer rod segment. Young and Bok (1969) demonstrated that the discs are intermittently detached from the apex of the rod's outer segment and end up in the pigment epithelium, where they are apparently disposed of.

Electron microscopy has been used to show that membranes are frequently organized into globular subunits. For example, this organization has been reported for kidney tubular cells, for pancreatic cells, and also for outer rod segments in the frog (Blasie, Dewey, Blaurock, & Worthington, 1965; Nilsson, 1964, 1965). The significance of this organization is not yet fully understood. However, a close similarity between the calculated number of rhodopsin molecules per outer segment and the estimated number of globules per outer segment suggests that each globular subunit is associated with a single molecule of the photopigment. This would mean that the rhodopsin is part of the membrane structure of the discs.

## Visual transduction

### *Photochemistry of vision*

Light energy entering the eye excites the photoreceptors by causing changes in their chemical pigments. As shown in the previous section, the rods of the retina contain a red pigment called visual purple, or *rhodopsin*. Rhodopsin is bleached by light, breaking it down into *retinene* and *opsin* (a protein). In the dark, retinene and opsin recombine to form rhodopsin. This reversible process is symbolized as follows:

$$\text{rhodopsin} \underset{\text{dark}}{\overset{\text{light}}{\rightleftharpoons}} \text{retinene} + \text{opsin}$$

The rate and amount of the bleaching of rhodopsin depends on the intensity and duration of exposure to light. Because of this relationship, the bleaching

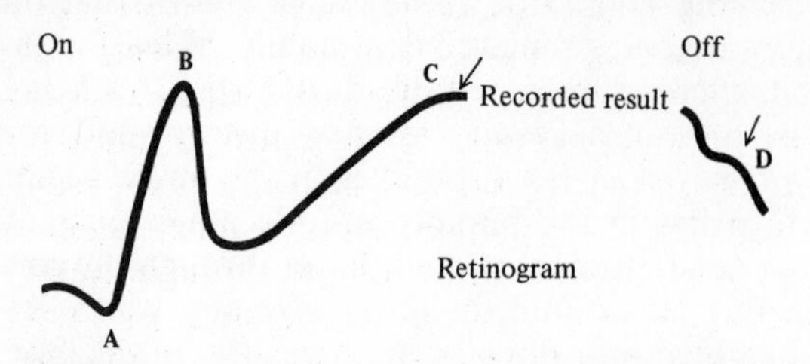


**Figure 3.15** The four main components of the electroretinogram: the initial negative deflection, or the *a* wave (A); the positive *b* wave that follows (B); the slower *c* wave (C); the off-response (D). (From Bartley, 1939.)

of rhodopsin is believed to contribute to light and dark adaptation.

The breakdown of rhodopsin by light is a rapid reaction. Slower chemical reactions also occur in the complete rhodopsin cycle, such as the synthesis of rhodopsin from vitamin A which involves retinene as an intermediate step.

The identification and analysis of the cone photopigments have proved to be more difficult and elusive than that of rhodopsin. However, the pigment *iodopsin* has been shown to be present in the cone cells. Iodopsin breaks down upon exposure to light into retinene and *photopsin*. Although photopsin is a protein, it is different from the opsin found in the rods; the retinene, however, appears to be the same in rods and cones. In fact, all photopigments, regardless of the animal species, are composed of the same retinene and a specific protein or opsin for each pigment (Wald, 1961).

There is now good evidence that the human retina has three different cone pigments, with absorption maxima at 440 (blue), 540 (green), and 590 (red) nanometers (Rushton, 1957; Wald, 1964). The cone pigments are discussed in Chapter 7.

### *The electroretinogram and receptor potentials*

The *electroretinogram (ERG)* is a complex potential recorded from two electrodes, one on the cornea and the other elsewhere on the body. The potential appears as a response to light shone into the eye. Figure 3.15 shows a typical ERG. The *a* wave is more marked in cone-rich retinas and most likely arises from the region of the photoreceptors. The *b* wave presumably reflects activity in the layer of bipolar cells. The *c* wave comes from the cells in the pigment layer of the retina.

In 1961, Davis noted that receptor potentials had not yet been recorded from photoreceptors. A year later, Brown and Watanabe (1962) used an intraretinal electrode to record what is now known as the *late receptor potential*. Brown and Murakami (1964a, 1964b) then discovered a new potential, the *early receptor potential (ERP)*, when they stimulated the eye with short, intense flashes of light. The ERP is a biphasic response with no detectable latency of onset; the peak of the first wave ($R_1$) occurs in less than 25 microseconds. The second wave ($R_2$) comes slightly after $R_1$ and lasts from 3 to 7 msec. These potentials arise from the photoreceptor layer of the retina (Brown, Watanabe, & Murakami, 1965). The largest amplitudes of wave $R_2$ of the ERP and of the late receptor potential are recorded at a depth of about 70 microns below the pigment layer.

The $R_1$ phase of the ERP is more directly related to the photochemical reaction of the photopigment to light. Of the two waves, $R_2$ is more temperature sensitive, and can be abolished by cooling the eye to freezing temperatures (Pak & Cone, 1964). The ERP has been extensively studied in the rat retina which contains only rhodopsin. There, the light wavelength to which rhodopsin is most sensitive also elicits the largest ERP. The ERP amplitude bears a linear relationship to the number of rhodopsin molecules excited by the light stimulus (Cone, 1964). The ERP's very short latency, less than 0.5 microseconds, suggests that it is triggered by a rapid change in molecular form, rather than by the much slower splitting of the photopigment molecule which occurs in the bleaching process. Thus the $R_1$ wave may signal the initial event in transduction—light altering the form of the rhodopsin molecule.

The evidence that separate molecules of rhodopsin are incorporated into the globular subunits of the disc membrane of the rod's outer segment suggests that the molecules are uniformly oriented within the membrane. The orientation of the rhodopsin molecule affects the ERP. Cone and Brown (1967) showed that heating an excised eye to 58° C disorients the rhodopsin, as if it were put into solution, and abolishes the ERP. Below 48° C, temperature has no effect on either the ERP or the orientation of rhodopsin. Between these two end-points, ERP amplitude and amount of pigment disorientation are highly correlated.

Many aspects of visual transduction are not yet understood. If the $R_1$ wave does signal the initial alteration of the photopigment by light, then what do the $R_2$ and the late receptor potentials signal? Most likely, the ERP, which is generated in

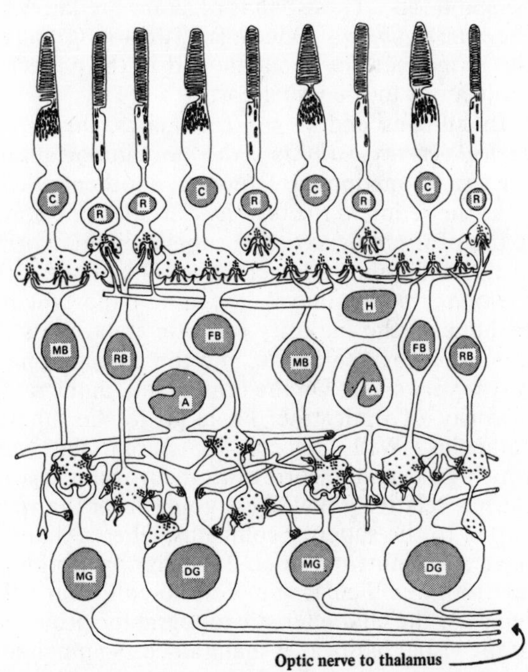


**Figure 3.16** A summary diagram of the synaptic contacts in the retina. R, rod; C, cone; MB, midget bipolar; RB, rod bipolar; FB, flat bipolar; H, horizontal cell; A, amacrine cell; MG, midget ganglion; DG, diffuse ganglion. See text for discussion. (From Dowling & Boycott, 1966.)

the outer segment of the rods and cones, triggers the late receptor potential, which is generated in the inner segment. How this effect is transmitted is not known, but it is almost certainly different from normal conduction in an axon. The cilium that connects inner and outer segments of the photoreceptor is presumably involved in this transmission. The late receptor potential may be a manifestation of the interaction between photoreceptor and bipolar cells.

## The visual pathway

### *Retinal connectivity*

Figure 3.16 summarizes the neural interconnections in the retina. An impulse is transmitted from the photoreceptor to the brain via first the bipolar and then the ganglion cell. The axons of the ganglion cells form the optic nerve which terminates in the thalamus. The optic nerve contains only around 1 million axons to serve the estimated 131 million photoreceptors. This convergence indicates complex interactions within the retina among the various cell types.

The cones connect in distinctly different ways with two types of bipolar cells, *midget* and *flat*. The connection with the midget bipolar is made within an invagination of the cone *pedicle* (the enlarged basal area of the cell) and is surrounded on each side by additional synaptic contacts with horizontal cells. The connection with the flat bipolar cell is superficial; that is, it is made on an uninvaginated portion of the cone pedicle. Each flat bipolar contacts many cone cells, and then synapses with the diffuse ganglion cells.

In the central foveal region, each of the many midget bipolar cells connects firmly to only one cone. Each midget bipolar cell, in turn, makes many synaptic contacts with a single midget ganglion cell (see left-hand column of cells in Figure 3.16). Amacrine and diffuse ganglion cells also form part of the synaptic network of connections between midget bipolar and midget ganglion cell.

The rod photoreceptors connect only with the rod bipolar cell. The horizontal cells receive inputs from cones and make contacts with rods, but they do not connect with each other. The amacrine cells make synaptic contact with all types of bipolar and ganglion cells, as well as with other amacrine cells. Because of amacrine-amacrine interactions, this cell appears to be the main one for spreading stimulus effects across the retina.

Moreover, the synaptic contacts that the amacrine cells make with the bipolar cells appear to be reciprocal; that is, the bipolars send axons to the amacrines and vice versa. This reciprocity allows adjacent bipolar cells to affect one another by means of the amacrines. It also makes possible feedback loops between the bipolars and amacrines, loops that could play a role in the adaptation recorded in the ganglion cells. Such feedback loops have been described in other sensory systems and in other species (Rall, Shepherd, Reese, & Brightman, 1966; Trujillo-Cenoz, 1965).

### *The neural pathway for vision*

Figure 3.17 shows the afferent neural pathway for vision. An important anatomical feature of the visual pathway is its topographic projection. The spatial arrangement of the retina is maintained throughout the system. For example, in the optic nerve the upper portions of the retina are located dorsally and the lower portions are located ventrally. The axons of the ganglion cells exit from the retina at the *optic disc,* which is on the nasal side of

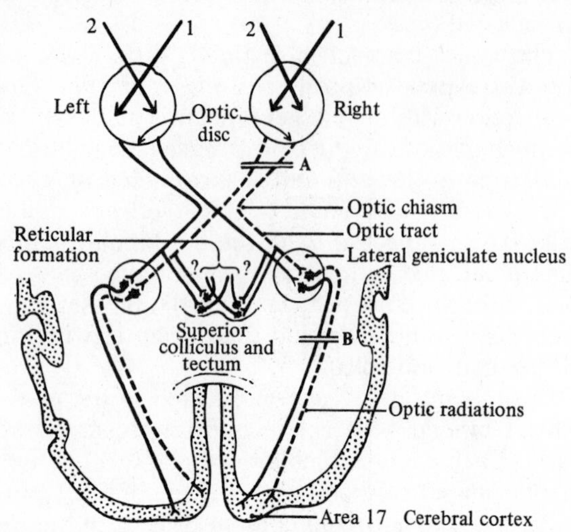


**Figure 3.17** Schematic diagram of the visual pathway. (From Gardner, 1968.)

each eyeball. That section of the retina has no photoreceptors and is popularly referred to as the *blind spot*. The optic nerves from the two eyes proceed in a postero-medial direction and meet at the *optic chiasm*, where half the nerve fibers cross over to the other side of the brain. This occurs immediately in front of the *infundibulum*, the stalk which connects the brain and pituitary gland. Fibers that have arisen from the temporal half of each retina remain uncrossed, whereas fibers that have originated in the nasal half of each retina cross over to the other side. Thus, posterior to the optic chiasm, the afferent pathway (now referred to as the *optic tract*) has a left and a right portion. The right optic tract is made up of axons from ganglion cells in the right half of each retina, that is, in the temporal half of the right retina and the nasal half of the left retina. The left optic tract is made up of axons from ganglion cells in the left half of each retina.

The optic tract terminates in the *lateral geniculate nucleus* of the thalamus, which serves as the primary relay station in vision. In humans and in most higher primates, it consists of six layers of cells numbered 1 to 6 from bottom to top. Layers 1, 4, and 6 receive fibers from the ganglion cells of the contralateral eye, and layers 2, 3, and 5 from the ipsilateral eye. Thus, in the right lateral geniculate nucleus, layers 1, 4, and 6 receive fibers from the ganglion cells of the left eye, and layers 2, 3, and 5 receive fibers from the right eye. The neurons which originate in the lateral geniculate nucleus send their axons to the visual sensory cortex in the occipital lobe. These bands of axons are known as the *optic radiations*. Once again, the topography of the retinal surface is maintained in the pattern of projections to the visual cortex.

In humans and in most primates, this *retino-geniculo-cortex pathway* is the more important one for visual functioning. However, another pathway links the retina to the *superior colliculus* (the homologue of the *optic tectum* in submammalian forms) in the midbrain. In lower animals like the rat, this *collicular pathway* may be the more important one. In humans the majority of optic tract fibers terminate in the geniculate, and the collicular pathway is very small. On the other hand, in the rat the majority of optic tract fibers go to the superior colliculus. With respect to efferent pathways, which go from the cortex to subcortical levels, the rat has relatively few fibers going from the visual cortex to the superior colliculus, whereas humans have a prominent cortico-collicular projection. In all retino-collicular or cortico-collicular fiber bundles, the characteristic topographic projection of the visual pathway is maintained. So much so in fact, that retino-collicular and cortico-collicular fibers project onto the same neurons of the superior colliculus (Garey, 1965).

## Physiology of visual neurons

### *Ganglion cells*

The *receptive field* of a retinal ganglion cell is defined by the area of the retina whose stimulation fires the cell. Such receptive fields tend to be organized in concentric circles which Kuffler (1953) has described as either center-on, surround-off or center-off, surround-on. A center-on cell is excited by light falling on the center of its receptive field, and is inhibited, that is, stops emitting action potentials, by light falling on the peripheral portions of the field. The diameter of a receptive field changes as a function of retinal locus. The center of the field is smaller, the closer the ganglion cell is to the foveal region. At the fovea, the center of the field can be as small as the diameter of a single cone (Hubel & Wiesel, as cited in Dowling & Boycott, 1966).

An anatomical feature of the ganglion cell may account for the observed differences in physiologically determined receptive field size. That feature is the distance over which the dendrites of the ganglion cell spread laterally. In the cat retina, this spread was found to be less than 15 microns in the central area, and to range from 18 to 710 microns in the periphery (Leicester & Stone, 1967). For example, because the midget ganglion cell connects with only one midget bipolar cell in the central area of the fovea, its dendritic field is small, and therefore it has a small receptive field. On the other hand, the diffuse ganglion cell, whose dendritic branches are longer, receives excitatory inputs from a larger number of bipolar cells and therefore has a large receptive field. Brown and Major (1966) proposed that the size of the center-on portion of the receptive field is a function of the spread of the ganglion cell dendrites.

The excitatory center of the field may therefore be the result of the connections within the direct photoreceptor-bipolar-ganglion cell pathway. The inhibitory surround probably results from light stimulating photoreceptors in a neighboring area of the retina. The pathway for inhibition would then be an indirect one of photoreceptor-bipolar-amacrine-ganglion cell. The inclusion of the amacrine interneuron means that the inhibitory pathway has one more synapse than the excitatory pathway, and so the latency of the off-effect should be longer than that of the on-effect. Such a longer latency has been reported in the rabbit (Barlow, Hill, & Levick, 1964).

Other features of ganglion cell physiology appear to build upon the concentric arrangement of the receptor field organization. For example, Gouras (1968) has shown that the ganglion cells of the monkey are color coded. He has described two types of cells. *Phasic* cells are excited by both red and green in the center of their field and are inhibited by red and green in the periphery. They adapt rapidly and merely signal the presence of red or green. *Tonic* cells are excited by either blue, green, or red in the center of their field and are inhibited by one of the other two colors in the periphery. They discharge continuously to steady stimuli of appropriate wavelength. Tonic cells tend to be more numerous toward the fovea, and phasic cells are more numerous toward the periphery, although both are found throughout the retina.

### *Lateral geniculate neurons*

The physiological responsiveness of single neurons in the lateral geniculate nucleus of the monkey has been extensively studied by De Valois and his colleagues (De Valois, 1965; De Valois, Jacobs, & Jones, 1963). Using diffuse illumination of the retina, they found two types of neurons in the lateral geniculate. The *broad-band* cell is always either excited or inhibited by all stimuli. It probably mediates information about light intensity. The

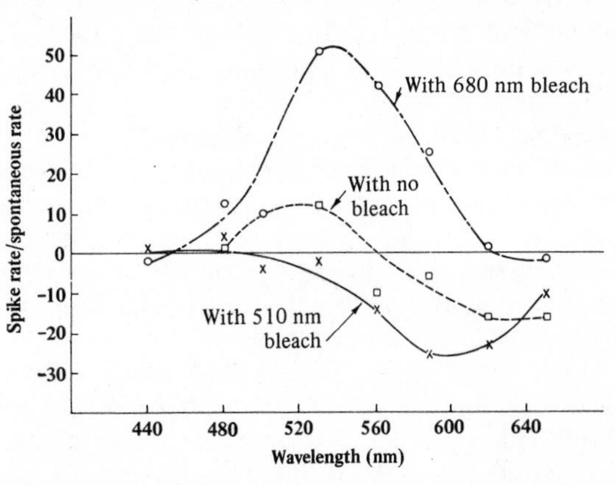


**Figure 3.18** Response to monochromatic light of a thalamic neuron that is excited by green and inhibited by red. Responses were measured during dark adaptation (dashed line) and during chromatic adaptation. Selective adaptation to a light in the red part of the spectrum (680 nm) leaves only an excitatory response curve. Adaptation to a light in the green part of the spectrum (510 nm) leaves only an inhibitory response curve. (From De Valois, Jacobs, & Jones, 1963.)

*spectrally opponent* cell is excited by one wavelength and inhibited by .another. For example, some cells are excited by red and inhibited by green, whereas other cells react in the opposite manner. De Valois (1965) found about equal numbers of broad-band and spectrally opponent cells in the lateral geniculate of the macaque.

Figure 3.18 indicates the effects of chromatic adaptation on the responsiveness of lateral geniculate neurons. The no-bleach condition indicates the response curve of a green-on, red-off cell. Its peak of excitation is at 510 nanometers (nm) and its peak of inhibition is at 620 nm. Adapting the eye to 510 nm virtually eliminates the excitatory phase of the response curve, leaving only an inhibitory response across a wide spectral range with the peak shifted from 620 nm to about 585 nm. Adapting the eye to 680 nm eliminates the inhibitory phase, leaving a broad range of excitatory responses with the peak shifted from 510 to 540 nm. A red-on, green-off cell presents the reverse picture of exitation and inhibition when adapted to lights at the peaks of its response curve.

### *Visual cortical neurons*

The response patterns of single neurons in the visual cortex are probably already known to many readers because of the popularity of the work of Hubel and Wiesel on the cat (1962, 1963, 1965) and on the monkey (1968). They have classified cortical neurons into four types—*simple, complex, hypercomplex,* and *higher-order hypercomplex*. Cells which have a simple receptive field have a center-on, surround-off field like the ganglion cell, but the field is not circular. Instead, the center of the field is elongated so as to resemble a slit or a narrow rectangle. It presumably receives inputs from cells with overlapping center-on fields.

Cells which have complex fields rarely respond to diffuse light, and their receptive fields are best described by a stimulus pattern in a specific orientation, such as a vertical line. Usually the effective stimulus for such a cell is a line or slit, although other effective stimuli have been contours or edges. The criterion of specific orientation is always present for complex cells. Hubel and Wiesel (1962) suggested that the complex cortical cell, one that responds to vertical lines, for example, receives excitatory inputs from a number of cells with simple fields. The simple cells that project to the complex cell presumably have receptive fields with an excitatory region to the left and an inhibitory region to the right of a vertical straight-line boundary. The boundaries of the simple fields are spread across the larger receptive-field area of the complex cell. Any vertical-edge stimulus falling within this area, regardless of its position within the area, would excite some of the simple cells, resulting in excitation of the complex cell.

To be excited, hypercomplex cells require more specific stimulus features than complex cells. Hypercomplex cells require that the stimulus line be orientated at a certain angle and have a certain length. Figure 3.19A shows how the response of a hypercomplex cell depends on the orientation and length of a line of light on its receptive field. Figure 3.19B shows two possible sets of neural connections between complex and hypercomplex cells that could account for the cell's responses. Hypercomplex cells receive both excitatory and inhibitory inputs from complex cells. The interaction of these inputs can account for the organization of the hypercomplex receptive field. The fields of the hypercomplex cells do have definite inhibitory regions, which are frequently referred to as either single-stopped or double-stopped depending on whether they are bounded by one or two adjacent inhibitory regions.

Hubel and Wiesel (1965) also described a small number of higher-order hypercomplex cells. These cells respond to an edge that moves anywhere across the receptive field, provided the edge is of the proper width. Some of these cells respond to two edges that form a 90° angle, and hence may be labeled *corner detectors*.

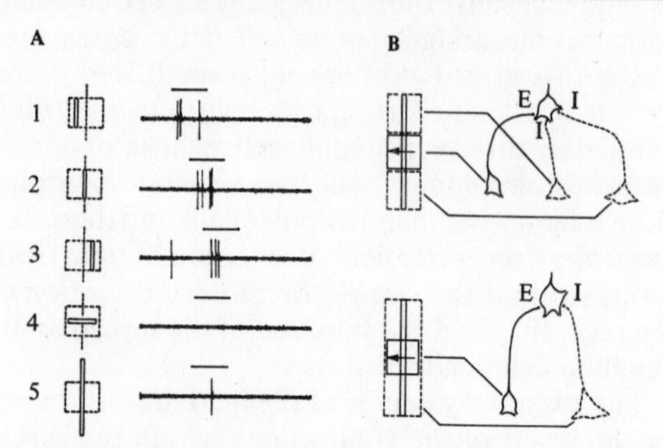


**Figure 3.19** Panel A: Responses of a hypercomplex cell, whose receptive field is represented by the outlined rectangle. The hypercomplex cell responds to an optimally oriented slit anywhere within the field as indicated in (1), (2), and (3), but does not respond if the slit is presented at 90° relative to optimum orientation as shown in (4). Even at optimum orientation, if the slit extends beyond the borders of the receptive field, the neural response is inhibited as in (5). Panel B: Two different sets of presumed neural connections to account for the responses of the hypercomplex cell shown in panel A. (After Hubel & Wiesel, 1965.)

Moreover, Hubel and Wiesel (1963, 1968) have shown that functionally the visual cortex is organized into columns. If the cortex is penetrated with a microelectrode that is perpendicular to the surface, the cells lying in the path of the microelectrode all respond to stimuli of the same orientation. Stimulus edges of different orientation are responded to by cells in a nearby column. This description of the behavior of single cortical units holds for both the cat and the monkey. However, the monkey's receptive fields are, on the average, smaller, and they exhibit a greater sensitivity to changes in stimulus orientation. Also, the monkey has two independent systems of vertical columns. One, as in the cat, contains cells whose receptive fields all have the same orientation. The second system is one of ocular preference, or eye dominance. In the monkey there is a marked tendency for successively recorded cells to have the same eye preference; for example, they may be stimulated by the inputs from only the contralateral eye. Of the two types of columns, those associated with eye dominance seem to be larger, often comprising several orientation columns. The two systems apparently have entirely independent borders (Hubel & Wiesel, 1968).

Hubel and Wiesel, in their analyses of the behavior of single neurons, may have unveiled the basic units of our perceptual world. Just how the millions of simple, complex, hypercomplex, and higher-order hypercomplex cells interact with one another, as well as with a color-coded system (Gouras, 1970), to permit us to view and enjoy the infinitely complex world around us is far from resolved, but Hubel and Wiesel seem to have made a good start. See Pollen, Lee, and Taylor (1971) for an initial attempt to extend the single-cell analysis to the complicated problem concerning the functional organization of the striate cortex.

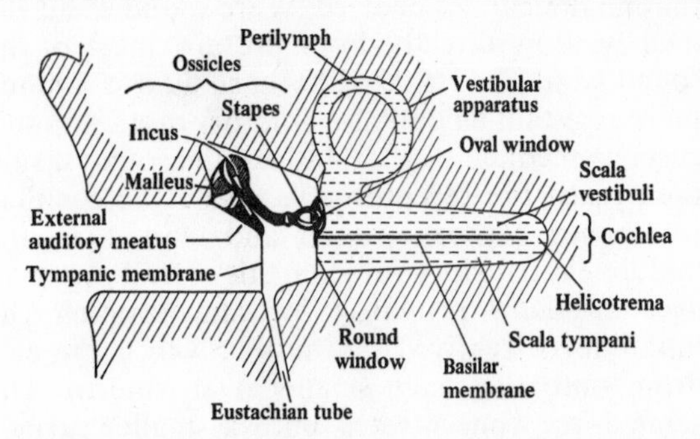


**Figure 3.20** Schematic drawing of the human ear. The coiled cochlea has been unrolled to give a clear view of the basic anatomical relationships. (From von Békésy & Rosenblith, 1951.)

## THE AUDITORY SYSTEM

### The structure of the ear

The ear is divided into three parts. The *outer ear* gathers the sound; the *middle ear* transmits the sound; and within the *inner ear*, the sensory receptor cells transduce the sound from mechanical to neural energy. From surrounding air to receptor cells, the route is complex, but it thereby provides maximum efficiency in getting the important sounds to the receptor cells and also protects those cells from disease and injury.

#### *Outer ear*

The outer ear comprises the *pinna,* the flappy structure on each side of the head which we commonly call the ear, and the *external auditory meatus,* or ear canal. Some animals can move their pinnae, orienting them so as to collect more of an impinging sound, whereas most humans have lost that ability.

In humans the external meatus is about 2.5 cm long. Stretched across the inner end of the meatus is the rather taut *tympanic membrane,* or eardrum (see Figure 3.20). The eardrum, the membrane that divides the outer from the middle ear, has an area of 69 mm$^2$ and is shaped like a cone with its apex directed inward. The height of the cone is 2 mm. Sound waves passing down the meatus strike against the eardrum and set it into vibratory motion. Being suspended between two bodies of air at equal pressure, the membrane vibrates rather freely, and its vibration pattern faithfully reproduces the pattern of the sound waves.

#### *Middle ear*

The middle ear is a small air-filled cavity behind the eardrum. Its total volume has been reported to vary from 2.0 cc (Gulick, 1971) to as much as 8.5 cc (Zwislocki, 1962). Air enters the middle ear from the mouth via the *Eustachian tube* which opens during swallowing. By this means, the air pressure on both sides of the eardrum can be kept equal. A difference in air pressure across the membrane impairs hearing because it hampers the vibratory motion of the membrane.

The middle ear includes three small bony ossicles, the *malleus,* the *incus,* and the *stapes,* which transmit sound from the eardrum to the inner ear. (The middle ear also includes two small muscles that affect sound transmission. They are discussed in Chapter 4.) The malleus is attached to the inner side of the eardrum by its armlike extension, the *manubrium;* vibration of the membrane initiates movement in the malleus. The head of the malleus is joined to the incus, which in turn is attached to the head of the stapes via the lenticular process. The stapes has the form of a stirrup. Its *footplate* fits up against the *oval window,* a membrane-covered opening in the bony external wall of the inner ear. Thus all three ossicles are set in motion by the vibratory action of the eardrum. As they vibrate, the ossicles push the footplate in and out against the oval window.

The inner ear comprises the coiled bony structure called the *cochlea* and the vestibular canals, which are not involved in hearing. Within the cochlea are the auditory receptor cells. It is primarily because the cochlea is filled with fluid that the middle ear has evolved. Were sound to hit the oval window directly from the air, most of the sound would be reflected because fluid is a much more resistant medium to vibratory motion than a gaseous medium like air; little of the sound would then reach the receptor cells inside the cochlea. Interposed between the air and fluid, then, the middle ear ossicles overcome this so-called *impedance mismatch* primarily by concentrating the initial force received by the relatively large eardrum onto the much smaller oval window. The same force concentrated onto a smaller surface becomes a much larger pressure (pressure equals force divided by area), and so the fluid can be set into motion with a minimum of reflection and energy loss. This system works so well because the force is also transmitted with maximum efficiency by the three ossicles; indeed at some sound frequencies, the ossicles amplify the sound pressure (see Chapter 4 for further details). Moreover, the form of the sound wave is faithfully reproduced in its passage through the middle ear. Mechanically, the middle ear is a beautifully engineered device.

*Inner ear*

The cochlea is a spiral structure which resembles a snail shell. The human cochlea has two and a half to two and three quarter turns, and is about 5 mm in diameter at its base. In cross section (see Figure 3.21), the tubelike structure of the cochlea can be seen to consist of three distinct tubes or canals: the *vestibular canal* (or scala vestibuli), the *tympanic canal* (or scala tympani), and the *cochlear canal* (or scala media). *Reissner's membrane* separates the vestibular canal from the cochlear canal, and the *basilar membrane* separates the cochlear canal from the tympanic canal. At the apex of the cochlea is a small opening, the *helicotrema,* which joins the vestibular and tympanic canals (see Figure 3.20). The cochlear canal is completely enclosed and separate from the other two canals. Since the trapped fluids of the inner ear are virtually incompressible, they could not transmit pressure waves from the oval window if the *round window* did not provide a relief point (see Figure 3.20). Facing the middle ear cavity, the round window is a membrane-covered opening in the cochlea located below the oval window in the base of the tympanic canal. When the oval window membrane moves in, the round window membrane moves out and vice versa. Thus, the stapes is able to push into the cochlear fluid.

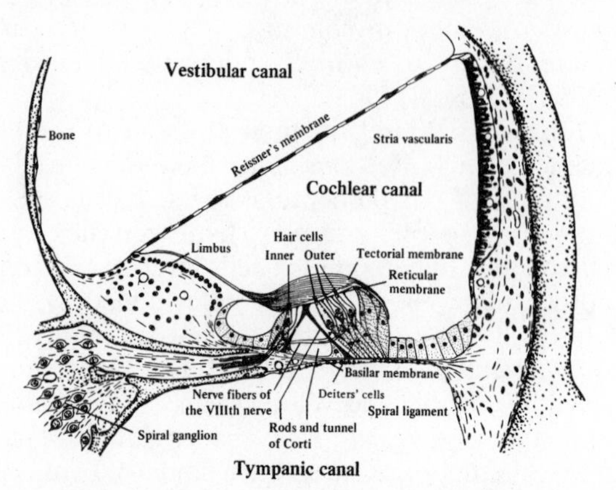


**Figure 3.21** Cross section of the cochlear partition of the guinea pig, showing the general features of the mammalian structure. (From Davis & Associates, 1953.)

From the direct observations of von Békésy (1960), it is known that the vibratory motion of the stapes causes a pressure wave to travel along the basilar membrane from the oval window to the helicotrema. As the wave moves along, it displaces the basilar membrane which moves up and down. Where the displacement is maximal depends on the frequency of the stimulating tone (see Chapter 4). In this manner, frequency is translated into spatial location on the basilar membrane. Low frequencies have their maximal effect toward the apex of the cochlea and high frequencies toward the oval window. Recently, Rhode (1971), using a technique quite different from von Békésy's to measure traveling waves, has fully supported von Békésy's observations. Among the many kinds of indirect evidence that corroborate these direct observations are the studies of the effect on hearing of selective damage to the basilar membrane. The closer the damaged section of the basilar membrane lies to the oval window, the higher the frequency at which the animal shows hearing loss (Schuknecht, 1960; Walzl & Bordley, 1942).

**Auditory receptors**

Resting on top of the basilar membrane is the *organ of Corti,* a complex structure in which are located the receptor cells for hearing. These are the *hair cells,* lined up in four or five rows as shown in Figure 3.21. The row which is located closest to the central axis of the cochlea comprises the *inner hair cells,* and the other three rows comprise the *outer hair cells*. The organ of Corti contains a number of structures besides the hair cells, including the *rods of Corti,* the *tunnel of Corti, Deiters' cells,* and the *reticular membrane*. These structures serve to support the hair cells and provide a stable connection to the basilar membrane.

The inner hair cells form a regular row that parallels the tunnel of Corti. Their hairs, or *stereocilia,* form almost one continuous line from the base to the apex of the cochlea. The three rows of outer hair cells form a definite geometric mosaic. Each cell in the second row is situated directly midway between two cells of the first row. Each cell in the third row occupies a similar position with respect to cells in the second row.

Figure 3.22 shows the fine structure of the hair cells. Both the inner and outer hair cells have a *cuticular plate* and a *basal body* at their apex. A number of fine stereocilia project out from the cuticular plate. At the base of each cell are various nerve endings and synapses. Thus the hair cell is, in a sense, polarized. At the top are the stereocilia, cuticle, and basal body, which are the cellular structures thought to be the site of the transducing process. At the bottom are synapses by which the receptor cell interacts with the sensory neurons.

Generally, the inner hair cells are longer (12 microns) than the outer hair cells (8 microns), have fewer projecting stereocilia, and are less sensitive to damage by drugs and intense sounds. The stereocilia of the inner hair cells vary in length, and form three or four irregular lines. The 120 or so stereocilia of the outer hair cells form a clear W pattern (Engström, Ades, & Hawkins, 1965). The differences in the arrangement of the stereocilia on the inner and outer hair cells are vividly revealed in the electron micrographs of Bredberg, Lindeman, Ades, West, and Engström (1970), one of which is shown in Figure 3.23. The hair cells also differ with respect to their contact with the *tectorial membrane* which lies above them (see Figure 3.21). Recent evidence based on electron microscopy shows that only the stereocilia of the outer hair cells make contact with the tectorial membrane; the stereocilia of the inner hair cells are free-standing (Lim, 1971).

The nerve endings at the base of the hair cells are of two types, $NE_1$ and $NE_2$. The $NE_1$ nerve endings are probably afferent terminals in which the generator potentials arise upon excitation of the hair cell. The $NE_2$ endings are probably efferent terminals bringing nerve impulses from the cochlear nucleus (see following discussion).

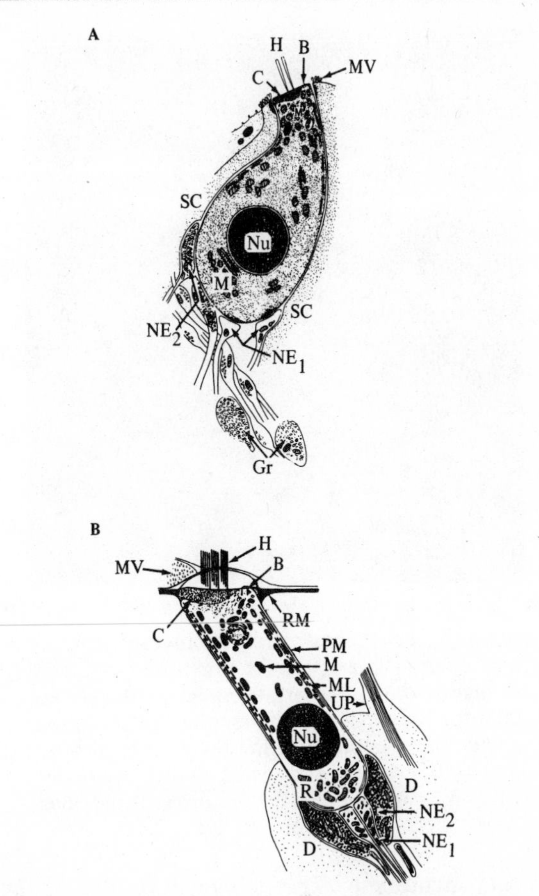


**Figure 3.22** Schematic drawing of an inner hair cell (A) and an outer hair cell (B). C, cuticular plate; H, hairs; B, basal body; MV, microvilli; M, mitochondria; Nu, nucleus; $NE_1$, afferent nerve ending; $NE_2$, efferent nerve ending; Gr, granulated structure; SC, supporting cell; RM, reticular membrane; PM, plasma membrane; ML, parietal membrane; D, Deiters' cell; UP, phalangeal process; R, Retzius' body. (From Engström, Ades, & Hawkins, 1965.)

*Auditory transduction*

Auditory transduction occurs at the hair cells as a result of the *shearing* of stereocilia by a pressure wave in the cochlea. This shearing action comes about in the following manner. A pressure wave in the cochlea sets the basilar membrane into vibratory motion. The tectorial membrane also moves up and down, but not in quite the same way as the basilar membrane. The difference in their motions causes the tectorial membrane to slide across the

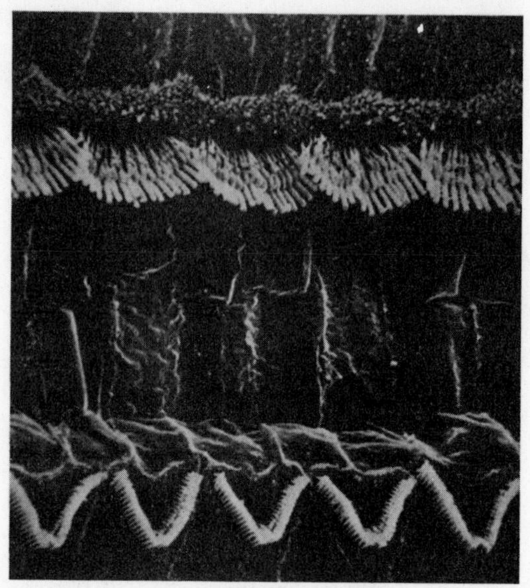

**Figure 3.23** Scanning electron micrograph of inner and outer hair cells in the organ of Corti. Top of figure shows the arrangement of the stereocilia for the single row of inner hair cells. Bottom shows the innermost of the three rows of outer hair cells, with the stereocilia in their characteristic W pattern. (From Bredberg, Lindeman, Ades, West, & Engström, 1970.)

basilar membrane. This slippage results in the bending of the stereocilia of the outer hair cells which are embedded in the tectorial membrane. The shearing movement on the stereocilia excites the hair cell to evoke a generator potential in the afferent nerve endings ($NE_1$) at its base. If the generator potential reaches threshold, a nerve action potential is elicited and propagated along the sensory nerve toward the brain.

The bending of free-standing stereocilia of the inner hair cells would result from the viscous forces of the endolymph fluid which surrounds them. The forces themselves are determined by the velocity with which the basilar membrane moves. The response of the outer hair cells would depend primarily on the amplitude of displacement of the basilar membrane; that of the inner hair cells would depend on the velocity of the displacement (Dallos, Billone, Durrant, Wang, & Raynor, 1972). Current hypotheses concerning the transduction of the hair cells have not as yet distinguished between these two modes of stimulation. Those that are presented in the following paragraphs assume only the manner of stimulation of the tectorial membrane. The stimulation of the inner hair cells could be essentially the same as that of the outer hair cells, with the endolymph having the same final result as the tectorial membrane.

One hypothesis is that the stereocilia function as microlevers in transmitting mechanical energy via the cuticular plate to the cell's basal body, which is assumed to be an excitable structure (Engström, Ades, & Hawkins, 1965). The position of the hair cells is such that the basal body, or *centriole,* faces toward the *stria vascularis* which lines part of the cochlea's inner surface, as shown in Figure 3.21. The stereocilia are situated directly behind the centriole. Possibly, bending the cilia toward the centriole leads to depolarization, while bending the cilia away leads to hyperpolarization, as happens in the lateral line system of the fish (Flock, 1965). Thus, the mechanical energy would be transduced to electrical and neural energy.

Spoendlin (1968) rejects the hypothesis that the basal body is involved in transduction. Instead, he suggests that the cilia act as transducers by virtue of possible piezoelectric (electricity resulting from mechanical pressure on a substance) properties. He points out that the spaces between the cilia are filled with acid mucopolysaccharides which have a regular molecular arrangement. Supposedly, bending the cilia alters this arrangement, thereby releasing a relatively large amount of energy and producing a potential change.

Davis (1961) proposed still a third hypothesis about auditory transduction. The shearing action on the stereocilia results in a change in electrical resistance across the hair-cell membrane. The hair cells therefore act as a variable resistor in regulating current flows. The current could either directly affect the afferent nerve terminal or release a transmitter substance at the base of the hair cells. Davis' proposal contradicts neither Spoendlin's nor Engström's since the changes in the variable resistor could be produced by a mechanism based on a piezoelectric effect, either on the basal body or on the mucopolysaccharide molecules, or by some other unspecified process.

## The auditory pathway

The neural pathway from the cochlea to the auditory cortex is perhaps the most complicated of all sensory pathways. The ascending and descending connections are shown in Figure 3.24. The cell bodies of the afferent neurons, whose dendritic terminals are at the base of the hair cells, lie in the spiral ganglion in the center of the cochlea (see

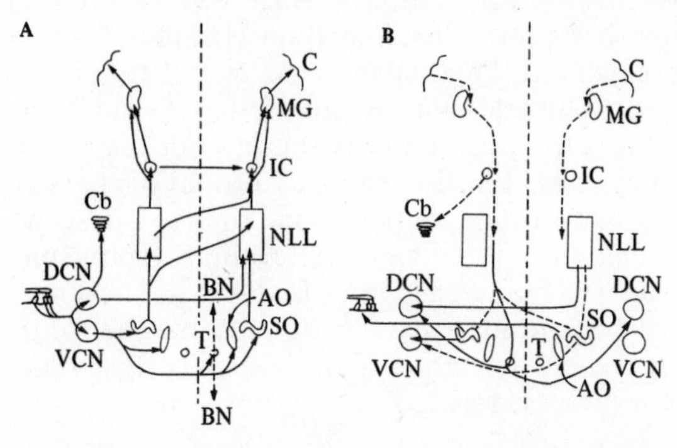


**Figure 3.24** Ascending, or afferent (A), and descending, or efferent (B), pathways of the auditory nervous system. Connections not firmly established anatomically are shown by dashed lines. DCN, dorsal cochlear nucleus; VCN, ventral cochlear nucleus; Cb, cerebellum; AO, accessory olive; SO, lateral olivary nucleus; T, nucleus of the trapezoid body; BN, brainstem motor nuclei; NLL, nuclei of the lateral lemniscus; IC, inferior colliculus; MG, medial geniculate nucleus; C, cortex. (From Whitfield, 1967.)

Figure 3.21). The axons of these nerve fibers form the auditory component of the *VIIIth cranial nerve* and enter the cranial cavity to terminate in the *dorsal* and *ventral cochlear nuclei.* Each axon sends a collateral branch to each of the two nuclei, and within the nuclei each collateral gives off finer processes that make contact with several hundred cells. In humans, the auditory nerve contains 30,000 axons, all of which terminate in the cochlear nuclei. Separate fiber systems proceed from the two cochlear nuclei. Fibers from the dorsal nucleus cross the midline of the brainstem and ascend toward the cortex in the nerve tract known as the *lateral lemniscus*. These fibers end in the *inferior colliculus* in the midbrain. Fibers that leave the ventral nucleus synapse in both the ipsilateral and contralateral nuclei of the *superior olivary complex* in the brainstem. The region in the brainstem where the crossover of fibers from both cochlear nuclei to the olivary complex on each side occurs is known as the *trapezoid body,* so named for the area's general outline.

The superior olivary complex is a cluster of five cell groups, or nuclei. It is also the first place in the auditory pathway where binaural interactions occur. Such interactions are known to take place in the *accessory olivary nucleus,* whose neurons are responsive to small differences in time of arrival of inputs from each cochlear nucleus. These neurons thus appear to have an important role in the localization of sound in space (see Chapter 4). From the superior olivary complex, these fibers ascend toward the cortex via the lateral lemniscus to the inferior colliculus.

Fibers from the inferior colliculus project to the *medial geniculate nucleus* in the thalamus. This fiber bundle is called the *brachium of the inferior colliculus.* From the medial geniculate, fibers go to the auditory cortex.

Figure 3.24B shows the efferent auditory fiber system which descends from the auditory cortex to the primary receptor cells in the cochlea. The dashed lines in the descending pathway are inferred from electrophysiological measurements but have not been identified anatomically, whereas the solid lines represent known anatomical connections. The *olivo-cochlear bundle*, which originates in the olivary complex (Rasmussen, 1946), is represented in Figure 3.24B by the arrow that begins just above the accessory nucleus and ends at the hair cells in the contralateral cochlea.

### Physiology of auditory neurons

The two predominant features of auditory neurons seem to be their *tuning curves* and their *tonotopic organization.* Throughout the auditory system the response of a single neuron to a tone is a function of the tone's intensity and frequency. The tuning curve represents the cell's threshold over a range of frequencies and intensities. It is sometimes referred to as the response area of the neuron (Katsuki, 1961). Tuning curves can be obtained by keeping either the intensity or the frequency constant and systematically varying the other over a wide stimulus range. Both methods yield highly similar functions, as shown in Figure 3.25. The tip of the tuning curve is that frequency having the lowest intensity threshold and is called the *characteristic,* or *best,* frequency of an individual cell. For example, unit 14 in Figure 3.25 has a best frequency of around 1.2 kHz, whereas the best frequency of unit 16 is slightly above 10 kHz.

Tonotopic organization refers to the fact that units with different best frequencies are arranged in a systematic order throughout a given nucleus or level of the afferent auditory pathway. Such organization begins at the basilar membrane, as noted earlier, and is maintained throughout the system, although tonotopic organization at the level of the auditory cortex is in doubt at the present time. Electrophysiological studies of single auditory neurons have shown that the cochlear nuclei (Rose,

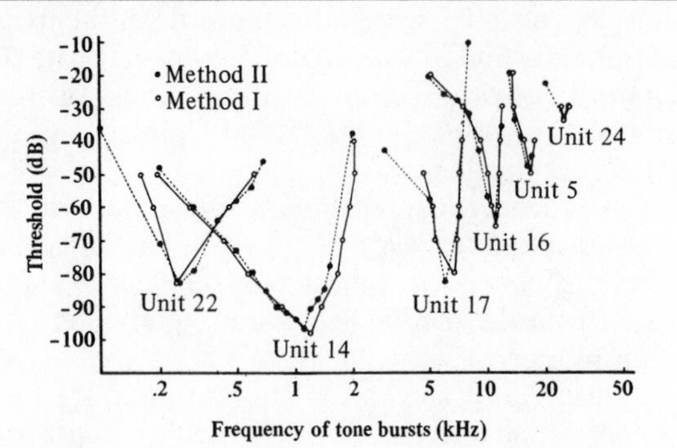


**Figure 3.25** Tuning curves for six auditory nerve fibers. The threshold curves for each unit were obtained by two different methods. In method I, the frequency is varied while intensity is held constant. In method II, the frequency is held constant while intensity is varied. (From Kiang, 1965.)

1960), the lateral olivary nucleus (Tsuchitani & Boudreau, 1966), the nucleus of the lateral lemniscus (Aitkin, Anderson, & Brugge, 1970), and the inferior colliculus (Rose, Greenwood, Goldberg, & Hind, 1963) exhibit definite tonotopic organization. So far, measurements have failed to uncover a clear tonotopic organization at the next highest neural level, namely, in the medial geniculate nucleus of the thalamus.

Tonotopic organization in the auditory cortex had appeared to be well established by earlier studies of gross potentials evoked in the cortex by tonal stimulation of an animal's ear. These measurements, however, have proved to be misleading, probably because the gross evoked potential reflects the activity of an unknown, but large, number of neurons. More recent studies of single cortical neurons have revealed, in the cat, for example, virtually no systematic arrangement of cells according to their best frequencies (Evans, Ross, & Whitfield, 1965). One is as likely to find a neuron that responds best to a frequency below 9000 Hz in one part of the auditory cortex as in any other. Still, high-frequency neurons do tend to be more numerous in the anterior portions of the auditory cortex. Nevertheless, whatever tonotopic organization may exist in the cortex is probably not functional. This position receives support from those studies which have shown that ablation of the auditory cortex does not disrupt frequency discrimination (e.g., Brown, Gedvilas, & Marco, 1967; Goldberg & Neff, 1961).

The auditory cortex is necessary for the detection of auditory patterns since lesions there do abolish pattern discrimination (Diamond, Goldberg, & Neff, 1962; Diamond & Neff, 1957). Moreover, Whitfield and Evans (1965) found many auditory cortical neurons that do not respond to steady tones but do respond to tones of changing frequency. Some units respond only to a descending change in frequency, while others respond only to an ascending change in frequency. These neurons behave in a manner directly parallel to the orientation detectors of the visual cortex, which were discussed earlier.

## The vestibular system

The sensory receptors of the vestibular system lie within the *labyrinth* of the inner ear. The entire labyrinth, as shown in Figure 3.26, includes the vestibular apparatus and the cochlea, which is part of the auditory system. The vestibular part of the labyrinth consists of the three *semicircular canals,* the *utricle,* and the *saccule.* The semicircular canals are the primary receptors for rotational movements, as they are affected by angular accelerations and decelerations. The utricle responds chiefly to gravity and to linear acceleration. The function of the saccule is not understood, but its anatomical similarity and position with respect to the axes of the head suggest that it functionally complements the utricle. However, it may also have some role as a vibratory receptor.

### *Semicircular canals*

The three membranous semicircular canals lie approximately at right angles to each other, one representing each major plane of the body. When both sides of the head are considered, the six canals form three pairs. The two lateral canals are in the same horizontal plane. In the other two pairs, the canals are parallel to each other. The six canals thus form a three-coordinate system to which accelerations and decelerations of the head are referred. The anterior and posterior canals on each side are in the vertical plane at 45° angles with the midline of the head.

The approximate lengths of the canals are 15 mm for the lateral, 20 mm for the anterior, and 22 mm for the posterior. The overall width of the bony labyrinth is 0.8 mm, whereas that of the membranous labyrinth is only 0.2 mm. A fluid, *perilymph,* fills the space between the bony and membranous labyrinths. The membranous labyrinth is also filled with a fluid, *endolymph.*

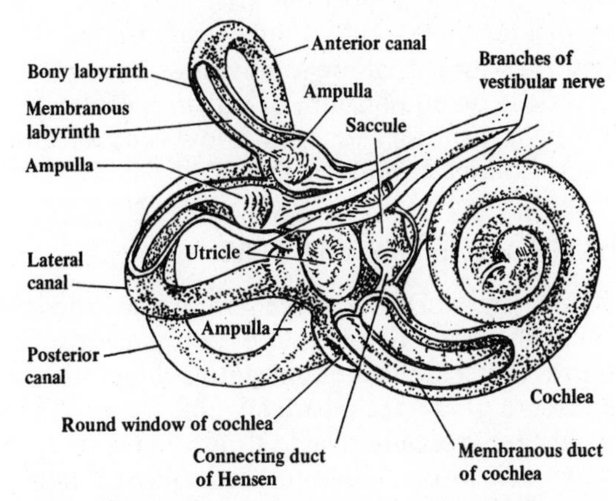


**Figure 3.26** Diagram of the labyrinth of the inner ear, showing the semicircular canals, utricle, and saccule and their relation to the cochlea. Large portions of the protecting bone have been cut away to reveal the membranous canals and sacs inside. The semicircular canals are approximately at right angles to each other. (From Geldard, 1972.)

The *ampulla,* an enlargement of each canal just before the utricle, houses the *crista* which contains the receptor cells (see Figure 3.27A). Attached at one end of the ampulla, the crista is an epithelial tissue containing not only the sensory cells but also supporting cells. The receptor cells have hairlike projections like those of the auditory hair cells. These cilia project into a gelatinous substance called the *cupula,* which is like a flap that fits over the crista and extends across the width of the ampulla. In a cross section of the cupula, a number of canals are seen in the gelatinous substance. The cilia of the sensory cells fit into these canals. This probably is the mechanism for the bending of the cilia. Histochemical evidence indicates that the cupula consists of sulfomucopolysaccharides which are probably supported in a protein matrix (Plotz & Perlman, 1955).

The cupula is fixed at its base (where the hair cells are), but is free to move at the distal end in response to hydraulic pressures created within the endolymph. Pressure is created whenever the head, and therefore the semicircular canals, moves. The heavier endolymph does not move as quickly as the head so that pressure waves arise within the canal, displacing the cupula. The displacement of the cupula results in a bending of the cilia of the receptor cells, stretching those on the side away from the bending and slackening those on the side toward it.

The bending of the cilia is the stimulus for the receptor cells, just as in the cochlea. The direction of bending determines whether the cell will increase or decrease its firing rate relative to its spontaneous level, as has been shown in the skate (Löwenstein & Sand, 1940) and in the cat (Gernandt, 1949). Gernandt (1949) showed that vestibular nerve fibers increased their firing when a cat was rotated to the side from which the neural recording was being made; that is, rotation to the left increased the firing rate in the left vestibular nerve, whereas rotation to the right inhibited these same nerves. Flock (1965) has shown that similar hair cells in the cristae of fish are depolarized when the cilia are bent in one direction and hyperpolarized when bent in the opposite direction. Presumably the same basic mechanism operates in the human.

*Nerve pathway*

The cell bodies of the nerve fibers that innervate the base of the hair cells are located in the vestibular ganglion just outside the labyrinth. The main axonal portions of these fibers enter the vestibular part of the VIIIth nerve, which in turn enters the brain just below the pons and terminates in the four vestibular nuclei which are located just below the fourth ventricle. Efferent fibers from the vestibular nuclei project to the spinal cord and cerebellum, from where the most important pathway leads to the oculomotor nuclei. It is uncertain whether the labyrinth receptors have a cortical projection.

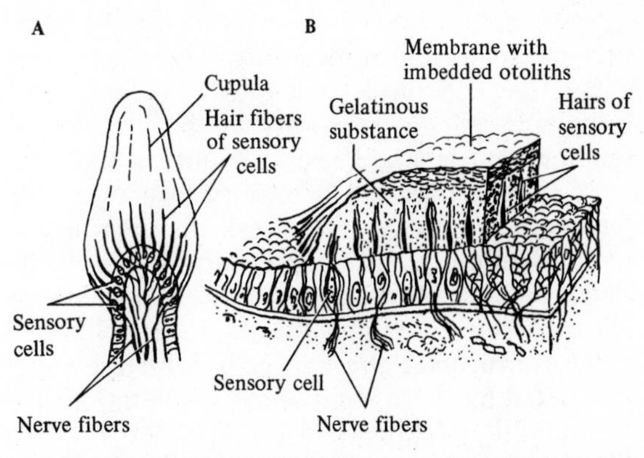


**Figure 3.27** Receptors of the labyrinth: the crista (A) and the macula (B). (From Geldard, 1972.)

### *Nystagmus*

Nystagmus, the involuntary eye movements that accompany and follow rotation of the head, provides a convenient means for studying the effects of the semicircular canals. As a subject is rotated about a vertical axis, his eyes move slowly in the direction opposite that of the rotation; as soon as rotation stops, the eyes return rapidly in the direction of the rotation. The nystagmus ceases if the rotation is maintained at a constant velocity for about 20 to 30 seconds, the time necessary for the cupulae to return to their normal position.

Besides eye movements, rotation evokes a number of reflexive responses. During the initial acceleration, the head may make slow sweeping motions and rapid returns just as the eyes do in nystagmus. If the rotation is vigorous, its abrupt cessation elicits compensatory movements of the head, arms, and legs, which are all responses that tend to prevent the subject from falling over.

Caloric stimulation is also an effective way to induce nystagmus. Irrigation of the external ear with either hot or cold water immediately elicits a reflex nystagmus. Hot water produces nystagmus with the rapid phase toward the stimulated side; cold water has the opposite effect. Presumably the nystagmus is induced by convection currents set up in the endolymph.

### *The utricle and saccule*

Within the utricle and saccule the sensory receptors are found in structures known as the *maculae* (see Figure 3.27B). The macula of the saccule lies in a plane approximately at a right angle to that of the utricle. In the human, the utricle itself lies in the same plane as the lateral canal. The receptor cells have cilia like those in the semicircular canals that project into a gelatinous substance. The stimulus for exciting the receptor cells is, as with all the receptors in the labyrinth, a bending of their cilia. The utricle and saccule, however, have a different accessory structure. The gelatinous substance into which the cilia project contains tiny crystals, called *otoliths*. Hence, the utricle and saccule are known as the otolith organs. The substance containing the otoliths is believed to weigh down upon the hair cells, which are then stimulated by gravity and linear acceleration. The inertia of the otoliths results in the bending of the cilia and excitation of the receptor cells. Vestibular nerve fibers have been found that respond to gravity, linear acceleration, and tilting of the head out of its normal position (Adrian, 1942). The stimulus for the saccule is not clearly understood. Since the saccule can be removed without noticeable effect on equilibrium or posture, it may possibly be a vibratory or even a low-tone auditory receptor, at least in lower animals.

## THE OLFACTORY SYSTEM

Smell and taste are generally classified as chemical senses because, for both, a sensation requires that a molecule come into contact with the membrane of the receptor cell. Olfactory cues for animals are typically related to feeding and reproductive behaviors. Although the biological importance of olfactory stimuli for humans is greatly reduced, olfactory sensations usually have strong emotional connotations.

### Olfactory receptors

The olfactory receptor cells lie in the upper reaches of the nasal cavity. They are found in only one relatively small area, called the *olfactory epithelium,* or *mucosa,* which covers about 10 cm$^2$ in humans. In what is referred to as the golden age of comparative neuroanatomy (the late 1800s and early 1900s), many histological descriptions of the cells of the olfactory epithelium were presented. As early as 1856, Schultze described three distinct

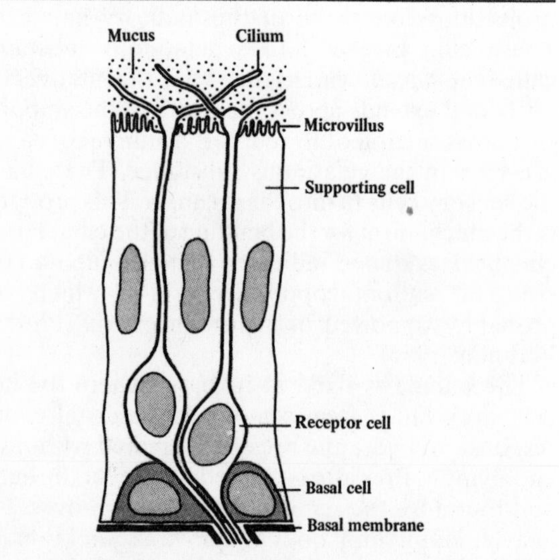


**Figure 3.28** Schematic representation of the vertebrate olfactory epithelium. (From Steinbrecht, 1969.)

**Table 3.2 Number of Cilia per Olfactory Receptor Cell**

| Animal | Cilia | Reference |
|---|---|---|
| Minnow | 4–6 | Bannister, 1965 |
| Frog | 6–12 | Hopkins, 1926 |
| Rabbit | 9–16 | Le Gros Clark, 1956 |
| Rat | 15–20 | von Brettschneider, 1958 |
| Cat | 40 | Andres, 1968 |
| Dog | 100–150 | Okano, Weber, & Frommes, 1967 |
| Human | 6–8 | von Brunn, 1892 |

types of cells in the vertebrate olfactory epithelium: receptor, supporting, and basal (see Allison, 1953). These cells are shown in Figure 3.28.

One hundred years later Le Gros Clark (1956), using the light microscope, described the receptor cell bodies as generally oval, measuring approximately 5 microns across and 10 microns in length. The cells are *bipolar,* having a fine proximal process which is the beginning of the axon and a coarser or thicker distal process labeled the *olfactory rod.* The rods, although thicker than the axons, are less than 1 micron in diameter and vary in length from 20 to 90 microns. This variation may provide an efficient means to increase the density of receptor cells in the epithelium (Moulton & Beidler, 1967). The rod extends beyond the external surface membrane of the epithelium and expands to form a terminal swelling, or *knob*. The knob bears one to twenty olfactory cilia; the number varies between and within species and is probably correlated with olfactory sensitivity. Table 3.2 shows cilia counts for various species.

The olfactory cilia are generally considered to be the parts of the cell that are actually stimulated by odorous molecules. However, the transduction mechanism is not yet understood, and its exact locus on the receptor cell has not been conclusively demonstrated. Most investigators assume that the initial events in olfactory stimulation occur along the cilia membrane. But stimulation could begin on the membrane of the terminal knob, which is also exposed to the odorous molecules in the nasal cavity. The question remains unresolved.

If the cilia are the sites of the molecule-membrane interaction, their length becomes an important factor in determining where they lie in the nasal cavity and how they may then be stimulated. The cilia could be either completely immersed in the mucous secretion covering the epithelium or located at the air-mucus interface. Because they are extremely fragile, the cilia are difficult to measure; the many different estimates of their length are probably due to artifacts in fixing and staining nasal tissues for microscopic examination. Another complicating feature is presented in the interesting study by Shibuya and Takagi (1963). The authors reported that the cilia of newts living in water remained a constant length of 4 to 6 microns; but when the animals were transferred to land, the cilia lengthened to 22 microns, later becoming gradually shorter. When the animals were returned to water, the cilia shortened to the original 4 to 6 microns. Although this dramatic change in the cilia resulting from the environmental change could be interpreted as clear evidence that the cilia are the sites of olfactory stimulation, the finding is also amenable to another interpretation. The cilia could be ancillary in function and serve only to facilitate the contact of the stimulus molecule on the membrane of the terminal knob.

Each receptor cell has only one axon. These axons are among the smallest in the brain, with an average diameter of 0.2 microns (de Lorenzo, 1956; Gasser, 1956). They leave the olfactory epithelium in small bundles of up to 1000 axons and enter the cranial cavity through the *cribriform plate.* They then spread out over the surface of the *olfactory bulb* which lies directly behind the cribriform plate.

The other types of cells in the olfactory epithelium are supporting and basal cells (see Figure 3.28). Both types are usually considered to have little or no direct role in olfactory transduction. However, the electron microscope has shown that the supporting cells have small projections, called *microvilli,* that are interspersed among the cilia of the receptor cells (de Lorenzo, 1960; Gasser, 1956). Their proximity to the cilia suggests that the microvilli may affect transduction.

A characteristic feature of the olfactory epithelium in land vertebrates, including humans, is the presence of *Bowman's glands,* which are found nowhere else within the nasal cavity. These glands possess short ducts which open onto the surface of the epithelium and bathe it continually with watery secretions. Such a mucous covering most likely plays a role in olfactory processes. It perhaps forms, between the stimulus molecule and the receptor cell membrane, a layer of mucus that influences the arrival of the odorants at the layer of receptor cells. The precise role depends, of course, on the exact length and location of the olfactory cilia.

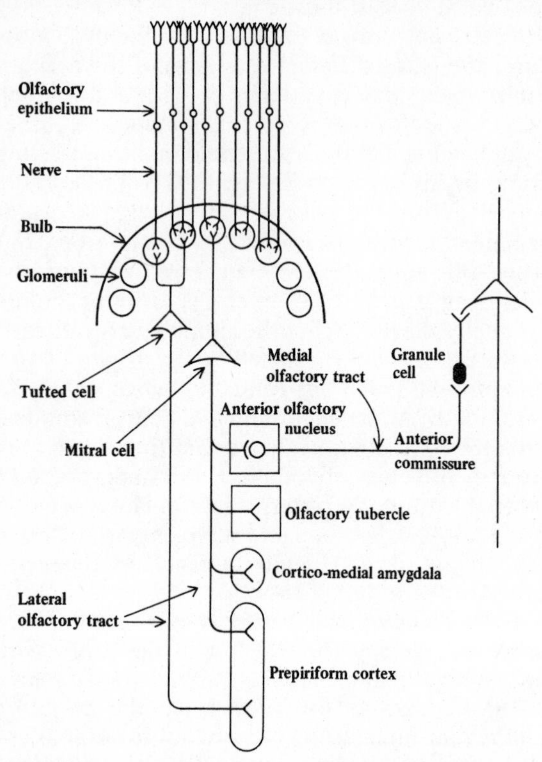


**Figure 3.29** Schematic diagram of the olfactory pathway.

## The olfactory pathway

The axons of the receptor cells form the *olfactory nerve* which goes directly to the olfactory bulb (see Figure 3.29). Since each receptor cell possesses its own axon, the excitation pattern in the receptor cells is the same as at the synapses in the olfactory bulb. The axons of the olfactory nerve spread out over the surface of the bulb to form a complex network of widely scattered *glomeruli.* An olfactory glomerulus is a spherical cluster of olfactory nerve axon boutons and dendritic processes of *mitral* and *tufted* cells. The glomeruli form a definite layer just below the surface of the olfactory bulb, and are the site of the first synapse in the olfactory system.

In vertebrates, the olfactory bulbs lie in front of the main forebrain mass to which they are connected by the *olfactory tracts.* Throughout the phylogenetic levels, from fish to human, the relative size of the bulb becomes smaller as the cerebrum becomes larger. The general structure of the bulb, however, remains approximately the same, as does the synaptic sequence from the olfactory epithelium to the brain.

The detailed anatomy of the olfactory bulb was described years ago by Cajal (1901–2), but only a few of the synapses need concern us. The important synapses are those of the mitral cells, whose cell bodies look like bishops' miters and lie deep in the bulb. Their apical dendrites extend to the glomerular layer, where they branch profusely into vast dendritic brushes. The axons of the mitral cells leave the olfactory bulb in the *lateral olfactory tract.* This tract, on its way to the brain, gives off collaterals to the *anterior olfactory nucleus,* a cluster of neurons at the posterior end of the olfactory bulb. The main axons of the lateral olfactory tract continue to the brain and terminate in the *olfactory tubercle,* the *cortico-medial nuclei of the amygdala,* and the *prepiriform cortex.* In higher primates, including humans, the prepiriform cortex is located on the medial side of the temporal lobe, extending to the *rhinal sulcus;* it is thought to be the primary sensory cortex for olfaction.

The axons of the *medial olfactory tract* arise from cell bodies in the anterior olfactory nucleus. These axons cross over to the other side of the brain, where they terminate in the anterior olfactory nucleus and olfactory bulb.

The afferent projections of the tufted cells are still not completely known. Valverde (1965) maintains that the axons of these cells remain within the bulb. Other investigators present both anatomical (Lohman & Mentink, 1969) and physiological (Nicoll, 1970) evidence that the axons of the tufted cells, like the axons of the mitral cells, leave the bulb in the lateral olfactory tract, as suggested in Figure 3.29.

## Physiology of olfactory neurons

Research in the chemical senses has often sought to determine the primary qualities of smell and taste, and then to account for differences in quality by finding differences in the structure of the receptors. For example, Le Gros Clark (1956) suggested that differences in length of the olfactory rod may serve as a basis for olfactory discrimination. Thus, the physiological investigations of the olfactory system (and of the taste system) have tended to focus on the problem of response specificity.

Ottoson (1956) was the first to investigate extensively the gross potential of the olfactory epithelium evoked by a puff of odorized air of known concentration. The measured epithelial potential was monophasic, first rising rapidly to a peak and then decaying slowly and with much variability to its original resting level. Examples of the epithelial response, which Ottoson called the *electro-olfactogram (EOG),* are shown in Figure 3.30.

Ottoson (1956) described a number of properties of the EOG. Originating at the surface of the olfactory epithelium, the EOG becomes progressively smaller as the tip of the recording electrode is advanced through the epithelium from the surface to the basement membrane (see Figure 3.28). Its amplitude is roughly proportional to the logarithm of the odor intensity and, for a constant odor concentration, to the volume of the stimulating air. But, if odor concentration is allowed to vary by distributing equal amounts of odorous material in different volumes of air, then the amplitude of the evoked response does not change as a function of air volume; that is, the product of volume and concentration necessary to evoke a given response is constant.

With continuous stimulation, the amplitude of the EOG declines from its peak to a level somewhere above the baseline, where it remains for the duration of the stimulation. The greater the intensity of the stimulus, the lower the maintained relative level of the potential. There is a progressive decline in the amplitude of the EOG when the epithelium is repeatedly stimulated at short intervals. However, this fatigue effect is selective. For example, after the epithelium has been repeatedly stimulated with butanol so that the EOG has virtually disappeared, a puff of amyl acetate will elicit a full-blown EOG.

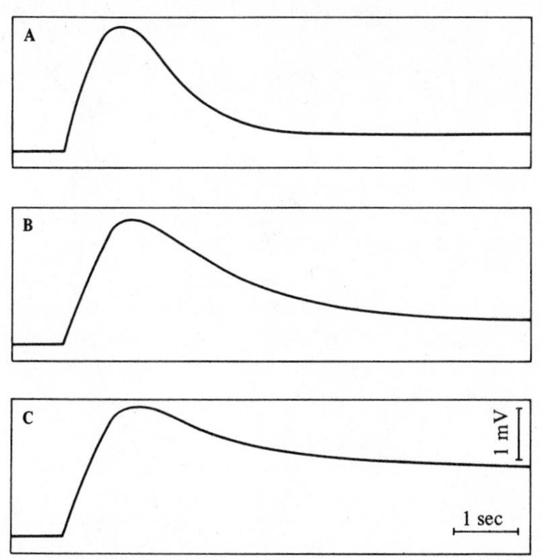


**Figure 3.30** Responses of the olfactory epithelium to amyl acetate (A), butanol (B), and oil of cloves (C). Volume of the stimulating air is 1 cc. (From Ottoson, 1956.)

Ottoson's (1956) extensive series of investigations indicates that the EOG arises from the region of the receptor cell cilia when the odorous molecules come into contact with the receptor cell membrane. The amplitude of the epithelial response depends on the number of stimulating molecules. The data from the selective fatigue experiments suggest that molecules of distinct substances may stimulate the receptor at different sites along the membrane. Ottoson proposed that the EOG potential is the generator potential in olfaction. Although this proposal remains to be proved and is somewhat controversial (cf. Mozell, 1962; Ottoson & Shepherd, 1967; Shibuya, 1964), it appears quite reasonable. Accordingly, in the schema of Figure 3.9 the EOG potential would be both the receptor and generator potential since the olfactory receptor cells generate nerve impulses and their axons form the olfactory nerve.

Gesteland and his associates (Gesteland, Lettvin, & Pitts, 1965; Gesteland, Lettvin, Pitts, & Rojas, 1963) were the first to record responses from single olfactory receptor cells. Although each cell responds to stimuli of all primary qualities, a given cell responds more strongly to some stimuli than to others. Its specificity is expressed by differential rates of firing when stimulated by different classes of odorants. Figure 3.31 gives a representative example of the type of response spectrum for a single receptor. No two neurons seemed to respond alike. Yet receptors did tend to fall into classes, but ones with extensive overlap. Neither chemical names nor odor properties describe the classes very well. For example, Gesteland et al. (1963) noted that one group responds to butyric acid, valeric acid, mercaptoacetic acid, and cyclohexanol; another group responds to limonene, camphor, pinene, and somewhat less to carbon disulfide. The general conclusion is that each receptor cell reacts to many stimuli, although it may react slightly differently from its neighbor on the other side of the supporting cell. Gesteland et al. interpret their data as indicating that a number of different types of receptor sites are distributed over each cell. The ratio of the different types is assumed to vary from cell to cell. In this way, the variation in individual cell responses could be accounted for by assuming that a given cell has more receptor sites for the molecule that elicits its maximal

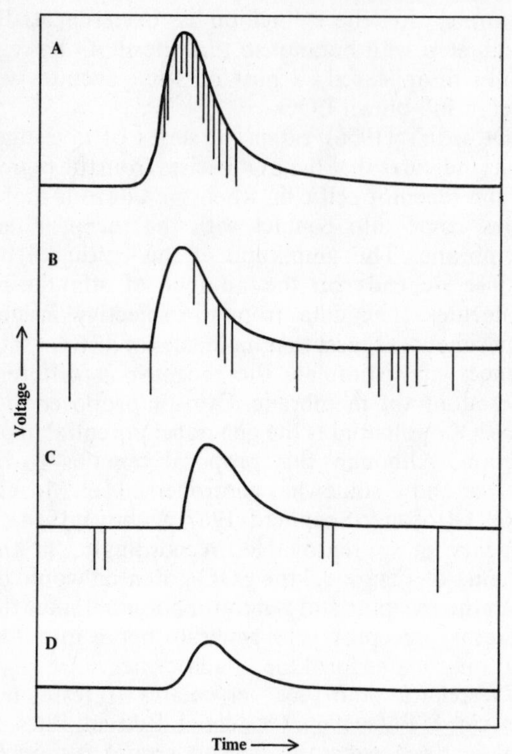


Figure 3.31 A unit that responds strongly to musk xylene (A), slightly to nitrobenzene (B), hardly at all to benzonitrite (C), and not at all to pyridine (D). Sweep length is 10 sec. (From Gesteland, Lettvin, Pitts, & Rojas, 1963.)

response than for molecules that elicit weaker responses.

Electrophysiological investigations of smell and taste have focused, for the most part, on the primary afferent fibers. No studies of single cortical neurons, comparable to studies in vision and audition, have been reported for smell and taste.

## THE TASTE SYSTEM

The sensory system of taste is normally always stimulated in conjunction with tactual stimuli in the oral cavity and with olfactory stimuli. However, for experimental purposes, taste sensations are considered to arise only when the specialized receptor cells are stimulated. Moreover, research workers usually restrict their investigations to the four basic taste qualities—sweet, sour, salty, and bitter.

### Taste receptors

Taste receptor cells are distributed on the dorsal aspect of the tongue and on the laryngeal aspect of the epiglottis, pharynx, and soft palate. They are found in the *fungiform, foliate*, and *circumvallate papillae*. Figure 3.32 shows the spatial distribution of papillae on the human tongue. Within each papilla are six to eight goblet-shaped structures called *taste buds*. A taste bud comprises twenty to thirty cells and is about 50 to 60 microns in diameter. Taste buds were first described by Leydig in 1851 (see Graziadei, 1969). Since that time, investigators have sought to determine the number of cell types within a taste bud. The early common description indicated at least two types—receptor and supporting cells. Parker (1922) suggested, however, that all cells within a taste bud are receptor cells that differ in appearance merely because they are in different stages of development. The demonstration by Beidler and Smallman (1965) that cells within the taste bud are continually being replaced indirectly supported Parker's suggestion. However, this evidence is inconclusive, since both cell types could be undergoing renewal.

The first electron microscopic study of taste

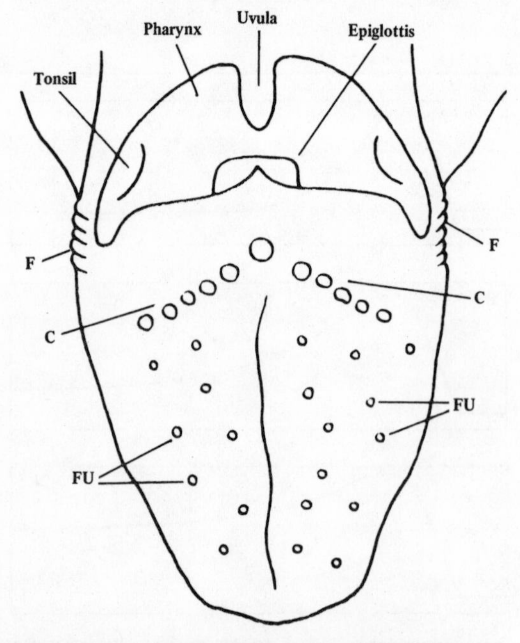


Figure 3.32 Arrangement of taste papillae on the human tongue. F, foliate; C, circumvallate; FU, fungiform papillae. (From Kalmus & Hubbard, 1960.)

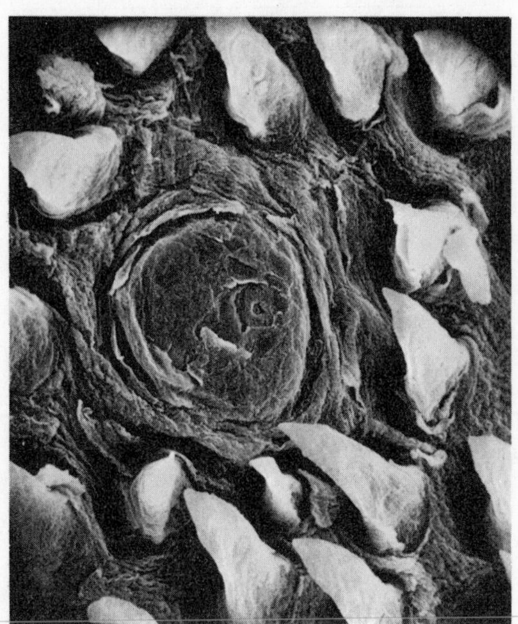

**Figure 3.33** Scanning electron micrograph of a papilla showing the taste pore. (Courtesy of P. P. C. Graziadei.)

buds and taste cells was reported by Engström and Rytzner (1956a, 1956b). They observed cells with different morphological characteristics in the buds, but interpreted them as cells in different stages of development. These findings have now been repeated many times so that a common description of taste-bud structure is possible. The buds are composed of slender epithelial cells with microvillilike structures at their apical end. The apical end of these cells lies in the region of the *taste pore*, which is an opening onto the surface of the tongue. Figure 3.33, which is a micrograph made with the scanning electron microscope, shows a fungiform papilla from the rat tongue with its taste pore. A beltlike system of tight junctions is situated at the apical pole of the taste cells, sealing off the intercellular spaces of the taste bud from the environment.

The structure and integrity of the taste bud depend on its innervation by nerve fibers that enter the bud through its basement membrane. When the nerves to the taste buds are severed, the taste buds disappear; the taste buds reappear after the nerve fibers have regenerated. The studies have been summarized by Farbman (1965) in a paper on the development of the taste bud in the rat.

## The taste pathway

As shown in Figure 3.34, the nerve supply to the tongue and other areas of the mouth is composed of fibers from the *lingual* (VII), *glossopharyngeal* (IX), and *vagus* (X) nerves. The lingual nerve to the anterior two thirds of the tongue subserves touch, temperature, pain, and taste. The afferent taste fibers leave this nerve in a strand called the *chorda tympani.* Taste fibers from the posterior third of the tongue travel in the glossopharyngeal nerve, and those from the pharynx, larynx, epiglottis, and so forth, travel in the vagus nerve. These three nerves terminate in the nucleus of the *solitary tract* in the medulla. From there, fibers ascend in the *medial lemniscus* to the *ventral posteromedial nucleus* of the thalamus. The most medial tip of this nucleus exclusively relays afferent information of taste. Neurons in the ventral nucleus send fibers to the somatic face region on the postcentral gyrus.

## Physiology of taste neurons

Beidler (1969) has extensively examined the neural innervation of the fungiform papilla of the rat. Although each papilla contains only one taste bud, he found that as many as fifty fibers may enter

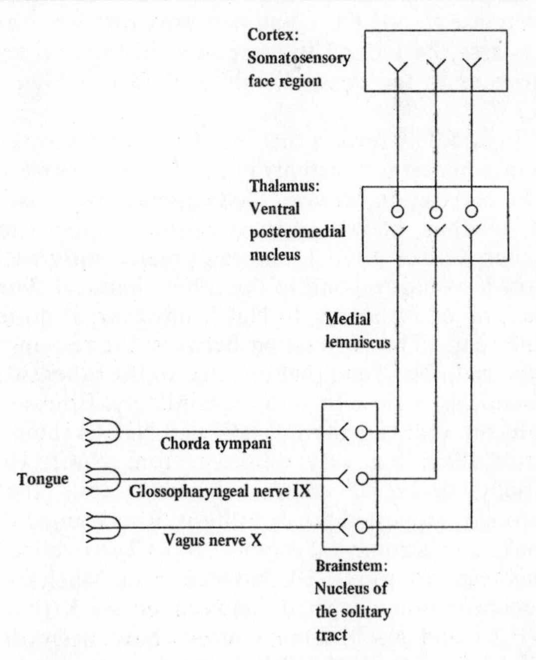


**Figure 3.34** Schematic diagram of the afferent pathway for taste.

a single bud. These fibers, in turn, may branch into just over two hundred fibers, resulting in over five hundred contacts with various cells. Also, the same chorda tympani axon may send collaterals to a number of different taste buds. Clearly, the transmission of afferent information regarding taste quality may be highly complex. These findings provide the anatomical basis for the results obtained in the study of single axons from any of the three afferent nerve bundles. Many such studies (e.g., Ogawa, Sato, & Yamashita, 1968) show, in general, that every afferent fiber transmits impulses initiated by any sort of taste stimulus, but at different rates. This generalization also applies to the responses of the taste receptor cells recorded by Kimura and Beidler (1961), who found that individual cells respond to all four basic taste qualities.

Erickson (1963), following a suggestion by Pfaffmann (1955) that the neural code for taste quality may be in the relative amount of activity in many fibers, presented what may be termed an *across-fiber pattern* analysis of information for taste quality. Erickson determined the response rate of thirteen chorda tympani neurons to three taste stimuli, 0.1 *mole (M)* ammonia chloride ($NH_4Cl$), 0.3M potassium chloride (KCl), and 0.1M sodium chloride (NaCl). A mole is a unit of gram-molecular concentration. He then rank-ordered the thirteen neurons from highest to lowest on the basis of their response to $NH_4Cl$. Using that rank order on the abscissa, he plotted the responses of the thirteen neurons to the three stimuli as shown in Figure 3.35.

Figure 3.35 reveals that $NH_4Cl$ and KCl evoke similar patterns of activity in the thirteen neurons. The correlation between the two sets of responses is .83; thus, knowing how a neuron responds to either KCl or $NH_4Cl$, one can predict fairly well how it would respond to the other chemical. The pattern of responses to NaCl, however, is quite different. The correlation between the response pattern to NaCl and that to either of the other two chemicals is close to zero. Accordingly, Erickson inferred that, for the rat, KCl and $NH_4Cl$ should taste alike, but very different from NaCl. He briefly described some behavioral tests that strongly supported the hypothesis. Rats trained to make an instrumental response to KCl generalized this response to $NH_4Cl$, and vice versa. Much less generalization occurred between either KCl or $NH_4Cl$ and NaCl. Similar results have been obtained by Marshall (1968) with the guinea pig.

The across-fiber pattern analysis has been extensively studied at the first synapse in the afferent pathway (Doetsch, Ganchrow, Nelson, & Erickson, 1969), where the axons of the chorda tympani terminate in the nucleus of the solitary tract (see Figure 3.34). Doetsch et al. investigated the responses of both chorda tympani axons and solitary tract neurons to chemical stimulation of the rat tongue. They found that some aspects of the afferent information for taste remain unchanged across the synapse. For example, the cells at both levels are sensitive to a relatively broad range of chemical stimuli typically representing more than one of the four basic taste qualities. Another common feature of both chorda tympani axons and solitary tract neurons is that the response patterns across neurons for individual stimuli are essentially the same.

Nevertheless, certain features of the sensory input are modified in synaptic transmission so as to produce more stable patterns of activity in the second-order nerve cells of the solitary tract. Doetsch et al. found that in the higher-order cells the average rate of response to all stimuli increased by a factor of slightly more than four. Moreover, in these neurons, the initial evoked burst of activity was attenuated relative to the steady-state response. The neural responses to different stimuli were less distinctive; that is, correlations between response patterns were higher for the neurons of the solitary tract than for those of the chorda tympani.

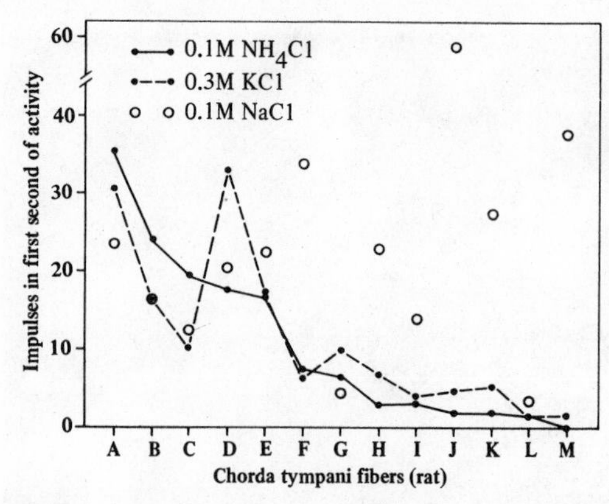


**Figure 3.35** Across-fiber patterns for thirteen axons (A–M) of the chorda tympani nerve in the rat. Fibers are arranged along the baseline in decreasing order of responsiveness to $NH_4Cl$. The KCl pattern is similar to the $NH_4Cl$ pattern, but neither of these patterns is similar to the NaCl pattern. (From Erickson, 1963.)

Across-fiber pattern analysis has been extended to the rat thalamus by Scott and Erickson (1971), who reported several interesting differences in these neurons in comparison to the lower-order cells. The authors noted a decrease in the average evoked discharge rate to about 25 percent of that recorded in the neurons of the solitary tract. They also found that chemically complex stimuli, such as sucrose, were relatively more effective in eliciting responses from thalamic neurons. This effect could be considered analogous to the response to the more complex stimuli by higher-order visual and auditory neurons.

## THE SOMATOSENSORY SYSTEM

The skin is man's largest sensory system measured in terms of area of the receptor surface. Yet its sensory functions have not been as extensively investigated as those of the eyes and ears. The skin, of course, is not solely a sensory system; it has several important survival functions. It prevents the loss of vital body fluids and is an integral part of the system that maintains body temperature. Heat regulation is aided by the sweat glands, which control the amount of water available for evaporation at the surface, and by the many fine cutaneous blood vessels, which control the flow of blood. Protection against solar radiations is afforded by the dark pigment, *melanin*, produced by *melanocytes,* which are special cells located in the skin. As a sensory system, the skin's most important function is probably to signal the presence of potentially harmful stimuli. Consider the extra caution that must be exercised in everyday life by the individual who lacks the normal ability to feel pain.

### Anatomy of the skin

The body is covered by several distinct types of skin. The skin with the simplest structure is the *mucous membrane*. This tissue lines the orifices and canals of the body that communicate with external air, such as the alimentary tract, the respiratory tract, and the urogenital tract. It participates in the interchange of nutritive or excretory substances in these regions and secretes digestive and lubricating fluids. Most of the body is covered by *hairy* skin (see Figure 3.36), even though it does not always look hairy. In some places the hair is long and tough, as on the scalp, while on other sites it is soft and downy (vellus). A subtype of skin, called *mucocutaneous,* is found at the junctions of hairy skin and mucous membrane, and covers the lips, the glans penis, the prepuce, the clitoris, the tongue, the inner margins of the eyelid, and the perianal region. Perhaps the most complex skin is *glabrous* skin (see Figure 3.37), found only on the palms of the hands and soles of the feet. Glabrous skin is thick, richly innervated, and deeply furrowed, thus providing protection, high sensitivity, and good gripping qualities to the manipulative surfaces of the body.

The *epithelium* is the coat of cells that covers both the internal and external surfaces of the body, whereas the term *skin,* or *common integument,* is usually reserved for the covering of the external surfaces of the body. Skin is composed of several relatively distinct layers of cells (see Figures 3.36 and 3.37) which are listed in Table 3.3.

The major layer divisions are the *epidermis* and the *dermis*. The innermost layer of the epidermis is the *stratum germinativum,* which rests upon a fibrous membrane called *lamina basilaris* and is composed of a single layer of columnar cells which are constantly dividing. All other layers of the epidermis are derived from these cells. As the cells divide, they begin an upward migration to the surface, passing first through the *stratum spinosum,* so named because of cytoplasmic processes called intercellular bridges which pass between the cells. In histological preparations, these processes look like spines. The cells increase in size as they ascend and gradually flatten to form the *stratum granulosum.* The cells then pass through the *stratum lucidum,* which has a translucent appearance under the microscope and serves as a barrier to prevent many noxious chemical agents from entering the body. The final stage in the transformation of epidermal cells is completed at the *stratum corneum,* where the cells die and flatten into a tough, pliable, protective covering. The major component of cells in the corneum is *keratin,* a stable protein impervious to most chemicals. As new cells migrate from below, the cells on the surface are shed with the help of friction encountered in everyday life. The entire cycle, from basal layer to corneum, is complete in about 27 days. The thickness of the epidermis ranges from 0.07 mm over most of the body to about 1.5 mm over the palms of the hands and soles of the feet. It is important to note that the organ we know as skin is a dynamic, evolving system and that an ongoing process is taking place throughout the life of the animal or human. The ultimate goal of that process is to provide the organism with a covering that both protects against

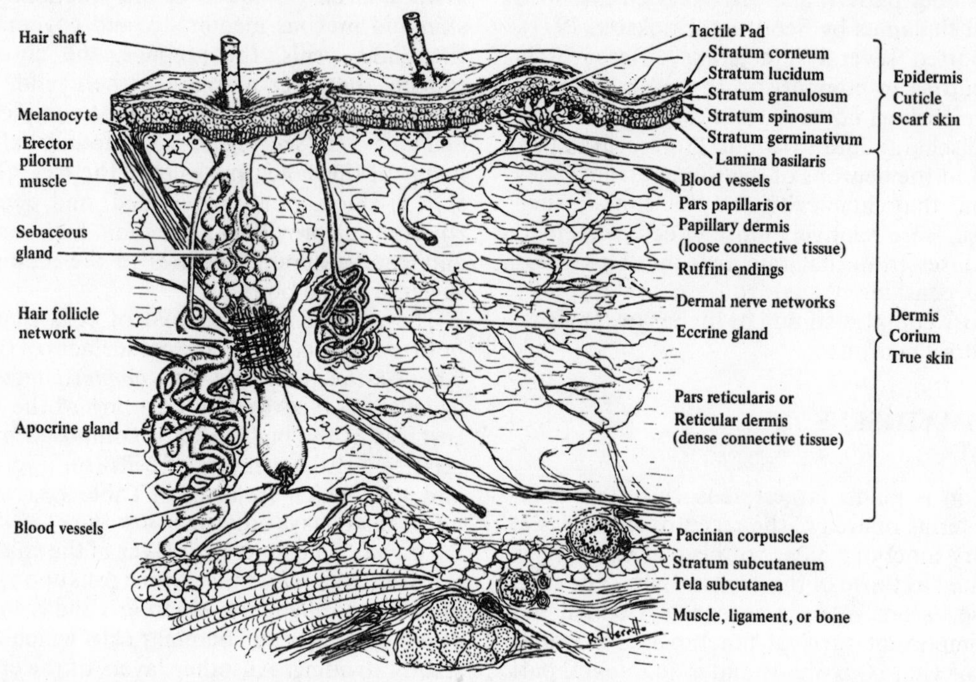


Figure 3.36 Representation of hairy skin showing various layers, glands, and structures.

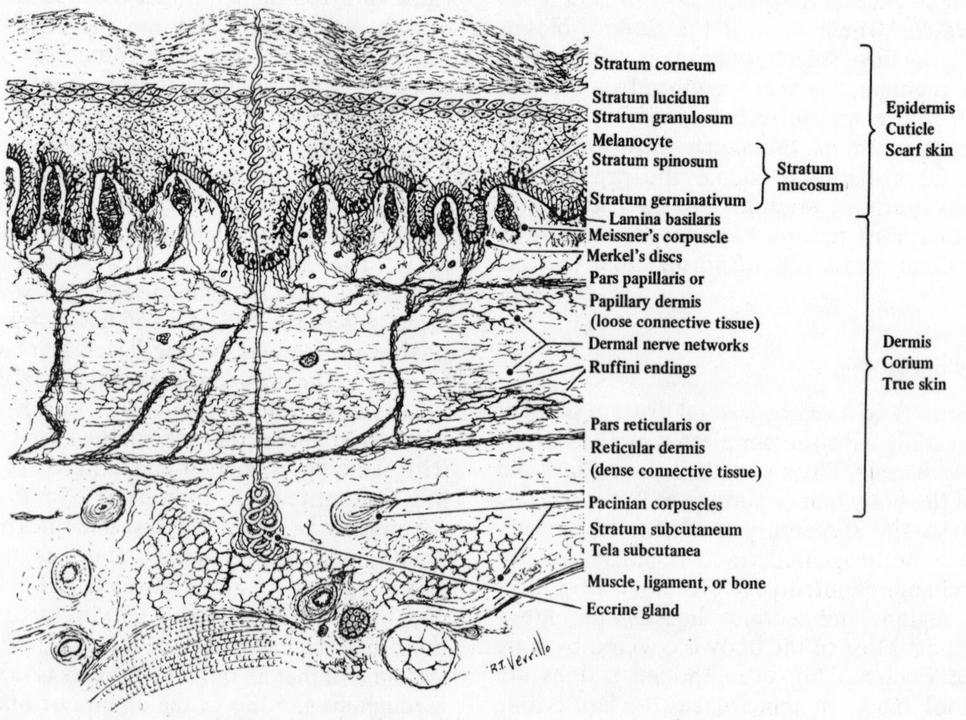


Figure 3.37 Representation of glabrous skin showing its layers and structures.

**Table 3.3 The Basic Structure of the Skin**

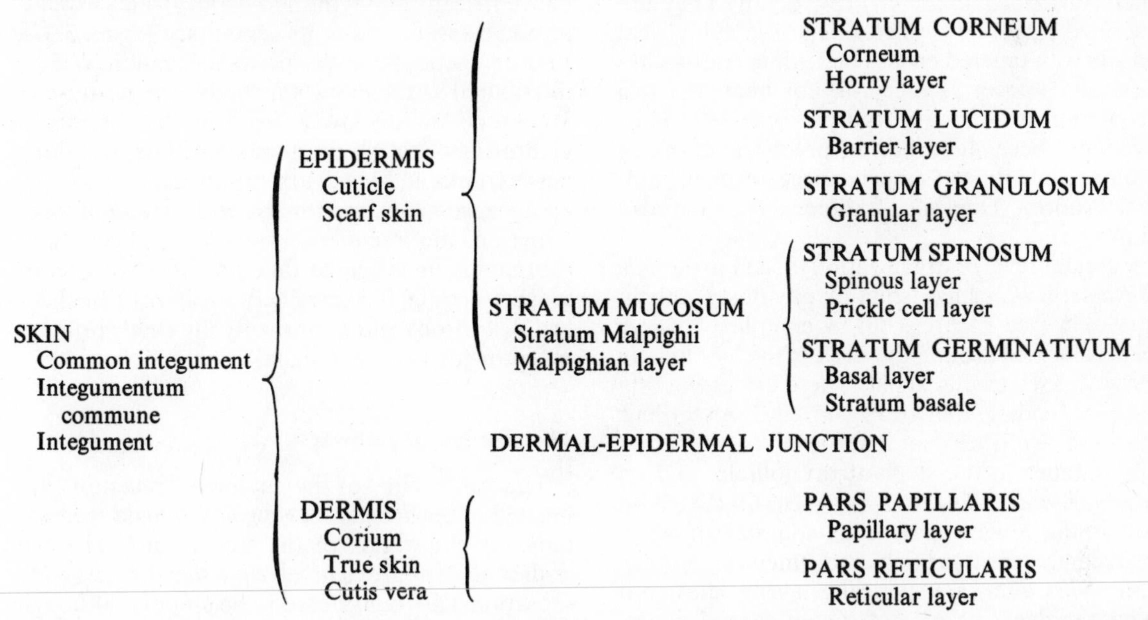

| | | | |
|---|---|---|---|
| SKIN<br>Common integument<br>Integumentum commune<br>Integument | EPIDERMIS<br>Cuticle<br>Scarf skin | | STRATUM CORNEUM<br>Corneum<br>Horny layer |
| | | | STRATUM LUCIDUM<br>Barrier layer |
| | | | STRATUM GRANULOSUM<br>Granular layer |
| | | STRATUM MUCOSUM<br>Stratum Malpighii<br>Malpighian layer | STRATUM SPINOSUM<br>Spinous layer<br>Prickle cell layer |
| | | | STRATUM GERMINATIVUM<br>Basal layer<br>Stratum basale |
| | DERMAL-EPIDERMAL JUNCTION | | |
| | DERMIS<br>Corium<br>True skin<br>Cutis vera | | PARS PAPILLARIS<br>Papillary layer |
| | | | PARS RETICULARIS<br>Reticular layer |

R. T. Verrillo

bodily injury and functions as a channel of communication.

The neural units involved in the transduction of environmental energies into neural signals are located primarily in the dermis. In the dermis are also located the hair *follicles,* from which the shaft of the hair grows, and the *erector pilorus* muscles, whose contraction causes the hair to stand erect. The action of these muscles is controlled by the hypothalamus in response to cold or danger. The dermis is not clearly stratified, although the connective tissue of the *pars papillaris* is less compact than the tissue of the deeper *pars reticularis.* In glabrous skin, the lower margin of the epidermis is marked by deep intrusions of the dermis which are called *papillae.* The interface between dermis and epidermis in hairy skin takes the form of gentle undulations. Over most of the body, the dermis is 1 mm to 2 mm thick; over the palms and soles, it can be 3 mm or more in depth.

### Cutaneous receptors

The most widely distributed sensory nerve endings in the skin are the *free endings* that make up the dermal nerve networks found in all types of skin (Montagna, 1960; Winkelmann, 1960). These nerves enter the dermis from subcutaneous tissues as myelinated fibers and pass upward through the dermis to the epidermis. As they ascend through the dermis, they send out numerous collaterals which form a dense, irregular network, or *rete.* Myelin is gradually reduced as the fibers near the epidermis until, at the most superficial dermal levels, the network consists of thinly myelinated fibers. In thick glabrous skin, some fibers penetrate the epidermis and course upward between the cells as far as the granular layer. It is a matter of contention whether or not such intraepidermal fibers are found in hairy skin. There is no apparent organization to the dermal nerve networks. Sensations of touch, pain, heat, and cold have been ascribed to these endings, but there is little direct evidence of their exact functions in skin.

The first step in the organization of cutaneous nerves into a recognizable organ is the *mucocutaneous end-organ.* This ending has the appearance of a loosely wound ball of yarn, with loops of nerve fibers rolled on one another, and since it is found only in the papillary dermis of mucocutaneous tissue it does not appear in Figure 3.36 or 3.37. Older textbooks refer to this ending as the *Krause end-bulb* or *Dogiel's body.* It was once thought that these endings were cold receptors, but this hypothesis has been rejected in recent years.

On a similar level of organization are the neural units known as *Ruffini endings.* There had been some dispute as to whether these endings exist;

some anatomists did not find them at all, while others described them in great detail. They are described as loosely rolled fibers in a cylindrical capsule with tapered ends. The Ruffini endings are classically known as receptors for heat, but this speculation is no longer regarded seriously. They have now been described in precise anatomical detail and identified as mechanoreceptors (Chambers, Andres, Duering, & Iggo, 1972; see also Chapter 5).

A greater level of organization is seen in the *hair follicle network,* which is found, obviously, only in hairy skin (see Figure 3.36). A complex of nerve fibers is located around the neck of the hair follicle below the sebaceous gland. These are essentially free nerve endings that are organized about the hair follicle in two layers: an inner layer of fibers that runs parallel to the shaft of the follicle, and an outer network that runs in a circular fashion around the follicle shaft. This complex of fibers is extremely sensitive to any movement of the hair.

*Merkel's discs* are typically found clustered about the deep margins of the epidermal ridges, which extend into the papillary layer of the dermis (see Figure 3.37). The leaflike hederiform enlargements at the ends of the nerve fibers appear as tiny buttons on and between the cells of the basal layer of the epidermis in glabrous skin. In the hairy skin of mammals, Merkel's discs accumulate along the basal layer of cells in units that appear on the surface as small, round, flattened hemispheres between the hairs. In this form, they are known as tactile pads (*haarscheibe, hair discs,* or *Pinkus endings*). These units exist in humans, but their function has not yet been conclusively demonstrated. They may be associated with the sense of touch (Iggo, 1962; Lindblom & Tapper, 1967; Tapper, 1965).

A much higher degree of organization is exhibited by *Meissner's corpuscles,* which are contained only in the dermal papillae of glabrous skin. Within an enveloping capsule composed of connective tissue, the nerve fibers coil and spiral upon themselves. The anatomy of this ending has been extensively investigated, but little is known about its response characteristics or its exact role in skin sensitivity. There is evidence that it is a mechanoreceptor, responding to deformations of the skin surface.

The most highly developed receptors associated with cutaneous tissue are the *Pacinian corpuscles.* These are the largest endings found in human skin. In its simplest form the Pacinian corpuscle is roughly football-shaped and is composed of alternate layers of connective tissue and fluid built up concentrically about the nerve stalk, which extends into and terminates in its center (see Figure 3.37). In cross section, it looks like a sliced onion. Widely distributed throughout the body, the corpuscles are found in the lower layers of the dermis in glabrous and hairy skin, about the joints, and along nerve trunks and many arteries. Because it is large, easily accessible in animals, and of unique construction, the Pacinian corpuscle has been more thoroughly investigated than any other cutaneous sensory ending. It is extremely sensitive to mechanical distortions and is probably the skin's primary receptor for vibratory signals.

### The anatomical pathway

The cell bodies of the cutaneous receptors are located in the *dorsal root ganglia* arranged segmentally on either side of the spinal cord. The cell bodies of all neurons involved in *somesthesis* (body sensations) are considered to be unipolar although they have a peripheral and a central process which become fused before entering the cell body (see Figure 3.2). The neural pathways within the central nervous system are organized into two great afferent systems, the *medial-lemniscal* and the *spinothalamic.*

#### *The medial-lemniscal system*

Upon entering the spinal cord over the medial bundle of the dorsal root, the large myelinated fibers of the medial-lemniscal system enter the *dorsal white columns,* or *posterior funiculi.* There they immediately divide, sending a short process caudally through several segments of the cord, and a long process rostrally toward the brain. Ascending fibers from the legs and lower trunk travel within a bundle of fibers known as the *fasciculus gracilis,* while fibers from the arms and upper trunk reach the brainstem by way of a bundle called the *fasciculus cuneatus.* These first-order neurons synapse in the *nucleus gracilis* and the *nucleus cuneatus,* which are aggregates of cells in the dorsal part of the medulla.

The axons of the second-order neurons cross to the contralateral side of the medulla and then ascend in a bundle of fibers known as the *medial lemniscus,* from which the system derives its name. Within the medial lemniscus, fibers pass through the region of the pons and midbrain and terminate in the *ventral posterolateral nucleus* of the thalamus. This region of the thalamus is referred to as the *ventrobasal complex.* The thalamic neurons project

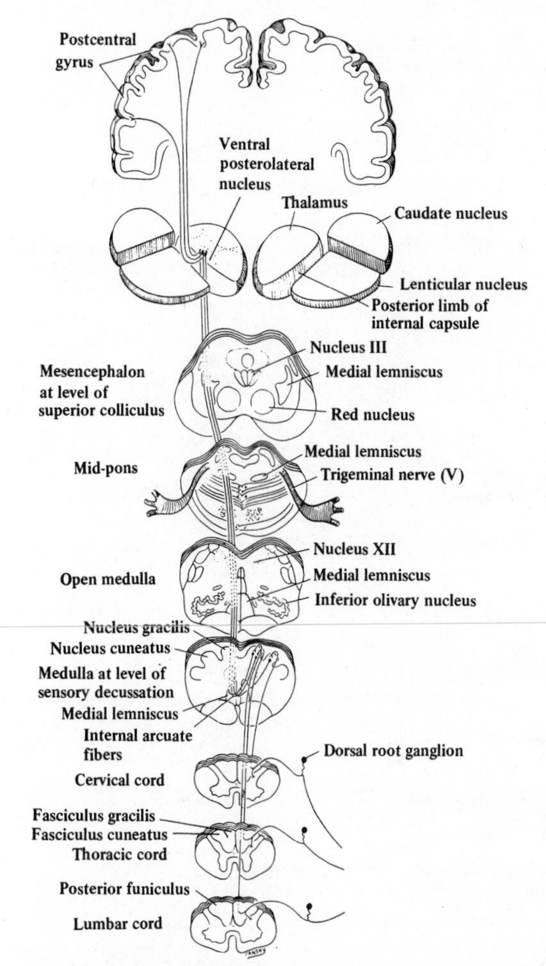


**Figure 3.38** The medial-lemniscal pathway of the somatosensory system. (From House & Pansky, 1967.)

their axons to the somatosensory cortex on the *postcentral gyrus*.

It is believed that the end-organs served by this system include the Pacinian corpuscles, Meissner's corpuscles, and the neuromuscular and neurotendinous spindles. The latter two receptors are involved in the neural control of motion and posture by signaling mechanical activity in muscles and tendons. Damage to the dorsal columns results in the loss of two-point discriminations, loss of the ability to perceive vibration and loss of the ability to locate where the skin is touched or to know the position of the limbs without looking.

*The spinothalamic system*

Although it may be considered a single system, the spinothalamic system travels over two special tracts conveying impulses from the peripheral receptors to the brain. These are the *anterior,* or *ventral, spinothalamic tract* and the *lateral spinothalamic tract*.

The small myelinated axons of the anterior spinothalamic tract enter the spinal cord from the dorsal root ganglia via the lateral bundle (see Figure 3.39A). There they penetrate the gray matter and synapse in the *proper nucleus* (*nucleus centrodorsalis*), a group of large cells located in the dorsal horn. Most of the axons originating in the proper nucleus cross to the contralateral side of the cord through the *anterior white commissure.* They then ascend in the contralateral *anterior spinothalamic fasciculus* to the ventrobasal complex of the thalamus. The axons of these third-order neurons then project to the postcentral gyrus. The exact nature of the information transmitted through the anterior spinothalamic system is uncertain. Although tactile thresholds are raised by injury to the system, sensitivity is not completely lost and sometimes recovers.

The first-order axons of the lateral spinothalamic tract (see Figure 3.39B) also enter the cord over the lateral bundle of the dorsal horns, and, as in the anterior spinothalamic tract, they are fibers of small diameter. They enter the *zone of Lissauer* (also called the *fasciculus dorsolateralis*), where they may send collateral fibers a short distance up and down the cord. Some of these fibers terminate in the proper nucleus and some in the *substantia gelatinosa*. The second-order fibers sweep across the cord through the anterior white commissure and ascend to the brain by way of the *lateral spinothalamic fasciculus*. They synapse in the ventral posterolateral nucleus of the thalamus. From there, third-order axons project to the somatosensory cortex.

Despite the close correspondence in certain parts of the two spinothalamic pathways, they appear to be quite distinct in function. Injury to the lateral spinothalamic tract results in a loss of sensitivity to pain and temperature, whereas no such loss occurs if the anterior spinothalamic tract is severed.

The areas of the body are represented on the cortex along the long axis of the postcentral gyrus, which lies just posterior to the central sulcus. The body is represented inversely; that is, the lower portions of the body make connections along the

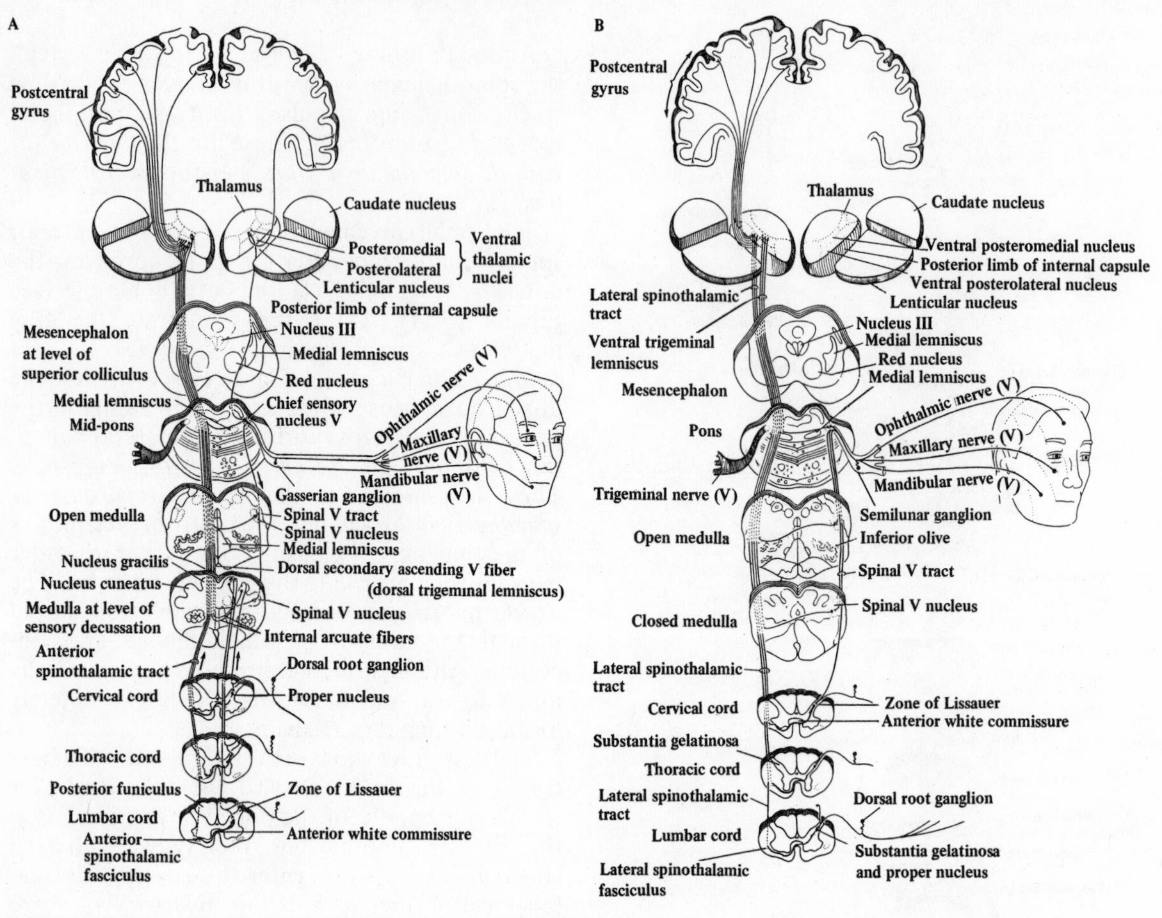


**Figure 3.39** The spinothalamic pathways of the somatosensory system: lateral (A) and anterior (B). The original figure showed fibers in the three lowest sections as crossing the spinal cord in the gray matter instead of in the anterior white commissure, as in this redrawing. (After House & Pansky, 1967.)

medial aspect and at the top of the somatosensory cortex, while the upper portions are represented along the lower lateral portion near the Sylvian fissure. The size of area receiving fibers from each part of the body is directly proportional to the neural innervation and, hence, to the sensitivity of that part: The denser the innervation and sensitivity for a given part, the larger the cortical representation. Thus, the face and tongue far outweigh the back of the head in neural elements, and the hand occupies a greater amount of cortical space than the rest of the arm.

The innervation of the body surface is organized in a sequence determined by the segments of the spinal cord from which the peripheral nerves originate. This arrangement is laid down during embryological development when each pair of *somites* receives one pair of spinal nerves. As a result of this organization, the entire surface of the body can be mapped for the sensations carried by each pair of spinal nerves. The areas thus defined, known as *dermatomes,* are important in locating pathologies of the spinal cord and in the understanding of *referred pain* (see Chapter 5).

A word of caution about sensory pathways is in order. The various somatosensory systems have been depicted, for the sake of clarity, in a manner that implies a sequence of wires strung out along well-defined pathways, with clearly circumscribed couplings along the way. This picture is a gross outline of complicated structural interrelationships within the cord and at higher centers that are largely unknown. *Reflex arcs* are established at all levels within the cord, and short collaterals are sent from the main pathways to other regions, such as the reticular activating system, not included in the general description. The bulk of research has been performed with animals, supplemented by scanty evidence derived from clinical descriptions of diseases and injuries in humans. There has been distressingly little high-quality electrophysiological investigation of this system in humans. The formulation of an adequate physiological model of perception for the cutaneous sensory systems is directly dependent upon such research.

## SUMMARY AND CONCLUSIONS

We receive information from the world around us by means of our sensory receptor systems. Each sensory system consists of specialized receptor cells and an afferent nerve pathway to the specific sensory neocortex in the brain. The receptor cells transduce the physical stimulus energy into biological nerve potentials, but just how sensory transduction occurs in any sensory system is not yet understood. The information contained in the energy pattern of the stimulus is encoded in the pattern of nerve impulses elicited in the afferent nerve fibers. This neural code undergoes changes at each synaptic transfer point along the pathway from receptor cell to sensory cortex.

The human eye contains 131 million photoreceptor cells, of which 6 million are cones and the rest are rods. The cones code information about color and fine detail, whereas the rods function mainly at low light levels but are color blind and insensitive to fine detail. Within the retina are the ganglion cells of the 1 million optic nerve fibers upon which all the photoreceptors converge. These ganglion cells have receptive fields made up of concentric rings of excitation and inhibition. Visual cortical neurons elaborate the relatively simple receptive fields of the ganglion cell into highly organized fields. For example, the so-called hypercomplex cells respond to a line stimulus only if the line has a certain length and is oriented at a particular angle.

The human ear is expertly constructed to bring sound from the air to the delicate receptor hair cells in the inner ear. Mechanical pressure exerted by the fluids of the inner ear bends or shears the fine stereocilia of the hair cells, thereby evoking neural impulses in the auditory nerve. The auditory pathway is tonotopically organized especially in its subcortical components where different stimulus frequencies are represented by different groups of neurons. Whereas neurons in the lower centers respond more readily to simple stimuli such as steady tones, cortical neurons respond more readily to complex stimuli such as tones ascending or descending in frequency.

In both chemical senses, smell and taste, physiological and chemical evidence suggests that specific molecules may be receptor sites in the nose and on the tongue for the appropriate stimuli, which are themselves molecules. The complexes formed by receptor molecules and stimulus molecules are probably intermediate steps in the stimulation of receptor cells in the chemical systems. A promising approach to the understanding of the neural codes in smell and taste is the analysis of neural firing patterns across many afferent fibers. Little is known about cortical activity for these two senses.

The skin includes several distinct types, and each type is composed of many layers of different cells. Located mainly within one of these layers, the dermis, are the receptor cells for touch, vibration, heat, cold, and pain. However, of the rich variety of possible receptors, it is not known which cells transduce which stimuli. Only the Pacinian corpuscle appears to have been clearly identified as the transducer of vibratory stimulation. Passing through the spinal cord, the afferent nerve fibers from the skin do not go directly to the cortex but make two or three synapses, and there is some crossing of fibers to the other side of the brain. Despite these complications, the entire surface of the body can be identified with specific parts of the somatosensory areas in the parietal lobes of the cortex.

# REFERENCES

**Adrian, E. D.** Discharges from vestibular receptors in the cat. *Journal of Physiology,* 1942, **101,** 389–407.

**Aitkin, L. M., Anderson, D. J., & Brugge, J. F.** Tonotopic organization and discharge characteristics of single neurons in nuclei of the lateral lemniscus of the cat. *Journal of Neurophysiology,* 1970, **33,** 421–40.

**Allison, A. C.** The morphology of the olfactory system in the vertebrates. *Biological Reviews,* 1953, **28,** 195–244.

**Andres, K. H.** Neue Befunde zur Feinstruktur des olfaktorischen Saumes. *Journal of Ultrastructure Research,* 1968, **25,** 163. (Abstract)

**Baker, P. F., Hodgkin, A. L., & Shaw, T. I.** Replacement of the protoplasm of a giant nerve fibre with artificial solutions. *Nature* (London), 1961, **190,** 885–87.

**Bannister, L. H.** The fine structure of the olfactory surface of teleostean fishes. *Quarterly Journal of Microscopical Science*, 1965, **106,** 333–42.

**Bargoot, F. G., Williams, T. P., & Beidler, L. M.** The localization of radioactive amino acid taken up into the outer segments of frog rods. *Vision Research,* 1969, **9,** 385–91.

**Barlow, H. B., Hill, R. M., & Levick, W. R.** Retinal ganglion cells responding selectively to direction and speed of image motion in the rabbit. *Journal of Physiology,* 1964, **173,** 377–407.

**Bartley, S. H.** Some factors in brightness discrimination. *Psychological Review,* 1939, **46,** 337–58. Figure 5, p. 347, Copyright 1939 by the American Psychological Association, and reproduced by permission.

**Beidler, L. M.** Innervation of rat fungiform papilla. In C. Pfaffmann (Ed.), *Olfaction and taste III.* New York: Rockefeller University Press, 1969. Pp. 352–69.

**Beidler, L. M., & Smallman, R. L.** Renewal of cells within taste buds. *Journal of Cell Biology,* 1965, **27,** 263–72.

**Békésy, G. von.** *Experiments in hearing.* E. G. Wever (Ed.) New York: McGraw-Hill, 1960.

**Békésy, G. von, & Rosenblith, W. A.** The mechanical properties of the ear. In S. S. Stevens (Ed.), *Handbook of experimental psychology.* New York: Wiley, 1951. Pp. 1075–115.

**Bennett, M. V. L.** Electroreceptors in mormyrids. *Cold Spring Harbor Symposia on Quantitative Biology,* 1965, **30,** 245–62.

**Blasie, J. K., Dewey, M. M., Blaurock, A. E., & Worthington, O. R.** Electron microscope and low-angle x-ray diffraction studies on outer segment membranes from the retina of the frog. *Journal of Molecular Biology,* 1965, **14,** 143–52.

**Bodian, D.** The generalized vertebrate neuron. *Science,* 1962, **137,** 323–26. Figure 1, p. 325, Copyright © 1962 by the American Association for the Advancement of Science, and reproduced by permission.

**Bodian, D.** Development of fine structures of spinal cord in monkey fetuses (Macaca irus): I. The motoneuron neuropil at the time of onset of reflex activity. *Bulletin of the Johns Hopkins Hospital,* 1966, **119,** 129–33.

**Bredberg, G., Lindeman, H. H., Ades, H. W., West, R., & Engström, H.** Scanning electron microscopy of the organ of Corti. *Science,* 1970, **170,** 861–63. Figure 2, p. 862, Copyright © 1970 by the American Association for the Advancement of Science, and reproduced by permission.

**Brettschneider, H. von.** Electronmikroskopische Untersuchungen an der Nasenscheimheit. *Anatomischer Anzeiger,* 1958, **105,** 194–204. Cited by Moulton & Beidler, 1967.

**Brown, J. E., & Major, D.** Cat retinal ganglion cell dendritic fields. *Experimental Neurology,* 1966, **15,** 70–78.

**Brown, K. T., & Murakami, M.** A new receptor potential of the monkey retina with no detectable latency. *Nature* (London), 1964, **201,** 626–28. (a)

**Brown, K. T., & Murakami, M.** Biphasic form of the early receptor potential of the monkey retina. *Nature* (London), 1964, **204,** 739–40. (b)

**Brown, K. T., & Watanabe, K.** Isolation and identification of a receptor from the pure cone fovea of the monkey retina. *Nature* (London), 1962, **193,** 958–60.

**Brown, K. T., Watanabe, K., & Murakami, M.** The early and late receptor potentials of monkey cones and rods. *Cold Spring Harbor Symposia on Quantitative Biology,* 1965, **30,** 457–82.

**Brown, T. S., Gedvilas, G., & Marco, L. A.** Effect of auditory cortical lesions on a test of frequency discrimination in the cat. *Proceedings of the 75th Annual Convention of the American Psychological Association,* 1967, **2,** 101–2.

**Brunn, A. von.** Beiträge zur mikroskopischen Anatomie der menschlichen Nasenhöhle. *Archiv für Mikroskopische Anatomie* (Bonn), 1892, **39,** 632–51. Cited by Moulton & Beidler, 1967.

**Cajal, Ramón y, S.** *Trabajos del Laboratorio de investigaciones biológicas de la Universidad de Madrid,* Tomo I, 1901–2. (Translated in L. M. Kraft, *Studies on the cerebral cortex.* Chicago: Year Book Publishers, 1955.)

**Caldwell, P. C., & Keynes, R. D.** The utilization of phosphate bond energy for sodium extrusion from giant axons. *Journal of Physiology* (London), 1957, **137,** 12P–13P.

**Chambers, M. R., Andres, K. H., Duering, M. von, & Iggo, A.** The structure and function of the slowly adapting Type II mechanoreceptor in hairy skin. *Quarterly Journal of Experimental Physiology,* 1972, **57,** 417–45.

**Cohen, A. I.** Vertebrate retinal cells and their organization. *Biological Reviews,* 1963, **38,** 427–59. Figure 2, p. 435, reproduced by permission of the Cambridge University Press.

**Cone, R. A.** Early receptor potential of the vertebrate retina. *Nature* (London), 1964, **204,** 736–40.

**Cone, R. A., & Brown, P. K.** Dependence of the early receptor potential on the orientation of rhodopsin. *Science,* 1967, **156,** 536.

**Dallos, P., Billone, M. C., Durrant, J. D., Wang, C.-Y., & Raynor, S.** Cochlear inner and outer hair cells: Functional differences. *Science,* 1972, **177,** 356–58.

**Davis, H.** Some principles of sensory receptor action. *Physiological Reviews,* 1961, **41,** 391–416.

**Davis, H., & Associates.** Acoustic trauma in the guinea pig. *Journal of the Acoustical Society of America,* 1953, **25,** 1180–89, Figure 1, p. 1182, reproduced by permission of the American Institute of Physics and the author.

**DelCastillo, J., & Katz, B.** Biophysical aspects of neuromuscular transmission. *Progress in Biophysics and Biophysical Chemistry,* 1956, **6,** 121–70.

**de Lorenzo, A. J.** Electron microscopy of the hippocampus and olfactory nerve. *Anatomical Record,* 1956, **124,** 328.

**de Lorenzo, A. J.** Electron microscopy of the olfactory and gustatory pathways. *Annals of Otology, Rhinology, and Laryngology,* 1960, **69,** 410–20.

**De Robertis, E.** *Histophysiology of synapses and neurosecretion.* Oxford: Pergamon Press, 1964. Figure 3–5, p. 36, reproduced by permission.

**De Robertis, E., & Bennett, H. S.** Some features of the submicroscopic morphology of synapses in frog and earthworm. *Journal of Biophysical and Biochemical Cytology,* 1955, **1,** 47–58.

**De Robertis, E., & Vaz Ferreira, A.** Submicroscopic changes of the nerve endings in the adrenal medulla after stimulation of the splanchnic nerve. *Journal of Biophysical and Biochemical Cytology,* 1957, **3,** 611–14.

**De Valois, R. L.** Behavioral and electrophysiological studies of primate vision. In W. D. Neff (Ed.), *Contributions to sensory physiology.* Vol. 1. New York: Academic Press, 1965. Pp. 137–78.

**De Valois, R. L., Jacobs, G. H., & Jones, A. E.** Responses of single cells in primate red-green color vision system. *Optik,* 1963, **20,** Heft 2, 87. Figure 4, p. 93, reproduced by permission.

**Diamond, I. T., Goldberg, J. M., & Neff, W. D.** Tonal discrimination after ablation of auditory cortex. *Journal of Neurophysiology,* 1962, **25,** 223–35.

**Diamond, I. T., & Neff, W. D.** Ablation of temporal cortex and discrimination of auditory patterns. *Journal of Neurophysiology,* 1957, **20,** 300–315.

**Doetsch, G. S., Ganchrow, J. J., Nelson, L. M., & Erickson, R. P.** Information processing in the taste system of the rat. In C. Pfaffmann (Ed.), *Olfaction and taste III.* New York: Rockefeller University Press, 1969. Pp. 492–511.

**Dowling, J. E.** Foveal receptors of the monkey retina: Fine structures. *Science,* 1965, **147,** 57–59.

**Dowling, J. E., & Boycott, B. B.** Organization of the primate retina: Electron microscopy. *Proceedings of the Royal Society of London,* Series B., 1966, **166,** 80–111. Figure 23, p. 104, reproduced by permission of The Royal Society and the authors.

**Eccles, J. C.** The synapse. *Scientific American,* 1965, **212**(1), 56–66. Figure, p. 66, Copyright © 1964 by Scientific American, Inc. All rights reserved. Reproduced by permission.

**Engström, H., Ades, H. W., & Hawkins, J. E.** Cellular pattern, nerve structures, and fluid spaces of the organ of Corti. In W. D. Neff (Ed.), *Contributions to sensory physiology.* Vol. 1. New York: Academic Press, 1965. Pp. 1–37. Figures 8, p. 11, and 13, p. 16, Copyright © 1965 by Academic Press, Inc., and reproduced by permission.

**Engström, H., & Rytzner, C.** The fine structure of taste buds and taste fibers. *Annals of Otology, Rhinology, and Laryngology,* 1956, **65,** 361–75. (a)

**Engström, H., & Rytzner, C.** The structure of taste buds. *Acta Oto-Laryngologica,* 1956, **46,** 361–67. (b)

**Erickson, R. P.** Sensory neural patterns and gustation. In Y. Zotterman (Ed.), *Olfaction and taste I.* Oxford: Pergamon Press, 1963. Pp. 205–13. Figure 4, p. 210, reproduced by permission.

**Evans, E. F., Ross, H. F., & Whitfield, I. C.** The spatial distribution of unit characteristic frequency in the primary auditory cortex of the cat. *Journal of Physiology,* 1965, **179,** 238–47.

**Faber, D. S., & Korn, H.** A neuronal inhibition mediated electrically. *Science,* 1973, **179,** 577–78.

**Farbman, A. I.** Electron microscope study of the developing taste bud in rat fungiform papilla. *Developmental Biology,* 1965, **11,** 110–35.

**Fatt, P., & Katz, B.** Spontaneous subthreshold activity at motor nerve endings. *Journal of Physiology,* 1952, **117,** 109–28.

**Flock, Å.** Transducing mechanisms in the lateral line canal organ receptors. *Cold Spring Harbor Symposia on Quantitative Biology,* 1965, **30,** 133–45.

**Flock, Å.** Transduction in single hair cells in the lateral line organ. In L. M. Beidler & W. E. Reichardt, Sensory transduction. *Neurosciences Research Program Bulletin,* 1970, **8**(5), 492–96. Figure 13, p. 496, reproduced by permission of the Neurosciences Research Program and the author.

**Gardner, E.** *Fundamentals of neurology.* (5th ed.) Philadelphia: Saunders, 1968. Figure 117, p. 206, Copyright © 1968 by W. B. Saunders Company, and reproduced by permission.

**Garey, L. J.** Interrelationships of the visual cortex and superior colliculus in the cat. *Nature* (London), 1965, **207,** 1410–11.

**Gasser, H. S.** Olfactory nerve fibers. *Journal of General Physiology,* 1956, **39,** 473–96.

**Geldard, F. A.** *The human senses.* (2nd ed.) New York: Wiley, 1972.

**Gernandt, B.** Response of mammalian vestibular neurons to horizontal rotation and caloric stimulation. *Journal of Neurophysiology,* 1949, **12,** 173–85.

**Gesteland, R. C., Lettvin, J. Y., & Pitts, W. H.** Chemical transmission in the nose of the frog. *Journal of Physiology* (London), 1965, **181,** 525–59.

**Gesteland, R. C., Lettvin, J. Y., Pitts, W. H., & Rojas, A.** Odor specificities of the frog's olfactory receptors. In Y. Zotterman (Ed.), *Olfaction and taste I.* Oxford: Pergamon Press, 1963. Pp. 19–44. Figure 13, p. 30, reproduced by permission.

**Goldberg, J. M., & Neff, W. D.** Frequency discrimination after bilateral ablation of cortical auditory areas. *Journal of Neurophysiology,* 1961, **24,** 119–28.

**Gouras, P.** Identification of cone mechanisms in monkey ganglion cells. *Journal of Physiology,* 1968, **199,** 533–47.

**Gouras, P.** Trichromatic mechanisms in single cortical neurons. *Science,* 1970, **168,** 489–92.

**Gray, E. G.** Axosomatic and axodendritic synapses of the cerebral cortex: An electron microscope study. *Journal of Anatomy* (London), 1959, **93,** 420–33.

**Gray, E. G.** Electron microscopy of excitatory and inhibitory synapses: A brief review. In K. Akert & P. G. Waser (Eds.), *Progress in brain research.* Vol. 31. *Mechanisms of synaptic transmission.* Amsterdam: Elsevier, 1969, Pp. 141–55.

**Graziadei, P. P. C.** The ultrastructure of vertebrate taste buds. In C. Pfaffmann, (Ed.), *Olfaction and taste III.* New York: Rockefeller University Press, 1969, Pp. 315–30.

**Grillo, M. A., & Palay, S. L.** Granule-containing vesicles in the autonomic nervous system. In S. S. Breese, Jr. (Ed.), *Electron microscopy.* Vol. 2. New York: Academic Press, 1962. Pp. U–1.

**Grundfest, H.** Electrical inexcitability of synapses and some of its consequences in the central nervous system. *Physiological Reviews,* 1957, **37,** 337–61. Figure 2, p. 343, reproduced by permission of The American Physiological Society and the author.

**Gulick, W. L.** *Hearing: Physiology and psychophysics.* New York: Oxford University Press, 1971.

**Hodgkin, A. L.** Ionic movements and electrical activity in giant nerve fibres. *Proceedings of the Royal Society of London,* Series B, 1958, **148,** 1–37.

**Hodgkin, A. L., & Huxley, A. F.** A quantitative description of membrane current and its application to conduction and excitation in the nerve. *Journal of Physiology,* 1952, **117,** 500–544. Figure 17, p. 530, reproduced by permission.

**Hodgkin, A. L., Huxley, A. F., & Katz, B.** Ionic currents underlying the activity in the giant axon of the squid. *Archives des Sciences Physiologiques,* 1949, **3,** 129–50.

**Hodgkin, A. L., & Katz, B.** The effect of sodium ions on the electrical activity of the giant axon of the squid. *Journal of Physiology,* 1949, **108,** 37–77.

**Hodgkin, A. L., & Keynes, R. D.** Active transport of cations in giant axons from *Sepia* and *Loligo. Journal of Physiology* (London), 1955, **128,** 28–60.

**Hopkins, A. E.** Olfactory receptors in vertebrates. *Journal of Comparative Neurology,* 1926, **41,** 253–89.

**House, E. L., & Pansky, B.** *Functional approach to neuroanatomy.* (2nd ed.) New York: McGraw-Hill, 1967. Figures 8–2, p. 155, 8–10, p. 166, and 8–13, p. 170, Copyright © 1967 by the McGraw-Hill Book Company, Inc. Used with permission of McGraw-Hill Book Company.

**Houssay, B. A., Lewis, J. T., Orías, O., Braun-Menéndez, E., Hug, E., Foglia, V. G., & Leloir, L. F.** *Human physiology.* (2nd ed.) New York: McGraw-Hill, 1955. Figure 411, p. 934, Copyright, 1951, 1955, by the McGraw-Hill Book Company, Inc. Used with permission of McGraw-Hill Book Company.

**Hubel, D. H., & Wiesel, T. N.** Receptive fields, binocular interaction and functional architecture in the cat's visual cortex. *Journal of Physiology*, 1962, **160**, 106–54.

**Hubel, D. H., & Wiesel, T. N.** Shape and arrangement of columns in the cat's striate cortex. *Journal of Physiology*, 1963, **165**, 559–68.

**Hubel, D. H., & Wiesel, T. N.** Receptive fields and functional architecture in two nonstriate visual areas (18 and 19) of the cat. *Journal of Neurophysiology*, 1965, **28**, 229–89. Figures 16, p. 250, and 38, p. 280, reproduced by permission of The American Physiological Society and the authors.

**Hubel, D. H., & Wiesel, T. N.** Receptive fields and functional architecture of monkey striate cortex. *Journal of Physiology*, 1968, **195**, 215–43.

**Iggo, A.** New specific sensory structures in hairy skin. *Acta Neurovegetativa*, 1962, **24**, 175–79.

**Judd, D. B., & Wyszecki, G.** *Color in business, science, and industry*. (2nd ed.) New York: Wiley, 1963.

**Kalmus, H., & Hubbard, S. J.** *The chemical senses in health and disease*. Springfield, Ill.: Charles C Thomas, 1960. Figure 2(a), p. 27, Courtesy of Charles C Thomas, Publisher, Springfield, Illinois.

**Kandel, E. R., Frazier, W. T., Waziri, R., & Coggleshall, R. E.** Direct and common connections among identified neurons in *Aplysia*. *Journal of Neurophysiology*, 1967, **30**, 1352–76.

**Katsuki, Y.** Neural mechanism of auditory sensation in cats. In W. A. Rosenblith (Ed.), *Sensory communication*. Cambridge, Mass.: M.I.T. Press, 1961. Pp. 561–83.

**Kiang, N. Y.** *Discharge patterns of single fibers in the cat's auditory nerve*. Cambridge, Mass.: M.I.T. Press, 1965. Figure 7.2, p. 86, reprinted by permission of the M.I.T. Press, Cambridge, Massachusetts. Copyright © 1965 by The Massachusetts Institute of Technology.

**Kimura, K., & Beidler, L. M.** Microelectrode study of taste receptors of rat and hamster. *Journal of Cellular and Comparative Physiology*, 1961, **58**, 131–39.

**Kuffler, S. W.** Discharge patterns and functional organization of mammalian retina. *Journal of Neurophysiology*, 1953, **16**, 37–68.

**Le Gros Clark, W. E.** Observations on the structure and organization of the olfactory receptors in the rabbit. *Yale Journal of Biology and Medicine*, 1956, **29**, 83–95.

**Leicester, J., & Stone, J.** Ganglion, amacrine and horizontal cells of the cat's retina. *Vision Research*, 1967, **7**, 695–705.

**Lim, D.** Morphological relationship between the tectorial membrane and the organ of Corti: Scanning and transmission electron microscopy. *Journal of the Acoustical Society of America*, 1971, **50**, 92.

**Lindblom, U., & Tapper, D. N.** Terminal properties of a vibrotactile sensor. *Experimental Neurology*, 1967, **17**, 1–15.

**Ling, G., & Gerard, R. W.** The normal membrane potential of frog sartorius fibers. *Journal of Cellular and Comparative Physiology*, 1949, **34**, 383–96.

**Lohman, A. H. M., & Mentink, G. M.** The lateral olfactory tract, the anterior commissure and the cells of the olfactory bulb. *Brain Research*, 1969, **12**, 396–413.

**Löwenstein, O., & Sand, A.** The mechanism of the semicircular canal: A study of the responses of single-fibre preparation to angular accelerations and to rotation at constant speed. *Proceedings of the Royal Society of London*, Series B., 1940, **129**, 256–75.

**Marshall, D. A.** A comparative study of neural coding in gustation. *Physiology and Behavior*, 1968, **3**, 1–15.

**McLennan, H.** *Synaptic transmission*. (2nd ed.) Philadelphia: Saunders, 1970.

**Montagna, W. (Ed.)** *Advances in biology of the skin*. Vol. 1. *Cutaneous innervation*. Oxford: Pergamon Press, 1960.

**Moulton, D. G., & Beidler, L. M.** Structure and function in the peripheral olfactory system. *Physiological Reviews*, 1967, **47**, 1–52.

**Mozell, M. M.** Olfactory and neural responses in the frog. *American Journal of Physiology*, 1962, **203**, 353–58.

**Nicoll, R. A.** Identification of tufted cells in the olfactory bulb. *Nature* (London), 1970, **227**, 623–25.

**Nilsson, S. E. G.** A globular substructure of the retinal receptor outer segment membranes and some other cell membranes in the tadpole. *Nature* (London), 1964, **202**, 509–10.

**Nilsson, S. E. G.** The ultrastructure of the receptor outer segments in the retina of the leopard frog. *Journal of Ultrastructure Research*, 1965, **12**, 207–31.

**Ogawa, H., Sato, M., & Yamashita, S.** Multiple sensitivity of chorda tympani fibers of the rat and hamster to gustatory and thermal stimuli. *Journal of Physiology* (London), 1968, **199**, 223–40.

**Okano, M., Weber, A. F., & Frommes, S. P.** Electron microscopic studies of the distal border of the canine olfactory epithelium. *Journal of Ultrastructure Research*, 1967, **17**, 487–502.

**Østerberg, G. A.** Topography of the layer of rods and cones in the human retina. *Acta Ophthalmologica* (Køjbenhavn), Suppl. 6, 1935, **61**, 1–102.

**Ottoson, D.** Analysis of the electrical activity of the olfactory epithelium. *Acta Physiologica Scandinavica*, 1956, **35** (Suppl. 122), 1–83. Figures 20, p. 48, and 23C, p. 57, reproduced by permission of the publisher.

**Ottoson, D., & Shepherd, G. M.** Experiments and concepts in olfactory physiology. In Y. Zotterman (Ed.), *Progress in brain research*. Vol. 23. *Sensory mechanisms*. Amsterdam: Elsevier, 1967. Pp. 83–138.

**Pak, W. L., & Cone, R. A.** Isolation and identification of the initial peak of the early receptor potential. *Nature* (London), 1964, **204**, 836.

**Pappas, G. D., & Bennett, M. V. L.** Specialized junctions involved in electrical transmission between neurons. *Annals of the New York Academy of Sciences*, 1966, **137**, 495–508.

**Parker, G. H.** *Smell, taste and allied senses in vertebrates*. Philadelphia: Lippincott, 1922.

**Pfaffmann, C.** Gustatory nerve impulses in rat, cat and rabbit. *Journal of Neurophysiology*, 1955, **18**, 429–40.

**Plotz, E., & Perlman, H. B.** A histochemical study of the cochlea. *Laryngoscope*, 1955, **65**, 291.

**Pollen, D. A., Lee, J. R., & Taylor, J. H.** How does the striate cortex begin the reconstruction of the visual world? *Science*, 1971, **173**, 74–77.

**Rall, W., Shepherd, G. M., Reese, T. S., & Brightman, M. W.** Dendrodendritic synaptic pathway for inhibition in the olfactory bulb. *Experimental Neurology*, 1966, **14**, 44–56.

**Rasmussen, G. L.** The olivary peduncle and other fiber projections of the superior olivary complex. *Journal of Comparative Neurology*, 1946, **84**, 141–219.

**Rhode, W. S.** Observation of the vibration of the basilar membrane in squirrel monkeys using the Mössbauer technique. *Journal of the Acoustical Society of America*, 1971, **49**, 1218–31.

**Rose, J. E.** Organization of frequency sensitive neurons in the cochlear nuclear complex of the cat. In G. L. Rasmussen & W. F. Windle (Eds.), *Neural mechanisms of the auditory and vestibular systems*. Springfield, Ill.: Charles C Thomas, 1960. Pp. 116–36.

**Rose, J. E., Greenwood, D. D., Goldberg, J. M., & Hind, J. E.** Some discharge characteristics of single neurons in the inferior colliculus of the cat: I. Tonotopical organization, relation of spike counts to tone intensity, and firing patterns of single elements. *Journal of Neurophysiology*, 1963, **26**, 294–320.

**Rushton, W. A. H.** Physical measurement of cone pigments in the living human eye. *Nature* (London), 1957, **179**, 571–73.

**Schuknecht, H. F.** Neuroanatomical correlates of auditory sensitivity and pitch discriminations in the cat. In G. L. Rasmussen & W. F. Windle (Eds.), *Neural mechanisms of the auditory and vestibular systems*. Springfield, Ill.: Charles C Thomas, 1960. Pp. 76–90.

**Scott, T. R., & Erickson, R. P.** Synaptic processing of taste-quality information in the thalamus of the rat. *Journal of Neurophysiology*, 1971, **34**, 868–84.

**Shibuya, T.** Dissociation of olfactory neural response and mucosal potential. *Science*, 1964, **143**, 1338–40.

**Shibuya, T., & Takagi, S. F.** Electrical response and growth of olfactory cilia of the olfactory epithelium of the newt in water and on land. *Journal of General Physiology*, 1963, **47**, 71–82.

**Sjöstrand, F. S.** The ultrastructure of the outer segments of rods and cones of the eye as revealed by the electron microscope. *Journal of Cellular and Comparative Physiology*, 1953, **42**, 15–45.

**Spoendlin, H.** Ultrastructure and peripheral innervation pattern of the receptor in relation to the first coding of the acoustic message. In A. V. S. DeReuck & J. Knight (Eds.), *Hearing mechanisms in vertebrates*. Boston: Little, Brown, 1968. Pp. 89–125.

**Steinbrecht, R. A.** Comparative morphology of olfactory receptors. In C. Pfaffmann (Ed.), *Olfaction and taste III*. New York: Rockefeller University Press, 1969, Pp. 3–21. Figure 1A, p. 5, reproduced by permission of The Rockefeller University Press and the author.

**Tapper, D. N.** Stimulus-response relationships in the cutaneous slowly adapting mechanoreceptor in hairy skin of the cat. *Experimental Neurology*, 1965, **13**, 364–85.

**Tauc, L.** Polyphasic synaptic activity. In K. Akert & P. G. Waser (Eds.), *Progress in brain research*. Vol. 31. *Mechanisms of synaptic transmission*. Amsterdam: Elsevier, 1969. Pp. 247–57.

**Tauc, L., & Gerschenfeld, H. M.** Cholinergic transmission mechanism for both excitation and inhibition in Molluscan central synapses. *Nature* (London), 1961, **192**, 366–67.

**Thompson, R. F.** *Foundations of physiological psychology*. New York: Harper & Row, 1967.

**Trujillo-Cenoz, O.** Some aspects of the structural organization of the arthropod eye. *Cold Spring Harbor Symposia on Quantitative Biology*, 1965, **30**, 371–82.

**Tsuchitani, C., & Boudreau, J. C.** Single unit analysis of cat superior olive S-segment with tonal stimuli. *Journal of Neurophysiology*, 1966, **29**, 684–97.

**Uchizono, K.** Characteristics of excitatory and inhibitory synapses in the central nervous system of the cat. *Nature* (London), 1965, **207**, 642–43.

**Valverde, F.** *Studies on the piriform lobe*. Cambridge, Mass.: Harvard University Press, 1965.

**Wald, G.** Retinal chemistry and the physiology of vision. In *Visual problems of color*. New York: Chemical Publishing Co., 1961. Pp. 15–68.

**Wald, G.** The receptors of human color vision. *Science*, 1964, **145**, 1007–17.

**Walzl, E. M., & Bordley, J. E.** The effect of small lesions of the organ of Corti on cochlear potentials. *American Journal of Physiology*, 1942, **135**, 351–60.

**Wertheim, T.** Über die indirekte Sehschärfe. *Zeitschrift für Psychologie*, 1894, **7**, 172–87.

**Westrum, O. E.** Synaptic contacts on axons in the cerebral cortex. *Nature* (London), 1966, **210**, 1289–90.

**Whitfield, I. C.** *The auditory pathway*. (Monographs of the Physiological Society.) London: Edward Arnold, 1967. Figure 1.5, p. 12, reproduced by permission of the author and the publisher.

**Whitfield, I. C., & Evans, E. F.** Responses of auditory cortical neurons to stimuli of changing frequency. *Journal of Neurophysiology*, 1965, **28**, 655–72.

**Winkelmann, R. K.** *Nerve endings in normal and pathologic skin*. Springfield, Ill.: Charles C Thomas, 1960.

**Woodbury, J. W., & Patton, H. D.** Action potential: Cable and excitable properties of the cell membrane. In T. C. Ruch & J. F. Fulton (Eds.), *Medical physiology and biophysics*. (18th ed.) Philadelphia: Saunders, 1960. Pp. 32–65. Figure 12, p. 39, Copyright © 1960, by W. B. Saunders Company, and reproduced by permission.

**Woodson, W. E.** *Human engineering guide for equipment designers*. Berkeley: University of California Press, 1954. Figure, p. 2–15, originally published by the University of California Press; reprinted by permission of The Regents of the University of California.

**Young, R. W., & Bok, D.** Participation of the retinal pigment epithelium in the rod outer segment renewal process. *Journal of Cell Biology*, 1969, **42**, 392–403.

**Young, R. W., & Droz, B.** The renewal of protein in retinal rods and cones. *Journal of Cell Biology*, 1968, **39**, 169–84.

**Zwislocki, J.** Analysis of the middle-ear function: I. Input impedance. *Journal of the Acoustical Society of America*, 1962, **34**(2), 1514–23.

# 4

# AUDITION

**Bertram Scharf**
**Northeastern University**

When sensory psychologists study hearing, they often call their discipline *psychoacoustics,* the study of the relation between the subjective response and the physical (acoustical) stimulus. What are the limits of hearing? What is the weakest sound we can detect and the strongest sound we can tolerate? What are the lowest and highest frequencies we can hear? And how easily can we tell when a sound has been changed? The measurement of auditory thresholds, both absolute and differential thresholds, has long occupied psychoacousticians. But most of the time we hear sounds easily, indeed too easily as people living near airports can testify. So, psychoacoustics is also about how sounds are heard at levels well above threshold. How do the pitch, loudness, size, location of sound depend on stimulus and subject variables? One must look at both the stimulus—sound in all its forms from rustling leaves to roaring jets—and the receiver—the listener with highly specialized ears and a marvelously complex nervous system. This chapter deals with all these questions, but in order to understand how people hear sounds, first we must know something about sound, what it is and how it is generated, controlled, and measured in the experimental study of hearing.

## SOUND

Sufficiently large and rapid displacement of the eardrum gives rise to sensations of sound. The eardrum's back-and-forth motion is transmitted over the three small bones of the middle ear into the inner ear where a traveling wave along the basilar membrane causes the cilia of the hair cells to bend, thus exciting the auditory nerve to fire. This transmission process and the ensuing neural events will be discussed after consideration of the physics of sound.

Sound is the result of motion. The source of the motion is usually a solid body activated by its own displacement or by impact, e.g., a vibrating string, shoes hitting the floor, or the turning blades of a fan. For the sound to be heard, the vibration of the solid body must be transmitted to the eardrum. The role of air as a common medium of transmission was recognized by the Greeks, but its importance was not

Preparation of this chapter was supported in part by a grant from the U.S. Public Health Service, National Institute of Neurological Diseases and Stroke. The author wishes to thank Ms. Rhona Hellman, Dr. Ronald Hinchcliffe, and Professor W. J. Remillard for their many helpful suggestions.

demonstrated until the invention of the air pump in the seventeenth century. Using the air pump, Boyle took the air out of a chamber containing a bell. In the resulting vacuum, the bell could barely be heard when rung. By letting some air back into the chamber, Boyle could plainly hear the bell again. Boyle thought he had clearly proved that air is needed to transmit sound. Subsequent analyses (Lindsay, 1966) have shown that the lack of air made it difficult to get the sound out of the bell into the air (owing to a so-called impedance mismatch), so that Boyle had not really tested sound transmission. Nevertheless, his conclusion was correct; air or some elastic medium is necessary for sound transmission.

## Sound transmission

Since sound is the result of motion, its transmission from one place to another means that motion is transmitted. Consequently, something must first be set in motion. As a solid body vibrates, it impresses a regular motion on nearby air molecules which are easily moved and, in fact, are already constantly in motion. These particles, in turn, set in motion particles next to them. In this way the original motion is transmitted far afield, as long as there are free air and sufficient energy. Note, however, that no molecules are transported with the sound; only the disturbance moves or is propagated through space. This transmission of energy without transportation of particles is called a *wave motion*. When Boyle showed that sound depends on the presence of air, he also refuted the alternative theory that the sound source emits particles that move through space and are collected by the ear.

### *Inverse-square law*

If the vibrating source is spherical, the disturbance will radiate in all directions, and the volume of air set in motion will increase with distance. Clearly then, the local disturbance cannot remain as strong when more air must be moved, and the disturbance of each particle is weaker far from the source where many more particles are set in motion than close to the source where relatively few particles are involved. The decrease in the strength of the disturbance is governed by the *inverse-square law*. The strength, or intensity, of a sound decreases inversely with the square of the distance from the sound source. This law is valid because the area of disturbance is equal to the surface of a sphere, which is proportional to the square of the sphere's radius. The radius is the distance from the vibrating source to the area or surface of disturbance; so as the distance increases, the surface being set in motion increases as the square of the distance. If the distance is doubled, the surface is quadrupled, as is the number of molecules that must be set in motion. The intensity of the sound at any point on the surface is then reduced to one-fourth.

### *Velocity of sound*

In air, sound travels approximately 331 meters (1100 feet) per second at 0° C (32° F), but its velocity increases with temperature. Higher temperature results in greater velocity by reducing the air's density, its compressibility, or both. In general, sound travels faster through less dense or less compressible (i.e., more elastic) media. Thus, although fluids and solids are denser than air and other gases, they are so much less compressible that they transmit sound more rapidly than air does. Sound velocity plays an important role in localization of sounds (as discussed later in the chapter) and when listening in large enclosed areas.

## Pure tones

The simplest acoustic motion and the kind most often used in the laboratory, although seldom met in nature, is *simple harmonic motion*. The sound associated with harmonic motion is called a *pure tone*. Lending itself to a simple mathematical expression, harmonic motion occurs when the displacement of the air particles is proportional to the applied force. Under this condition the particles move back and forth in a repetitive pattern. This motion continues as long as force is applied by the vibrating source. Usually the source does not stop vibrating abruptly, but rather its displacements gradually become smaller until finally the motion stops altogether. The air particles follow this change. During the starting and stopping of the vibratory motion, however, certain complications arise that will be dealt with later in a discussion of transients.

Harmonic motion produces a continuous change in the speed of the air particles. The particles move most rapidly as they cross the place where they were originally located; they slow down as they move out to their maximum distance where they stop and start moving back. Thus, the particle's velocity changes as a function of displacement. The change from maximum speed to zero speed is a smooth process, as is the reverse change from zero to maximum speed. Velocity is a simple sinusoidal function of time ($t$), as shown in Figure 4.1A. Of course, no sound ever started with an instantaneous shift from zero velocity (on the average) to maximum velocity as Figure 4.1A would seem to indicate, but this simplification does not alter the basic process.

Although particle velocity is one important measure of simple harmonic motion, particle displacement and pressure are even more important in hearing. Displacement refers to the particle's distance from its original location, or average resting place. Figure 4.1B gives the function for displacement: At the onset of the motion, when $t = 0$, displacement is 0 since the particle is at its resting place, but velocity is maximum. Otherwise displacement changes as a function of $t$ in exactly the same way as velocity. The equation for the displacement is

$$d = A \sin \omega t, \quad [1]$$

where $d$ is the displacement, $A$ is the maximum displacement, or *amplitude*, $t$ is time, and $\omega$ is angular velocity. (Angular velocity may be thought of as the rate of change in the size of an angle, and is measured as degrees or radians per second.) The meaning of $\omega$ is made clearer by relating the sinusoidal function to circular motion in Figure 4.2.

Panel A represents a vibrating particle as it moves back and forth along a path drawn as a dashed line in the vertical plane. The particle's original position, $O$, is the center of a circle drawn with radius equal to the amplitude, $A$, of displacement, which is the same in both directions along the vertical path. The circle can help clarify the trigonometric meaning of sinusoidal motion.

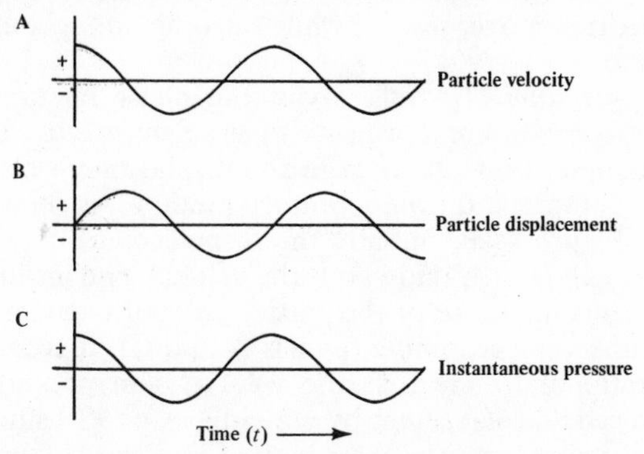


**Figure 4.1** Curves showing the various aspects of a sinusoidal sound wave. (After Stevens & Davis, 1938.)

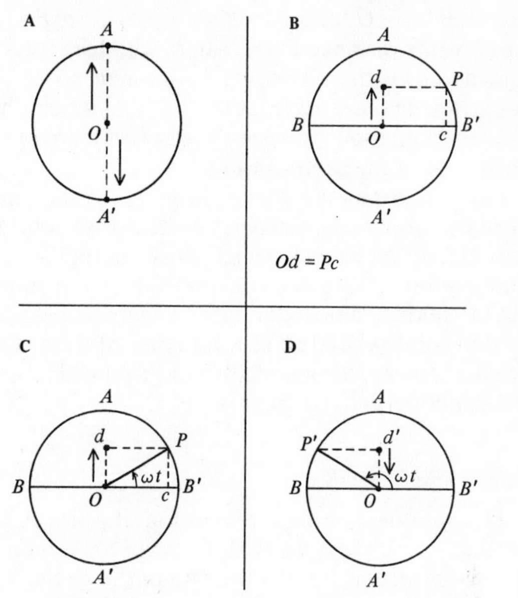


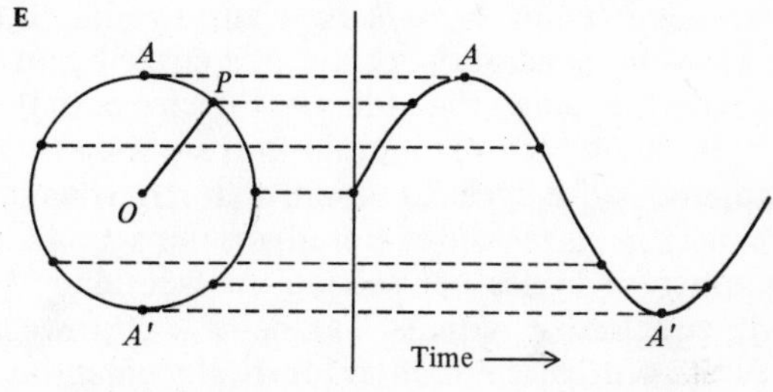


**Figure 4.2** Derivation of the sinusoidal function from the projection of the position of a particle undergoing simple harmonic motion onto a circle. See text for discussion.

In Figure 4.2B, the particle is shown at a locus, $d$, between $O$ and $A$, which represents the displacement of the particle from its original position at a given moment. The projection of $d$ onto the circle at point $P$ is such that the vertical distance from $P$ to point $c$ on the horizontal diameter, $\overline{BB'}$, is always equal to the distance between $d$ and $O$. In simple harmonic motion, the projected point $P$ moves around the circle at a constant angular velocity, $\omega$. To show that $d$, or equivalently $\overline{Pc}$, is a sinusoidal function of $\omega$ and time, we construct a right triangle between points $O$, $c$, and $P$ in Figure 4.2C. Angle $POc$ is changing with time, $t$, at rate $\omega$, since $\omega$ is the angular velocity of the moving point, $P$. Since $\angle POc/t = \omega$, the value of the angle is equal to $\omega t$ and is so labeled in the figure. The sine of the angle $\omega t$ is equal to $d/P$, where $d$ is the distance from $O$ to $d$ (and equivalently from $P$ to $c$), and $P$ is the distance from $O$ to $P$, which is equal to the radius of the circle, $A$. So we can write the equation, $\sin \omega t = d/A$, as $d = A \sin \omega t$, which is the same equation given for the displacement of the particle as a function of time.

Panel D shows the projected point, $P'$, at a new position which corresponds to the position of the particle, $d'$, on its way back from $A$. Panel E shows that a point moving at a constant velocity around a circle yields a sinusoidal curve when the position of the point is plotted as a function of time. This graphic construction is equivalent to the algebraic construction derived from panel C.

### *Period and frequency*

During one complete revolution of point $P$, the particle completes one cycle, moving to $A$, then to $A'$, and returning to $O$ at the end of the cycle. The duration required to complete one full cycle is called a *period.* During one period, point $P$ moves through 360°, or $2\pi$ *radians,* where 1 radian is the angle subtended at the center of a circle by an arc of length equal to the radius of the circle. In these terms, a quarter of a cycle corresponds to $\pi/2$ radians, half a cycle to $\pi$, and so forth. If angular velocity, $\omega$, is measured in radians per second, the number of cycles per second, or frequency ($f$), will equal $\omega/2\pi$ radians. Taking $\omega = 2\pi f$, we can rewrite our basic equation for displacement as

$$d = A \sin 2\pi f t. \qquad [2]$$

Frequency is measured in *Hertz (Hz),* which is an international unit equal to 1 cycle per second. This equation means that the size of displacement, $d$, at any given moment in time depends on the maximum displacement, $A$, during that particular motion and the frequency, $f$, with which it occurs. $A$ and $f$ are independent of each other: If $f$ increases, $A$ remains unchanged; the particle simply reaches $A$ more often.

### *Pressure*

Although displacement and velocity are basic aspects of particle motion, they are much more difficult to measure than the pressure exerted by the particle as it moves. Pressure is a force applied to an area, and a force is applied whenever a moving object changes speed (accelerates), as a vibrating particle does continuously (see Figure 4.1A). The unit of force used in acoustics is the *dyne,* which is the force that causes a mass weighing 1 gram to accelerate 1 centimeter per second in a period of 1 second:

$$1 \text{ dyne} = 1 \text{ gm} \times 1 \text{ cm/sec}^2. \qquad [3]$$

The unit of pressure used is dyne per square centimeter (dyne/cm$^2$).[1] The atmospheric pressure normally exerted on the eardrum is about $10^6$ dynes/cm$^2$, but this pressure is, of course, balanced by air on the inside of the eardrum. Sounds are changes in this constant pressure. While the human auditory system is totally insensitive to a constant, unchanging pressure, a periodic pressure change may be as small as 0.0002 dynes/cm$^2$ and still be detectable as sound. When the particle velocity changes sinusoidally, so does the pressure. Figure 4.1C gives the instantaneous acoustic or sound pressure as a function of $t$:

$$P_1 = P_{max} \sin (\omega t + \Theta), \qquad [4]$$

where $P_{max}$ is the maximum pressure exerted, and $\Theta$ is the *phase* of a sound.

### *Phase*

Phase indicates on which part of the cycle a sinusoidal motion falls at a given instant relative to some arbitrary reference point in time, and is measured in degrees or radians. Interest usually centers on *phase relations* between sounds rather than on absolute phase. An example of phase relations is the comparison of a tone arriving at the two ears: If the tone is at the same part of the cycle upon its arrival in both ears, it is said to be *in phase*. If displacement is zero in the right and is maximum in the left, then the tone in the left ear leads the first by 90°, or $\pi/2$ radians. The tone is then said to be partially in phase. If the difference between the two ears is 180°, the tone is *out of phase:* One eardrum moves inward while the other moves outward.

One may also talk about the phase relations between different aspects of a single wave. For example, pressure change and displacement may be compared during vibratory motion. As shown in Figure 4.1B, initially the displacement of the particle is zero. However, the velocity and instantaneous pressure of the particle are both maximal at the very beginning (panels A and C). It is conventional to say that the velocity and pressure precede displacement by $\pi/2$ radians, or 90°, since if the sine functions were plotted backward in time the former would be at zero on the ordinate 90° sooner.

[1] This unit is being replaced by the Newton per square meter, which equals 10 dynes/cm$^2$.

### *Subjective counterparts of intensity, frequency, and phase*

We have touched upon the three most important physical aspects of a sound stimulus: intensity, frequency, and phase. Intensity is a measure of the strength of the physical stimulus and is most often expressed as a change in pressure. *Sound pressure* is the main physical variable upon which loudness depends: The greater the sound pressure, the louder the sound. But sound pressure is not loudness; loudness is subjective intensity—the intensity of the sound perceived directly by the listener without the use of measuring instruments, as determined by neural events in the brain. Sound pressure is a purely physical attribute of a sound that may initiate events in the auditory system that lead to a sensation of loudness. However, sound pressure on the eardrum is no guarantee that a sound will be heard. The frequency with which the sound pressure is changing over time also determines the loudness. At a given sound pressure, the loudness of a pure tone can be changed radically by changing only frequency. Although loudness changes with frequency, an even more noticeable change that accompanies changes in frequency is a change in *pitch*. Although not always honored, psychologists make the same distinction between pitch and frequency as between loudness and sound pressure: Pitch is the subjective phenomenon, frequency the physical measure. Pitch is based on biological events and must be distinguished from the stimulus events to which the subjective event is related but not identical.

A sound's location in space seems to be the most important subjective counterpart of phase differences, but both ears must be involved.

## Complex sounds

Thus far only pure tones have been considered. Sounds such as speech, noise, and even music are not pure tones, but they can be analyzed into sinusoidal components. Thus, not only does the pure tone provide a simple laboratory example of sound, it also is relevant in specifying the composition of natural sounds. Let us see first how two tones combine, at similar and different frequencies, in and out of phase. Then we shall look closely at how a complex sound can be analyzed into sinusoidal components.

Figure 4.3A shows two tones at the same frequency and in phase. Since pressures are equal and

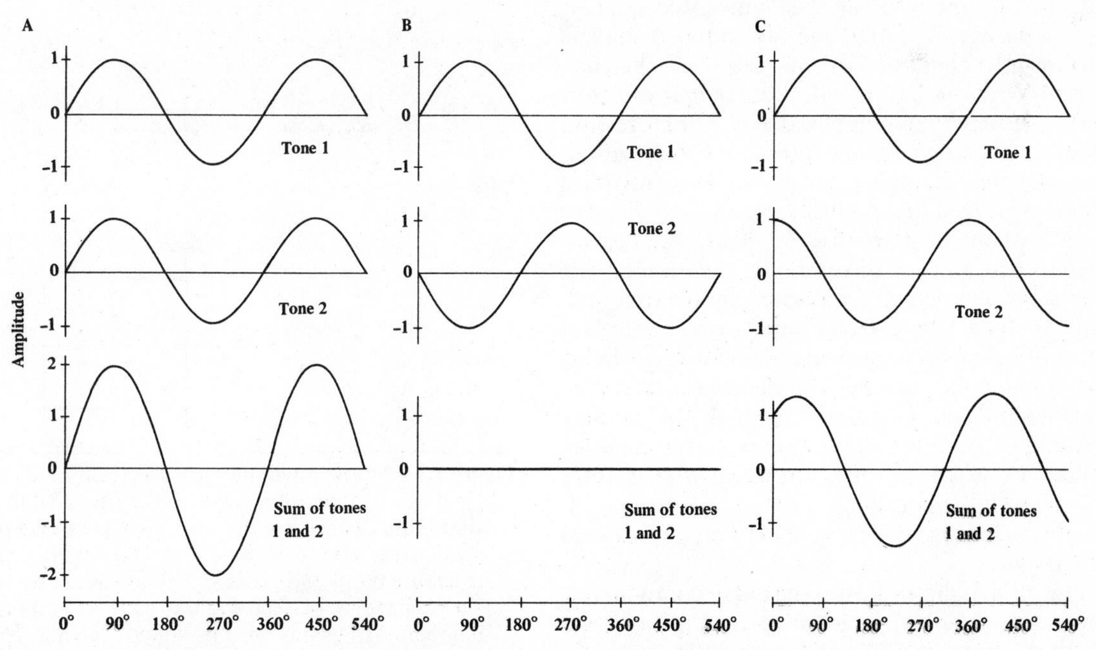


**Figure 4.3** The summation of tones of equal frequency and amplitude but in various phase relations. In panel A the two tones are in phase; in panel B they are 180° out of phase; and in panel C they are 90° out of phase. The waveform of the complex sound formed by combining the two sinusoids is their simple algebraic sum.

positive at the same time, when sounded together the two tones reinforce each other. If the two tones are 180° out of phase, as in Figure 4.3B, then the pressures have opposite signs and equal values, and they cancel each other. Intermediate phase relations yield patterns lying between those for 0° and 180° as, for example, when the phase difference is 90° (Figure 4.3C). If the frequencies are different, the summed pattern takes on various shapes depending on the difference in frequency; phase differences then become rather meaningless unless one frequency is an integral multiple of the other. When the frequencies are close, they *beat:* The tones pass from a momentary in-phase condition to a momentary out-of-phase condition with a waxing and waning in between. The number of beats always corresponds to the number of Hertz by which the tones differ. For example, the summed pattern for the frequencies 1000 Hz and 1003 Hz has three maximum displacements per second, resulting in three beats per second. Beats are quite audible when the original frequencies are themselves audible, and the beats do not exceed about ten per second. Beyond ten beats per second the ear cannot follow them, and the sound takes on a rough quality. The sound is then more like a noise, although noises arise in many other ways as well.

The definition of noise is arbitrary, often denoting an unpleasant or at least unwanted quality. Even a pure tone, if loud and high pitched, may be unpleasant. Therefore, let us drop for the time being the term *noise* and talk about *complex sounds,* that is, those sounds composed of two or more pure tones, in contrast to single pure tones. Any sound, no matter how complex, can be analyzed into pure tones. Although first published in 1822 by Fourier in a mathematical treatise on heat, the *Fourier analysis* (the analysis of a periodic function into its sinusoidal components) was soon applied to sound. This analysis had a strong impact on subsequent developments in acoustics and theories of hearing, for it is not simply a mathematical exercise. Instruments and, to a limited extent, the ear may respond to the sinusoidal components of a complex sound, as when we pick out each of two notes played simultaneously on a piano. *Ohm's law* explicitly states that the ear is able to make this kind of analysis.

Figure 4.4 shows how sinusoidal components, when added together in proper amplitude and phase relations, can sum to form a *square wave* (see bottom waveform on the right). A perfect square wave has 90° corners, meaning first an instanta-

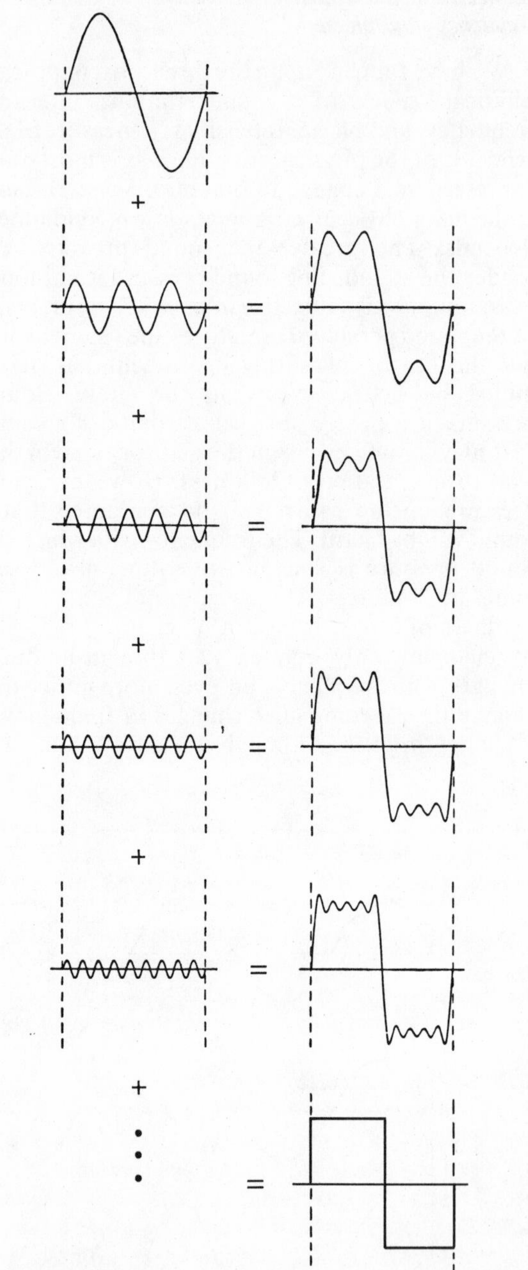

**Figure 4.4** The first two sine waves on the left sum to yield the first complex wave on the right. Adding sinusoidal waves to the first two components yields the complex waves on the right that resemble more and more closely a square wave. To achieve a perfect square wave an infinite number of sinusoids must be added together. The sinusoids used in this series are all odd harmonics, i.e., odd multiples, of the first sinusoid which is called the fundamental. (After Newman, 1948.)

neous change from zero to maximum amplitude, and then at the end of the wave an instantaneous change back from maximum to zero amplitude. An infinite number of sinusoids is needed to duplicate exactly a square wave, but just five sinusoids, as on the left side of Figure 4.4, can sum to give a close approximation of the proper form. Similarly, pure tones can be added to yield any kind of function that repeats itself in time, that is, a *periodic* function.

Fourier analysis (and integration) can also be carried out with nonperiodic functions if the period of the function is assumed to be infinitely long. Although any sound can indeed be said to be made up of sinusoidal components, a complex sound wave is not necessarily composed of many sinusoidal displacements, all occurring simultaneously. The displacement of the particles corresponds to the sum of sine waves, and all the particles in a given plane of the sound wave are moving together in the same way. Other kinds of movement are illustrated in Figure 4.5, which shows the waveforms (i.e., amplitude plotted as a function of time) for a *white noise,* which comprises all the audible frequencies and sounds somewhat like a waterfall, a violin note, and a spoken vowel. Particle displacement corresponds to the waves as shown. Where, then, are the sinusoids? Sinusoids are mathematical representations of how part of the energy in the sounds is distributed.

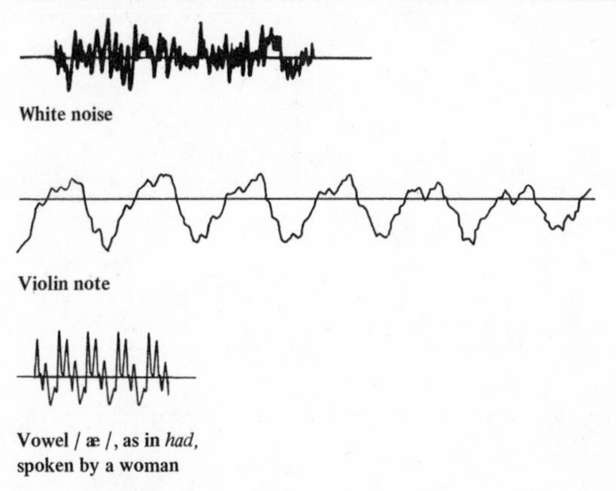


**Figure 4.5** Waveforms for a white noise, a violin note, and a spoken vowel. Displacement is plotted against time. (N.B.: The scales are not the same for the three waveforms.)

The presence of sinusoids can be shown not only mathematically but also mechanically and electronically. A mechanical resonator, such as the sounding board of a violin, responds primarily to a relatively narrow band of frequencies. These frequencies are called the *resonant frequencies;* their value depends on the resonator's size, shape, material, and so forth. A complex sound impinging on the resonator evokes vibrations only at those frequencies in the complex that correspond to the resonant frequencies. If the complex does not contain energy at those frequencies, then the resonator responds little or not at all. The concept of resonance plays a crucial role in modern theories of hearing and is important in the analysis of the sensitivity of the auditory mechanism.

Resonance is also important in the electronic production of sound. A *wave analyzer* is an electronic device that can be tuned to resonate at a very narrow band of frequencies, for example, a 3-Hz band, centered at any desired frequency. Thus, if a complex wave composed of, say, three sinusoids at 500, 1000, and 2000 Hz is led to the analyzer, the analyzer can be set to measure a 3-Hz band centered first on 500 Hz, then on 1000 Hz, and finally on 2000 Hz. In this manner, the sinusoidal components are independently measured. Such measurements are acoustically meaningful because the complex electrical wave usually corresponds very closely to the complex sound wave. This correspondence will be discussed later.

Thus far we have talked about sound waves, such as those presented in Figures 4.3, 4.4, and 4.5. The sound wave shows how amplitude changes as a function of time. A discussion of resonance and Fourier analysis, however, lends itself more easily to a different graphical representation of sound, the *spectrum*. In the spectrum, the amplitude of a sound or electrical wave is plotted as a function of frequency instead of as a function of time. In effect, the spectrum is a graph of the frequency components of a sound. Unless special techniques are used, the spectrum does not convey phase information. Figure 4.6 presents the spectra for a pure tone, a white noise, a violin note, and a square wave. Each line stands for a different sinusoidal component; plotted as a waveform, each line would yield a pattern like that in Figure 4.3A. A pure tone (panel A) is represented by a single vertical line whose location on the abscissa gives the frequency of the tone and whose height gives the amplitude. A white noise (panel B) is represented by a single horizontal line since all audible frequencies are present at equal amplitude. All frequencies are not present simultaneously, but over a long enough period of time every frequency has an equal chance of occurring. The term *white*

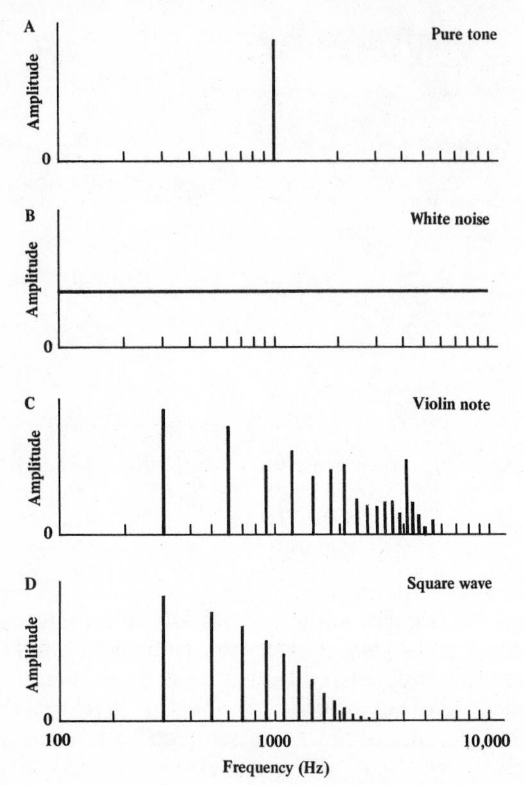


**Figure 4.6** Spectra for a pure tone (A), a white noise (B), a violin note (C), and a square wave (D). Amplitude (arbitrary scale) is plotted against frequency.

*noise* comes from the analogy with white light, which contains all the visible wavelengths (frequencies). The spectrum for white noise is thus continuous, with equal, and very small, amplitude at all frequencies. Figure 4.6C shows a violin note as represented by many vertical lines at 300-Hz intervals, since the note is composed of a number of pure tones all harmonically related (i.e., all frequencies are integral multiples of the component with the lowest frequency). Panel D shows the spectrum for a square wave, in which many frequencies are represented. These frequencies arise in the sudden onset and offset of the pulse.

## Acoustic measurements

A great advantage in the study of hearing is the precise measurement of sound stimuli that is possible, and the relatively simple means for their production. As previously mentioned, frequency is measured in Hertz, or the number of times per second an air particle undergoing simple harmonic motion completes one full excursion in both directions. A complex sound has energy at two or more frequencies. If harmonically related, the frequencies are integral multiples of each other. The lowest frequency is called the *first harmonic* or *fundamental,* the next frequency is the *second harmonic,* and so on. For example, if the fundamental is 800 Hz, then the second harmonic is 1600 Hz, and the third harmonic is 2400 Hz. The violin note shown in Figure 4.6 is an example of a series of harmonics with the fundamental at 300 Hz. The harmonic content determines quality, or *timbre,* of musical sounds. Indeed, a note played on two different musical instruments, for example, the flute and the oboe, may have the same fundamental frequency, but the other harmonics or overtones differ enough to give to each instrument its distinctive quality. Harmonics are also common and unwanted by-products in the laboratory generation of sound.

The measurement of the intensity of a sound is somewhat complicated. As noted earlier, the strength of a sound wave may be expressed in terms of particle displacement, velocity, or pressure. Pressure is the quantity most easily and, therefore, most often measured. Since the pressure of a sound wave varies between positive and negative values with zero as the average (see Figure 4.1), it is necessary to measure over at least one full period and to avoid a simple average. The measure used is the *root-mean-square* (*RMS*) value. The instantaneous pressure values are squared before they are averaged, and the square root of the average is taken. An RMS value is used because it is directly proportional to the square root of the energy in the sound wave. Thus $P^2/rc = J$, where $P$ is the root-mean-square value of the pressure, $J$ is intensity (energy per unit time per unit area), $r$ is the average density of air, and $c$ is the velocity of the sound wave. This simple relation between energy and pressure holds in most circumstances for a *plane progressive* sound wave.[2]

Recall that pressure is measured in dynes per square centimeter. In hearing, however, measures of pressure are almost always expressed in *decibels*

[2]The plane progressive sound wave is the simplest type of wave because at all points on any given plane perpendicular to the line of propagation, the acoustic pressures, particle displacements, etc., have common phases and amplitudes. The uniformity of the plane wave is possible only in a *plane sound field* where surfaces do not reflect the wave; such reflections produce patterns of reinforcement and cancellation called *standing waves.*

($dB$), which are derived from the ratio of quantities of energy. Decibels are readily used with pressure (and also voltage and current) as well as energy because of the simple exponential relation between energy and pressure:

$$\begin{aligned}\text{Number of dB} &= 10 \log E_1/E_2 \\ &= 10 \log P_1^2/P_2^2 \\ &= 20 \log P_1/P_2\end{aligned} \quad [5]$$

where $E$ is energy and $P$ is acoustic pressure. Most often the decibel is used to specify *sound pressure level* (*SPL*), where $P_2 = 0.0002$ dynes/cm², a pressure close to the lowest sound pressure level audible. Thus the threshold is close to 0 dB. (On a logarithmic scale such as the decibel scale, 0 equals the log of 1 so that the quantity is not absent at 0 dB but is equal to the reference value, in this case 0.0002 dynes/cm².) The highest SPL that can be sustained without permanent and rapid damage to the human ear is about 130 to 140 dB. Figure 4.7 gives the SPLs that correspond to real sounds between 0 and 180 dB. One advantage of the decibel scale is that it avoids numbers like 0.0002 and units of measurement like dynes per square centimeter, while covering a huge range of values (e.g., from 0.0002 to 200,000 dynes/cm² in Figure 4.7). It has the added convenience that decibels are always added or subtracted, never divided or multiplied, since addition and subtraction represent multiplication and division on a logarithmic scale. A third advantage is that decibels are independent of the unit of measurement, provided the same unit is used throughout any single series of measurements. In dealing with sound pressure, it is convenient to remember that a tenfold change in sound pressure equals a 20-dB change, and a twofold change equals a 6-dB change. Table 4.1 gives the ratio between two sound pressures (or voltages) and the corresponding difference in decibels.

| Decibels | Sound pressure level | Typical sounds |
|---|---|---|
| | 180 | Space rocket |
| | 160 | Wind tunnel |
| | 140 | Jet at takeoff |
| | 120 | Thunder |
| | 100 | Subway train |
| | 80 | Vacuum cleaner |
| | 60 | Conversation |
| | 40 | Residential neighborhood at night |
| | 20 | Leaves rustling in a breeze |
| | 0 | Threshold of hearing |

**Figure 4.7** Sound pressure levels in decibels of typical sounds.

**Table 4.1 The Number of Decibels That Corresponds to a Given Pressure (or Voltage) Ratio**

| Pressure ratio (voltage ratio) | Decibels |
|---|---|
| 1 | 0.0 |
| 2 | 6.0 |
| 3 | 9.5 |
| 4 | 12.0 |
| 5 | 14.0 |
| 6 | 15.5 |
| 7 | 17.0 |
| 8 | 18.0 |
| 9 | 19.0 |
| 10 | 20.0 |
| 20 | 26.0 |
| 50 | 34.0 |
| 100 | 40.0 |
| 1000 | 60.0 |

## Producing sounds in the laboratory

Until the 1920s the sounds used in laboratory studies of hearing were mostly produced mechanically by striking a tuning fork or by rotating a perforated disc. A great deal was learned with this equipment, but the advent of the vacuum tube and the amplifier made experiments easier to perform and to control. Especially difficult had been the control of intensity, which now became simple. The following paragraphs deal with common pieces of electronic equipment used to generate, control, transduce, and measure sounds.

### *Sound generation*

One apparatus for producing sounds in the laboratory is the *oscillator,* or tone generator. The oscillator produces sinusoidal currents that, impressed on a loudspeaker, yield pure tones. Many oscillators can be tuned to produce oscillations at frequencies from 20 to 20,000 Hz covering the entire audible range, but only one frequency is produced at a time. For experiments with complex sounds, the outputs of two or more oscillators are combined. Another common sound source is the white-noise generator, which produces a noise with all the audible frequencies equally represented (see Figure 4.6B).

*Sound control*

Since the output of these generators is often not intense enough to produce sounds as loud as desired, an amplifier may be required. The ideal amplifier increases the amplitude of the sinusoidal output without introducing any new frequency components. Once the required maximum output can be obtained, the problem of precise control of intensity may arise. The most convenient way to control intensity is by means of an *attenuator*. An audio attenuator is usually calibrated in decibels and consists of *resistors* which convert part of the electrical signal to heat, thereby reducing the signal amplitude. An attenuator is a good device for reducing intensity because its decibel scale simplifies the measurements. Moreover, an attenuator, regardless of its setting, is a constant electrical load on the sound-generating source. If the load, or *impedance,* is suitable to the sound source, the least amount of sound other than at the desired frequency will be produced.

Frequency is usually controlled directly on the tone generator by means of one or two *condensers* and can be changed continuously. One can also speak of frequency control for a white-noise generator. A particular *band* of frequencies is selected from the total range available by means of a *filter,* which lets through some frequencies and blocks others. An ideal *low-pass* filter lets through all frequencies below a certain value and none above; a *high-pass* filter allows through all frequencies above, and none below, a cutoff value; a *band-pass* filter permits the passage of the frequencies between two values and none outside. In practice, there is no abrupt transition from complete to zero transmission at the cutoff frequency; rather, the transition is more or less gradual. A filter never completely suppresses frequencies outside the pass band but attenuates them, the amount of attenuation depending on the construction of the filter. Commercial filters are available that permit continuous variation of the cutoff frequencies, but if sharp transition and large attenuation are desired, then filters with fixed cutoff frequencies are usually necessary.

Filters are used not only to select frequencies from a white-noise generator or other source of a continuous spectrum, but also to eliminate unwanted frequencies (noise) that arise when, for example, the output of a tone generator is turned on and off. Inevitably, changing the amplitude of a pure tone produces *transient* frequencies other than that of the tone. If the change in amplitude is large and abrupt, as when an ongoing tone is interrupted completely, then these transients become audible as clicks. A click can be largely eliminated by passing the interrupted tone through either a low-pass filter, since the click contains mostly high frequencies, or through a band-pass filter centered at the frequency of the pure tone.

Another way to eliminate clicks is by turning the tone on and off relatively slowly, that is, by allowing the tone to increase slowly to full amplitude and to decrease slowly from full amplitude. An interval of 25 to 50 msec is considered slow, and can be achieved by means of an electronic switch which permits variation of the speed with which the tone can be turned on and off. Such a switch also permits precise control of the cycling and timing of signal presentation when used with *pulsing equipment*. Pulsing equipment tells the electronic switch when to turn the tone on and off; tone bursts lasting only a few milliseconds can be generated.

All the functions of such equipment may be replaced by computers which can be programmed to produce almost any kind of electrical waveform. Because of advances in computer technology, it is feasible to set up and run hearing experiments using electrical signals produced by a computer.

*Transducers*

Whether the electrical signals are produced by programming a computer or by turning knobs on generators and attenuators, the electrical current must be converted to airborne acoustic waves by a transducer. Loudspeakers and earphones (a small loudspeaker) are transducers in which an electrical current sets a stretched diaphragm vibrating. Although the transducer is the weakest link in the chain of sound production, a loudspeaker can vibrate in proportion to the electrical input very well over a wide frequency range. Earphones are somewhat more restricted, usually not operating efficiently above approximately 7000 Hz. In the laboratory, earphones are used more frequently than loudspeakers in order to avoid the problems imposed by sound being reflected by walls, furniture, and listeners' bodies. To use a loudspeaker and still avoid these problems, the speaker and the listener are located in an *anechoic* room whose walls, floors, and ceiling, usually made of fiberglass wedges, absorb most of the sound energy; but an anechoic room is expensive and therefore seldom available.

*Measurement and calibration*

The SPL is usually not measured directly during an experiment, but the voltage level of the electrical input to the transducer can be readily measured with a *voltmeter*. From the voltage level across the earphone the SPL can be computed if the earphone has been *calibrated*. The frequency of a sinusoid into the earphone is most readily measured with a *frequency counter*, which gives the number of Hertz as a digital readout. If more than one frequency is present, then a wave analyzer can be used. A wave analyzer is, in effect, a filter which may be tuned to a very narrow band of frequencies. This device is used to examine small sections of the frequency domain.

Fourier components may also be seen on an *oscilloscope*, in which an electric waveform is presented visually. Although an oscilloscope would be difficult to use for analysis of complex sounds, it is well suited for measurements in the time domain. An oscilloscope presents a visual image of the electrical signal and not of the sound wave itself. A sinusoid, as represented in Figure 4.1, is seen on the screen of an oscilloscope so that it is possible to measure amplitude and frequency, but voltmeters and frequency counters are more convenient and accurate. Oscilloscopes are best used for measuring signal duration, intervals between signals where two or more signals follow each other, and the *rise* (onset) and *fall* (offset) times, but they can also be used to measure phase relations between two sinusoids. Perhaps its most common use in the hearing laboratory is as a monitoring device that permits the experimenter to see what electrical input is going to the listener's earphone and to detect the occurrence of distortions and noise.

Thus far we have considered only the electrical signal. What do we know about the acoustical signal, the sound wave? How well does the loudspeaker follow the electrical input and what are the sound pressures produced? These questions can be answered by taking the acoustical output of the speaker and converting it back to an electrical signal via a microphone. To be sure of the microphone's performance and to know that it is a faithful reproducer of the acoustic signal, a microphone is used that has been *absolutely calibrated* in some standardized manner. Then all the electrical apparatus can be applied in the following manner to correlate the electrical input to the earphone and the electrical output from the microphone.

A known voltage is impressed across the earphone and held constant while the frequency is varied. The sound from the earphone travels through the air to the calibrated microphone which, in turn, produces a small current that is then amplified and measured. Note that a voltage measurement is made at the beginning and end of the procedure. In order to determine the sound pressure of the sound wave that intervened between the electrical input and output, the calibration chart of the microphone is used to give the SPL at each frequency that produces a given voltage. From this voltage, the sound pressure produced by the earphone can be calculated. One difficulty is the mechanical *coupling* of the two phones. The larger the volume of air between them, the smaller the sound pressure at the microphone, since the surface of the microphone then represents a smaller portion of the whole sphere of the sound wave from the earphone. In the United States the practice is to use a metal coupler with a cavity containing 6 $cm^3$ of air. This amount of air is about the same as the air trapped between the earphone and the eardrum of the average listener and therefore is a fair approximation, but still only an approximation, of the sound pressure generated by the earphone at the eardrum. At frequencies below 300 Hz the sound pressure in the ear is usually less than the calibrated pressure because some energy is lost through leakage in the coupling between the earphone and ear, but not in the coupling between the earphone and microphone. Nevertheless, the 6-$cm^3$ coupler is a standard reference that permits cross-experimental comparisons of data even though the absolute sound pressures reported may not be completely accurate.

Automatic techniques yield a continuous written record of the response of the microphone as a function of frequency for a given voltage input to the earphone. The response of the microphone is converted to SPL, and the calibration chart for the earphone is complete. Although measurements are made without changing the voltage across the earphone, the chart is applicable to all voltages because the SPL and voltage are directly proportional: Since halving the voltage halves the sound pressure, the decibel changes in voltage level correspond exactly to the decibel changes in SPL. Given the SPL produced at one voltage level, the calibration for all other usable voltage levels is known.

One final point about the use of calibration curves may be noted: Calibrations are generally made with a bare earphone, whereas the earphone is almost always used in an *ear cushion* (unless it is a special, small phone that is inserted into the ear canal). An ear cushion permits a comfortable coupling between the head and earphone, and it also attenuates unwanted external sounds. But not all types of ear cushions enclose the same volume of air between the earphone and eardrum. The ear canal, between the entrance and the eardrum, contains about 1 $cm^3$ of air. The volume of air between the entrance to the ear canal and the earphone depends largely on the cushion used. Often, the cushion used lies on top of the pinna and gives a total air volume, including that of the canal, equal to about 6 $cm^3$. (The MX-41/AR cushion is the most common one of this type used in the United States.) So a standard 6-$cm^3$ calibration chart may be safely used with this cushion. Other cushions, which fit over the pinna and rest on the head, usually enclose larger volumes of air. Rather than trying to compute the differences in air volume and the expected sound pressure at various frequencies, a simpler and more accurate method of determining the sound pressure with a particular type of cushion is used. Thresholds are measured at various frequencies for listeners using the same earphone with the standard MX-41/AR and with the unknown cushion. Of course the measures must be counterbalanced and properly conducted, but threshold measures under standard conditions are reliable enough to provide a good comparison of the effect of the two cushions. Most cushions, being larger than the MX-41/AR, will result in a smaller sound pressure at the eardrum, and therefore the thresholds computed on the basis of the 6-$cm^3$ calibration will appear higher. If other factors, such as practice effects, have been properly counterbalanced between the two cushions, then the difference between the thresholds with the MX-41/AR and with the other cushion at each frequency shows the effect of the difference in the cushions as a function of frequency. (See Jerger & Tillman, 1959, for established measurements for three different cushions.)

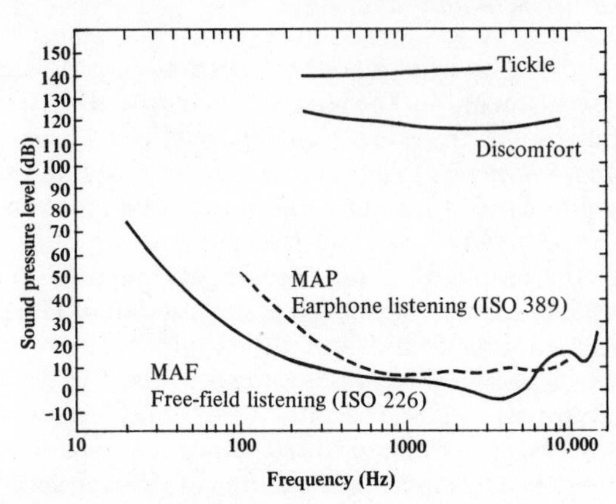


**Figure 4.8** Threshold as a function of frequency. Bottom curves represent the minimum audible pressure (MAP) that young adults with normal hearing can hear in an earphone and the minimum audible field pressure (MAF) that can be heard binaurally in a free field. Thresholds for discomfort and tickle are also shown. (After ISO Recommendations 226, 1961, and 389, 1964; and Licklider, 1951.)

## THRESHOLDS

### The limits of hearing

Not all acoustic vibrations can be heard by all listeners. Even with normal hearing a person cannot hear vibrations whose sound pressure is too weak or whose frequency is too high or too low. The minimum audible sound pressure, the hearing threshold, varies with frequency—no single SPL, is *the* threshold. Both the SPL and the frequency must be specified.

Figure 4.8 shows the minimum sound pressure, as a function of frequency, audible to young adults. Two lower curves are shown, one labeled *MAP* (minimum audible pressure) for measurements made with an earphone, the other labeled *MAF* (minimum audible field) for measurements made in a *free field* with the sound coming from a loudspeaker. (In a free field, no sounds are reflected from surrounding surfaces such as objects and walls. A free field occurs naturally outdoors over an open field of fresh-fallen snow or high grass; indoors, an anechoic room is needed.) Both bottom curves are taken from recommendations of the International Organization for Standardization (ISO R226, 1961; ISO R389, 1964) and are based on many experiments that used various procedures in different countries. (The MAP curve has been extrapolated to lower and higher frequencies not contained in the ISO recommendation.) The sound pressure from the earphone was measured in the standard coupler used in the United States. In the free field, the sound pressure was measured with a calibrated microphone placed where the listener's head had been. Differences between free-field and earphone thresholds are ascribed to very soft noise produced under the ear cushion (especially at low frequencies) which makes the tone signal harder to hear; to the effect of the head which tends to reflect the higher frequencies; and to the fact that both ears were stimulated in the free field, but only one ear by the single earphone.

Figure 4.8 shows that the MAP hovers around a level of 8 dB between 600 and 8000 Hz. The rather sharp dip in the MAF curve near 4000 Hz and the rise near 8000 Hz reflect changes in the sound field caused by the listener's head. Sounds may be audible beyond the frequency limits of these curves, that is, 20 and 15,000 Hz, but not below 2 Hz nor above 20,000 Hz. Very low frequencies are difficult to produce, especially at high SPLs, so few threshold measurements have been made below 20 Hz. Above 15,000 Hz, listeners differ greatly as to the highest frequency they can hear. Figure 4.8 also shows the upper pressure limits beyond which sounds become uncomfortable and begin to tickle. People disagree about how intense a sound must be before it no longer is a "sound," but most studies show that the discomfort and tickle levels are independent of frequency and lie between 100 and 140 dB. Above approximately 140 dB SPL, the inner ear is likely to suffer permanent damage from even a brief exposure. Long exposure to sound at levels between 90 and 140 dB may damage some people's ears.

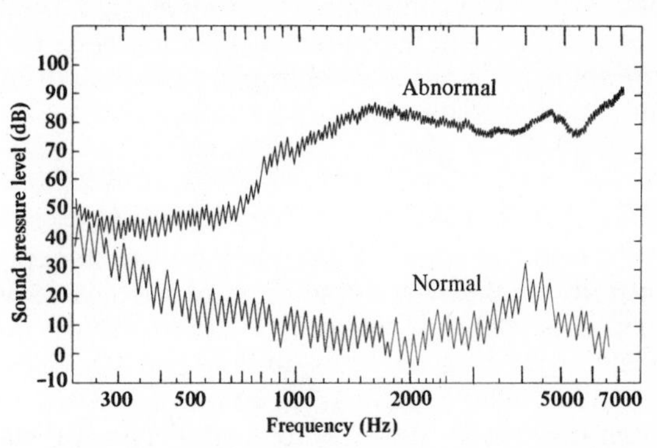


**Figure 4.9** Threshold curves obtained by the von Békésy tracking procedure. The bottom curve is from a young adult with normal hearing. The top curve is from a listener with a severe sensorineural hearing loss.

### Measuring the limits

A host of psychophysical procedures are available for measuring thresholds (see Chapter 2), especially to the psychoacoustician and audiometrist who can precisely and easily control frequency and intensity, as well as stimulus sequences.

In the past two decades, von Békésy's (1960) *tracking* procedure and the *forced-choice* procedure have become popular. Tracking is widely used both in the clinic and in the laboratory because it is fast and it helps distinguish different auditory pathologies. Forced-choice procedures are long and tedious. They are used in the laboratory to measure thresholds very accurately, to study motivational variables such as reward and feedback, or to test implications of signal detection theory.

#### *Tracking*

In this procedure, the subject controls sound intensity with a two-position switch, one position to increase the intensity until the sound is just detectable, and the other position to decrease the intensity until the sound just disappears. A motor-driven attenuator changes the intensity and a pen records it on a moving sheet of paper. The subject alternately increases and decreases the intensity, producing a zigzag curve like the ones in Figure 4.9. The SPL is plotted against sound frequency, which increases continuously as the subject tracks the sound. Frequency is controlled by a second motor that turns both the paper and the frequency dial on an oscillator. A whole threshold curve is obtained in one session that lasts from 5 to 20 minutes depending on how fast the frequency is changed. Threshold is the midpoint of the excursions. In effect, tracking is an automated combination of the methods of limits and adjustment. The rate of change of attenuation is usually about 2 dB per second, but faster or slower speeds are possible without altering the threshold. The sound may be either on continuously or turned on and off intermittently. Judgments are somewhat easier with intermittent stimuli, but in the clinic some patients produce narrow excursions at high frequencies when they track a continuous tone; their tracing resembles the one at the top of Figure 4.9. Such patients have poorer absolute thresholds but better differential thresholds at the higher frequencies when they change direction more rapidly than normal to produce the narrow excursions. These results are diagnostically important because they usually indicate that the patient has an impairment of the sensorineural structures of the inner ear rather than of more centrally located neural structures or auditory conductive mechanisms.

A variation of the von Békésy procedure is to hold the frequency constant while the subject or patient tracks his threshold as a function of time. This simplifies the measurement of time-dependent variables, such as recovery from prior stimulation, fatigue, and adaptation.

### *Forced choice*

Perhaps the chief disadvantage of the tracking procedure, like most of the classical procedures, is that each subject chooses his own criteria for deciding when a sound is audible and when it is inaudible. The experimenter has no easy way to determine what those criteria are. The forced-choice procedure avoids this problem by asking the subject not whether he heard a sound, but when he heard it. Judgments can then be scored right and wrong. In one version of the procedure, for example, the subject reports which of two time intervals contains the sound. The experimenter presents the sound in only one interval. Since guessing alone would yield 50 percent correct judgments, the sound intensity that yields 75 percent correct judgments is commonly taken as the threshold value.

This procedure can yield accurate and stable thresholds. Certain disadvantages, however, restrict it primarily to the laboratory. The experimenter must set the sound to a level where the subject will neither always hear it nor always miss it. To pinpoint the 75 percent level, he must make many measurements at various levels that yield percentages of correct judgments between 50 and 100 percent. This means hundreds of trials at each frequency and intensity. During all these trials, it is essential to keep the subject's motivation high, for if his attention wanders, his threshold increases. Although signal detection theory permits separating certain motivational variables from sensitivity, shifts in motivation during a block of trials are not easily analyzed (see Chapter 2 for further discussion). Moreover, shifts in attention cannot be distinguished from shifts in sensitivity, for the two seem inseparable. (Lack of attention is quickly noticed in a tracking record where the excursions suddenly widen.)

Generally, the tracking method or a classical procedure is used when a fast threshold measurement is desirable and when criteria are expected to remain stable and not to interact with the experimental conditions. A forced-choice procedure is used when highly accurate (within a decibel) measures are needed, when criteria are expected to vary, or when motivation is to be manipulated.

## Physiological basis of the threshold curve

Regardless of how the threshold is measured, the results show that humans hear frequencies between approximately 600 and 8000 Hz better than low and high frequencies. Why? The answer can be found by looking at the auditory system. To simplify matters, a distinction is made between what happens in the auditory system before it converts sound energy into neural energy and after. Up to the hair cells, sound moves through the middle and inner ear in the form of mechanical energy, ending up as displacements of the basilar membrane (see Chapter 3 for more detailed discussion of the anatomy of the auditory system). The hair cells then convert or transduce these displacements to neural energy. Threshold must vary with frequency in the way it does, either because the middle frequencies are favored as the sound energy is transmitted to the hair cells, or because the hair cells and other neural elements respond better to those frequencies. Zwislocki (1965) has shown that both transmission characteristics and, to a lesser extent, neural factors determine how threshold depends on frequency.

### *Transmission characteristics*

The free-field SPL, it has been pointed out, is measured with a microphone placed where the listener's head had been. The head's absence, however, introduces an error, since the pattern of sound waves is different with the head in the field than without it. For example, a sound pressure that was constant across frequency, when measured at the microphone with the head absent, now has a maximum near 2000 Hz when measured at the entrance to the ear canal.

The external ear canal also amplifies some frequencies relative to others. Frequencies near the resonant frequency, 4000 Hz, are amplified about 10 dB between the canal's entrance and the eardrum. Frequencies far from 4000 Hz are only slightly amplified and those below 1000 Hz hardly at all.

The middle ear ossicles do not handle all frequencies in the same way. Their main function is to concentrate the sound pressure at the eardrum onto the oval window. Since the eardrum's area is some twenty-five times larger than the oval window's, the pressure greatly increases between the two. Increased pressure is needed at the oval window in order to move the cochlear fluid, which is much heavier and less elastic than the air at the eardrum. The increase in pressure is greater at low than at high frequencies; above about 1000 Hz, it decreases with increasing frequency.

In the cochlea itself, the displacement of the basilar membrane, which initiates the neural response, increases with frequency given a constant pressure at the oval window.

This section has so far traced the acoustic signal through the outer, middle, and part of the inner ear right to the basilar membrane, where the hair cells convert mechanical into neural energy. Given the various changes in sound pressure that depend on frequency, and given the response of the basilar membrane, the original question can now be succinctly posed. Starting with a free-field sound pressure that is the same at all frequencies, how does displacement of the basilar membrane depend on frequency? Displacement of the basilar membrane is the penultimate "stimulus" in hearing. If the neural events, in the hair cells and beyond, are all alike regardless of the part of the basilar membrane involved, then differences in the displacement produced by different stimulus frequencies should be reflected in the psychophysical threshold curve. The shape of the threshold curve would be predicted when all the transmission effects are included. Zwislocki (1965) made the necessary calculations, showing that the transmission characteristics of the auditory system do determine most of, but not the whole, relation between threshold and frequency. With increasing frequency, the threshold decreases more rapidly up to 1000 Hz, and then above 4000 Hz it increases more slowly than predicted on the basis of the transmission characteristics alone. This discrepancy, amounting to 3 dB per octave, can be explained by reference to auditory neural processes.

### *Neural processes*

Specifically, Zwislocki (1965) ascribes the discrepancy between predicted and measured threshold curves to *temporal summation,* which means that not only the amplitude of displacement of the basilar membrane, but also the frequency of displacement, is important to the nervous system. Each displacement gives rise to responses in the neural pathways, and these responses summate over time up to about 200 msec (see following discussion). The higher the frequency, the larger the number of neural responses; doubling the frequency doubles the number of responses, which corresponds to a change of 3 dB per octave. Corrected for temporal summation, the predicted and measured threshold curves almost coincide.

It appears that threshold varies with frequency because the vibratory motions do not get to the hair cells with the same ease at all frequencies, and because the nervous system summates *neural impulses* over time. Thus we may reasonably assume that the hair cells respond to all frequencies in about the same way (excluding the role of temporal summation). Moreover, neural responses beyond the hair cell also seem to be independent of frequency and the particular hair cells that give rise to the impulses. No known anatomical or physiological data seem to contradict this assumption of neural equivalence.

### **Temporal summation**

What is the evidence indicating that at threshold the ear summates nerve impulses that occur within about 200 msec? As sound duration is increased up to 200 msec, the threshold intensity can be reduced. Beyond 200 msec, the intensity must be held constant if the sound is to remain just audible. The product of intensity and duration, $I \times t$, is a measure of energy. In these terms, up to about 200 msec the energy just sufficient to evoke a response remains constant. (See discussion of the corresponding laws in vision, the Bunsen-Roscoe law and Bloch's law, in Chapter 7.) Stated another way, the threshold energy can be packaged in a variety of ways in time, all within 50, 100, or 200 msec, just so long as 200 msec is not exceeded. Just how energy is packaged doesn't matter to the ear as far as detection is concerned.

Although the ear seems to summate energy over time, such a statement needs to be qualified. To summate stimulus energy, the ear would have to store it, as a *condenser* stores electrical energy or as a light-sensitive pigment accumulates light energy. However, none of the ear's structures seems capable of doing so. It is more likely that the auditory nervous system does the summating, perhaps a summating of neural energy. The final response in the nervous system that leads a subject to say that a tone is audible seems to depend on the total number of neural events occurring within 200 msec. Repeated tone bursts show the same effect: Two bursts have a lower threshold than either one alone when they occur within 200 msec of each other (Zwislocki, 1960).

### Summation over frequency

The ear summates not only over time, but also over frequency. Two tones at different frequencies are easier to hear than either one alone. Presented together, each tone can be made one-half as intense as either one alone in order to reach threshold. In other words, the threshold intensity for each of two simultaneous tones is one-half the threshold intensity for either one by itself; similarly, the threshold for each of four tones is one-fourth that of any one of them alone, and so on. However, if the tones are too far apart in frequency, they do not summate at threshold. The maximum frequency separation within which summation takes place is called the *critical band* (Scharf, 1961, 1970).[3] Two tones separated by less than a critical band can be detected when each is at, for example, 5 dB SPL; moved more than a critical band apart the tones must be set at 8 dB, their threshold level when presented individually. Just how far apart the tones can be and still summate depends on their frequencies. Low-frequency tones must be closer together than high-frequency tones. For example, when the average, or *center*, frequency (usually taken as the geometric mean) of two tones is 500 Hz, the critical band is 100 Hz; when the center frequency is 4000 Hz, the critical band is 700 Hz. Figure 4.10 indicates the value for the critical band as a function of the center frequency. The critical band also sets a limit in other kinds of auditory measurements which will be discussed later.

With respect to thresholds, the listener may be able to detect only one critical band at a time. If so, two 100-msec tones presented one after the other would summate over time only when within the same critical band. Another prediction is that a subject instructed to listen for a known frequency would detect other frequencies from the same critical band equally well, but would detect frequencies outside that band less well. Greenberg and Larkin (1968) reported just such results, supporting the notion that we detect one critical band at a time.

### Binaural summation

Summation over time and frequency is true for both monaural and binaural stimuli. With regard to summation across the two ears, do we hear better with two ears than with one? The answer

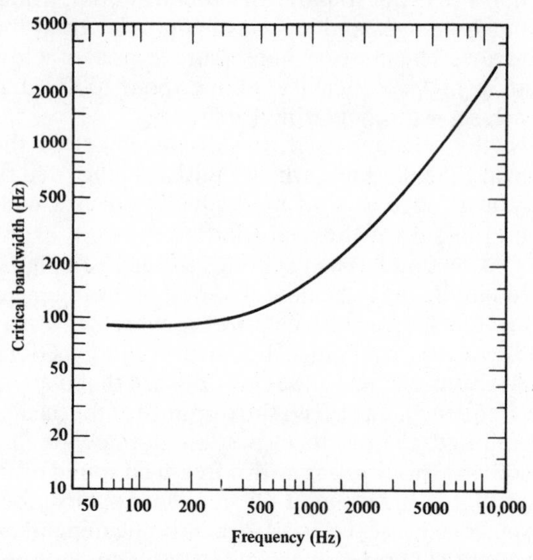


**Figure 4.10** The width of the critical band as a function of its center frequency. (After Zwicker, Flottorp, & Stevens, 1957.)

is yes, since the threshold intensity for a sound led to only one ear is twice that for the same sound led to both ears. It has been suggested that two ears are twice as good as one simply because two ears have twice as much chance of detecting a sound. Chocholle (1962), however, has shown that the whole psychometric function, relating the percentage of detected stimuli to sound intensity, shifts in binaural listening. His observers detected all the binaural signals at an intensity that monaurally produced less than 100-percent detection. If only probabilities were summing, the function would stay below 100 percent until at least one of the monaural functions reached 100 percent, because the listener must sometimes miss both sounds in a binaural presentation when neither one alone has a 100-percent chance of being detected.

As in temporal summation, somewhere in the nervous system the neural events from both ears are summed. Moreover, Schenkel (1967) has shown that temporal summation can take place across the two ears within 200 msec. The threshold for a tone which is first led for 20 msec to one ear and then led for 20 msec to the other ear is 3 dB lower than that for a tone which is led to only one ear for 20 msec. Since a 3-dB decrease means that intensity is halved, as mentioned earlier, this finding means that the threshold intensity can be halved when

[3]Obtaining a value for the critical band from measurements of the threshold for each of two simultaneous tones is difficult; some experiments have succeeded, while others have not.

the duration is doubled even though the tone is in one ear one-half of the time and in the other ear the other half.

## Masking

Pure tones are the rare exception, not the rule, in nature. Our ears are usually besieged by a variety of sounds with many component frequencies. We sometimes synthesize these sounds, as when hearing chords played on a piano; at other times we analyze them, as when listening for the cello in a quartet or attending to a friend's voice at a large party. *Masked thresholds* are measured when the masked sound (e.g., the friend's voice) is listened for in the presence of the masking sound (e.g., the party hubbub). The amount of masking in decibels is the threshold increase caused by the masking sound, or *masker*. Thus, the amount of masking equals the threshold for a sound in the presence of the masker minus the threshold for the same sound in the quiet. Measurements of masking reveal much about interactions within the auditory system.

Figure 4.11 shows how a narrow band of noise centered on 1200 Hz, or 1.2 kHz (frequency limits near 1100 Hz and 1300 Hz), affects the threshold for pure tones. Threshold is plotted against frequency for tones presented in the quiet and against a noise set at various SPLs. As indicated in the figure, the more intense the noise band, the more it masks tones within its frequency limits and at

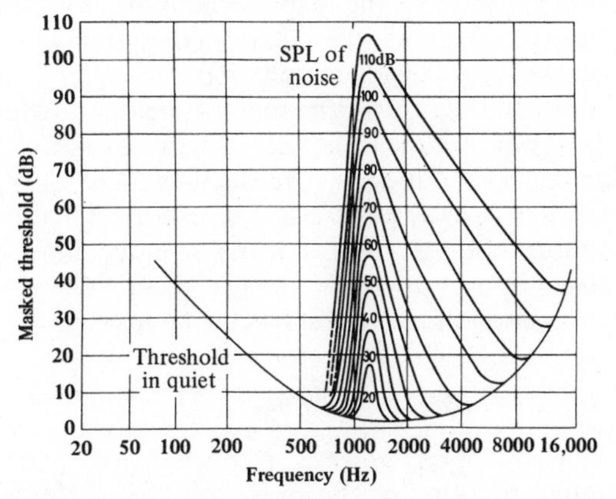


**Figure 4.11** Masking of pure tones by a narrow band of noise centered at 1200 Hz. The SPL of the noise is given on each curve. The frequency of the masked tone is given on the abscissa. (From Zwicker & Scharf, 1965.)

higher frequencies. Frequencies below the noise band are hardly affected, even by an unpleasantly loud, 110-dB noise. Noise bands centered at low and high frequencies mask tones in a similar fashion and produce similar masking patterns.

Note that the threshold for a tone at the noise's center frequency rises in direct proportion to the noise intensity at levels above 20 dB. When the masker's intensity increases 10 dB, so does the threshold for the masked tone. The signal-to-noise ratio at threshold remains constant at about −4 dB; the tone at the center frequency, here 1200 Hz, is just barely heard when it is 4 dB weaker than the noise.

A pure-tone masker produces the same masking patterns as a noise band (Figure 4.11), except that the curve dips sharply at those frequencies where the masked tone equals, or is an integral multiple of, the masker frequency (Wegel & Lane, 1924). At those frequencies, beats reveal the masked tone's presence. Nevertheless, whether produced by pure tones or by noise bands, masking is greater at frequencies higher than the masking frequency than at lower frequencies.

### *Cochlear patterns*

To understand why low frequencies mask high frequencies better than the other way around, it is necessary to follow the sound wave beyond the middle ear into the cochlea. A sound sets the stapes vibrating, alternately pushing in and pulling out the oval window. This motion gives rise to a pressure differential inside the cochlea between the scala vestibuli and the scala tympani (see Chapter 3, Figure 3.20). The pressure differential then causes a deformation, called a *traveling wave,* that travels along the basilar membrane from the oval window toward the helicotrema. The displacement or deformation of the basilar membrane is needed to produce neural activity in the auditory system.

Georg von Békésy (1960), who won the Nobel Prize for this work, observed the displacements of the basilar membrane that followed stimulation by tones of different frequencies. The observed amplitude of displacement was not the same all along the basilar membrane; usually, one region of the membrane was displaced more than other regions. The displacement patterns observed by von Békésy are plotted in Figure 4.12. These patterns represent not the traveling wave, but the *maximum displacement* a given tone produces at each point on the basilar membrane.

Two important points should be made about

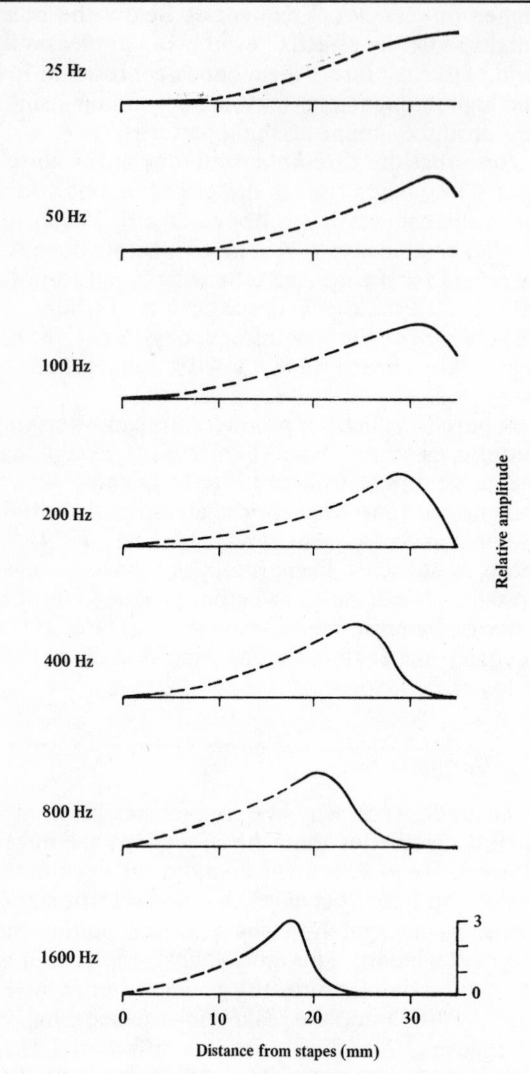


**Figure 4.12** Pattern of displacement of the basilar membrane when stimulated by pure tones at various frequencies. These patterns were observed in a cadaver specimen. (From von Békésy, 1960.)

these displacements. First, as the stimulus frequency increases, the place of maximum displacement shifts from near the helicotrema toward the oval window and stapes. Second, the place of maximum displacement is not a sharply localized point, but falls off gradually, especially toward the oval window. At higher intensities, both the longitudinal spread along the basilar membrane and the amplitude of displacement increase. The spatial representation of frequency on the basilar membrane is perhaps the single most important piece of physiological information about the auditory system, clarifying many psychophysical data, including the masking data and their asymmetry. We assume only that a masked tone becomes just audible when intense enough to override the ongoing activity on the basilar membrane produced by a masking noise or tone. According to the von Békésy data, the activity is much greater at points on the basilar membrane that mediate frequencies above the masking frequency than at points below. Thus to become just audible, a tone at a higher frequency must be made more intense than a tone at a lower frequency.

Neural responses reflect the asymmetry of activity on the basilar membrane. By measuring the minimum SPL needed to elicit a criterion response in single auditory nerve fibers, physiologists map the relation between the electrophysiological threshold and frequency (e.g., Galambos & Davis, 1943; Kiang, 1965). Most fibers have a *characteristic frequency* at which the minimum SPL or threshold is lower than at any other frequency. At higher stimulus frequencies, the minimum SPL increases rapidly; at lower frequencies, it increases slowly. This is just what is expected if the fiber terminates at a single place on the basilar membrane. The neural fiber responds to displacement at place *P*, regardless of the stimulus frequency, as long as the displacement is large enough to trigger the fiber. When the stimulus frequency gives rise to a pattern whose maximum displacement is at *P*, then the minimum required displacement may be obtained with the weakest stimulus. As the frequency increases, the displacement quickly diminishes at *P* (and the threshold quickly rises) because the displacement spreads very little toward the region of the membrane that mediates the lower frequencies (see Figure 4.12). With decreasing frequency, the displacement at *P* diminishes slowly, as does the threshold. This result supports the assertion that masking asymmetry is caused by asymmetry in the spread of displacement and excitation along the basilar membrane.

### *The critical band in masking*

Narrow-band noise and pure tones produce similar masking patterns, except for differences caused by audible beats when pure tones mask other pure tones, provided the bandwidth of the noise does not exceed the critical band. Extended beyond the critical band, a noise produces masking patterns that are wider at the top and that spread over a larger frequency range. At the same time, the threshold for a tone at the center of the band decreases (unless the sound pressure of the original critical band is held constant and the overall level of the whole noise increases). Energy added to a noise by extending it beyond the critical band does not help mask a tone at the center frequency. This result was predicted and first partially demonstrated by Fletcher (1940).

The spatial representation of frequency on the basilar membrane suggested to Fletcher that when a wide-band noise masks a pure tone, only a small band of frequencies around the tone, called the critical band, actually does the masking. He thought that at the tone's masked threshold, the tone and the masking band were equally intense. Although in fact the critical band of noise must be about 4 dB more intense, the basic notion of a critical band of masking has been amply borne out (Scharf, 1970).

Since critical bands are wider at high than at low frequencies (see Figure 4.10), the critical bands that are centered at the high frequencies in a white noise, which has a constant spectrum level (SPL per Hertz) throughout the audible frequency range, are more intense. Consequently, a white noise masks high frequencies better than low ones. To eliminate this difference and raise all the frequencies to the same masked threshold level, the wider and more intense critical bands in a white noise must be attenuated. Passing a white noise through a filter that attenuates frequencies above 1000 Hz at an increasing rate gives a *uniform masking noise* consisting of equally intense critical bands.

### *Interaural masking*

Although masking is mostly determined by interference in the cochlea, certain interaural phenomena show that interference also may occur at a higher level in the auditory nervous system where the inputs from the two ears have already joined. (However, the possibility that events in one ear influence, via efferent fibers, events in the other ear's cochlea has not been excluded.)

Perhaps the most striking interaural phenomenon is when a listener sets a tone so that he just barely hears it against an intense background noise. Both the tone and the noise are led to the same ear. When the noise is led to the other ear as well, twice as much noise is going to the listener. One would expect that the tone, which was just barely audible in monaural noise, would now disappear altogether in binaural noise. Instead the tone is clearly audible. To set the tone again to threshold, the listener must reduce the tone's intensity. This phenomenon, which is most apparent around 300 Hz, is not entirely understood, but it does depend on the phase relations between the two ears (Hirsh, 1948).

To reduce the threshold for the monaural signal, the noise must be added to the other ear in phase with the noise in the first ear. Subjectively, phase relations affect the apparent location of the sound in our heads. At low frequencies, sounds in phase are perceived as a single sound in the center of the head; sounds out of phase are perceived as being more spread out. When the phase difference is between 0° and 180°, the sound seems to come from the direction of the leading ear, that is, the ear which is stimulated at an earlier part of the signal cycle. In the preceding example, the monaural tone is, of course, heard at the stimulated ear; the binaural, in-phase noise is perceived as being in the center of the head. A binaural, out-of-phase noise would be heard at both ears, and the threshold for the tone would be about the same in the binaural as in the monaural noise. As the phase of the noise is changed from 180° (out of phase) to 0° (in phase), the threshold for the tone slowly decreases. With the binaural noise now in phase, if the tone were added in phase to the other ear, the threshold for the tone would increase; if the tone were added out of phase to the other ear, the threshold would probably decrease somewhat. The general rule is that threshold decreases when the masking noise and masked tone are localized in different places in the head. Thus, for a binaural noise and a binaural signal, threshold increases when their phase relations are the same and decreases when their phase relations are different.

Some masking also occurs between the two ears, and an intense noise in one ear can mask a tone in the other. Care must be taken to prevent noise from reaching the test ear through the skull. A noise from an external earphone at one ear gets to the other ear, but is attenuated by approximately 50 dB. A tiny earphone inserted in the external ear canal increases the interaural attenuation to 70 or 80 dB, permitting the measurement of true central masking by sounds as intense as 70 or 80 dB SPL. *Central masking,* as the term implies, is thought to be caused by interference in the central nervous system, at or beyond the point where the neural pathways from the two ears meet. Central masking is 50 or 60 dB less effective than *peripheral masking:* A monaural masker that raises the threshold for a signal in the same ear by 70 dB raises it in the other ear by only 20 dB. In central masking, a narrow-band noise masks lower frequencies just as well as higher ones, producing a symmetrical masking pattern (Zwislocki, Damianopoulos, Buining, & Glantz, 1967). The absence of the asymmetrical pattern found in peripheral masking (masking and masked sounds in the same ear) supports the notion that peripheral masking depends primarily on the pattern of activity on the basilar membrane. However, the neural pathways of the auditory system are too complex to allow simple inferences.

Interaural and central masking suggest that not all masking is based on cochlear events. Some interference may occur in the central nervous system, at least when the masker exceeds 50 dB SPL. Whether exclusively monaural stimulation also involves some central masking is not clear.

## Subject variables

Individuals usually have similar masked thresholds, but their absolute thresholds often differ greatly. Thresholds depend on the state of the subject: his recent auditory experience, his age, his motivation and experience in the task, and the condition of his auditory system.

### *Residual masking and fatigue*

Depending on the intensity and duration of the masking sound, thresholds may stay above normal for as long as 1 second after the masking sound stops. Threshold measurements at various frequencies and times after cessation of a brief, narrow-band masker yield masking patterns that look like those obtained under simultaneous masking, except that the amount of masking, i.e., the threshold increase, rapidly decreases with time (cf. Harris, 1959). This *residual* masking is so similar to simultaneous masking that it, too, probably results from ongoing excitation in the peripheral auditory system.

Usually residual masking ceases within a second or two, but thresholds may stay high as a result of *fatigue*. Fatigue is most noticeable after prolonged stimulation at high intensities. Recovery from fatigue is slow; thresholds decrease to their normal levels in proportion to the logarithm of the post-exposure time (Ward, Glorig, & Sklar, 1959). Fatigue causes the greatest threshold shift, not at the center frequency of the masker, as in residual and simultaneous masking, but one-half to one octave higher. For example, a fatiguing tone at 1000 Hz causes the largest threshold shift near 1500 Hz. Why fatigue is not greatest at the stimulus frequency is an unanswered and intriguing question.

Auditory fatigue has been intensively studied because the *temporary threshold shift (TTS)* may provide clues about permanent threshold shifts, i.e., irreversible hearing loss. Such information is needed in setting criteria for the maximum levels of industrial and other noise to which people may be exposed for long periods.

### *Age*

Older people generally hear less well than younger people, although we do not know precisely why. How much *presbyacusis* (hearing loss in old age) results from exposure to noise—the older a person, the more noise he has heard—and how much results from natural degeneration of the hair cells and auditory neural pathways have not been determined. Some measurements indicate little hearing loss in members of primitive tribes who live without jet planes, automobiles, air conditioners, gun powder, etc., and so are exposed to little noise. Since these people also differ in many ways other than noise exposure, we cannot be sure that reduced presbyacusis results only from less noise exposure, but it certainly must be a factor.

Whatever the cause, the relation is clear. As we age beyond 25 or 30 years, our thresholds increase, especially at the higher frequencies. Women accrue smaller hearing losses than men, perhaps because they are generally exposed to less noise.

### *Motivation and practice*

Threshold judgments are like other tasks insofar as people tend to do better when well practiced and highly motivated. One experiment (Zwislocki, Maire, Feldman, & Rubin, 1958) measured a 6-dB reduction in threshold, apparently as the result of monetary reward, practice, and interpersonal factors (the experimenter got friendly with the subjects). While the effects of such factors are highly variable and difficult to pinpoint, they should not be ignored. Use of the forced-choice procedure and signal detection theory can help analyze but cannot eliminate them (see Chapter 2).

### *Pathology*

Abnormally elevated thresholds are usually the clearest, but seldom the only, symptom of auditory pathology. Nevertheless, threshold curves are often the only psychophysical data in the diagnostic file. They help determine whether there is pathology and where in the auditory system it is likely to be. Thresholds 16 dB or more above the average of the patient's age group may indicate pathology. On the basis of the probable locus of the pathology, the patient is put into one of two diagnostic groups, *conductive impairment* or *sensorineural impairment.* In conductive impairment, something is wrong with the conductive mechanism: the external ear canal, the eardrum, or the middle ear ossicles. A common type of conductive problem is *otosclerosis,* a disorder in which calcium deposits form around the stapes and impede its movement. In sensorineural impairment, on the other hand, the pathology lies in the hàir cells, the acoustic nerve (VIIIth cranial), or both. On occasion, the pathology may be located still higher in the nervous system; it is then called *central impairment.*

One good way to distinguish conductive from sensorineural impairment is to compare *air-conduction* with *bone-conduction* thresholds. Air-conduction thresholds are measured for sounds arriving at the eardrum through the air in the external ear canal. An earphone is usually the sound source. Bone-conduction thresholds are measured for sounds reaching the cochlea directly through the skull, thus bypassing the conductive mechanism of the middle ear. A vibrator placed on the mastoid bone behind the pinna is the bone-conduction sound source. Abnormally high air-conduction thresholds but normal bone-conduction thresholds indicate conductive impairment. Both high air- and high bone-conduction thresholds indicate sensorineural impairment. When, in addition, the patient makes very narrow excursions in tracking a continuous high-frequency tone by the von Békésy method, then the sensorineural damage is probably cochlear rather than more central. On the other hand, when the threshold for a single frequency rises rapidly the longer the patient listens (abnormal adaptation), the lesion is likely to be in the auditory nerve.

The shape of the threshold curve is also relevant. In otosclerosis, for example, thresholds are high at all the audible frequencies. In noise-induced deafness the threshold curve often is normal up to 3000 or 4000 Hz, above which point it then rises steeply.

Threshold measurements in pathological ears give the experimental psychologist and the psychoacoustician opportunities to test their theories about how the auditory system works. For example, if masking is mostly peripheral, then a lesion in the nervous system should not affect the masking patterns. Lilly and Thalmann (1964) measured the *masked audiogram* for patients with VIIIth-nerve lesions who rapidly adapt to a steady tone. (An audiogram is a graph of the difference between an individual patient's thresholds for pure tones and normal thresholds; the difference, called the *hearing loss,* is plotted as a function of frequency. The masked audiogram is a plot of the difference between thresholds measured in the presence of a masking sound and thresholds measured in the quiet.) The impaired ear was stimulated with a steady tone that was inaudible to the patient after adaptation. In the presence of the steady tone, thresholds were then measured for intermittent tones at various frequencies. The *inaudible masker* gave the same masked audiogram as an audible masker in normal ears. These results, showing that when the cochlea is normal, masking is also normal despite gross disturbance of the auditory nerve, support the notion that masking is mostly peripheral.

## PITCH

Thresholds are convenient boundaries, but hearing is concerned with suprathreshold, audible sounds. Audible sounds are almost infinitely variable: Consider the possible frequencies, intensities, durations, phase relations, and their combinations and permutations. Fortunately, the relation between the physical input and the sensation (output) is fairly orderly. Thus, as a pure tone's frequency increases, its *pitch* goes from low to high. Pitch is the subjective attribute of a sound that changes most readily when frequency changes. Pitch, however, is not the same as frequency, just as loudness is not the same as intensity, nor brightness the same as luminance, nor hue the same as wavelength. The subjective phenomenon is or is based on a neural event only remotely related via the sensory apparatus to the physical stimulus. Psychophysicists try to determine the relation between the subjective phenomenon and the physical input, while physiologists and physiological psychologists may contribute to this determination by measuring the relation between certain aspects of the neural event and the physical input. However, the precise physiological counterpart to subjective experience or sensation is unknown; there is no single place in the brain to hook the electrode and exclaim, "Aha, now I am measuring sensation!" Moreover, it seems unlikely that sensations are

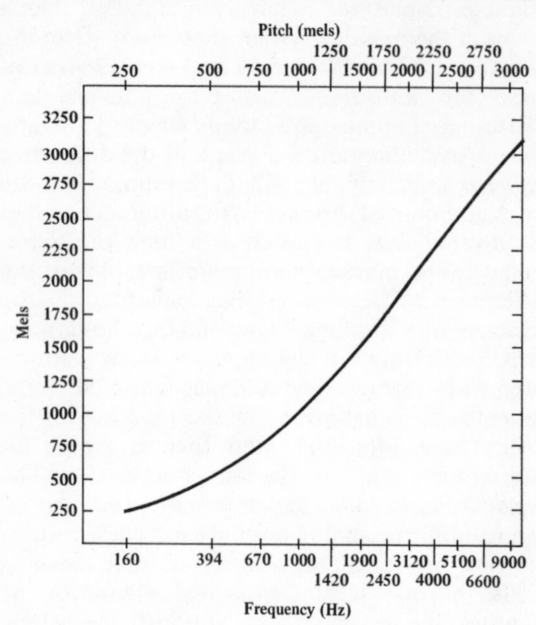


**Figure 4.13** The mel scale of pitch.

uniquely determined in the nervous system. Consequently, everything known about pitch and how it is related to frequency is based on behavioral responses by human subjects.

## Mel scale

Figure 4.13 gives pitch as a function of frequency. The unit of pitch is called the *mel*. One thousand mels is the pitch of a 1000-Hz tone at an SPL of 40 dB. Only at 1000 Hz does the number of mels equal the number of Hertz. Since pitch changes more slowly than frequency, for a given tone the number of mels is greater than the number of Hertz below 1000 Hz, and is less when above 1000 Hz. The difference increases as the frequency moves away from 1000 Hz. Like all units of measurement, the mel is arbitrary; any frequency could have been chosen to equal 1000 mels, but 1000 Hz is used as a standard in many applications.

The mel scale of pitch was constructed by two methods (Stevens & Volkmann, 1940). In the *method of fractionation,* listeners set a variable tone to one-half the pitch of a standard. The frequency of the standard was set at different values to cover most of the audible frequency range. In the *method of equisection,* the subject was given a low and a high frequency and asked to set three other tones at equal pitch intervals between the two extremes. Thus the subject set the middle three of the five tones—$S_1$, $S_2$, $S_3$, $S_4$, and $S_5$—so that the pitch intervals between neighbors $S_1$ and $S_2$, and $S_2$ and $S_3$, etc., were all equal. Three different pairs of tones served as the end stimuli in three sets of equisections. Agreement among these three sets and between the equisections and the fractionation judgments was very good. Moreover, the mel scale agrees with some basic physiological data relating frequency to its representation in the auditory system.

Pitch may also change as intensity changes. Stevens (1935) found for one subject that high frequencies tend to go up in pitch and low frequencies to go down when intensity increases. Cohen (1961) observed similar, but much less pronounced, tendencies among the two groups of ten and twelve subjects he studied.

## Difference limen

Although the mel scale of pitch is continuous, one cannot infer that the ear distinguishes infinitely small changes in frequency. Nevertheless, the human ear is remarkably sensitive to changes in frequency. Within the audible frequency range (20 Hz to 20,000 Hz), we can detect changes as small as 3 Hz when the absolute frequency is below 1000 Hz, and changes as small as 0.2 to 0.3 percent of the absolute frequency above 1000 Hz. Our sensitivity at the low frequencies is equivalent to being able to see a positional change of 1/7 inch in a total span of 87 feet.

The constancy of the *relative* frequency shift above 1000 Hz follows *Weber's law* according to which the just noticeable difference, jnd or $\Delta I$, in stimulus magnitude increases in direct proportion to the absolute magnitude, $I$ (see Chapter 2). Stimulus magnitude may be intensity, size, length, duration, frequency, and so on. When frequency is the stimulus magnitude, the jnd is expressed as $\Delta f$ and absolute magnitude as $f$. Above 1000 Hz, the Weber fraction, $\Delta f/f$, is constant at approximately 0.003. Below 1000 Hz, however, the Weber fraction increases as frequency decreases, meaning that the ear is relatively less sensitive at low frequencies. Sensitivity also decreases, in an absolute sense, at low intensities. As the SPL is reduced from approximately 30 dB above threshold, the jnd at all frequencies rises. In other words, regarding frequency, soft tones are more difficult to tell apart than are loud tones.

## Representation of frequency in the auditory system

Pitch changes with frequency in an orderly fashion and in small steps, as indicated by the size of the jnd. The human ear distinguishes well over 1000 different pitches at most SPLs. How are all these different sensations represented in the nervous system? How is frequency encoded by the auditory nervous system? The answer is complicated by the fact that we can hear more than one pitch at a time, so that a number of different frequencies must be simultaneously and separately encoded. Attempts to answer these questions are considered so fundamental that they constitute theories of hearing.

### *Place theory*

Earlier it was shown that mechanical action in the cochlea translates the frequency of an acoustic signal into a spatial configuration on the basilar membrane. High frequencies give rise to maximum membrane displacement near the stapes, and low frequencies near the helicotrema at the apex of the cochlea. This *place* theory is confirmed by von Békésy's (1960) direct observations under the microscope of the pattern of vibration of the basilar membrane and by the observations of Johnstone and Boyle (1967), who used the Mössbauer technique (involving measurements at the molecular level). The place theory receives much additional support from studies of clinical pathology, permanent deafness caused by intense sounds, cochlear models, experimental injury, embryological development of the inner ear, and cochlear microphonics. Spatial representation of frequency is a fact. What is not proven is the hypothesis that pitch and pitch discrimination are determined exclusively, or even primarily, by the place of maximum displacement on the basilar membrane. The hypothesis seems eminently reasonable because pitch would then depend on which neural fibers are stimulated.

However, the place theory poses some difficulties. A major difficulty is to reconcile the grossness of the displacement patterns on the basilar membrane with the purity of our pitch sensations (to pure tones) and with the fineness of our frequency discriminations. A pure tone gives rise to a definite unitary sensation without the interference of other sensations associated with stimulation on other parts of the basilar membrane which, however, are also being set in motion by the same pure tone. Additionally, a change of 3 Hz, which is just detectable below 1000 Hz, gives rise to a very tiny shift in the pattern of disturbance on the basilar membrane. Given the unreliability of neural transmission, it is unlikely that so tiny a shift in a large pattern of proximal stimulation could be maintained as a discriminable neural event at higher levels in the nervous system. Von Békésy (1960) has set out to show that the gross pattern of stimulation is sharpened in the peripheral nervous system, much as his analogous measurements on the skin and the eye have shown that a real stimulus spread over a large surface is "funneled" to give rise to sharply defined sensations. He postulates *lateral inhibition* (neural inhibition between adjacent sections) in the neural network at the receptor as the basis for this sharpening, but sharpening by lateral inhibition may not be sufficient to account for the ear's fine discrimination.

Another difficulty posed by the place theory is that the patterns of displacement are all alike for frequencies below 400 Hz. These low frequencies set the whole basilar membrane vibrating in phase, yet we can discriminate quite well below 400 Hz. A third difficulty is the similarity between the masking patterns produced by narrow-band noise and those produced by pure tones. This similarity implies that the patterns of displacement are similar, yet bands of noise and pure tones sound very different.

Finally, and perhaps presenting the greatest difficulty, there is *periodicity pitch*. A series of harmonically related tones presented simultaneously gives rise to a distinct pitch usually corresponding to that of the fundamental frequency, even when the fundamental is missing. Thus the tones 1200, 1400, and 1600 Hz may give rise to a pitch normally associated with a 200-Hz tone, along with a rough, high-pitched sound associated with the input frequencies. The pitch of the missing fundamental, or *residue,* is heard even when the tones are faint; the residue cannot then be a simple distortion product, since the necessary distortion is absent below a sensation level of 50 or 60 dB. Moreover, the residue does not beat with a neighboring tone (say, 202 Hz in our example) as it should if the fundamental frequency were present in the cochlea. Also, the residue cannot be masked by a low-pass noise which should normally mask a low-pitch sound like the residue; it can be masked only by a noise that masks the physical input frequencies. A similar phenomenon occurs when the stimulus is a series of pulses. A pitch corresponding to the pulse frequency may be heard. In both cases, the unexpected pitch corresponds to the period of the waveform rather than to any component frequencies. (The correspondence is not always exact, but this question is secondary to the present discussion.) Hence the name, periodicity pitch.

The main point of these phenomena is that we can hear a distinct pitch without stimulation at that place on the basilar membrane normally associated with the pitch. Consequently, pitch does not depend only on the place of maximum displacement, but may also depend on temporal characteristics of the stimulus.

### *Telephone theory*

The obvious temporal characteristic to which the ear may respond is frequency. Although the problem is still that of the relationship between pitch and frequency, it is possible that the nervous system directly encodes temporal information, such as frequency, which is transmitted to the brain and serves as the basis for the perception of pitch. Measurement of electrical activity in the cochlea shows that those pressure changes that initiate traveling waves also elicit electrical responses, most likely in the hair cells of the organ of Corti (see Chapter 3). These responses duplicate almost exactly the form of the acoustic stimulus and are therefore called the *cochlear microphonic*. Thus, a 1000-Hz tone gives rise to a cochlear microphonic with the same sinusoidal form and frequency. A complex sound gives rise to a microphonic with the same complex waveform. Since the stimulus retains its temporal characteristics right up to the receptor cells, information about frequency is available at that point. The *telephone* theory postulates that the neural firing rate matches the frequency of the acoustic stimulus, and in this sense the auditory nerve acts like a telephone line. This theory quickly became untenable, however, when it was shown that the auditory neural fibers, like other neural fibers, do not respond faster than 1000 times per second, needing at least a millisecond to recover after each response (the *refractory period*). Faced with a maximum rate of 1000 Hz, the telephone theory failed to account for the human's ability to distinguish frequencies up to at least 16,000 Hz. Even without these physiological measurements, it would be difficult to show how duplication of the "frequencies" of a complex sound could permit us to recognize its components as distinct pitches, which we often can do. The telephone theory is a dead line, but the basic idea appears in an altered and more acceptable form.

### *Volley theory*

Despite the limitations on neural firing rates set by the refractory period, the auditory nerve can fire in step with frequencies up to 4000 or 5000 Hz. Wever (1949) used this information as an important basis for his volley theory, stating that pitch is based on both place of maximum displacement and temporal encoding. *Volley* refers to the assumed mechanism by which groups of nerve fibers, stimulated at high frequencies, can fire synchronously at rates far beyond those of single units. Pitch is determined by which groups of fibers are firing and how fast: Which group fires depends on the place of maximum displacement, and the firing rate depends on the volley principle. According to the volley principle, while one group of fibers rests during its refractory period, a second group fires. If, for example, the stimulus is a 1000-Hz pure tone, one-half of the fibers could fire in response to every other cycle of the stimulus. Between firings the group would have almost 2 msec to rest. During those 2 msec the other half of the involved fibers would fire. In this manner, each cycle of the tone could evoke neural impulses from the two groups of fibers in alternation, and so impulses could be generated 1000 times per second.

Wever suggests that pitch is determined by the firing rate alone at frequencies below 400 Hz (where the whole basilar membrane vibrates to all frequencies), by rate and place together between 400 and 5000 Hz, and by place alone above 5000 Hz. This theory solves most of the problems unanswered by the place theory. The problem of fine discrimination is taken care of by firing rates so redundantly encoded that small changes in frequency can remain discriminable at higher levels in the nervous system. Since a number of fibers participate in a volley, lapses by several do not affect the group's frequency, as Wever (1949) theoretically demonstrated. The problem of periodicity pitch is also met. Where temporal and place information are discordant, both place and periodicity pitch are perceived, but the more regular periodicity pitch may predominate.

Basing pitch on both place and the subtle but necessary neural firing rate, the auditory system is able to make its fine frequency analysis and still maintain rapid responding. The apparent failure of the dual system at low and high frequencies has interesting implications in psychophysical experiments, but so far no data have indicated that, in Wever's postulated transition regions around 400 and 5000 Hz, there are discontinuities in the quality, detectability, or other subjective aspects of pure tones. The transitions are, no doubt, smooth, but are they smooth enough to escape detection by careful psychophysical measurements?

The volley theory by no means solves all the problems of auditory theory. It hardly touches upon those problems associated with dichotic listening—in which the signals at the ears are different—but it does handle many of the more usual difficulties.

## LOUDNESS

### The growth of loudness

An enormous range of intensities lies between the softest sound that humans can detect and the most intense sound that can be tolerated. The energy ratio of these two limits is 100,000,000,000,000:1. Because the loudness ratio between these extremes is relatively small, something like 100,000:1, the range of our subjective experience is greatly compressed. Nevertheless, from threshold to the loudest tolerable sound, loudness increases monotonically with intensity. Using such direct psychophysical techniques as magnitude estimation and production and ratio estimation and production (see Chapter 2), many laboratories have mapped out the relationship between loudness and intensity. Their results are summarized by a power function:

$$L = kP^{0.6}, \qquad [6]$$

where $L$ is loudness, $P$ is sound pressure, and $k$ is a constant of proportionality (Stevens, 1955). This relationship applies most closely for pure tones between 500 and 4000 Hz.

Figure 4.14 graphs the loudness in *sones* of a 1000-Hz tone as a function of *loudness level.* The sone is defined as the loudness value for a 1000-Hz tone at an SPL of 40 dB, which is the same as a loudness level of 40 *phons.* In general, loudness level is the SPL of an equally loud 1000-Hz tone; phon is substituted for decibel to keep clear the distinction between SPL and loudness level. Since a 1000-Hz tone is equal in loudness to itself, its SPL and loudness level have the same values. (Sometimes loudness is plotted as a function of *sensation level,* which is the difference in decibels

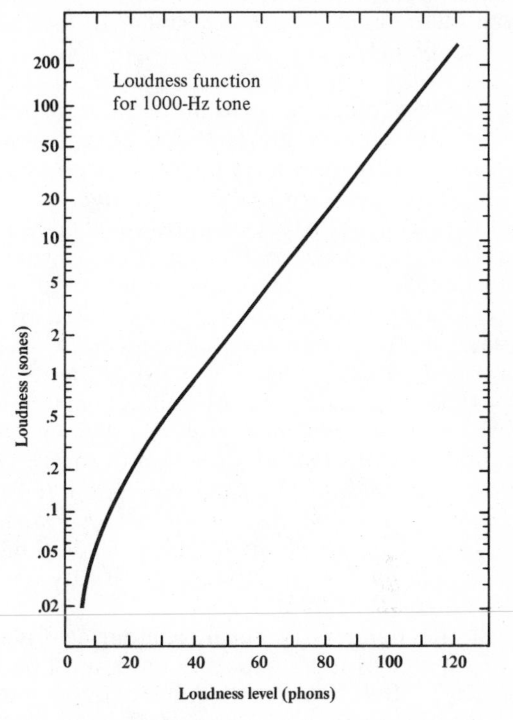


**Figure 4.14** Loudness of a binaural, 1000-Hz tone as a function of loudness level.

between a sound's SPL as presented and its SPL at threshold.) Figure 4.14 plots loudness on a logarithmic scale. Since loudness level is also a logarithmic scale, the graph is a log-log plot on which a power function is a straight line. The slope of the line is the exponent, here 0.6 (see Chapter 2). Figure 4.14 shows that above approximately 30 phons, each 10-phon increase in level doubles the loudness. Below 30 phons, loudness changes more rapidly, and the power function fails unless a correction such as the following is made:

$$L = k(P - P_0)^{0.6}. \qquad [7]$$

The value $P_0$ is the *effective threshold pressure.* Its introduction means that at threshold, where the stimulus first begins to have an effect, the stimulus is counted as zero at that point instead of at the true physical zero. (Some controversy exists about the best correction to use, since other ones are possible; intuitively, however, this one is the most reasonable.)

The loudness functions are steeper at low frequencies than at 1000 Hz (Hellman & Zwislocki, 1968). Loudness functions for high-frequency tones, although not directly measured, appear from loudness matches to be similar to the function at 1000 Hz.

Use of the term *direct measurements* to distinguish these procedures from *loudness matches* should not obscure the fact that both types of measurement involve matching. In the most commonly used direct procedure, *magnitude estimation,* the listener matches numbers and loudness (see Chapter 2). It is assumed that when the listener calls a 1000-Hz tone at one level "10" and at a second level "100," the tone is ten times louder at the second level. Judgments of tones presented at different levels yield functions like those in Figure 4.14. In loudness matching, two sounds are matched to each other by such methods as the *method of adjustment* or the *method of constant stimuli.* Matching data for free-field listening are shown as *equal-loudness contours* in Figure 4.15. Earphone listening yields similar curves, except for the differences already noted in the threshold curves.

All the tones on a single contour in Figure 4.15 are equally loud, but some tones must be set to a higher SPL than others. Each contour is at a different loudness level. From these contours and the loudness function of a 1000-Hz tone (see Figure 4.14), the loudness function at any frequency can be constructed. On the basis of the 1000-Hz loudness function, loudness level is converted to loudness in sones. Then, for a given frequency, the equal-loudness contours give the relation between loudness and SPL. Loudness is plotted against SPL to yield the desired loudness function for the frequency. Without going through the procedure, we can see from the bunching of the contours at the low frequencies that loudness increases more rapidly with intensity there than at the moderate or high frequencies.

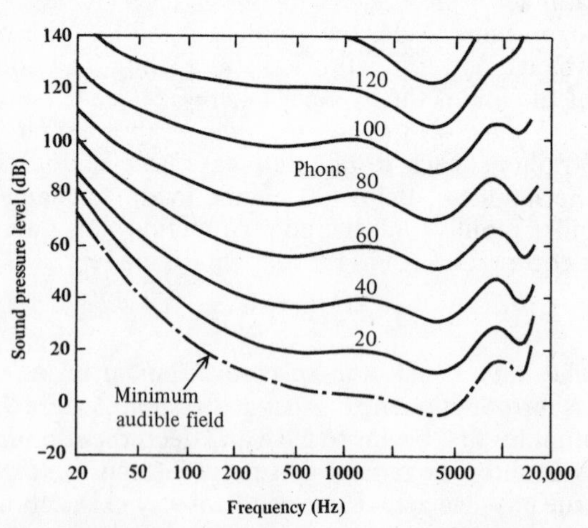


**Figure 4.15** Equal-loudness contours for free-field listening. The SPL required to yield the loudness levels, given on the curves, is plotted as a function of frequency. (From Robinson & Dadson, 1956.)

The rapid growth of the loudness of low-frequency tones is an example of *loudness recruitment*. Recruitment also occurs against noise backgrounds, in auditory fatigue, and in certain types of hearing impairment. The term *recruitment* is used whenever the loudness of a sound grows more rapidly as a function of SPL than that of a 1000-Hz tone presented in the quiet to a group of listeners with normal hearing. For example, a tone in noise may not be heard until it is 50 dB more intense than the same tone in the quiet. Yet, raised another 20 or 30 dB the tone in the noise is just as loud as an equally intense tone in the quiet, one 70 or 80 dB above its threshold. Thus, over a range of only 20 or 30 dB loudness increases as much in the noise as it does over a range of 70 or 80 dB in the quiet. Similarly, rapid loudness growth is characteristic of disturbed cochlear function, either of the temporary fatigue type that follows exposure to an intense sound, or the permanent pathology in some types of sensorineural deafness. A patient may have a 50-dB hearing loss (threshold shift) in his impaired ear, but 30 dB above his elevated threshold, loudness is the same as for his normal ear. Loudness recruitment is usually measured by matching tones in a masked and an unmasked ear or in a pathological and a healthy ear. Stevens (1966) suggested that these recruitment functions can be represented by two power functions; between threshold and the level where normal loudness is reached the exponent is large, whereas above that level the exponent has its usual value of 0.6.

Loudness recruitment is a quite general phenomenon, to be found nearly always when thresholds are elevated as they are at low frequencies, against noise, and in cochlear pathology. Another example is for white noise, whose threshold is about 10 dB higher than that for a 1000-Hz tone and whose loudness function is steeper at low levels. Higher thresholds, then, are accompanied by steeper loudness functions, and as a general rule, the higher the threshold, the steeper the function. (An exception is for thresholds raised by a conductive impairment; the loudness function is usually no steeper than normal.)

Of course, we are sensitive to changes in intensity as well as to absolute magnitude. Our sensitivity follows Weber's law above approximately 40 dB sensation level (SL), where we can just detect a 0.5-dB change in intensity at most frequencies. Below 40 dB SL, the jnd increases more rapidly for the low and high than for the middle frequencies; at 5 dB SL, it ranges from 2.5 dB to over 6 dB (see Stevens & Davis, 1938).

**Physiological basis for loudness**

Loudness seems to be directly related to the total number of neural impulses per unit of time. The more auditory fibers that fire and, to a lesser extent, the more often, the greater the sensation of loudness. Although intuitively reasonable that stronger stimuli elicit more neural activity and that loudness depends on the amount of that activity, inhibitory neural elements doubtless complicate these relationships. Recall that adding noise to a previously unstimulated ear may reduce the masked threshold for a low-frequency tone in the other ear; the noise also increases the loudness for the tone set a few decibels above threshold. Nevertheless, some neurophysiological measurements show good correlations between auditory activity and stimulus intensity. Measurements of action potentials produced by the whole auditory nerve, of slow-wave potentials in the superior olivary complex (see Chapter 3), and of EEG recordings from the scalp of human observers all show that the electrical activity in the nervous system increases with stimulus intensity. Moreover, the relation is often a power function, sometimes with the same exponent as the loudness function (Stevens, 1970). This and other evidence suggests that the nonlinear relation between loudness and intensity is determined peripherally, probably at the hair cells where acoustic energy is transduced to neural energy. Indeed, the nervous system would hardly be able to encompass a range of $10^{14}$ or $10^{7}$ by making a direct linear transformation of energy or pressure. It follows that the auditory neural pathways to the brain serve as simple relay stations which introduce no additional nonlinear changes in loudness. This corollary is supported by experiments on animals whose discrimination of sound intensity remains intact after removal of auditory areas of the temporal lobes (Raab & Ades, 1946).

How does an increase in stimulus intensity augment auditory activity? A stronger stimulus results in a larger amplitude of displacement on the basilar membrane. The larger amplitude may be coded in the nervous system in three ways: faster neural firing, more inner hair cells firing, and more neural fibers firing.

Generally, faster firing follows more intense stimulation (see Chapter 3), presenting a difficulty for the volley theory of pitch perception. The theory assumes that pitch depends, in part, on the frequency of neural firing, yet pitch hardly changes with stimulus intensity even though the rate of neural firing may change drastically. Wever (1949) has shown, however, that the faster rate of firing in single fibers does not alter the overall volley rate for a group of fibers; synchrony among individual fibers permits the group's firing rate to follow the stimulus frequency despite more impulses per unit time. Thus, volley rate is free to mediate pitch, while the total number of active neural units is free to help mediate loudness.

The inner hair cells lie on the basilar membrane toward the inner core of the cochlea, whereas the outer hair cells are located toward the outer bony shell (see Chapter 3, Figure 3.21). About 6000 inner hair cells form a single row along the membrane, and about 30,000 outer hair cells form three or four additional rows. The outer cells are more sensitive than the inner cells (intense acoustical stimulation and certain drugs damage them more easily), contain more hairs, and differ in shape and structure. Most important to the perception of loudness, the less sensitive inner hair cells first begin to fire when the stimulus is 50 or 60 dB above the absolute psychophysical threshold. Apparently the inner hair cells are less sensitive because they are in a less favorable position, and because displacement of the basilar membrane is smaller close to the cochlear core than toward the outer shell. Other structural and internal differences may also contribute to their reduced sensitivity. But whatever the reasons, the firing of large numbers of inner hair cells could in itself signal a more intense stimulus regardless of the total amount of neural activity. This explanation is a kind of place theory of loudness. It remains, however, in considerable doubt.

More intense sounds also stimulate more hair cells and thereby excite more neural fibers. With increasing stimulus intensity, the amplitude of displacement increases all along the basilar membrane, causing neural responses to appear at places where the displacement produced by weak intensities was too shallow to elicit a neural response. How excitation spreads with increasing intensity may be inferred from the masking patterns (see Figure 4.11), which reflect the amount of ongoing excitation in the auditory system: The higher the masked threshold, the greater the assumed amount of neural excitation. Procedures are available for calculating the loudness of all kinds of sounds from these masking patterns (Zwicker & Scharf, 1965). Excitation is calculated, converted to a loudness measure, and then the whole loudness pattern is integrated. The final result is an estimate of the loudness of the masker that produced the original masking pattern.

Measurements of loudness as a function of bandwidth also show that directly stimulating a larger area of the basilar membrane produces sensations of greater loudness (Zwicker & Scharf, 1965). The loudness of a band of noise or multitone complex increases with bandwidth even though the overall stimulus intensity is held constant (spectrum level is decreased). Loudness increases when the acoustical energy covers a wider range of frequencies, thereby more effectively stimulating a larger area of the basilar membrane. Supporting this theoretical approach is the fact that the loudness of a complex sound does not begin to increase until the critical band is exceeded. Sounds at the same center frequency are all equally loud when equally intense, provided they are subcritical. (Subcritical sounds, including a pure tone at the center frequency, produce similar masking patterns.) The masking pattern does not begin to expand until the sound's bandwidth exceeds the critical band; only then is more of the basilar membrane stimulated and does loudness begin to increase with stimulus bandwidth.

Since loudness appears to depend on the total amount of neural activity per unit of time, it is reasonable that loudness increases with duration of stimulation—up to between 100 and 150 msec. If loudness is to remain constant as duration is increased, then intensity must be decreased. The relation is such that intensity times duration is approximately a constant (corresponding to Bloch's law in vision; see Chapter 7). Since the product of intensity and time is a measure of energy, the same quantity of acoustic energy is needed to reach a given loudness level at 10 msec as at 50 msec.

What about the effect of the ear's transmission characteristics on loudness? The way in which these characteristics affect the dependence of the absolute threshold on frequency is similar to their effect at higher intensities. Thus the equal-loudness contours near threshold (see Figure 4.15) have the same shape as the threshold curve. The flattening of the curves at the low frequencies as intensity is increased reflects the reduced influence of an internal masking noise and the rapid increase in the spread of displacement that accompanies low-frequency stimulation. These low frequencies have the whole basilar membrane over which to spread, since they cause maximum displacement near the apex of the cochlea (Figure 4.12). Certain aspects of the transmission process, however, do depend on intensity. The *tensor tympani* and *stapedial* muscles of the middle ear contract at higher intensities, making the eardrum more tense and the stapes more difficult to move. Thus the ability of these structures to transmit sound energy is reduced, especially at low frequencies. These muscles serve to protect the delicate structures of the inner ear from the effects of overstimulation, but some evidence indicates that they also play a role at safe levels. Theirs may be a kind of tuning role, similar to that of the iris in vision, since at most frequencies their activity reduces loudness to some extent. Since their effect is not the same at all frequencies, the equal-loudness contours must be affected by their presence, but the effect is probably small.

An additional safety factor is provided by a change in the movement of the stapes during low-frequency, high-intensity stimulation. Such stimulation causes the stapes' normal push-pull motion against the oval window to become rotational around an axis perpendicular to the window. As a consequence, less pressure is transmitted to the cochlea.

### Binaural loudness

Thus far, the discussion of loudness has not differentiated between stimulation of both ears and stimulation of a single ear. Generally, stimulation of both ears results in greater loudness than stimulation of one ear. Binaural loudness is about one and three quarter times greater than monaural loudness except near threshold, where it is almost twice as great (Scharf & Fishken, 1970). Since the neural pathways from the two ears meet and mix, it is not surprising that some neural interference at high stimulus levels prevents a doubling of the experienced loudness.

In earphone listening, when the intensity is not the same at the two ears, the listener may hear the sound only in the more intense earphone (see following discussion of sound localization); he hears nothing in the other phone. Yet if the weaker, unheard sound is removed, loudness decreases. Clearly, the tone to the inhibited ear contributes to the overall, binaural loudness. This phenomenon is an example of what von Békésy (1967) called *funneling*, the process by which a stimulus is inhibited and is not detected as a separate entity but joins the inhibiting stimulus to produce a stronger sensation. (See Chapter 5 for examples of funneling on the skin.)

## OTHER SUBJECTIVE ATTRIBUTES

Pitch and loudness, the most salient attributes of sounds, especially of pure tones, have been the most thoroughly studied. Other subjective attributes include roughness, annoyance, pleasantness, and so on, but volume, density, and vocality have received more attention and will be considered briefly here.

### Volume

Loud sounds seem to fill a larger space than soft sounds, and low-pitch sounds seem larger than high-pitch sounds. The subjective size, or *volume*, of a sound depends almost equally on intensity and frequency. Sometimes volume and loudness are confused (as on some radio and television dials), but their independence can be demonstrated by keeping volume constant while varying loudness. Balancing an increase in intensity, which enhances the volume, with an increase in frequency, which diminishes the volume, we can keep volume constant while changing loudness (and pitch). The confusion between loudness and volume is not surprising since they both increase as a power function of sound pressure. Direct estimates of the volume of tones at various frequencies show that the exponent of the power function relating volume to sound pressure increases from 0.1 to 0.75 as frequency is increased from 100 to 5000 Hz. (Only near 3750 Hz is the exponent for volume and loudness the same, between 0.6 and 0.7.) The change in the value of the exponent with frequency means that the volume of low-frequency tones changes slowly as a function of sound pressure, whereas the volume of high-frequency tones changes much more rapidly. Low-frequency tones are already big at low SPLs and do not grow much bigger at higher levels. High-frequency tones start out small but, growing rapidly with SPL, at very high levels they are judged as big as low frequency tones. At 140 dB, all tones, regardless of frequency, may be perceived as being equal in volume. Since all tones appear about equally loud at 140 dB, a distinction between volume and loudness becomes meaningless at that point (Terrace & Stevens, 1962).

It has been suggested that subjective volume reflects the extent of excitation along the basilar membrane (von Békésy, 1963). Intense, low-frequency sounds are big, and they produce the largest spread of excitation, as shown by masking patterns.

### Density

Independently of its volume, loudness, and pitch, a sound can be judged to be more or less dense, compact, or hard. High-frequency, loud sounds are denser than low-frequency, soft sounds. Appropriate adjustments of frequency and sound pressure permit the experimenter to hold density constant while varying volume, loudness, and pitch (see Chapter 1). Density, like loudness and volume, is a power function of sound pressure (Guirao & Stevens, 1964): The exponent of density is larger at low than at high frequencies. The relation of density to loudness and volume may be even closer, since one set of measurements suggests that loudness is a product of volume and density (Stevens, Guirao, & Slawson, 1965).

### Vocality

Tones spaced at octave intervals are often judged as more similar than tones closer in frequency. For example, tones from the musical scale share a common quality when harmonically related. This quality of "C-ness" or "E-ness" is called *vocality*, or the degree of harmonic relationship. In terms of frequency, there seems to be some similarity between, for example, 500, 1000, and 2000 Hz, or 650, 1300, and 2600 Hz. Such similarities do not exist between, for example, 500 and 800 Hz or 1300 and 1600 Hz. Perhaps these affinities reflect no more than the presence of *aural harmonics* in the ear (see following discussion). Thus 500 and 1000 Hz, or 650 and 1300 Hz, seem to sound alike because they share a common set of harmonic frequencies produced by distortion in the ear itself. However, at low SPLs these aural harmonics are so soft that their role can be questioned. Whatever its cause, vocality is a real phenomenon of great importance in music.

## AUDITORY DISTORTION

Nonlinear distortion in the middle ear and inner ear produces frequencies not present in the original physical input. In any transmission system, sound is distorted when the resulting displacement is not proportional to the force applied. In the ear, two types of distortion products are generally distinguished: *aural harmonics* and *combination tones.* Aural harmonics arise when a single intense pure tone is introduced to the ear, whereas combination tones arise when two tones are introduced simultaneously.

### Aural harmonics

An intense tone (the *primary* tone) at frequency $f$ gives rise in the ear to frequencies at both the even harmonics ($2f$, $4f$, etc.) and the odd harmonics ($3f$, $5f$, etc.). For example, presented with a 500-Hz pure tone, a trained listener may detect a pitch corresponding to 1000 and 1500 Hz. In one study by Plomp (1966), however, only 17 percent of the listeners could detect harmonics when the primary was 100 dB SPL; below 100 dB even fewer listeners could hear them. Aural harmonics are difficult to hear, partly because they occur at higher frequencies and are therefore easily masked by the intense primary.

In attempts to measure aural harmonics indirectly, investigators introduced, along with the primary tone, a *probe* tone near the frequency of the expected harmonic (e.g., Fletcher, 1930). By adjusting the frequency and amplitude of the probe tone, the investigator supposedly caused it to beat with the aural harmonic. The *best beat* would occur when the amplitude of the probe tone matched that of the aural harmonic. However, it is now recognized that these beats may arise from interaction between the primary tone and a combination tone produced from the primary and probe tones. For example, if the primary is at 500 Hz and the probe is at 1001 Hz, a difference tone of 501 Hz could beat with the 500-Hz primary; the beating would not mean that the 1000-Hz harmonic was present. From the direct observations of Plomp, it would appear that aural harmonics are less important than indirect observations by the method of best beats had led us to believe.

### Combination tones

When two tones are presented simultaneously to the ear, nonlinear distortion may give rise to *difference* and *summation tones.* A lower frequency, $f_l$, and a higher frequency, $f_h$, may give rise to difference tones like $f_h - f_l$ and to summation tones like $f_l + f_h$. Few listeners can hear summation tones, perhaps because they lie at higher frequencies than the two primaries and are masked by the primary tones. Difference tones, however, are easily heard. The simple difference tone, $f_h - f_l$, is heard when the primary tones are at least 50 to 60 dB above threshold. For example, primary tones of 1700 Hz and 2000 Hz give rise to a difference tone of 300 Hz. The frequency separation between the primary tones can be varied without greatly affecting the minimum level at which they produce the difference tone. As the level of the primaries is increased above this minimum, the amplitude of the difference tone also increases, and more rapidly than the amplitude of the primaries; the relative distortion is then said to increase with the level of the primaries. Measurements of the amplitude of the difference tone are made by the *cancellation method* in which a probe tone at the same frequency as the difference tone, but opposite in phase, is varied in amplitude until it and the difference tone cancel each other. Cancellation requires the amplitude of the external probe tone to equal that of the internal difference tone.

Other more complex difference tones can also be heard. Goldstein (1967) has shown that we can hear $2f_l - f_h$, $3f_l - 2f_h$, and even $4f_l - 3f_h$. He showed that the *cubic difference tone*, that is, $2f_l - f_h$, could be heard at SLs as low as 20 to 30 dB. The amplitude of this difference tone was usually 20 to 30 dB below the level of the primary tones, regardless of their absolute level, so that the relative distortion was independent of the level of the primaries. For example, a 1000-Hz tone and a 1200-Hz tone at 30 dB SL gave rise to a cubic difference tone at 800 Hz (i.e., [2 × 1000 Hz] − 1200 Hz) whose amplitude, as determined by the cancellation method, was 20 dB below the level of the primaries. When the primaries were at 70 dB SL, the difference tone was 30 dB below their level. Another important relation noted by Goldstein and others (e.g., Zwicker & Feldtkeller, 1967) was that as the frequency separation between the two primary tones was decreased, the amplitude of the cubic difference tone decreased.

Some of the dissimilarities of simple and complex difference tones may be summarized as follows. Simple difference tones first arise at moderate to high stimulus levels, and their relative distortion increases with stimulus level but is independent of the frequency separation between the primaries. Complex difference tones may arise at very low stimulus levels, and their relative distortion is independent of level but decreases with frequency separation. These findings suggest that simple difference tones are caused by nonlinear distortion in the middle ear and that complex difference tones are caused by distortion in the inner ear where frequency separation, in particular, would first be expected to play an important role.

It is interesting to note that only the middle ear distortion products, which first appear at higher intensities, would be apt to be perceived as distortion by the listener. The other difference tones, being almost always present, would be a natural part of any complex auditory sensation and their absence would then seem strange.

## SOUND LOCALIZATION

Localizing a sound is as important to the listener, human or animal, as telling sounds apart. For example, hearing an approaching car may not help much if one can't judge its distance and direction. To react properly to an acoustic danger signal one must both recognize it as a danger signal and locate it in space. Since the auditory system has nothing like the eye's retina to map out in a one-to-one fashion the two-dimensional, spatial characteristics of the external world, it must resort to indirect procedures. These procedures depend mostly on differences in the sound input to the two ears. Because the ears are separated, the sound waves from a single source differ significantly at the two ears in *time of arrival,* in *phase* (at low frequencies), in *intensity* (at high frequencies), and in the *angle of incidence* of the waveforms on the pinna (at very high frequencies). These differences, however, do not uniquely specify the direction of a sound. For example, sound waves coming from a source in front of the listener may differ in exactly the same way at the two ears as waves from a source behind him. By moving his head, a listener removes this ambiguity and can readily distinguish front and back.

### Time differences

Sound travels through air at 1100 ft/sec. The length of the acoustic path between the ears of the average adult male is about 0.75 feet. Thus, a sound from the right arrives at the right ear about 0.7 msec sooner than at the left ear. As the sound source moves toward the median plane (directly in front of or behind the listener), the difference in the distance from sound source to each ear decreases and so, therefore, does the time difference. When the sound source is in the median plane, the sound waves arrive at the two ears simultaneously, and the interaural time difference is zero. Clearly, time difference may serve as a cue to a sound's direction, but does the auditory system actually make use of these temporal cues?

Tests with earphones show that an interaural time difference as small as 0.01 msec is detectable (Zwislocki & Feldman, 1956). But the listener does not hear one sound arriving 0.01 msec sooner in one ear than in the other. Instead, he hears a single fused sound whose location somewhere in his head or in one of the earphones depends on the time difference. When the difference is less than 0.01 msec the sound seems to be centered inside his head. As the interaural time difference increases, the sound image moves toward the *leading ear,* or the ear that receives the sound first. When the time difference becomes large, the sound breaks up into two distinct sounds, each in its own earphone. As expected, tests with loudspeakers as the sound source have shown that these time differences help a listener locate sounds in space.

These experiments have been carried out, for the most part, with clicks or bursts of noise. Pure tones are avoided because the initial difference between arrival times is soon outweighed by the ongoing phase difference at the two ears. As the sinusoid keeps coming, the crest of one wave continues to arrive at one ear before or after the crest of the wave at the other ear.

### Phase

A tone differs in phase between the ears when the sinusoidal waves are at different stages of a cycle. For example, a cycle that is partially completed in the leading ear is just beginning in the other ear. If the cycle is one-fourth completed, the phase difference is 90°, if it is one-half completed, it is 180°, etc., and the leading ear is said to lead by 90°, 180°, and so on. The size of the phase difference, like that of the interaural time difference, depends on the *azimuth,* the angle between a line projected perpendicular to the median plane directly in front of the head and a line from the head to the sound source. Unlike the interaural time difference, the phase difference also depends on the frequency of a pure tone coming from a distant source. The phase difference increases with frequency because as the wavelength (reciprocal of frequency) gets smaller, the wavefront reaches the second ear on a later part of the cycle. When the wavelength for a sound coming from the side is equal to the distance between the two ears, the phase difference equal to or greater than 360° is ambiguous; beyond 360° a source could be placed at positions either on the left or the right sides of the head to yield identical phase differences.[4] Since the acoustic distance between the two ears corresponds approximately to the wavelength of 1500 Hz in air, localization based on phase differences would be expected to deteriorate around that frequency. That it does has been shown in tests with pure tones presented in an anechoic room and in the outdoors (Mills, 1972).

However, the deterioration in phase discrimination is apparently not directly related to the distance between the two ears. For tones presented via earphones, the phase difference can be set electrically at the input to the two phones and is therefore independent of the distance between the ears. Yet phase discrimination still deteriorates around 1500 Hz. A neurophysiological explanation of this deterioration is often invoked. It is assumed that phase discrimination requires that a neural impulse represent each cycle of the wave. Such frequency-following would permit centers somewhere in the auditory nervous system to compare successive impulses from the two ears for a constant time difference. However, frequency-following would be less precise at high frequencies where a neural impulse might not follow every cycle, and so the *neural comparator* would become confused. Moreover, a given phase difference corresponds to a time difference that decreases with the frequency of the tone, so that the temporal comparisons between the two ears would become more difficult. Wever (1949) argues that phase discrimination favors his volley theory, even though the theory would predict phase discrimination up to 3000 or 4000 Hz. Nevertheless, the coincidence of the upper limit for phase discrimination in earphone listening with the upper limit set by the interaural distance is striking. Could it be that pitch perception follows a volley principle at lower frequencies in order to make better use of phase cues in localizing sounds? At higher frequencies the volley principle would then be discarded because localization can be based on intensity differences between the ears.

[4]Cues do not become ambiguous when the phase difference is 180°, because, as neurophysiological and psychophysical measurements have shown, the ear responds differently to the *rarefaction* and *condensation* parts of an acoustic wave. During rarefaction the air particles are moving away from each other, and the stapes pulls out. During condensation the particles are moving closer together, and the stapes pushes inward.

### Intensity

As the wavelength of a tonal stimulus decreases, the intensity difference between the two ears increases because the head acts as a better sound barrier for short wavelengths than for long ones. (The intensity also decreases as the sound travels from the near to the far ear, according to the inverse-square law, but the decrease is significant only for sources very close to the head.) At a given frequency above approximately 500 Hz, the intensity difference depends on the azimuth of the sound source; it is maximum when the azimuth is 90°, that is, when the sound source is opposite one ear. Our ability to use these intensity cues is shown by (1) the localization of pure tones above 1500 Hz, the upper limit for phase discrimination; (2) the *lateralization* of a binaural pure tone to the earphone in which the signal is more intense; and (3) the close agreement between the discrimination of interaural intensity differences between tones presented in earphones and the localization of pure tones in an anechoic chamber. This last point needs clarification: Above approximately 2000 Hz, localizing tones in free space requires the same minimal intensity difference as measured for interaural discrimination in earphone listening. Below 2000 Hz, localization becomes poorer because the interaural differences between the two ears goes below the discrimination threshold. (The dichotic intensity threshold hovers between 0.5 and 1.0 dB throughout the frequency range.) However, below 1000 Hz, localization improves again as phase cues become effective. Hence, localization of pure tones is poorest between 1000 and 2000 Hz where the system shifts from depending mostly on phase cues to depending mostly on intensity cues, providing clear evidence that localization below 1500 Hz is based on something other than intensity differences (see Mills, 1972). Naturally, the sound source is localized toward the more intense side.

### Trades between time and intensity differences

Since both time and intensity differences play a role in localization, the question arises as to how they interact. Sounds presented through earphones can be set so that the time and intensity differences oppose each other as cues to direction. For example, a click that reaches the right ear a few hundred microseconds before the left ear is perceived as being toward the right. If the sound is now made more intense in the left than in the right ear, the sound image may be centered between the ears or may even be moved to the left ear. Depending on sensation level and frequency content, a time difference of 0.03 to 0.2 msec compensates an opposite intensity difference of 1.0 dB.

Outside the laboratory, of course, time and intensity differences supplement each other; they seldom oppose each other. Moreover, sounds usually contain both low and high frequencies, so that time, phase, and intensity differences all may aid in localization. Under normal conditions, sounds have two added advantages for localization. First, the quality of a sound changes somewhat as its direction changes because interaural intensity and phase differences depend on the interaction of frequency and azimuth. For sounds from one direction low frequencies may be relatively emphasized, whereas for sounds from another direction high frequencies may be emphasized. Second, in enclosed areas a sound arrives at the ears directly from the source and also indirectly after being reflected by walls and other objects. These echoes or reverberations, usually arriving a few milliseconds later, are not heard separately, but blend with the direct sound to affect its quality. This effect, whereby the direct sound both preempts apparent direction and almost completely suppresses perception of the reverberations, is called the *precedence effect* (Wallach, Newman, & Rosenzweig, 1949). However, since the quality of the sound does depend on the total spatial configuration, including sound source, reflecting surfaces, and listener, sound quality can serve as a cue to location.

### Head movements and the pinna

Head movements provide cues to sound location by producing changes in the interaural intensity, phase, and time relations, all of which depend on the direction of the sound source. These changes help a listener tell whether a sound source is in front or back, above or below, discriminations that are otherwise very difficult. Turning the head also affects the absolute intensity at each ear, so that monaural cues are then available and a person with unilateral deafness, for example, can localize sounds fairly well. In both monaural and binaural listening, the perceived motion of his own head determines how the purely auditory cues influence the listener's localization of sound (Wallach, 1940).

The pinna also provides monaural cues. Frequencies above about 8000 Hz are reflected back and forth in the whorls of the pinna, especially in the *concha* (the large cavity surrounding the entrance to the ear canal), creating echoes whose pattern varies with the direction and distance of the sound source. The ability of listeners to use these cues was demonstrated by Batteau (1967), who recorded sounds picked up by a microphone through an artificial pinna. Presented to a listener via a single earphone, the sounds seemed to come from out in space. Sounds recorded with the same microphone without an artificial pinna were localized in the usual place—in the earphone. The artificial pinna apparently transformed the incoming sound enough to create some stimulus cues important to localization in free space.

### Special effects

#### *Stereophonic listening*

By picking up sounds via two or more microphones and reproducing the sounds through two or more loudspeakers, the audio engineer retains most of the cues to location and thereby provides a more realistic, spatially correct sound reproduction.

#### *Rotating tones*

At low frequencies a small difference in frequency between a tone in the left ear and a tone in the right ear yields a sound image that moves from one ear to the other at a rate equal to the frequency difference. Apparently the rotation is caused by the changing phase relation between the two tones. Sometimes this rotating tone is called a *binaural beat* because its loudness waxes and wanes as it moves back and forth. It is loudest when the two tones are in phase and centered inside the head.

#### *Split tones*

If these low-frequency tones differ by more than a few Hertz, they split into two simultaneous sounds, one in each ear. Higher-frequency tones, however, do not rotate, nor do they split up when the frequency difference between the two ears is small. They remain fused and centered up to fairly large frequency differences; for example, at a center frequency of 2000 Hz the tones may remain fused up to a difference between 200 and 900 Hz, depending on the listener. The dissimilarities at low and high frequencies with respect to rotation and fusion may be related to the different localization mechanisms for pure tones that operate at low and high frequencies.

### Distance

To localize a sound, we must specify its distance as well as its direction. One cue to distance derives from the inverse-square law: Intensity decreases as the square of the distance, so that the more distant source is softer. However, the first time a sound is heard its loudness cannot be related to distance. The sound must be familiar to the listener so that he knows how loud the sound is at a given distance. Nevertheless, even unfamiliar sounds tend to be judged closer when they are louder.

Timbre is a second cue to distance. As distance increases beyond approximately 5 feet, the high frequencies in a complex sound decrease in intensity more rapidly than the low because they are attenuated more by air. The sound must still be familiar in order for the listener to relate its timbre to distance.

Since intensity and phase differences between the two ears depend on distance as well as azimuth, accurate judgment of the distance of unfamiliar sounds is theoretically possible. Although the pattern of interaural intensity and phase differences could specify a unique distance, this possibility has not been demonstrated in the laboratory.

A fourth possible cue to distance requires familiarity with both the sound source and the surroundings. In an enclosed space, distance affects the reverberations and, thus, the quality of a sound as well.

Generally, humans judge auditory distance less well than direction. Only when sounds become familiar do distance judgments become consistent and valid.

## SUMMARY AND CONCLUSIONS

The acoustic stimulus, the ear and auditory nervous system, and the behavioral response constitute the content areas of hearing. This chapter emphasizes the relations between stimulus and response, tying them whenever possible to known physiological events.

Sound is vibratory movement. Normally we hear sounds in air, and it is the movement of air particles pushing against the eardrum that results in hearing. The dimensions of sound relevant to hearing are *frequency, intensity,* and *phase.* Frequency and intensity are most important, as together they determine the auditory threshold and the basic subjective attributes, including pitch and loudness. Phase is important in localizing sound in space and in hearing signals against noisy backgrounds.

*Frequency* is the number of times per second the air particles move back and forth through an initial or resting position. It is measured in *Hertz (Hz),* which stands for cycles per second. In the laboratory, sounds comprising only a single frequency, called *pure tones,* are readily produced electronically. The lowest frequency that humans can hear is around 20 Hz, and the highest is between 16,000 and 20,000 Hz; after the age of 30 years, the upper limit becomes steadily lower. Increases in frequency are heard as rises in *pitch,* from low to high, from bass to treble. Natural sounds, however, are not pure tones, but comprise many more than one frequency, and are called *complex sounds.* All the component frequencies together determine a complex sound's quality, or *timbre.*

Within the auditory system, frequency is represented both by the place of maximal stimulation and, except at high frequencies, by the time intervals separating successive neural impulses. Some auditory perceptions are best explained by a *place theory* of pitch, other perceptions by a time or *periodicity theory*. One difficulty for the place theory is our ability to detect frequency changes as small as 0.3 percent at frequencies above 1000 Hz; the spatial representation of frequency seems too gross to permit such fine discrimination.

Sound *intensity* is directly related to the amplitude, or distance, traversed by the air particles during a single cycle of a sound wave. A more common measure is *sound pressure,* which is proportional to the square of intensity and which is defined as the force exerted by the moving air particles on a cross-sectional area. The harder the particles push against the eardrum, the better we hear. Sound pressure is usually measured in dynes per square centimeter (dynes/cm$^2$), but is then transformed onto a logarithmic scale in order to encompass the enormous range of sound pressures to which the ear responds. On the logarithmic scale, the unit is the *decibel (dB).* The number of dB $= 20 \log P_1/P_0$, where $P_1$ is the measured pressure and $P_0$ is the reference value, 0.0002 dynes/cm$^2$. Measured on a decibel scale, sound pressure is referred to as *sound pressure level (SPL).*

*Thresholds* are expressed as the lowest SPL humans can detect. For the listener with normal hearing, the level at threshold depends largely on a sound's frequency and duration. At frequencies between approximately 500 and 4000 Hz, the normal threshold is close to 0 dB SPL, that is, close to 0.0002 dynes/cm$^2$. As frequency increases or decreases, the threshold increases until at the limits of 20 and 20,000 Hz, no matter how intense the sound, we hear nothing. Threshold also changes with duration. As the duration is shortened below 200 msec, the SPL at threshold must be increased. Specifically, for each halving of the duration, the sound pressure must be doubled.

Threshold varies with frequency in the way it does mainly because the ear transmits the middle frequencies to the receptor cells (the hair cells) better than the low or high frequencies. However, part of the insensitivity to low frequencies is caused by internal, physiological noise which masks low-frequency external sounds.

*Masking* is the increase in the threshold for one sound caused by the presence of another sound. It is commonly met in our noisy environments, as when we try to listen to a new acquaintance against the party hubbub or to a lecturer as a plane flies by. Laboratory studies have shown that a sound masks primarily other sounds at the same and higher frequencies, and that for sounds similar in frequency, masking increases in direct proportion to the intensity of the masking sound.

Closely related to sound pressure is *loudness*. Loudness, however, is a subjective attribute of sound and is distinct from sound pressure or intensity, which are physical aspects of a sound. The loudness of a 1000-Hz tone and of most other pure tones above 500 Hz increases as a power function of sound pressure (*Stevens' power law*). The formula is $L = kP^{0.6}$, where $k$ is a constant of proportionality, and $P$ is sound pressure. An exponent less than 1.0 means that loudness changes more slowly than pressure. Specifically, when pressure increases tenfold, loudness increases fourfold. However, loudness increases more rapidly under a number of conditions—near threshold, against a background noise, in certain types of deafness, at low frequencies, and after exposure to loud sounds. This rapid increase in loudness is called *loudness recruitment*. With respect to frequency, at fixed, low sound pressures, middle-frequency tones are loudest. At high sound pressures, the advantage of the middle frequencies over the low frequencies disappears, and the *equal-loudness contours* are flat at frequencies below approximately 5000 Hz.

Loudness is thought to depend primarily on how active the auditory nervous system is, that is, the more neurons firing and the faster, the louder the auditory experience. Physiological observations have shown that an intense pure tone excites a larger portion of the auditory system than does a weak tone. Likewise, a wide-band sound, covering a large range of frequencies, excites a much larger part of the auditory system than a narrow-band sound or pure tone, and is therefore considerably louder.

The third physical aspect of sound important to hearing is *phase*, which refers to how much of one full cycle a sound wave has covered. Phase is important mainly to the *localization* of sound. Thus if, in both ears, a sound is equally intense, starts at the same time, and is in phase, a listener hears it as coming from directly in front (or in back). When the same sound is out of phase at the two ears, it is heard as coming from the side that is leading in phase, that is, the side which is farther along through a cycle. Phase cues work, however, only up to about 1500 Hz.

Stimulus variables such as frequency, sound pressure, and phase are critical, but they are meaningless for hearing without reference to the listener. Age, sex, previous exposure to intense sounds, pathology of the auditory system, and so forth determine thresholds, loudness, pitch, and the ability to localize sounds. Even whether a person listens with one or two ears makes a difference. The threshold for binaural listening is 3 dB lower than for monaural listening. And a binaural sound is nearly twice as loud as a monaural sound. Both ears are used in localizing sound, not only by means of phase differences between the ears, but also by means of small interaural differences in intensity and time of arrival.

Many other interactions take place between the two ears, as well as within a single ear, and these are under intensive study both psychophysically and physiologically. Scientists are also seeking better ways to diagnose and treat deafness, to control and reduce noise pollution and thus prevent noise-induced deafness, to relate speech perception to the basic psychoacoustic parameters. Much is known about hearing, but many questions remain unanswered, and much of what is known remains to be applied to solving the problems of the deaf and the deafened.

# REFERENCES


**Batteau, D. W.** The role of the pinna in human localization. *Proceedings of the Royal Society of London,* Series B., 1967, **168,** 158–80.

**Békésy, G. von.** *Experiments in hearing.* E. G. Wever (Ed.) New York: McGraw-Hill, 1960. Figure 11–43, p. 448, Copyright © 1960 by the McGraw-Hill Book Company, Inc. Used with permission of McGraw-Hill Book Company.

**Békésy, G. von.** Hearing theories and complex sounds. *Journal of the Acoustical Society of America,* 1963, **35,** 588–601.

**Békésy, G. von.** *Sensory inhibition.* Princeton, N. J.: Princeton University Press, 1967.

**Chocholle, R.** Les effets des interactions interaurales dans l'audition. *Journal de Psychologie,* 1962, **3,** 255–82.

**Cohen, A.** Further investigation of the effects of intensity upon the pitch of pure tones. *Journal of the Acoustical Society of America,* 1961, **33,** 1363–76.

**Fletcher, H.** A space-time pattern theory of hearings. *Journal of the Acoustical Society of America,* 1930, **1,** 311–43.

**Fletcher, H.** Auditory patterns. *Review of Modern Physics,* 1940, **12,** 47–65.

**Galambos, R., & Davis, H.** The response of single auditory-nerve fibers to acoustic stimulation. *Journal of Neurophysiology,* 1943, **6,** 39–57.

**Goldstein, J. L.** Auditory nonlinearity. *Journal of the Acoustical Society of America,* 1967, **41,** 676–89.

**Greenberg, G. Z., & Larkin, W. D.** Frequency-response characteristic of auditory observers detecting signals of a single frequency in noise: The probe-signal method. *Journal of the Acoustical Society of America,* 1968, **44,** 1513–23.

**Guirao, M., & Stevens, S. S.** Measurement of auditory density. *Journal of the Acoustical Society of America,* 1964, **36,** 1176–82.

**Harris, C. M.** Residual masking at low frequencies. *Journal of the Acoustical Society of America,* 1959, **31,** 1110–15.

**Hellman, R. P., & Zwislocki, J. J.** Loudness determination at low sound frequencies. *Journal of the Acoustical Society of America,* 1968, **43,** 60–64.

**Hirsh, I. J.** The influence of interaural phase on interaural summation and inhibition. *Journal of the Acoustical Society of America,* 1948, **20,** 536–54.

**International Organization for Standardization.** Normal equal-loudness contours for pure tones and normal threshold of hearing under free-field listening conditions. Recommendation 226. Geneva, Switzerland: ISO, 1961.

**International Organization for Standardization.** Standard reference zero for the calibration of pure-tone audiometers. Recommendation 389. Geneva, Switzerland: ISO, 1964.

**Jerger, J. F., & Tillman, T. W.** Effect of earphone cushion on auditory threshold. *Journal of the Acoustical Society of America,* 1959, **31,** 1264.

**Johnstone, B. M., & Boyle, A. J. F.** Basilar membrane vibration examined with the Mössbauer technique. *Science,* 1967, **158,** 389–90.

**Kiang, N. Y.** *Discharge patterns of single fibers in the cat's auditory nerve.* Cambridge, Mass.: M.I.T. Press, 1965.

**Licklider, J. C. R.** Basic correlates of the auditory stimulus. In S. S. Stevens (Ed.), *Handbook of experimental psychology.* New York: Wiley, 1951. Pp. 985–1039.

**Lilly, D. J., & Thalmann, R.** The masking of interrupted pure tones by inaudible, continuous pure tones in pathological ears. Paper presented at the 40th Meeting of the American Speech & Hearing Association, San Francisco, November, 1964.

**Lindsay, R. B.** The story of acoustics. *Journal of the Acoustical Society of America,* 1966, **39,** 629–44.

**Mills, A. W.** Auditory localization. In J. V. Tobias (Ed.), *Foundations of modern auditory theory.* Vol. 2. New York: Academic Press, 1972. Pp. 301–48.

**Newman, E. B.** Hearing. In E. G. Boring, H. S. Langfeld, & H. P. Weld (Eds.), *Foundations of psychology.* New York: Wiley, 1948. Pp. 313–50.

**Plomp, R.** *Experiments on tone perception.* Soesterberg, The Netherlands: Institute for Perception RVO-TNO, 1966. Pp. 70–87.

**Raab, D. H., & Ades, H. W.** Cortical and midbrain mediation of a conditioned discrimination of acoustic intensities. *American Journal of Psychology,* 1946, **59,** 59–83.

**Robinson, D. W., & Dadson, R. S.** A redetermination of the equal-loudness relations for pure tones. *British Journal of Applied Physics,* 1956, **7,** 166–81. Figure 8, p. 171, Copyright 1956 by the National Physical Laboratory, Teddington, Middlesex, England. Adapted and reproduced by permission of The Institute of Physics and the authors.

**Scharf, B.** Complex sounds and critical bands. *Psychological Bulletin,* 1961, **58,** 205–17.

**Scharf, B.** Critical bands. In J. V. Tobias (Ed.), *Foundations of modern auditory theory.* Vol. 1. New York: Academic Press, 1970. Pp. 157–202.

**Scharf, B., & Fishken, D.** Binaural summation of loudness: Reconsidered. *Journal of Experimental Psychology,* 1970, **86,** 374–79.

**Schenkel, K. D. von.** Die beidohrigen Mithörschwellen von Impulsen. *Acustica,* 1967, **18,** 38–46.

**Stevens, S. S.** The relation of pitch to intensity. *Journal of the Acoustical Society of America,* 1935, **6,** 150–54.

**Stevens, S. S. (Ed.)** *Handbook of experimental psychology.* New York: Wiley, 1951.

**Stevens, S. S.** The measurement of loudness. *Journal of the Acoustical Society of America,* 1955, **27,** 815–29.

**Stevens, S. S.** Power-group transformations under glare, masking and recruitment. *Journal of the Acoustical Society of America,* 1966, **39,** 725–35.

**Stevens, S. S.** Neural events and the psychophysical law. *Science,* 1970, **170,** 1043–50.

**Stevens, S. S., & Davis, H.** *Hearing: Its psychology and physiology.* New York: Wiley, 1938.

**Stevens, S. S., Guirao, M., & Slawson, A. W.** Loudness, a product of volume times density. *Journal of Experimental Psychology,* 1965, **69,** 503–10.

**Stevens, S. S., & Volkmann, J.** The relation of pitch to frequency: A revised scale. *American Journal of Psychology,* 1940, **53,** 329–53.

**Terrace, H. S., & Stevens, S. S.** The quantification of tonal volume. *American Journal of Psychology,* 1962, **75,** 596–604.

**Wallach, H.** The role of head movements and vestibular and visual cues in sound localization. *Journal of Experimental Psychology,* 1940, **27,** 339–68.

**Wallach, H., Newman, E. B., & Rosenzweig, M. R.** The precedence effect in sound localization. *American Journal of Psychology,* 1949, **62,** 315–36.

**Ward, W. D., Glorig, A., & Sklar, D. L.** Relation between recovery from temporary threshold shift and duration of exposure. *Journal of the Acoustical Society of America*, 1959, **31,** 600–602.

**Wegel, R. L., & Lane, C. E.** The auditory masking of one pure tone by another and its probable relation to the dynamics of the inner ear. *Physical Review,* 1924, **23,** 266–85.

**Wever, E. G.** *Theory of hearing*. New York: Wiley, 1949.

**Zwicker, E., & Feldtkeller, R.** *Das Ohr als Nachrichtenempfänger*. Stuttgart: S. Hirzel Verlag, 1967.

**Zwicker, E., Flottorp, G., & Stevens, S. S.** Critical bandwidth in loudness summation. *Journal of the Acoustical Society of America,* 1957, **29,** 548–57. Figure 12, p. 556, adapted and reproduced by permission of the American Institute of Physics and the authors.

**Zwicker, E., & Scharf, B.** A model of loudness summation. *Psychological Review*, 1965, **72**, 3–26. Figure 2, p. 7, Copyright © 1965 by the American Psychological Association, Inc., and reproduced by permission.

**Zwislocki, J.** Theory of temporal auditory summation. *Journal of the Acoustical Society of America,* 1960, **32,** 1046–60.

**Zwislocki, J.** Analysis of some auditory characteristics. In R. D. Luce, R. Bush, & E. H. Galanter (Eds.), *Handbook of mathematical psychology*. Vol. 3. New York: Wiley, 1965. Pp. 1–97.

**Zwislocki, J., Damianopoulos, E. N., Buining, E., & Glantz, J.** Central masking: Some steady-state and transient effects. *Perception & Psychophysics,* 1967, **2,** 59–64.

**Zwislocki, J., & Feldman, R. S.** Just noticeable differences in dichotic phase. *Journal of the Acoustical Society of America*, 1956, **28,** 860–64.

**Zwislocki, J., Maire, F., Feldman, A. S., & Rubin, H.** On the effect of practice and motivation on the threshold of audibility. *Journal of the Acoustical Society of America,* 1958, **30,** 254–62.

CURRENT THEORIES
- Receptor Specificity
- Pattern Theory
- An Eclectic Approach

MECHANORECEPTION
- Instrumentation
- The Adequate Stimulus
- Threshold Measurements
- Suprathreshold Measurements
- Neural Basis of Vibrotaction

THERMORECEPTION
- Instrumentation
- The Adequate Stimulus
- Threshold Measurements
- Suprathreshold Measurements
- Theoretical Positions

PAIN
- The Adequate Stimulus and Definitions
- Theories
- Threshold Measurements
- Suprathreshold Measurements

SUMMARY AND CONCLUSIONS

# 5

# CUTANEOUS SENSATION

**Ronald T. Verrillo**
**Syracuse University**

By far the largest of our sensory systems, the skin has a surface area of about 2 square meters and contains a variety of specialized structures for transducing different forms of energy change (see Chapter 3). It lies open to scientific observation and experimentation and is much more accessible than the eye and ear. Nevertheless, the skin remains relatively neglected by the sensory scientist. To see and to hear are often considered miracles of nature, while to touch is commonplace. Perhaps this easy acceptance is part of the reason for our knowing so much less about cutaneous sensation than about vision and audition.

Since several forms of energy change elicit neural activity in receptor organs of the skin, it is not surprising that the phenomenal experiences resulting from this activity are more or less distinct. The skin mediates several sense modalities. Raise the temperature at the skin's surface, the subject says "warm"; lower the temperature, the subject says "cool"; mechanically deform the surface of the skin by pushing in or pulling out, the subject reports "touch," "light touch," "pressure," or "vibration." If any one of several types of energy is applied at a sufficient intensity, the resulting experience is usually pain.

The wealth of sensory experience from a single organ system has resulted in numerous theories and one of the longest-standing controversies in experimental psychology: the problem of receptor specificity, which concerns the extent to which each type of experience is mediated by its own specific receptor system within the skin.

Although individual parts or sectors of a system may be investigated for purposes of analysis, the ultimate goal of research is synthesis. To understand how a person is able to sense a cold object pressed against his hand involves a sequence of functionally related, complex structures and events at the periphery of the body and within the central nervous system. The goals of research are to determine what structures are involved and just how they interact to produce an observable response. Adequate understanding of a system requires that investigations be carried out on its parts and on the functioning of the system as a whole. It requires consideration of the contributions made by a number of seemingly diverse disciplines and the cooperative efforts of anatomists, electrophysiologists, and psychophysicists.

Preparation of this chapter was supported in part by Grant GB-5945 from the National Science Foundation and Grants NINDB–NS–03950 and NS–09940 from the National Institutes of Health, U.S. Department of Health, Education, and Welfare.

## CURRENT THEORIES

A detailed history of the many hypotheses concerning the mechanisms by which we perceive different sensations on the skin is beyond the scope of this chapter (see Boring, 1942; Sinclair, 1967). Because ideas are important, however, in the proper understanding of any system, three major theories of somatosensory experience will be presented. Two theories of somesthesis, one old and one relatively new, have achieved a classical status: *receptor specificity;* and *spatio-temporal patterning,* or *pattern theory.* A third formulation attempts to reconcile the classical theories by combining features of both.

### Receptor specificity

The human senses were first classified by Aristotle into the five modalities—vision, hearing, smell, taste, and touch. Touch was later expanded to include sensations originating in muscles, joints, and the viscera, and was given the name *general sensation.* Later, it was changed to *somesthesia,* or the consciousness of the body. Somesthesia has always been a problem since, unlike the four other senses, no special organs could be found to mediate the sensations so obvious to all.

Although many had speculated about the nature of cutaneous sense modalities, it was Charles Bell (1811) who first suggested that the nerves themselves were specific in the type of information they carried. Johannes Müller (1838) expanded this concept into a series of propositions which came to be called the *doctrine of specific energies.* Müller noted that excitation of a nerve by different stimuli always gave rise to the same sensation; that different sensory nerves activated by the same stimulus yielded sensory experiences in the modality of the stimulated nerve, and that an experience was the same regardless of where along its length the nerve was stimulated. He concluded that there was something intrinsically distinct about the nerves subserving the senses and that there were five different kinds of nerves. He located the site of specificity within the fibers of the sensory system or, possibly, at the neural termination in the cortex and spoke of the *specific irritability* of the sense organs (see Chapter 1).

Volkmann (1844) applied the ideas of Müller to the sense modalities subserved by the skin and postulated different nerves for each sensory experience. Forty years later, Blix (1884) in Sweden, Donaldson (1885) in the United States, and Goldscheider (1884) in Germany discovered, independently, that all the sense modalities could not be activated from the same spot on the skin and that different spots were sensitive to different stimuli. Thus, a mosaic of cold, warm, touch, and pain spots could be mapped over the surface of the skin.

The next logical step, considered by some to have been a leap, was taken by von Frey (1895), who suggested that beneath the skin surface under each sensory spot lay a morphologically distinct end-organ which responds exclusively to a single type of physical energy and which leads to a unique sensory experience. Von Frey went on, despite scanty evidence, to assign the known receptors to each sense modality: Krause end-bulbs for cold, Ruffini endings for heat, Meissner corpuscles and hair-follicle endings for touch, and free nerve endings for pain (see Chapter 3). This simple formulation, however, has been shown inaccurate with respect to temperature sensation and insufficient in explaining the complexities of mechanoreception. Only the assignment of pain to the free nerve endings was essentially correct.

A wholesale rejection of the position held by Müller and von Frey, however, overlooks the essential and lasting contribution they made to our understanding of the nervous system, namely, that the brain receives information about the external world over sensory (afferent) neural pathways, which are distinct from motor (efferent) nerves, and that receptors display a specific irritability with respect to environmental energies.

### Pattern theory

Nafe's (1927) pattern theory, later refined and extended by Weddell (1955), Sinclair (1955), and Kenshalo and Nafe (1962), maintains that there are neither nerve endings nor nerve fibers that respond to or carry information specific to a given form of stimulus energy or that produce a circumscribed sensation. Rather, "... what leaves the skin as a result of cutaneous stimulation is a complex, spatially and temporally dispersed pattern of impulses, and this, or something like it, appears to be what arrives at the sensory cortex of the brain ... [Sinclair, 1955, p. 609]." The whole concept of a receptor responding exclusively to one form of energy is rejected: "Thus activity in a given fiber could at one time contribute towards the experience of a sensation of touch, and at another, towards the experience of pain, cold, or warmth [p. 586]."

While there is no doubt that spatial and temporal patterns of neural activity having varying degrees of complexity do transmit information about the stimulus to the brain, the pattern theory fails to account for the manner in which these patterns are formed at the receptor. Furthermore, it fails to provide a precise definition of what is meant by a pattern.

### An eclectic approach

Melzack and Wall (1962) attempted a reconciliation between the specificity and pattern theories by incorporating some features from both and rejecting others. After a careful analysis of the ideas and experimental evidence for both positions, they advanced a series of eight propositions to explain somesthetic experiences. The eight propositions are organized around events taking place at three levels in the nervous system: at the receptor, in the presynaptic terminals, and within the cells of the central nervous system.

At the level of the receptor, they reject von Frey's notion of matching anatomical structures to psychological events. Thus, there are no "touch," "temperature," or "pain" endings. On the other hand, they reject the concept that all endings are alike except in the pattern of impulses they transmit. The concept of specificity is preserved insofar as the "receptors are specialized physiologically for the transduction of particular kinds and ranges of stimuli into patterns of impulses [Melzack & Wall, 1962, p. 342]." The presynaptic terminations of the peripheral fibers constitute a filter that blocks certain aspects of the neural pattern and passes others. The fate of the signal at the synapse is determined by the anatomy and the state of polarization of the terminal arborizations of the presynaptic neurons (see Chapter 3). Synchronous patterns have a higher probability of crossing the synapse than those patterns that are temporally or spatially out of phase.

The final level of activity is within the central nerve cells whose threshold, temporal and spatial summation, adaptation, and special connections determine the characteristic patterning of impulses. This patterning is the basis for the different somesthetic perceptions.

Melzack and Wall postulated an integrated somesthetic system with specialized component parts at the periphery and within certain central pathways. They maintain that specialization is physiological in nature and reject the concept of a separate transmission route for each specific modality. While detailed and explicit enough to permit systematic testing, this theory has been insufficiently investigated to draw any firm conclusions about its validity.

## MECHANORECEPTION

Mechanoreception refers to those neural events and sensations that result from mechanical distortion or displacement of cutaneous tissue, including the propagation of that distortion into deeper tissues. It includes repetitive displacements, such as vibration, and a single displacement, such as touch, pressure, or tangential movement of a stimulus along the surface of the skin. Mechanical stimuli may be considered as *static* (steady pressure) or *dynamic* (moving or vibrating).

### Instrumentation

Investigators at one time applied vibrations to the skin by modifying loudspeakers and phonograph crystals to suit their needs. Today, commercially available vibrators range in size from hand-held units to very large units able to shake objects the size of the human body and larger. These vibrators operate over a wide range of frequencies and intensities.

Not only is it necessary to produce the desired stimulus configuration, but an accurate method of measuring the resulting movements is necessary in order to define the stimulus quantitatively. Earlier attempts to monitor the displacement of the skin included systems that displayed the movement of the stimulator by means of light reflected from the moving element. These methods required the subject to remove his hand (or other body part) during the measurements. Without the mass of the hand upon it, the stimulator could very well move or vibrate quite differently than under the conditions of actual stimulation. Accurate measurements of the stimulus, therefore, were limited.

With the discovery and application of the electrodynamic qualities of *piezoelectric crystals,* the problem became simpler. Under mechanical stress some materials produce a measurable electrical output that is proportional to the amount of stress. Highly sensitive measuring devices, *accelerometers,* have been developed utilizing this principle, which permits the measurement of displacement at the actual time of stimulation. The effective use of this and other electrical properties (for example, *capacitance* and *inductance*) has taken much of the uncertainty out of the measurement of vibrotactile stimuli and has produced a great deal of accurate information.

### The adequate stimulus

One of the earliest controversies among scientists investigating touch revolved around the uncertainty over which dimension or parameter of the physical stimulus activates the receptor. Weber (1846) suggested that it was *pressure,* or force per unit area, to which the skin receptors respond. Von Frey (1896a) rejected this hypothesis because he found that when he attached a small object to the skin, he could evoke identical sensations by pressing the object into the skin (*positive* pressure) or by lifting the skin upward (*negative* pressure). Von Frey and Kiesow (1899) proposed *tension,* or the stretching of a length of skin, as the principal parameter involved in touch.

The familiar experience of feeling more pressure along the waterline when a finger or arm is placed in water led Meissner (1859) to propose the *gradient theory,* according to which a gradient of pressure along the surface of the skin constitutes the adequate stimulus. Von Békésy (1960) refined this hypothesis in a more sophisticated version a century later. Making an analogy to *Mach bands* in vision (see Chapter 7), he argued that the gradient and the curvature of displacement constitute the significant stimulus for mechanoreceptors. Verrillo (1963), in an experiment that carefully controlled the area as well as gradient and curvature, concluded that although gradient may be an important component in the touch experience, it does not take precedence over displacement of a given area. Gray and Sato (1953) successfully demonstrated that a sudden displacement of the membrane of nerve filaments within the Pacinian corpuscle was sufficient to cause the nerve to fire. They concluded that there is no reason to believe that displacement is not also the adequate stimulus for unencapsulated nerve terminals in the skin.

Nafe and Kenshalo (1958) added a dynamic component when they demonstrated on frog and rat skin that when the stimulus stops moving, the firing of the activated neuron ceases. Responses were elicited either by downward movement into the skin or withdrawal of the stimulating probe. This point of view was shared by Grindley (1936a, 1936b), who also showed rate of deformation to be an important parameter, and is supported by the fact that Pacinian corpuscles do not fire until some critical velocity of the displacement is reached (Sato, 1961). Psychophysical experiments show that at low frequencies which produce slow displacements, the response to differences in frequency disappears (Verrillo, 1963). It has also been demonstrated that thresholds remain constant regardless of the direction of the movement (Eijkman & Vendrik, 1960; Verrillo, 1965c). These findings can be accounted for by the physical structure of the Pacinian corpuscle itself (Loewenstein & Skalak, 1966). At low frequencies the nerve terminal, deep within the corpuscle, is not distorted. What appears to be a velocity-dependent phenomenon can be explained in terms of membrane distortion or displacement. In another sense modality, von Békésy (1951) has shown that the *cochlear microphonic* in audition (see Chapter 4) is proportional to displacement rather than velocity.

Although the problem has not been resolved conclusively, the evidence supports the position that membrane distortion is the adequate stimulus to elicit a sensation of touch. Thus, the current practice in tactile research is to use amplitude of displacement as the measure of stimulus magnitude. The unit of measurement in general use is the *micron* or *micrometer,* which is represented by the symbol $\mu$ ($1\mu = 0.001$ mm = approximately 0.00004 inch). Because of the wide range of amplitudes involved, the measurements are converted to a logarithmic scale and expressed in *decibels (dB)* (see Chapters 2 and 4). For amplitude measurements, the number of decibels ($n$) is given by twenty times the logarithm of the ratio between a measured amplitude ($d_m$) and an arbitrarily selected reference amplitude ($d_o$). The equation reads: $n = 20 \log (d_m/d_o)$. The decibel scale compresses a wide range of numbers into one of convenient size. For example, in tactile experiments the useful range of displacement is from less than $0.1\mu$ to more than $1000\mu$, a 10,000-fold ratio. Converted to the decibel scale with a reference amplitude of $1\mu$, this large range is reduced to from $-20$ to $+60$ dB. The decibel scale also facilitates the comparison of experimental results obtained from different sensory systems. The different units of intensity for each system are thereby converted to a common scale for cross-modality comparisons.

The frequency of sinusoidal vibrations (see Chapter 4) is another important parameter of the stimulus used in tactile research. Frequency is measured in cycles per second (cps), which by international agreement has been named *Hertz (Hz)* to honor the German physicist Heinrich Hertz (1857–94), the discoverer of electromagnetic waves.

## Threshold measurements

All experiments concerning the adequate stimulus for touch involve threshold measurements of one kind or another. Measurements of the lower limits of sensitivity of a sensory system are also useful in establishing the importance of the various physical components of the stimulus. For mechanoreception the stimulus parameters fall into two domains, the spatial and the temporal.

### *Spatial parameters*

Within the spatial domain are such aspects of the stimulus as its location on the body surface, the area and geometric configuration of the contactor, and the distance between two contact points (the two-point threshold). All of these parameters are relevant to the excitation of mechanoreceptors.

All parts of the body are not equally sensitive to tactile stimulation; regions such as the hands and face are more sensitive than the back or upper arm. A number of investigations have been reported, but it is difficult to compare them quantitatively because the different investigators used a variety of physical measures. Some report their results in *ergs,* others in milligrams or grams per square millimeter, and still others as displacement.

Wilska (1954) tested four parts of the body at five different frequencies using sinusoidal vibrations. Ranked from most to least sensitive, the body sites were finger, palm, back of hand, and forearm. Verrillo (1966, 1967), using the same mode of stimulation, verified the rank ordering of finger, palm, and forearm and also found the sole of the foot to fall between the palm and forearm in sensitivity to vibration at any frequency.

Weinstein (1968) determined touch and two-point thresholds for twenty body parts from head to toe. Motivated by the appearance in a textbook of physiology of a classic "sensory figure" that depicts the two-point thresholds over various regions of the body, Weinstein traced the origin of the illustration to Weber (1835), whose data from an experiment performed 133 years earlier and never repeated were still being accepted without question (see Boring, 1942, for a history of two-point threshold measurements). Although there is considerable agreement in the two sets of data, the two-point thresholds obtained by Weinstein tend to be smaller than those of Weber.

**Table 5.1 Rank Order of Body Parts for Sensitivity to Force and for Two-Point Discrimination**

| Touch thresholds | Two-point thresholds | mm |
|---|---|---|
| Nose | Middle finger | 2.5 |
| Upper lip | Index finger | 3.0 |
| Cheek | Thumb | 3.5 |
| Forehead | Ring finger | 4.0 |
| Belly | Little finger | 4.5 |
| Back | Upper lip | 5.5 |
| Shoulder | Cheek | 7.0 |
| Little finger | Nose | 8.0 |
| Ring finger | Palm | 11.5 |
| Upper arm | Hallux | 12.0 |
| Middle finger | Forehead | 15.0 |
| Forearm | Sole | 22.5 |
| Thumb | Belly | 34.0 |
| Breast | Breast | 36.0 |
| Index finger | Forearm | 38.5 |
| Thigh | Shoulder | 41.0 |
| Palm | Back | 44.0 |
| Calf | Upper arm | 44.5 |
| Sole | Thigh | 45.5 |
| Hallux | Calf | 47.0 |

(After Weinstein, 1968.)

Weinstein made measurements at twenty contralateral body sites of male and female subjects. He first measured the threshold for single, tactile stimuli using a calibrated set of modified von Frey hairs. Named for their originator, von Frey hairs consist of fine bristles or nylon filaments inserted into wooden handles. The filaments can be calibrated on a fine balance, and the force needed to bend them is measured in milligrams (mg). It is assumed that the same amount of force is exerted when these filaments are pressed onto the skin until they bend as when they are pressed upon the pan of the balance scale.

The rank order of sensitivity to touch for various parts of the body is shown in the left-hand column of Table 5.1. Values range from as high as 40 mg over the big toe, sole, and calf to as low as 0.5 mg on the nose. In general, females were found to be more sensitive than males. These data must be viewed with caution because the author does not provide a precise definition of the quantitative values obtained. The results shown in Table 5.1

may be different when the experiment is repeated under more precisely controlled conditions with methods of force and pressure measurement more modern than are possible with von Frey hairs.

The rank order of two-point thresholds for different parts of the body appears in the right-hand columns of Table 5.1. The two-point threshold is the minimum distance between two punctiform stimuli that can be felt as separate points. At lesser distances the two points are indistinguishable from a single point. This technique provides a measure of tactual acuity which varies over different parts of the body. On the calf, subjects could not distinguish as being separate two points that were less than 47 mm (nearly 2 inches) apart; on the fingertip, they could distinguish two points as little as 2.5 mm apart. These values are considerably reduced when the two points are vibrating stimuli instead of static stimuli. For example, the two-point threshold on the back drops from 44 mm for static pressure (Weinstein, 1968) to 17.8 mm when the points are vibrating at 60 Hz (Eskildsen, Morris, Collins, & Bach-y-Rita, 1969). No clear-cut sex differences were found in this measurement.

One may ask why measurements of sensitivity and two-point resolution at different parts of the body are important. There are several answers. For one, the establishment of sensory norms can be useful to clinicians who deal with deviations resulting from abnormalities of the nervous system. Another practical reason is that a considerable amount of effort has been and is being expended to develop ways of utilizing the skin as an additional channel of communication. Knowledge of the functional characteristics of the skin is essential in this endeavor. Finally, these functional characteristics can lead to a more complete understanding of how the nervous system is organized and how it works. For instance, Weinstein's data show that the ability to discriminate two points on a limb improves with distance from the torso: Sensitivity increases from shoulder to finger and from hip to toe. The greater acuity in the extremities suggests that the density of neural innervation increases along the limbs. This finding also agrees well with the mapping of sensory areas in the cortex, since more sensitive regions of the body are represented by larger areas of cortical tissue.

One of the more important spatial variables involved in the determination of thresholds is the size of the stimulator. However, since size has several aspects, it is essential to specify which one is meant—the circumference, the area, or the geometric configuration. Until recently, scientists have not agreed about the role of contactor area. Whereas von Bagh (1935), Nafe and Wagoner (1941), and Cosh (1953) did not find any effect of contactor area on vibrotactile thresholds, Holway and Crozier (1937) and Sherrick (1960) demonstrated that thresholds decrease as the area of stimulation increases.

Verrillo (1962, 1963, 1966a) also demonstrated the importance of contactor area in the determination of vibrotactile thresholds. Using specially designed stimulators whose area, circumference, and shape could be controlled, he found that area was the most important of these variables. Thresholds on the glabrous (hairless) skin of the hand remained unchanged so long as the area was the same, regardless of the circumference and shape of the contactor—whether round, a straightedge, or an annulus.

Another important feature of these findings was the amount of change in the threshold as the contactor area was varied. For every doubling of the area, the threshold dropped 3 dB, which means that the energy was reduced by one-half (Figure 5.1). This is an example of complete *spatial summation:* All of the energy increments delivered to the skin by increasing the area of stimulation are utilized by the receptors in the skin. The experiment was repeated on hairy skin with the same result (Verrillo, 1966e). There can be no doubt that the area of the contactor must be carefully controlled in touch experiments if the results are to be meaningfully interpreted.

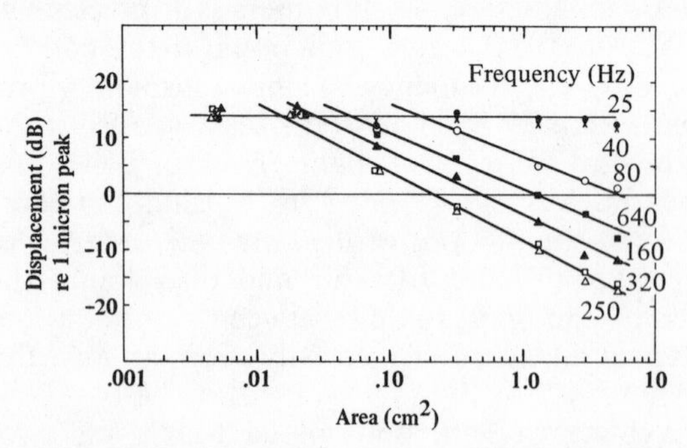


**Figure 5.1** Spatial summation of vibrotactile stimuli. As the size of the contactor increases, the sensitivity to vibration increases at a rate that shows perfect spatial summation, except at the two lowest frequencies. See Figure 5.4 for the comparison of decibels to a linear scale. (From Verrillo, 1963.)

Figure 5.1 shows also that at low frequencies (25 and 40 Hz) spatial summation does not occur; the threshold remains unchanged regardless of contactor area. Craig (1968) observed a similar effect when he tested with two contactors at a low frequency. These data suggest that the skin contains more than one mechanoreceptor system—that there is one system which is not capable of summating energy over space, as well as another system which apparently produces spatial summation at threshold. At low stimulating frequencies, the nonsummating system is activated; at higher frequencies, the summating system, which probably involves the Pacinian corpuscle, is activated. This hypothesis will be discussed in greater detail later in the chapter.

The effect of spatial summation can also be determined by measuring the combined effect of two stimuli applied to the skin at points adjacent to each other or on contralaterally identical sites. (Similar effects can be demonstrated for vision and audition.) Kietzmann (1927) obtained lower thresholds when the right and left index fingers were stimulated simultaneously than when either finger was stimulated alone. Von Békésy (1958) stimulated adjacent sites on the same surface and found that thresholds reached a minimum (applied energy was least) when the stimuli were separated by about 4.0 cm.

To determine where in the nervous system spatial summation occurs—at the periphery or at some level of the central nervous system—Craig (1968) measured spatial summation using two independently driven contactors located (1) at different distances along the thigh, (2) on two different fingers of the same hand, and (3) on the index finger of the right and left hands. The degree of spatial summation (approximately 2.0 dB) was the same under all conditions. Since the third condition involved bilateral summation, at least a portion of the summation must occur within the central nervous system. The summation (2.0 dB) between two contactors never equaled the summation (3.0 dB) obtained by Verrillo (1963, 1966a) over the area of a single contactor. Spatial summation is most likely due to the combined effects of peripheral and central events.

*Temporal parameters*

Important questions concerning the functional characteristics of the nervous system involve the temporal aspects of the stimulus. The responses of a sensory system to frequency, duration, and the repetition patterns of pulses are vital to understanding how the system works.

One of the earliest problems investigated was the response of the skin to different sinusoidal frequencies. The minimum detectable energy is measured over a wide range of frequencies. The analogous function has been long established for hearing (see Chapter 4). The investigators who have attempted to determine the function for skin are legion, but they have used different experimental procedures or inadequate equipment, or they have not specified the experimental conditions in sufficient detail, so that it is difficult to make quantitative comparisons of the results. In general, the measured functions are U-shaped and reach a maximum of sensitivity in the region of 200 to 300 Hz (von Békésy, 1939; Sherrick, 1953). Although the shape of the function has been fairly constant, the absolute threshold values at each frequency have varied considerably, probably due to the variety of contactor sizes used in the different studies and to the differences in the conditions under which the measurements were made.

Figure 5.2 illustrates the form of the vibrotactile threshold as a function of frequency, measured with a stimulator whose size was precisely controlled (Verrillo, 1963). These measurements were made on the glabrous skin of the hand, but are similar to those obtained on hairy skin of the forearm (Verrillo, 1966a) and on the sole of the foot (Verrillo, 1967). Only the absolute positions of the curves varied, reflecting

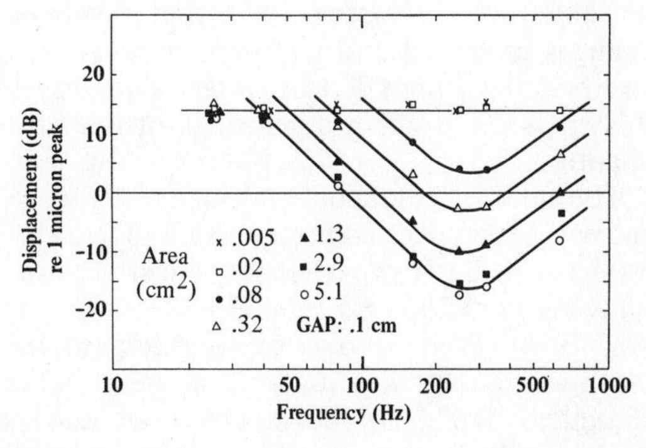


**Figure 5.2** Absolute thresholds measured for seven contactor sizes as a function of frequency of vibration. Threshold does not change below 40 Hz, and frequency has no effect on threshold for contactors smaller than 0.02 cm². See Figure 5.4 for the comparison of decibels to a linear scale. (From Verrillo, 1963.)

the differences in sensitivity of the various body sites. Clearly, then, cutaneous tissue contains a receptor system that is capable of summating energy over time and is also responsive to changes in the time pattern of the stimulus (different frequencies have different time patterns). The effects of time patterning were investigated in greater detail by substituting rectangular pulses for sinusoids (Verrillo, 1965a, 1965b, 1966c). The results support the findings shown in Figure 5.2.

Another question concerns the upper and lower frequency limits of vibratory sensation. These limits are well known for hearing (from about 20 to 20,000 Hz), but have been only partially determined for skin. Notice in Figure 5.2 that the threshold curves rise as frequency decreases below 250 Hz, but, depending on the size of the contactor, they stop rising at some low frequency and become horizontal. For the largest contactors, threshold stops rising and reaches a plateau in the vicinity of 40 Hz. It appears that the lower limit of sensitivity to sinusoidal vibration depends on the size of the contactor and that no contactor (regardless of size) can elicit frequency-dependent responses below approximately 40 Hz. This conclusion is supported by other similar psychophysical findings (von Békésy, 1939) and by physiological measurements of the response of the Pacinian corpuscle (Sato, 1961). The flattening of the threshold curves, coupled with the observation that the smallest contactors demonstrate no frequency response (0.005 and 0.02 cm$^2$ in Figure 5.2), brings to mind the question asked earlier: Is it possible that the skin contains more than one mechanoreceptor system—one that responds to changes in spatial and temporal parameters and another that responds to neither? The answer to this question is again deferred until later in the chapter.

The limit of cutaneous sensitivity at the upper end of the frequency continuum has not been firmly established. Early experiments placed the limit in the vicinity of 2500 Hz (von Gilmer, 1935; Knudsen, 1928). Weitz and Geldard (Geldard, 1962) managed to obtain sensations at frequencies of 10,000 to 20,000 Hz, but not without much difficulty, and the sensations appeared only in short bursts. Sherrick (1959) reported similar results and speculated that the sensation is evoked not by the high frequency at which the vibrator is driven, but by *subharmonics* (Sherrick, personal communication). Subharmonics are frequencies lower than the driven frequency (see Chapter 4). They arise when the skin cannot follow exactly the movement of the vibrator and consequently has only intermittent contact with it. This decoupling produces a complex waveform that contains not only the vibrator frequency, but also unwanted lower frequencies to which the mechanoreceptors may be sensitive. Moreover, the waveform produced is probably also irregular; hence, the intermittent nature of the sensations obtained by Weitz and Geldard.

Much is known about the effects of stimulus duration in vision and audition, but little is known about its effects in touch. We do know that as the duration of the stimulus increases, the intensity at threshold decreases. Zwislocki (1960) described in precise mathematical terms the quantitative relationship between time and intensity at the threshold of detection. His theory of temporal summation, although first formulated and verified for audition, applies equally well to vibrotaction. It predicts, among other things, the amount of change in the absolute threshold resulting from changes in the stimulus duration. Figure 5.3 shows the results of an experiment performed to test the theory (Verrillo, 1965a). The data show that, first, skin receptors are able to summate energy over time; as the duration of the burst of sinusoidal vibrations increases, the threshold decreases. Second, the observed temporal summation is not dependent on frequency, since all three frequencies tested showed the same decrease in threshold. (Both of these findings conform to the predictions of Zwislocki's theory.) Third, the effect is dependent on the size of the

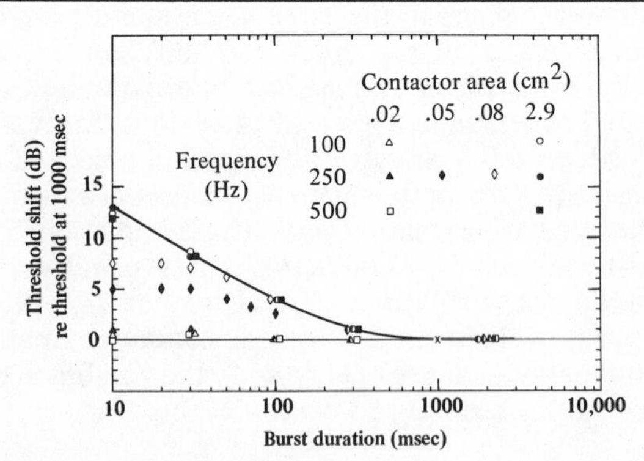


**Figure 5.3** Temporal summation of vibrotactile stimuli. The curve is theoretical. The symbols represent the differences between threshold at each duration and the reference duration of 1000 msec (X). (From Verrillo, 1965a.)

contactor. As the size of the contactor is decreased, the amount of temporal summation diminishes, until for the smallest contactor (0.02 $cm^2$) the threshold remains constant over all durations of the stimulus. This finding was predicted on the basis of the evidence, shown in Figure 5.2, that for small contactors threshold is independent of frequency; this raises again the possibility of more than one mechanoreceptor system in skin.

Adaptation refers to a decrease in sensitivity as a result of prolonged exposure to stimulation. It is a phenomenon observed in all sensory systems, and it is a useful one. Imagine the discomfort if you did not adapt to the pressure of shoes on your feet, the clothes on your body, or your own weight as you sit. A simple and direct demonstration of the phenomenon is produced by placing a weight on some part of the body and measuring the time that it takes for the sensation of pressure to disappear. Using such a method, Zigler (1932) measured the time course of adaptation for stimuli of different weight and area over the forehead, forearm, and dorsal surface of the hand. He found that adaptation time was longer for heavier stimuli and shorter for larger areas. Cohen and Lindley (1938) and Wedell and Cummings (1938) have used effectively the method of absolute threshold measurement to show adaptation to vibratory signals.

In another method of measuring adaptation, the subject matches the magnitude of the adapting stimulus and that of a second stimulus, which is introduced after a period of time. Von Frey and Goldman (1915) had subjects match the intensity of a static pressure and that of a test stimulus presented after various intervals over a period of 4 seconds. The apparent intensity of the constant stimulus decreased exponentially over the 4 seconds. Adaptation is very rapid in the first second of stimulation and then tapers off so that the subjective magnitude reaches some steady value. Von Békésy (1959a) used the matching procedure to determine the time course of adaptation to a 100-Hz vibration on the lip and forearm. Adaptation time for the lip, where the epidermis (outer skin) is thin, was much shorter than for the arm, which has a thicker epidermis.

The question must be asked, What causes adaptation? Does the stimulus fail to provide stimulation appropriate to the receptor system or does the receptor system fail to respond to an appropriate stimulus? Nafe and Wagoner (1941), addressing themselves to this question, demonstrated that subjects reported the disappearance of sensation as soon as the stimulus stopped moving into the skin. The sensation returned when the weight was removed. They termed the effect *stimulus failure*. In a further study of this effect, Nafe and Kenshalo (1958) recorded impulses from the dorsal cutaneous nerve of the frog and the femoral nerve of the rat using stimulus conditions closely paralleling those of Nafe and Wagoner. The results supported the earlier conclusions: When the stimulus stopped moving, the nerve ceased firing. The concept of stimulus failure rather than neural failure as the explanation for adaptation was supported also by Wall (1959, 1960), who found that the nerve ceased firing when the stimulating object stopped moving. On the other hand, several investigators suggested that adaptation is a genuine neural event in the central nervous system (e.g., Eijkman, 1959; Eijkman & Vendrik, 1960).

The controversy over the exact definition and location of adaptation has neither lessened its importance as a measurable event nor deterred its investigation. Hahn (1966) investigated adaptation to a sinusoidal vibration (60 Hz) by threshold measurement and intensity matching. He found that after 25 minutes, adaptation was still progressing regardless of the method, although the judged magnitude was less affected by the adapting stimulus than were the detection thresholds. The adaptation time of 25 minutes is considerably longer than the 30 seconds measured for static pressure by Nafe and Wagoner (1941). Adaptation to a prolonged vibratory signal is much slower than adaptation to sustained static pressure. Stimulus failure may account for adaptation to steady pressure, but other factors must be considered in the case of sinusoidal signals which are constantly changing. These factors may be related to the structure of the receptor (Loewenstein & Skalak, 1966) or to events taking place within the central nervous system. A definitive account of these factors is not possible at the present time.

### Suprathreshold measurements

We have thus far been concerned primarily with the effects of various physical parameters on the threshold of detectability. In this section we consider events at intensities above the absolute threshold.

#### *Intensity scaling*

The perceived loudness of a sound is related in an orderly fashion to the physical intensity of the stimulus delivered to the ear. The perceived magnitude of tactile sensations is similarly related to the physical intensity of the stimulus applied to the skin. These relationships have been extensively investigated in audition (see Chapter 4), and from these studies have been developed the modern methods for the direct scaling of sensory magnitude. The methods, called *magnitude estimation* and *magnitude production,* are among the most powerful techniques available for the investigation of suprathreshold phenomena (see Chapter 2).

The psychophysical functions, relating subjective magnitude to stimulus magnitude, have been established for a number of sensory continua by Stevens (1961) and his collaborators. For nearly every sensory system investigated, the subjective magnitude increases as a power function of the physical intensity of the stimulus—hence the name, *power law.* Stevens (1959), using magnitude estimation, determined the psychophysical function for vibrotactile stimuli. He demonstrated that his power law (Stevens, 1957) adequately describes the relationship between the amplitude of vibration on the skin and the magnitude of the sensation. Sherrick (1960) and Franzén (1966) used the same psychophysical method and obtained similar results. It has also been shown that the subjective intensity of vibrotaction increases more rapidly over areas of skin having a low density of innervation than over areas having a high density (von Békésy, 1955). The rapid increase in subjective magnitude is well known in auditory experiments as *loudness recruitment* (see Chapter 4).

More recent experiments, however, have shown that the rate of growth in subjective magnitude is more directly related to the number of sensory receptors activated by the stimulus than to the density of neural innervation (Verrillo, 1974; Verrillo & Chamberlain, 1972). The question of neural density versus number of units activated is important since it relates directly to the way in which the nervous system detects intensity changes (Zwislocki, 1973). Evidence suggests that near the detection threshold, subjective intensity may be dictated by the firing rates of individual neurons, and at higher levels by the combined responses of whole nerve bundles.

A different question concerns the effect of stimulus frequency on subjective magnitude. The subjective magnitude functions for ten vibration frequencies have been determined over a wide range of intensities (Verrillo, Fraioli, & Smith, 1969) by the method of *numerical magnitude balance* (Hellman & Zwislocki, 1963). This method is a modification of the direct scaling methods developed by Stevens and utilizes both magnitude estimation and magnitude production in order to counterbalance their individual biases. Verrillo et al. (1969) confirmed the findings of earlier studies, showing that the subjective magnitude of vibration obeys Stevens' power law. They found that the value of the exponent (0.89) is not dependent on frequency, except for very high frequencies. Stevens (1968), on the other hand, found the functions to be steeper at frequencies to which the skin is least sensitive. The discrepancy between the two sets of data remains unresolved, but is under investigation.

Another scaling procedure involves the matching of two frequencies for equal subjective magnitude. The results yield curves of equal subjective magnitude well known in hearing as *equal-loudness contours* (Fletcher & Munson, 1933) (see Chapter 4). Plotted against frequency, these contours indicate the sound intensities required to maintain a constant loudness over the range of frequencies used. One of the earliest attempts to establish similar contours for vibrotaction (Hugony, 1935) gave results at four suprathreshold levels. The contours look remarkably like those obtained for hearing. Stevens (1968) constructed a series of equal-sensation contours based on five frequencies between 20 and 320 Hz at seven levels of intensity. Verrillo et al. (1969) published a still more complete set of contours, shown in Figure 5.4. Data points and contours are shown for ten frequencies between 25 and 700 Hz at twelve sensation levels. (Sensation level is the number of decibels above threshold; see Chapter 4.) Although the data shown in Figure 5.4 were obtained by the method of numerical magnitude balance, they agree with those obtained by matching. The magnitude of sensation along a given curve is identical. Owing to technical difficulties, the points at frequencies above 500 Hz are unreliable and subject to change.

Since both direct scaling and matching yield measures based on subjective magnitude, their results can be compared on the same coordinates. Figure 5.5 shows contours at two suprathreshold levels obtained by the two methods (Verrillo et al., 1969). (The threshold curves were measured in corresponding sessions.) The results show that either method can be used to determine equal-magnitude contours of vibrotactile sensation, and they affirm the validity of direct scaling as a method

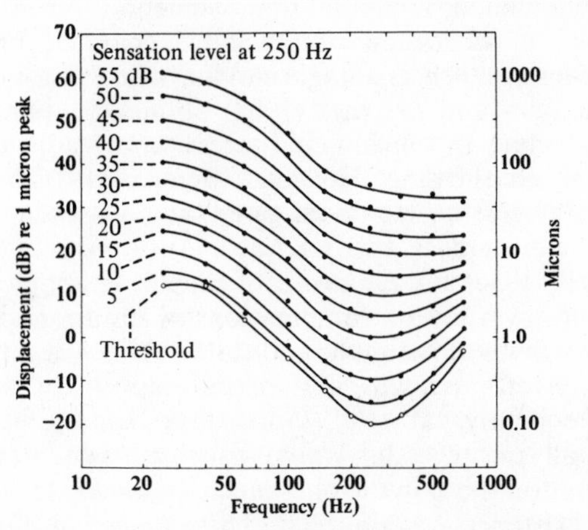


**Figure 5.4** Equal-sensation contours for vibrotaction. The subjective intensity is the same at all points along any given contour. The linear scale in microns is shown on the right-hand side of the graph. An increase of 20 decibels occurs for every tenfold increase on the linear scale. (From Verrillo, Fraioli, & Smith, 1969.)

for accurately measuring responses at suprathreshold levels of stimulation.

*Frequency discrimination and pitch perception*

The auditory system is superbly designed to detect differences in stimulus frequency or in its sensory counterpart, *pitch.* The skin, while able to function as a pitch discriminator, does the job much more crudely. Apparently, none of the skin's receptor systems is equipped to analyze frequency. Why, then, study its ability to analyze frequency if that is not one of the skin's normal functions? Answers may be given at two levels. At the theoretical level, the skin can be used very effectively as a substitute for the nerve supply on the basilar membrane in order to study auditory functions. Von Békésy (1960) has contributed much to the understanding of auditory phenomena by his experiments on the skin. At an applied level, knowledge about the skin's capabilities is important in the development of cutaneous communication systems.

The fusion of individual impacts into a smooth sensation of vibration occurs in the vicinity of 10 to 18 Hz (von Békésy, 1957b; Brecher, 1934). Judgments of vibratory "pitch" or perceived frequency become possible but are so difficult that few investigators have tried to measure pitch. Von Békésy (1962a, 1962b), however, measured a doubling of pitch when the number of clicks increased from 200 to 400 per second. No pitch change was felt when the click rate increased from 300 to 600 per second, and then pitch declined when the rate went from 400 to 800 per second. Von Békésy explains this lowering of pitch by reference to the *volley* concept (see Chapter 4). Assuming that the pitch depends on the rate at which neural discharges arrive at the relevant brain center, von Békésy suggests that the receptors are unable to respond to impulses coming in rapid sequence and so begin to skip some. Consequently, the neural discharge rate is reduced and the pitch lowered. Von Békésy calls it a *demultiplication* of the neural process.

The *Bezold-Brücke effect* in vision, in which hue changes with light intensity, and the slight change of pitch with intensity in audition have their counterpart in skin sensation. Figure 5.6 shows that the apparent pitch of vibrations on the skin first rises and then drops as the amplitude of the vibration is increased (von Békésy, 1957b). The pitch rises only near threshold, then drops over most of the intensity range. The effect is greatest at higher frequencies. Using a matching technique, von Békésy (1962a) was able to measure changes in pitch as a function of vibration frequency for the fingertip, palm, and upper arm. For regions with

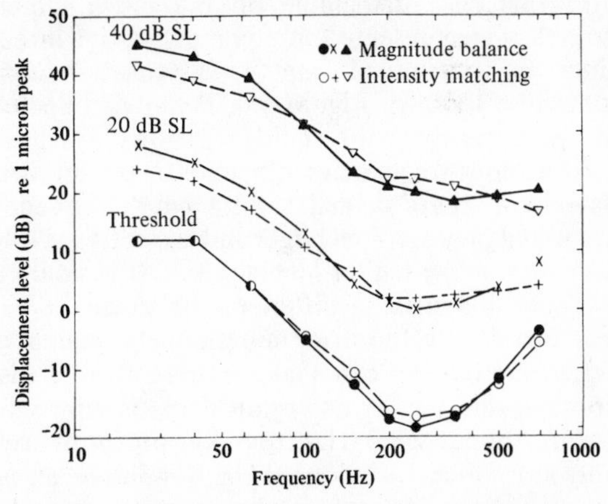


**Figure 5.5** Comparison of equal-sensation contours at two intensity levels obtained by the methods of magnitude balance and intensity matching. Corresponding threshold curves are also shown. The close similarity between the suprathreshold curves shows that either method can be used to determine the functions. (From Verrillo, Fraioli, & Smith, 1969.)

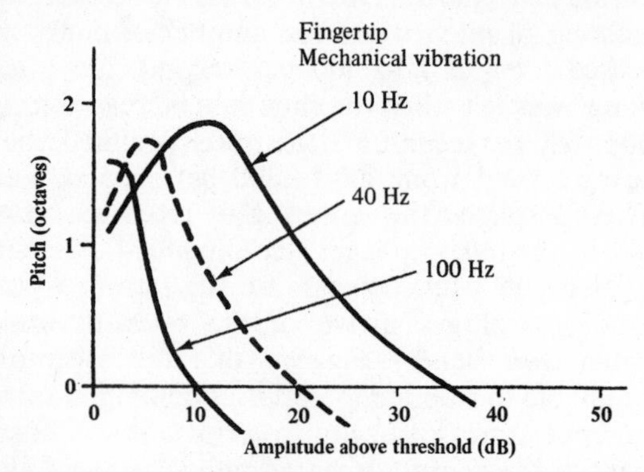


**Figure 5.6** "Pitch" perception on the skin (fingertip) as a function of amplitude above threshold. The pitch of high frequencies drops faster than that of low frequencies as intensity increases. (From von Békésy, 1962a.)

low neural density (upper arm), pitch rises with frequency up to about 20 Hz, beyond which it remains constant. At the fingertip, where neural density is high, pitch rises more sharply with frequency up to about 100 Hz before it levels off. Data for the palm lie between those for the fingertip and arm.

Goff (1967) studied the skin's ability to analyze frequency by measuring frequency discrimination. She measured the smallest change in frequency ($\Delta f$) that was detectable on the index finger. Stimuli were presented at equal subjective intensities, as determined from equal-sensation contours like those in Figure 5.4. Results, collected at two levels above threshold, are shown in Figure 5.7. At low frequencies (25 to 50 Hz) subjects detected changes as small as 5 Hz, but as frequency increased they required larger and larger $\Delta f$'s. Note also that at the higher intensity the $\Delta f$ is smaller.

There is a striking difference between the ear and the skin in the discrimination of frequency. Whereas the ear can make extremely fine discriminations out to its region of maximum sensitivity (about 2000 Hz), the skin performs well only at frequencies below 50 Hz. In relative terms, the difference is even greater since the ear can discriminate a 0.3 percent difference in frequency, but, according to Goff, the skin needs at least a 10 percent difference.

### *Effects of multiple stimulation*

The skin, like the ear, has its counterpart to the phi phenomenon of vision. In vision, the phi phenomenon, an apparent movement, is achieved when a succession of spatially separated light flashes are seen as a single moving light. For touch, von Frey and Metzner (1902) obtained apparent movement by touching in succession two adjacent spots on the skin. However, Benussi (1916) was less successful. He investigated tactual movement in an attempt to verify Korte's (1915) visual laws (Neff, 1936) for the sense of touch. Although he tried a variety of combinations of duration, distance between stimuli, and time between stimuli, his efforts yielded only partial movement and infrequently, at that. Other investigators were equally unsuccessful. Unlike visual apparent movement, on the skin the phenomenon was fickle, and its existence was doubted. The vague sensations of movement were relegated to the realm of the subject's imagination.

It was not until Bice (Geldard, 1961) substituted bursts of vibration for the impact stimuli of the earlier studies that the true character of apparent tactual movement was revealed. By adjusting the temporal patterning of six vibrators arranged around the chest, Bice was able to induce a sensa-

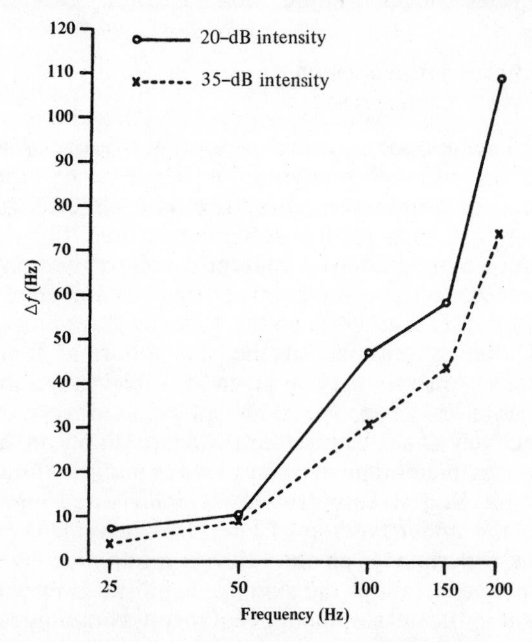


**Figure 5.7** Just detectable differences in the frequency of vibration as a function of frequency. Smaller differences can be detected at low frequencies than at high frequencies, and detection is improved by increasing the intensity level from 20 to 35 dB above threshold. (From Goff, 1967.)

tion of movement. The subject has the illusion of a single tactual sensation swirling around his chest. Easily perceived sensations of movement can also be induced between two vibrators delivering 200-msec bursts of vibration to the skin (Sumby, 1955). The effect is dependent on the time interval between the onsets of the successive stimuli, the *interstimulus onset interval*. The interval duration at which optimal movement is achieved depends, in turn, on the duration of the individual stimuli (Rogers, 1964). Other factors such as vibration frequency, body locus, sensation magnitude, interstimulus distance, direction of motion (proximal-distal or distal-proximal), and stimulus magnitudes are relatively unimportant (Sherrick, 1968).

Geldard and Sherrick (1972) obtained dramatic apparent movement when they delivered five mechanical pulses to each of three contactors equally spaced along the forearm. If all fifteen pulses are separated by the same time interval, the subject experiences not simple sensations under the three contactors, but rather a vivid hopping from wrist to elbow. The sensation runs up or down the arm depending on the sequence in which the stimulators are energized. This important phenomenon has been dubbed by its discoverers the *cutaneous rabbit*. At this time no adequate hypothesis explains it.

The success in achieving apparent movement on skin seems to depend on the use of vibrating stimuli rather than single impacts. Sherrick (1968) points out that vibrations have a unitary character similar to tone bursts and flashes of light, which are the stimuli used to achieve good apparent movement in audition and vision. Moreover, the physical effects of single impacts on the skin are probably more complex.

The effects produced by the interaction of stimuli presented simultaneously to the skin contribute to a better understanding of other sense modalities and also to understanding the action of the nervous system in general. The effects include summation, inhibition, and a product of the two, named *funneling* by von Békésy (1958, 1959b).

As the distance between two stimuli of equal intensity is increased, the sensation remains unitary at first and is more intense than that of either stimulus alone (von Békésy, 1957a). The energy of the two stimuli summates, just as the energy over increasing contactor areas summates (see earlier discussion of spatial parameters). When the two-point threshold is reached, two sensations are felt, and the intensity of each decreases considerably. The sudden weakness of the sensations is due to *reciprocal* inhibition between the two stimuli; the neural activity aroused at each point exerts an inhibitory action on the activity aroused at the other. As distance is further increased, the perceived magnitude at each point grows, and complete separateness is experienced.

Funneling occurs, for example, when the intensity of one of the stimuli is increased above that of the other. If the two points are far enough apart to be perceived separately when stimulated with equal intensity, then as one of the stimuli is intensified, the weaker of the two sensations disappears completely. At the same time, the magnitude of the remaining sensation increases so that it is perceived as being more intense than if presented alone (von Békésy, 1958). The activity from the weaker stimulus, although inhibited, seems to contribute to the subjective magnitude of the other stimulus. In effect, neural activity is funneled into the one stimulus that is able to inhibit the other. Similarly, auditory funneling may occur in earphone listening. When a tone is made more intense to one ear than to the other ear, it is heard only in the first ear; nevertheless, the audible tone is louder because of the contribution from the inhibited tone. Psychologically this interaural funneling is like funneling on the skin, but physiologically it may be quite different (see Chapter 4).

### *Tactile communication*

The visual and auditory systems are the primary channels of communication for human beings. The eye is best suited to processing spatial information, such as orientation, distance, direction, and size. It performs rather poorly when it must discriminate events in time. The ear, on the other hand, has no peer in handling messages that involve a rapid temporal sequence of events, such as occurs in speech and music. When a person is blind or deaf or must respond to a great many signals at once, as when piloting a spaceship, then channels other than the eye and ear have been sought to fulfill the role of information receiver. Because the skin can make both spatial and temporal discriminations, it has been under intense investigation as a supplementary channel for communicating both types of information.

An index of the magnitude of the problem posed by communication disorders may be appreciated by the fact that in the United States there are approximately 300,000 persons who are incapable of normal speech as a direct result of hearing loss and an additional 700,000 persons who suffer some degree of a combination of visual and hearing disorders. The annual cost of coping with disorders of communication is estimated to be at least $500 million, plus an annual deficit in earning power of about $2 billion. It is not possible to calculate the price in terms of personal tragedy and social misunderstanding.

Recognition of the skin's potential as a surrogate for the eyes and ears is by no means a modern development. Early in the sixteenth century, a Benedictine abbot devised a system for communicating through the skin (Gnudi & Webster, 1950), and in 1762 Jean Jacques Rousseau suggested that, properly used, the skin may become a supplement to sight and a substitute for hearing. (Geldard, 1966). Louis Braille in 1826 was the first to devise a practical and widely accepted system for communicating language to the blind through the skin. The Braille system utilizes a pattern of three pairs of dots embossed on heavy paper and read by scanning with the fingertips. Because the Braille system is relatively slow, difficult to learn, and requires prior transposition into the code, efforts continue to develop a method by which the blind may read printed material directly, using sophisticated light-sensitive devices. Some of these efforts reflect a gadgeteering approach to the problem and consequently result in disappointment. Meaningful solutions cannot be realized until fundamental research tells us more about the skin's capacity to utilize the information delivered to it.

Two lines of investigation have characterized the efforts to determine the skin's potential for mediating information. One early approach, attempting to force skin to perform like an ear, involved the application of auditory stimuli, through the appropriate stimulators, onto the surface of the skin (Gault, 1926). Although subjects could learn to use a new communication channel, their performances were poor and highly unreliable.

A second and more scientific approach to the problem emphasized the investigation of the skin's capacity to make discriminations on a number of stimulus dimensions (Bliss, 1970). Geldard (1957, 1960, 1962) and his colleagues have studied extensively the ability of the skin to discriminate locus, intensity, duration, and frequency. The development of a *tactile code* requires that the performance of the skin in these dimensions be known in considerable detail.

*Locus*. Nine tiny vibrators were placed in a variety of spatial configurations over the surface of the body in order to determine which pattern would minimize errors of localization (Geldard & Sherrick, 1965). The vibrators were distributed two to each arm, two to each leg, and one to the abdomen. Identical spots on the right and left sides were avoided in order to eliminate any contralateral masking effects. Geldard (1968) used these and many other experimental results to develop a system and code by which written material can be translated into symbols to be delivered to the body surface. Called the *optohapt* (Greek *optos,* seen; *haptein,* to touch), the system utilizes a photoelectric sensor to "read" printed characters. The sensor contains nine tiny photocells whose amplified electrical output controls nine small vibrators distributed over the body in the optimal arrangement determined by Geldard and Sherrick. Since the configuration of the letters of the alphabet often presents a confusing pattern of vibrations to the skin, Geldard selected symbols that yielded patterns more easily recognized on the skin.

Symbols and letters were matched in decreasing order of difficulty and frequency so that the most easily recognized symbol (●) represented the letter most often used (E), and the most difficult symbol (□) represented the letter least used (Q). Geldard emphasizes that his system is not offered as the solution for enabling the blind to read, but rather as a method for investigating the capacity of the skin to make useful pattern discriminations.

Another device, the *Optacon* (Bliss, 1969; Linvill & Bliss, 1966), stimulates the fingertips, which have low two-point thresholds, via a matrix of tiny vibrators. A small, hand-held array of phototransistors scans a printed page and converts the light patterns into electrical impulses. These impulses drive the vibrators and produce a replica of the image as a vibration pattern on the tip of the index finger. Still another system projects onto a person's back a vibratory display that is a close approximation of the light and dark patterns detected by a television camera (Bach-y-Rita, 1972; White, 1969). The claims made for these devices await confirmation by rigorous testing.

*Intensity*. Among the stimulus dimensions of locus, duration, and intensity, Geldard and Sherrick's (1965) subjects made most of their errors on the intensive continuum. Between the threshold of detectability and the threshold for pain, the average subject can make only three absolute judgments of intensity; that is, he can distinguish among only three widely spaced intensities. A code based on intensity would therefore be limited.

*Duration.* Estimations of the length of time that a stimulus lasts were not much better than those of intensity. Between 0.1 sec and 2.0 sec only four or five durations can be absolutely discriminated.

*Frequency.* Subjects are able to make fairly good judgments of rate when the frequency of vibration is below 50 Hz, but the capability drops off sharply above this frequency (Goff, 1967). The skin performs very poorly within the frequency range of voice communication. The difficulties in using frequency as a basis for cutaneous discriminations are compounded by the fact that perceived pitch on the skin is highly dependent on intensity (von Békésy, 1959a).

A problem which is closely related to frequency discrimination and which is important to design considerations of a tactile communication device involves the ability to distinguish stimuli separated in time. Gescheider (1966, 1967) determined the temporal resolution of brief stimuli for the auditory and cutaneous systems. Whereas the ear can distinguish two clicks separated by 1.8 msec, the fingertip requires a separation of at least 10 msec between stimuli. Moreover, tactile resolution depends much more on stimulus intensity than does auditory resolution. If a tactile communicator is to utilize successive, brief stimuli, it is important that intensity levels well above the threshold of detectability be used.

Although a number of laboratories have been actively seeking a suitable method of encoding language information for use by the skin, no system has as yet proved acceptable. Mechanical stimulators (Geldard, 1966, 1968; Linvill & Bliss, 1966; Pickett & Pickett, 1963), puffs of air (Bliss, Crane, Mansfield, & Townsend, 1966), and electrical stimulation of the skin (Gibson, 1963, 1968) have been tried. Each has its merits, but none satisfies enough of the requirements of a communication system to substitute for hearing or sight. The weakness lies not in the ability to develop clever devices, but rather in the gaps in our knowledge of the functional characteristics of skin as a sensory system and in the lack of systematic procedures when evaluating the effectiveness of the devices. At best, success in these endeavors must be considered limited.

## Neural basis of vibrotaction

The controversy surrounding the issue of receptor specificity in cutaneous sensation has been reviewed earlier. For most of the nerve endings found in skin, little can be said regarding their association with sensation. In recent years, however, the Pacinian corpuscle has become identified as the primary receptor for the perception of vibration.

Physiological studies have shown that the Pacinian corpuscle is ideally suited as a transducer of mechanical vibrations (Loewenstein & Skalak, 1966) and that it does indeed respond with great fidelity to vibrations (Sato, 1961). It has also been shown that the Pacinian corpuscle, while responding well to mechanical deformation, is quite unresponsive to changes in temperature (Loewenstein, 1961).

To show that a receptor can respond to a given form of energy in an electrophysiological experiment does not prove that it mediates the sensation. Behavioral evidence must also be obtained. Such evidence has been provided by a series of experiments designed in part to examine the role of the Pacinian corpuscle in vibrotaction (Verrillo, 1966b, 1966d, 1968).

The threshold of detectability for vibration depends on frequency and contactor size, except at low frequencies and for small contactor sizes (Figures 5.1 & 5.2). This dual mode of operation, flat at low frequencies and U-shaped at higher frequencies, suggests that more than one receptor system subserves the sense of touch. One system functions at low frequencies and apparently does not summate energy over time and space. The other system, involving the Pacinian corpuscle, is frequency sensitive and therefore produces the U-shaped portion of the threshold curves. The U-shaped curve is found for any cutaneous tissue, such as the glabrous skin of the hand and foot and hairy skin. Both types of skin are known to contain Pacinian corpuscles. Hence, frequency sensitivity is a distinctive feature of such tissue. On the other hand, the top surface of the tongue, which is devoid of these endings, yields a flat threshold function, that is, one that does not change with frequency; it also lacks the capacity for spatial and temporal summation. Figure 5.8 compares psychophysical measures of the vibrotactile threshold to physiological measures of the frequency response of the Pacinian corpuscle. The physiological data (●) were obtained by recording directly from corpuscles subjected to mechanical

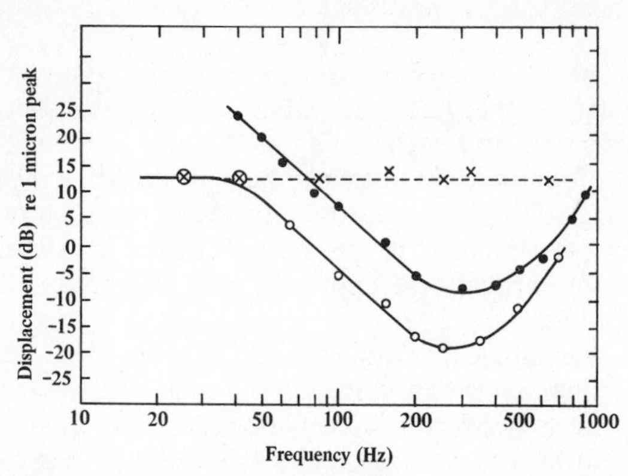


**Figure 5.8** Absolute thresholds for vibration obtained by the psychophysical testing of humans (unfilled circles) compared to electrophysiological data obtained directly from Pacinian corpuscles in the cat (filled circles). Note the similarity in the shape of the two functions. The psychophysical curve flattens at low frequencies where Pacinian corpuscles no longer respond. The flat curve (X) is typical of psychophysical data obtained over areas lacking the corpuscles or in response to stimulation by very small contactors.

stimulation at a number of different frequencies. The psychophysical data were obtained on skin lacking Pacinian corpuscles (X) and on skin containing them (○). The psychophysical data that involved Pacinian corpuscles and the physiological data show a remarkable degree of correspondence. There can be little doubt that the Pacinian corpuscle and its associated neural structures form a sensory system subserving vibrotaction in humans. These results were later confirmed by experiments in which human psychophysical results were compared with data obtained by recording from the cutaneous nerves of monkeys (Talbot, Darian-Smith, Kornhuber, & Mountcastle, 1968). Further studies showed that the threshold curves for vibrotaction are similar in human and monkey and that both correlate closely with the results from single-unit, peripheral nerve recordings (Mountcastle, LaMotte, & Carli, 1972).

The response characteristics of mechanoreceptors other than the Pacinian corpuscle are less well known. Most of the data are recorded from nerve fibers remote from the site of stimulation, and the neural response patterns are associated by inference with specific terminal structures. Reasoning from such data has led to the hypothesis that in glabrous skin the flat portion of the threshold curve at low frequencies is the product of activity in Meissner corpuscles served by fast-adapting fibers (Talbot et al., 1968), and in hairy skin it may be the result of activity in large fast-adapting fibers from the hair-basket endings (Merzenich & Harrington, 1969).

In addition to the fast-adapting fibers which innervate the Pacinian and Meissner corpuscles and the hair-basket endings, a class of slow-adapting, large-diameter fibers appear also to be associated with receptors responsive to mechanical distortions of the skin (Harrington & Merzenich, 1970). Tapper (1965) and Lindblom and Tapper (1967) provided details of the response of the *haarscheibe,* or *tactile domes* (see Chapter 3), in the skin of cat and monkey. A receptor closely resembling the classical Ruffini ending (see Chapter 3) has also been described in precise anatomical detail and shown to be a cutaneous mechanoreceptor (Chambers, Andres, Duering, & Iggo, 1972; Chambers & Iggo, 1967). Both the tactile dome and the Ruffini ending adapt slowly and respond to static indentations of the skin by firing steadily as long as the displacement is maintained. They also will respond to low-frequency sinusoidal stimulation. The exact function of the various types of fibers and receptors found in cutaneous tissue awaits correlative studies in which electrophysiological and psychophysical techniques and information are combined. We are dealing with a sensory system and must therefore approach the problem of function through a systematic integration of seemingly isolated bits of information.

## THERMORECEPTION

Among its other functions, the skin provides information about external temperature, that is, information vital to the maintenance of internal temperature. The survival of a person depends on the capacity of the body to maintain its temperature within rather narrow limits around approximately 37° C (98.6° F). Too large a deviation in either direction would prove fatal. Part of the mechanism that maintains body core temperature near its optimum is located in the skin. It includes such peripheral mechanisms as sweating, shivering, and modulation of the blood supply to the cutaneous vascular system. Under normal conditions, these mechanisms respond to variations in the external temperature. As an adjunct to the homeostatic mechanisms, which are largely reflexive, there is a sensory system by which the thermal state of the environment is brought to awareness.

## Instrumentation

The literature on the sensitivity of the skin to external temperature describes a plethora of methods for producing temperature changes and for recording skin temperature. These methods include plunging the hand into hot and cold water baths, pressing hot and cold brass cylinders against the skin, and applying sophisticated electronic devices. Most methods involve the transfer of heat by conduction, in which an object is placed in contact with the skin. Since the resulting sensation may be a blend of touch and temperature, radiant heat, such as that produced by infrared lamps, is sometimes used to eliminate the sensation of touch. Kenshalo (1963) adapted to sensory research an electronic solid-state device known as the *Peltier refrigerator*. The device consists of two dissimilar electrical conductors whose temperature is a function of the amount, rate, and direction of the current passed through it. The temperatures obtained range from 0.05° C to 20° C, with the rate of change continuously variable between 0° C and 2° C per second. The precise temperature control provided by this instrument surpasses anything previously available for the investigation of thermal sensitivity.

## The adequate stimulus

The physical stimulus necessary to evoke a thermal sensation is a change in the temperature of the skin at a depth of 150 to 200$\mu$ below the surface (Hensel, 1950), the level at which receptive elements subserving thermoreception are believed to be located (Hensel, Ström, & Zotterman, 1951). The temperature at this level can be calculated if the skin temperature at the surface is known (Hensel, 1952). This calculation poses a problem because the cutaneous vascular system is also located at this depth and the flow of blood affects the temperature. Investigators of thermal sensitivity generally use the skin temperature measured at the surface as the significant variable.

The total area of skin exposed must be specified, since the change in temperature beneath the skin is a function of the total heat incident on the skin. The rate of temperature change also enters into the equation since rapid shifts are more easily detected than slow shifts. Thus, available data (Hensel, 1950) indicate that the temperature of the skin, the size of the area stimulated, and the rate of change in skin temperature are the three variables directly related to the threshold of detectability for thermal sensations.

## Threshold measurements

### *Skin temperature*

It is impossible to discuss threshold measurements for temperature without the concepts of *physiological zero* and the *neutral zone.* Within a narrow range of temperatures, the thermoreceptors adapt completely, and sensations are aroused only by a departure from the adapting temperature. Physiological zero refers to that skin temperature at which subjects report no thermal sensation. The value of physiological zero is different for different parts of the body, ranging from approximately 28° C at the earlobe to as high as 37° C on the forearm. An average value may be set at approximately 33° C (Kenshalo & Nafe, 1962). The neutral zone is a narrow range above and below physiological zero within which the temperature can change without producing a change in sensation. The size of the neutral zone varies from 0.01° C to 8° C depending on the value of physiological zero, the size of the area stimulated, the rate of temperature change, and the body site stimulated.

The sensation of temperature is determined largely by the temperature to which the skin has been adapted just prior to stimulation. Figure 5.9 shows the results of an experiment in which subjects reported the just noticeable difference (jnd) in sensation on an area of 6 cm$^2$ over the dorsal surface of the forearm, and also reported whether the sensation was "warm" or "cool" (Kenshalo, Nafe, & Brooks, 1961). The smallest change in stimulator temperature that led to a perceived change in thermal sensation was the jnd, and the temperature at which "warm" or "cool' was first reported identified the absolute threshold. Over most of the adapting temperatures, difference thresholds and absolute thresholds were the same. At adapting temperatures below 33° C, the subjects always reported a sensation of "cool" and could detect increments as small as 0.4° C, which they reported as "less cool." A report of "warm" required considerably greater increments. At adapting temperatures above 33° C, decrements of 0.6°C could be detected and were reported as "less warm." Larger decrements were required to evoke a response of "cool." The results show

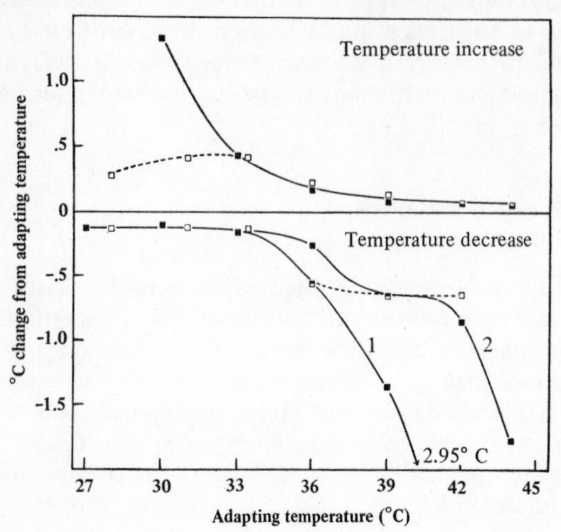


**Figure 5.9** The size of the absolute threshold (filled squares) and of the just noticeable difference (unfilled squares) as a function of the temperature to which the skin was adapted. Male and female subjects showed the same thresholds to both increments and decrements in the adapting temperature except as shown by curves 1 (males) and 2 (females). (From Kenshalo, Nafe, & Brooks, 1961.)

that temperature sensations are correlated with the direction of temperature change, that the reports of sensation depend on the temperature to which the skin is adapted, and that sensitivity to changes in temperature is greatest at the extremes of the adapting temperature range. Complete sensory adaptation occurred at a higher temperature for females (41° C) than for males (36° C). The dependence of absolute threshold on adaptation temperature has also been demonstrated by Hensel (1950) and Lele (1954).

*Spatial parameters*

In general, the intensity of the experience of warmth or cold increases with the area stimulated. For areas up to 14 $cm^2$ the absolute threshold for detection is reduced by one-half for every doubling of the area (Hardy & Oppel, 1937; Kenshalo, Decker, & Hamilton, 1967). As in mechanical stimulation, the summation of energy is complete. The results were the same for radiant and conducted heat, indicating that spatial summation does not depend on the way in which the temperature of the skin is changed. This finding contradicts the notion of Jenkins (1951) and Woodworth and Schlosberg (1954) that the sensations produced by conducted heat are confused by interactions between thermo- and mechanoreceptors.

The question of the locus, peripheral or central, of spatial summation exists for thermal sensitivity as it does for touch. Hardy and Oppel (1937) found that the absolute threshold was 30 percent lower when the backs of both hands were warmed simultaneously than when only one hand was warmed. Stimulation of hand and forehead, however, failed to produce summation. The two-hand results suggest that the summation process is taking place in the central nervous system. Kenshalo and Gallegos (1967) demonstrated summation over space in peripheral nerve fibers of monkeys. Recording from fibers that respond to cooling, they found the rate of neural firing to be directly proportional to the number of individual spots stimulated on the skin. The effect was produced by spot stimuli separated by up to 16 mm. Apparently, spatial summation cannot be attributed exclusively to peripheral or central mechanisms.

*Temporal parameters*

Adaptation to thermal stimulation refers to the reduction in the sensation produced by a constant stimulus over a period of time. For temperatures not too different from physiological zero, the sensation of temperature may disappear entirely in time. The research literature has yielded a wide range of results. Holm (1903) determined that adaptation occurred up to 152 sec at 45° C and 210 sec at 5° C. These temperature limits were reduced by Gertz (1921) who showed that the effects of adaptation can be observed only at temperatures between 12° C and 42° C. Hensel (1950) found even narrower limits, from 19° C to 40° C.

The most thorough determination of the temporal course of thermal adaptation (Figure 5.10) shows that complete adaptation to temperatures between 28° C and 37.5° C occurs within approximately 25 minutes (Kenshalo & Scott, 1966). At lower and higher temperatures, a sensation of cold or warmth persists regardless of the duration of the stimulus. A Peltier device covering approximately 14.5 $cm^2$ stimulated the subjects, who adjusted the temperature so that a just detectable sensation of warmth or cold was maintained over a 40-minute period. Above normal skin temperature, adaptation occurs at a more rapid rate than below normal skin temperature. Within the range of adapting temperatures the direction

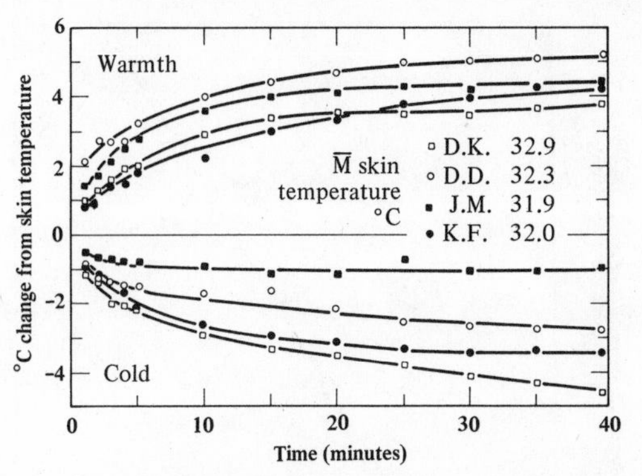


**Figure 5.10** The temporal course of warmth and cold adaptation for four subjects. Each point on the curves represents the amount by which the subject had changed the temperature of the stimulator from the initial skin temperature in order to maintain a just detectable sensation. Also shown are the means of eight measurements of skin temperature taken on each subject just prior to adaptation measurements. (From Kenshalo & Scott, 1966.)

of the temperature change determined the thermal sensation; a rise in temperature felt warm and a drop in temperature felt cold. Below the lower limit of complete adaptation any change in temperature is detected as "more cool" or "less cool," and above the upper limit any change is "more warm" or "less warm." The narrow temperature range for complete adaptation found by Kenshalo and Scott was probably due to improved control of the stimulus and subject conditions, a more stringent criterion for complete adaptation, and the size and location of the stimulated area.

Within the limits of complete thermal adaptation, the appreciation of temperature changes can be achieved only when the change exceeds some minimal rate. Hensel (1950) determined that a rate of at least 0.007° C/sec is necessary for a thermal sensation to occur within the range of 29° C to 36° C. At slower rates, no thermal sensation occurs. A more complete evaluation of the effect of the rate of temperature change was provided by Kenshalo, Holmes, and Wood (1968). They measured the rate of change from physiological zero necessary to produce a thermal sensation and found the minimal rate to be approximately 0.1° C/sec (Figure 5.11), indicating that neither warmth nor cold absolute thresholds are affected when the rate of change is 0.1° C/sec or greater. Rates slower than 0.1° C/sec had a greater effect on the sensation of warmth than on the sensation of cold. Kenshalo et al. suggest that the difference may be due to the fact that the first minute of adaptation to a warm sensation occurred at a more rapid rate than to a cool sensation (see Figure 5.10).

## Suprathreshold measurements

### *Intensity scaling*

The degree of comfort or discomfort that we experience in our environment is largely determined by how we perceive the temperature of that environment. Clothing and housing are designed, in part, to maximize thermal comfort. Early attempts to study the relationship between comfort and temperature were undertaken by the heating and ventilating industry, for very practical reasons, about fifty years ago. Subjective reactions to various combinations of dry-bulb temperature, humidity, and air motion were studied, and standards of comfort were established which are still used (Gagge & Stevens, 1968). Subjects described their experiences in these early experi-

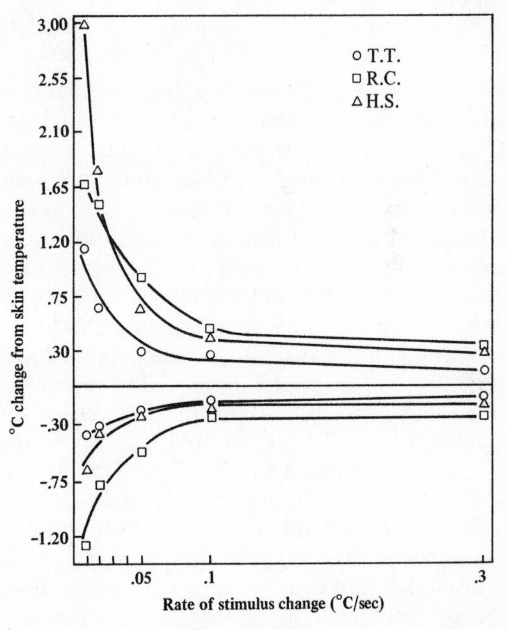


**Figure 5.11** The effect of the rate of the stimulus temperature change on the warm and cool thresholds of three male subjects. The ordinate shows the change from normal skin temperature necessary to reach threshold at each of the rates of change in temperature. (From Kenshalo, Holmes, & Wood, 1968.)

ments by selecting words from a seven-point continuum ranging from "cold" to "hot" with "comfortable" in the middle. Comfort was thus defined as the absence of thermal sensation. The result was a rather crude index of thermal comfort, and precisely measured estimates of thermal sensations were not obtained, partly because adequate techniques of measurement were not available.

The development of direct scaling methods (Stevens, 1960) provided a powerful tool for the investigation of temperature sensations. Using the method of magnitude estimation, Stevens and Stevens (1960) were able to assess quantitatively the sensations of warmth and cold. Using a contact stimulator, they found that the sensations of warmth and cold on an area (3.14 cm$^2$) of the forearm grow as power functions of thermal departure from physiological zero. The rate of growth, however, was different for cold and warmth. Cold sensations increase in direct proportion to decreases in temperature (a slope of 1.0) below physiological zero, whereas warmth grows at a faster rate (a slope of 1.6) than the increases in temperature.

What happens when a large area of the body is exposed to temperature variations rather than to the localized stimuli used in the experiments just described? Stevens and Marks (1967) irradiated an area of the back (1248 cm$^2$) with heat lamps and obtained a power function with a slope of 0.7 when subjects estimated the magnitude of thermal sensation. Using the method of magnitude estimation with complete exposure of the ventral body surface, Gagge and Stevens (1968) and Stevens, Marks, and Gagge (1969) asked subjects to scale the amount of discomfort they experienced as the temperature was shifted above and below that point at which they felt comfortable. The results, shown in Figure 5.12, show that: (1) power functions were obtained with slopes of 0.8 for warm and 1.7 for cold stimuli, which means that discomfort increased much more rapidly when the temperature dropped than when it rose; (2) close to the comfortable level, small increases in temperature produced more discomfort than small decreases; and (3) temperatures at 14° above or below the comfortable level produced the same amount of discomfort. The similarity of the slopes obtained by Stevens and Marks for warmth (0.7) and by Gagge and Stevens for discomfort (0.8) indicates that apparent warmth and discomfort grow at about the same rate.

In the same experiments, Gagge and Stevens

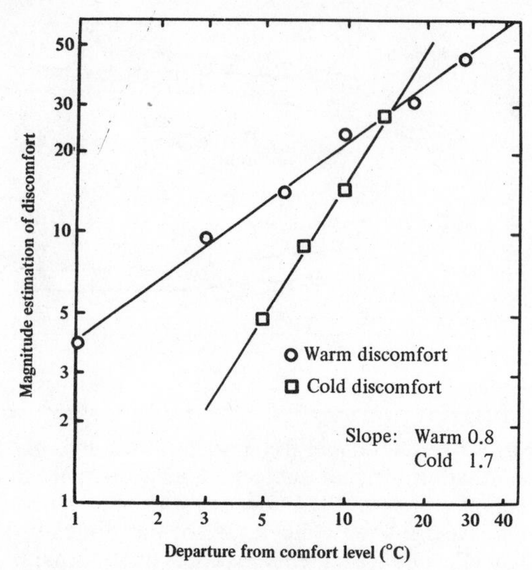


**Figure 5.12** The growth of discomfort as a function of the change in temperature above and below the effective comfort level (22° C). Discomfort due to falling temperatures develops more rapidly than discomfort due to rising temperatures. The ambient air temperature in the chamber was 4° C. (From Gagge & Stevens, 1968.)

asked subjects to adjust their own skin temperature by changing the voltage to an overhead bank of infrared lamps (radiant heat). With the ambient air or room temperature set to various levels by the experimenter, the subject adjusted the irradiated temperature until he felt comfortable. The combined measures of radiant heat absorbed by the body and ambient air temperature yielded an index of comfort called the *operative temperature.* Subjects did not always select a neutral value; some preferred slight sweating or slight body cooling.

The effect of stimulus duration on perceived warmth was studied by Marks and Stevens (1968). They showed that irradiation of the ventral surface of the body for durations of 2 to 12 seconds produced little change in the rate of growth or in the magnitude of the sensation. This lack of effect seemed strange since at the surface of the skin and at several levels below the surface the temperature increased with duration. After rejecting rate of temperature change, thermal gradients, and temperature difference between skin layers as possible correlates of perceived warmth, Marks and Stevens concluded that the increase in skin temperature over time was counterbalanced by the adaptation of thermoreceptors; adaptation appeared to cancel the effect of duration on the perceived magnitude of the thermal sensation.

*Phenomenal effects*

*Paradoxical sensations.* Very early in the era of mapping sensory spots on the cutaneous surface, cold spots were found to occasionally elicit cold sensations in response to very warm stimuli (von Frey, 1895). The effect was named *paradoxical cold.* The temperatures required to produce paradoxical cold (45° C to 50° C) were below the threshold for pain, but well above those necessary to produce warm sensations. Hair movements and low-frequency alternating currents also arouse cold sensations. The counterpart to paradoxical cold is *paradoxical warmth,* which is produced by the application of a cold stimulus to a warm spot. Although widely reported in the literature, the existence of paradoxical sensations is attended by some controversy. Jenkins (1938) was able to arouse warmth and cold inversions only 27 times in 9000 stimulations, and von Gilmer (1942) reported only one paradoxical sensation (warmth) from 13,000 trials. Jenkins and Karr (1957) noticed that paradoxical warmth is produced only when the inappropriate cold stimulus follows the application of a warm stimulus to the same warm spot.

A third illusory sensation called *paradoxical heat* (not warmth) can be aroused by an alternate pattern or grid of warm (42° C to 44° C) and cold (12° C to 15° C) stimuli (Burnett & Dallenbach, 1927). The pattern of warmth and cold produces a burning sensation that stings and often elicits a quick withdrawal reaction when experienced for the first time. Alrutz (1908) attributed the sensation to the simultaneous stimulation of nearby warmth and cold receptors.

These observations have been widely interpreted as strong support of the view that sensory nerve fibers give rise to specific sensations regardless of the mode of excitation (doctrine of specific nerve energies, discussed earlier in this chapter and in Chapter 1). The stinging sensation of paradoxical heat has been ascribed to the excitation of mechanoreceptors by the stimulus object (Herget & Hardy, 1942).

## Theoretical positions

A variety of models have been proposed to explain temperature sensations. The controversy over the specificity of receptors is, after more than half a century, still a focal issue, and the question is still asked: Are we dealing with a single system for temperature detection or with two distinct systems, one for mediating sensations of warmth and another for cold?

The classical theory was formulated by von Frey (1895) as part of his general ideas on the specificity of end-organs. Knowing that sensations of heat and cold could be elicited from discrete spots on the skin (Blix, 1884), von Frey proposed that the sensation of heat was mediated by the Ruffini cylinders, and cold by the Krause end-bulbs. He based his proposal on the observation that body areas having high thermal sensitivity were richly endowed with these endings, and that the time from the onset of the stimulus to the perception of warmth and cold was roughly correlated with the depths at which the receptors were found. This position was supported by histological studies that found a high correlation between psychophysically determined warmth and cold spots and the existence of Ruffini cylinders and Krause end-bulbs in the underlying tissue (Bazett, McGlone, Williams, & Lufkin, 1932; Strughold & Karbe, 1925). Most damaging to the theory, however, is the fact that hairy regions of the body are highly sensitive to thermal changes, but contain Ruffini cylinders and no Krause end-bulbs. Moreover, careful histological examinations of the tissue under warmth and cold spots have failed to turn up the appropriate endings. Nevertheless, without identifying the end-organs, a vast literature details the physiological evidence showing nerve fibers that have a high degree of specificity with respect to stimulating temperature (Zotterman, 1959). Although the association of Krause and Ruffini end-organs with cold and warmth sensations is no longer seriously entertained, the idea that the two sensations are mediated by functionally different receptor systems is still considered.

Bazett (1941) offered an alternative theory based on his finding that a *spatial thermal gradient* exists in the tissues underlying the surface of the skin. He and his co-workers inserted tiny *thermocouples* into the skin and measured the temperature at varying depths below the surface. They found that the normal temperature of the tissue changes as a function of distance from the surface. Theoretically, any upset of this gradient causes the sensation of warmth or cold; when heat is lost from the surface to a cold stimulus, the normal gradient is disturbed, thermal equilibrium breaks down, and the sensation of cold is produced. A warm stimulus disturbs the gradient at a different depth, and the sensation of warmth is produced. The theory makes no attempt to explain sensation in terms of neural elements, but concentrates on the conduction rates of heat transfer through cutaneous tissue.

The gradient theory is contradicted by a number of experiments, including some by Bazett and his collaborators. They applied warm and cold stimuli to the surface of the human prepuce, stretched out for the experiment, and measured conduction times of heat transfer via a thermocouple located on the undersurface. They also measured reaction times for the thermal sensations. On the basis of these experiments, they determined that cold receptors lie about 0.1 mm and warmth receptors about 0.3 mm beneath the surface of the skin. These estimates are in agreement with the average depth at which Krause and Ruffini endings are found. The difficulty for the gradient theory lies in the fact that the same results were obtained from either side of the prepuce. When the stimulus was applied to the underside of the fold, the gradient should have been affected in the reverse direction and the results should have reflected this change, but they did not.

Additional difficulty for the gradient theory is that the latency in the firing of cold fibers in the cat's tongue is not affected by cooling the top or the bottom of the tongue (Hensel & Witt, 1959; Hensel & Zotterman, 1951). Moreover, it is possible to compare the effects of warming the skin with and without upsetting the temperature gradient. The use of a *microwave source* (radar) permits increased temperatures to be distributed uniformly to a predetermined depth below the surface of the skin which, presumably, does not produce a gradient. An infrared source heats from the surface inward, which does produce a gradient. One would therefore expect lower thresholds for an infrared source than for a radar source. However, both heat sources yield the same thresholds (Vendrik & Vos, 1958). The threshold appears to be determined by the temperature at the site of stimulation rather than by the production or alteration of a thermal gradient.

Another attack on the concept of receptor specificity is embodied in the *neurovascular theory*. First articulated by Nafe (1934) and further developed by Kenshalo and Nafe (1962), this theory states that sensations of warmth and cold are produced by the mechanical stimulation of undifferentiated free nerve endings embedded in the walls of the cutaneous vascular system and the hair-erector muscles. The mechanical stimulation is provided by expansion or contraction of smooth muscle in the walls of the blood vessels upon warming or cooling. The smooth muscle of the arterioles, venules (tiny veins), and hairs constitute the receptor end-organ, a thermomechanical transducer. The emphasis is not on the nerve terminals, which are supposedly all alike, but on the mechanical action of the tissues in which the nerves terminate. Warmth and cold sensations are produced by different spatiotemporal patterns of nerve impulses or by the terminal sites of the nerve fibers within the central nervous system. Although no area of the cortex has been experimentally identified with thermal stimulation at the periphery, the mechanoreceptive region of the postcentral gyrus is assumed to subserve this function.

Several lines of evidence are inconsistent with the neurovascular theory. If the same fibers are excited by warming or cooling the vascular smooth muscle, temperature-sensitive fibers should respond in some way to both increases and decreases in skin temperature. The neurophysiological literature, however, abounds with reports of fibers that respond specifically to either warming or cooling but few fibers that respond to both (Zotterman, 1959). The neurovascular theory depends directly on the action of vasoconstriction and vasodilation on nerves in the vascular walls to explain temperature sensations. These nerve fibers, however, contain many synaptic vesicles, which are subcellular structures found in presynaptic but generally not in postsynaptic terminals (Rhodin, 1962). If their terminals are presynaptic, then the nerves in the vascular walls are probably sending signals to the muscles and not from them as postulated by the neurovascular theory. The function of these nerve fibers may be to control the motility of the vascular walls; they may have nothing at all to do with signaling changes in the walls caused by temperature shifts. Furthermore, the psychophysical evidence shows a dual set of functional relations for warmth and cold sensitivity: Their time parameters appear to differ, and the subjective magnitudes of warmth and cold are markedly different functions of stimulus temperature (Gagge & Stevens, 1968; Stevens, Marks, & Gagge, 1969; Stevens & Stevens, 1960).

Only three of the many theories that attempt to explain the mechanism of thermal sensitivity have been presented. None of them alone is adequate, and only the specific-receptor theory and the neurovascular theory are seriously considered by present-day investigators.

## PAIN

Much of the literature and research concerning pain has been motivated and organized around the controversy regarding the nature of pain or its adequate stimulus. The emphasis in more recent years has shifted from threshold measurements, whose meaning depends on the theoretical orientation of the author, toward the measurement of clearly felt, suprathreshold pain. There has also been a reaffirmation of an earlier position that pain must be regarded within the context of its meaning to the individual, which implies multiple determinants rather than solely neurosensory ones.

Disagreement over the nature of pain reaches across centuries of medical and scientific literature. Pain has always seemed a more personal sensation and more difficult to communicate than sensations in the other modalities. Light, sound, temperature, and other stimuli are *out there*—they can be shared and can be used to tag the sensation. But pain is felt *in here* and defies such ease of definition or the same level of sharing. The problem is due partly to the difficulty in defining the stimulus that gives rise to pain.

Two schools of thought have developed concerning the nature of pain. These may be characterized as the *sensory* and *intensive* points of view (Dallenbach, 1939). The sensory viewpoint, which traces its origin at least back to Avicenna in the eleventh century A.D, maintains that pain is a separate and distinct sense modality. The intensive definition states that pain is the product of excessive stimulation of any sense modality and does not exist as a separate modality. The two positions have implications for the specificity-nonspecificity controversy already discussed.

A second disagreement dates from the time of Aristotle, who emphasized the *affective* (*pleasant-unpleasant*) nature of pain over its sensory qualities. Most of the scientific writings of the nineteenth and twentieth centuries have taken the position that pain is a sensation, regardless of whether an intensive or sensory viewpoint was adopted. An effort has been made in recent years to reject the position that pain is simply another sensory system and to take into account complicating factors, such as environmental situations, that influence the perception of pain (Melzack & Casey, 1968; Sternbach, 1968).

### The adequate stimulus and definitions

If an object is pressed against the skin, the resulting sensation is touch or pressure, depending on the force and duration of application. It may also be sensed as cool or warm, depending on its temperature. If the force is increased or the temperature changed substantially, the sensation quickly turns to pain. The fact that pain can be elicited by a variety of mechanical, chemical, thermal, and electrical stimuli is the essence of the difficulty and the core of the controversy. Is pain a separate sense modality or is it the result of overstimulation in any sense modality? Is it mediated by a specific pain-receptor system or by nonspecific endings?

The classical viewpoint defines the stimulus for pain as any form of energy sufficiently intense to cause tissue damage. Hardy, Wolff, and Goodell (1952) showed that a skin temperature of 45° C, within the range where tissue damage begins to occur, was sufficient to cause pain. Needle pricks deep enough to cause pain will almost always produce redness of the skin, which indicates damaged tissue (Lewis, 1942). Stoll and Greene (1959) showed that pain intensity is directly related to the logarithm of the rate of tissue damage on the skin. The threshold for pain in audition is reached at a sound pressure level of about 140 dB (von Békésy, 1952); at higher levels damage to the receptors for hearing becomes imminent (see Chapter 4).

The definition linking pain to tissue damage was later modified to include potentially damaging stimuli, since pain is usually felt before actual damage occurs. Even this modification has limitations because many stimuli can cause damage without giving rise to painful sensations, and some forms of energy, such as ultraviolet radiation, cause pain (sunburn) long after the damage has occurred.

Some investigators have turned their attention away from the damaging aspects of pain stimuli to find what parameter of the stimulus causes the pain. Thus, von Frey (1896b) linked pain sensations to the amount of pressure exerted on the skin. Since applying pressure to the skin involves the stretching of tissue, Bishop (1949) concluded that stretch applied to nerve terminals constitutes the effective stimulus for the arousal of pain. Going to even finer levels of analysis, several investigators have proposed that chemical agents, released when tissue is injured or diseased, constitute the adequate stimulus for pain. Lim (1968) proposed that chemicals, released as a consequence of tissue damage, act upon somesthetic chemoreceptors which signal pain. Benjamin (1968) pointed out that the release of potassium always accompanies tissue injury, and that any stimulus that can produce pain leads to the release of intracellular potassium. He demonstrated that concentrations of potassium administered experimentally will produce pain, and that agents which inhibit the release of potassium are effective in reducing pain. Rosenthal (1968), on the other hand, provided considerable evidence that *histamine*, a chemical found in all animal tissues, is the mediator of cutaneous pain and of pain *referred* from the viscera to cutaneous tissue (see discussion of referred pain later in the chapter).

Over the past decade emphasis has shifted away from pain as a purely sensory experience toward the position that pain is the combined result of sensory, affective, motivational, and central nervous system determinants (Melzack & Casey, 1968; Sternbach, 1968). For example, severe battle wounds may produce little pain response, whereas an inept vein puncture elicits bitter complaints from the same patients (Beecher, 1959). The influence of nonsensory factors is revealed in a study showing that *placebos* (dummy pain relievers) reduce pain in only 3 percent of subjects in experimental situations, but bring relief to 35 percent of patients in clinical studies (Beecher, 1960).

The current trend is toward including the response to pain in any definition of pain (Sternbach, 1968). The response may be verbal (ouch!), a facial expression, or a body movement in the form of avoidance or withdrawal. The response to pain may also be measured by physiological reactions (heart rate, blood pressure, sweating, etc.) or by the activity in specific nerves. All of these responses have served to indicate the presence of pain, but no one of them in itself is a sufficient measure of pain.

The definition of pain and its adequate stimulus is difficult and complex. No single category of determinants seems adequate to specify what pain is and what conditions are necessary for its arousal. Sternbach (1968) suggested a definition that may satisfy our experimental knowledge and clinical experience:

> Pain is an abstract concept which refers to (1) a personal, private sensation of hurt; (2) a harmful stimulus which signals current or impending tissue damage; (3) a pattern of responses which operates to protect the organism from harm [p. 12].

The measurement of pain is made in terms of verbal, behavioral, physiological, and neurological responses.

## Theories

Current theories of pain fall into three major categories: (1) *specificity theory,* which gives to pain the status of a sense modality with specific neural units designed expressly for the mediation of pain; (2) *pattern theory,* in which pain is a function of the spatio-temporal patterning of impulses in nonspecific nerve fibers; and (3) *duplex theories,* which combine some features of both specificity and pattern positions. The general tenets of these positions have been given earlier in this chapter.

### *Specificity theory*

Pain is considered to result from the stimulation of specific pain receptors, widely held to be free nerve endings located in cutaneous and subcutaneous tissues. According to this theory, the neural impulses are carried by specific peripheral fibers within the *A-delta* (1 to 6 $\mu$ diameter) and *C* (0.4 to 1.2 $\mu$ diameter) categories (Bishop, 1946) via the lateral spinothalamic tract (Sweet, 1959) to a *pain center* in the thalamus (Head, 1920; Mark & Yakovlev, 1955) and on to the cortex.

Goldscheider (1885) noted that pain could be aroused with a fine needle at specific spots over the skin's surface and not at other spots. These studies were verified and greatly expanded by the detailed explorations of the skin by von Frey (1894). There is almost universal acceptance of free nerve endings as the end-organ mediating pain sensations (Weddell & Sinclair, 1953). Areas of human skin from which only pain sensations could be aroused contained only simple, free nerve endings (Sinclair, 1967; Sweet, 1959; Woolard, Weddell, & Harpman, 1940).

A number of experiments have attempted to correlate pain with nerve-fiber size, but many of them are difficult to interpret because they were performed on animals. Collins, Nulsen, and Randt (1960) overcame this problem by testing conscious patients undergoing spinal surgery. They found that the sensation of pain did not appear unless *A-delta* fibers were stimulated, and that the pain became unbearable when *C* fibers were also involved. They concluded that conscious appreciation of pain in humans is mediated by small fibers. Weddell and Verrillo (1972) concur that pain is mediated by small fibers which end in free arborizations. They suggest, however, that pain is related to the normal degeneration-regeneration cycle of the "free nerve ending," and that pain arises from the chemical stimulation of those terminals during the regeneration phase. The following sequence of events, based on the work of Lewis (1960, 1963) and others, has been proposed by Mountcastle (1968) and Weddell and Verrillo (1972) as a speculative but probable peripheral mechanism for the initiation of pain: Cell injury releases proteolytic enzymes which act upon the globulin in the intercellular fluids. These enzymes produce polypeptides which are powerful stimulators of small-diameter, unmyelinated free nerve endings, the nociceptive afferents. Some research supports these propositions and more is in progress.

Attempts to identify specific spinal cord tracts with the conduction of pain impulses have yielded mixed results. Sectioning the lateral spinothalamic tract (Schwartz & O'Leary, 1942) affects pain responses more than any other cutaneous sensations, but the results of many experiments indicate that while pain can be appreciably diminished by cord sectioning, it is rarely extinguished completely (Sinclair, 1967).

The picture is clearer in the thalamus where well-defined nuclei have been identified with the perception of pain. There is a *somatotopic* representation of the body for pain sensation in the thalamic nuclei. (Somatotopic representation refers to the duplication of the spatial relationships among parts of the body within a group of cells in the central nervous system.) Lesions in the *parafascicular* and *intralaminar* nuclei of the thalamus result in the abolition of pain while not affecting the appreciation of touch, temperature, or pinprick (Mark, Ervin, & Yakovlev, 1963). Patients showed no changes in emotional status. The experiment delimits a specific central neural center for the appreciation of pain and supports the separation of pain from the other sense modalities. The thalamus appears to be the highest center at which such a clear distinction can be made. Attempts to relieve pain by *lobotomy,* the transection of fibers linking frontal cortical areas to lower brain centers, most often result in the continued presence of pain, but an indifference on the part of the patient toward the pain (Sternbach, 1968). An undesired side effect is the drastic personality modification that such operations usually produce (Sweet, 1959).

The finding that pain sensations are carried over two sets of fibers (*A-delta* and *C*) has stimulated renewed interest in the phenomenon of *double,* or *second,* pain. When the skin is punctured by a needle or a toe is stubbed, the first sensation is that of sharp, bright pain followed by a longer-lasting, dull ache. The difference in the conduction velocity of *A-delta* fibers (19 to 45 m/sec) and *C* fibers (less than 2 m/sec) has been used to explain double pain (Sweet, 1959). Although the phenomenon is commonplace, it has been disappointingly difficult to reproduce in the laboratory. The two sensations tend to merge if the stimulus intensity is too high, and the effect fails to occur at weak intensities (Sinclair & Stokes, 1964). A study by Lewis and Pochin (1937) supports the hypothesis of two sets of fibers with different conduction rates. They showed that the time interval between first and second pain decreased as the site of stimulation was advanced along the limbs toward the torso.

*Pattern theory*

The pattern theorists reject the notion that pain results from stimulating specific receptors and that the impulses are transmitted over separate neural pathways (Nafe, 1927; Sinclair, 1955; Weddell, 1955). Instead, they propose that the sensory information is contained in the spatio-temporal code carried over nonspecific fibers coming from nonspecific nerve endings. Unfortunately, more space is devoted to attacking the evidence for specificity than to providing examples of spatio-temporal patterns that can be associated with sensory experiences. A vast amount of information, supporting a position of specificity, was too often simply ignored by early advocates of the pattern theory.

One of the earliest attempts to explain pain by nonspecific nerves suggested that *reverberating circuits* are set up in the spinal cord by intense pathological stimulation of the body (Livingston, 1943). A reverberating circuit is a system of neurons in a complex circular arrangement that once activated continues to excite itself and so perpetuates its own activity. Once established, these circuits can be activated by normally harmless stimuli which thereby produce pain. A similar mechanism located at the cortical level has been proposed by Hebb (1949) and Gerard (1951).

Today, few investigators adhere strictly to the rigid concepts of the early pattern theorists. The evidence for stimulus specificity in peripheral nerves is difficult to ignore. Several attempts have been made to reconcile specificity with pattern concepts. The common features of these duplex theories is that all of them explain sensations as an interaction of two systems of nerves.

### *Duplex theories*

The common ancestor of the duplex theories is that of Henry Head (1920). In the early 1900s Head severed a peripheral nerve in his own arm and then noted carefully the sequence of the return of sensations as the nerve regenerated. Based on the differential rates of regeneration, he concluded that there were two anatomically distinct systems of nerve fibers subserving the cutaneous sensations. He gave the name *protopathic* to the system that regenerated first and mediated pain and temperature extremes. The *epicritic* system regenerated more slowly and was associated with light touch, touch localization, and temperature discrimination.

Modern counterparts of Head's theory resulted from the development of techniques for recording from single nerve fibers. Mountcastle (1961, 1968) proposes two distinct systems. One is highly specific and fast; its impulses travel over the spinal cord's dorsal column medial-lemniscal pathway (see Chapter 3). This pathway seems to mediate pressure, touch, and vibration. The second system, which is not as highly organized as the first, conducts slowly over the lateral spinothalamic tract (see Chapter 3). This system contains fibers mediating pain as well as thermal sensations.

Noordenbos (1959) regards pain not as a specific modality, but the result of excessive stimulation of any nerve ending. He suggests that potentially harmful stimuli activate a slow, multisynaptic system that serves as a nonspecific system for alerting the organism. Detailed, quantitative information is conveyed by a fast, more specific set of fibers. Pain is the result of patterns of impulses traveling over either pathway. Noordenbos deemphasizes the concept of modality and stresses the pattern of activity produced by the interaction of fast and slow fiber impulses.

The *gate control theory* proposed by Melzack and Wall (1965) attempts to reconcile the specificity and pattern approaches by integrating the facts concerning specialization, central summation patterning, and spinal-cord mechanisms. Impulses from receptors that respond optimally to either mechanical or thermal stimuli are transmitted to the spinal cord over both large and small fibers. The type of stimulus is encoded in the temporal patterning of the impulses. In the region of the *substantia gelatinosa* within the spinal cord (see Chapter 3) and the first central transmission cells in the dorsal horn of the spinal cord, the large and small fibers produce a pattern of excitatory-inhibitory activity. The relative balance of activity from large and small fibers determines whether a message signaling pain is transmitted to higher centers over the anterolateral spinothalamic pathways. When the input from large fibers dominates, the small-fiber activity is inhibited and nonpainful sensations result. As the balance of activity shifts from large to small fibers, inhibition of small-fiber impulses is reduced and the sensation shifts to one of pain. In addition, the entire gate control system can be modulated by a central control mechanism that influences the experience of pain.

Proponents of this theory have shown that intense pain can be relieved by bombarding the cutaneous afferent systems with nonpainful stimuli that excite the large afferent neurons (Wall & Sweet, 1967). The domination of small-fiber activity by large-fiber activity presumably "closes" the gate temporarily to painful impulses. As the relative proportion of small-fiber activity increases, the gate is "opened" and pain returns. A later paper (Melzack & Casey, 1968) demonstrates the usefulness of the gate control theory in explaining many of the sensory, motivational, and cognitive determinants of pain. The argument that pain is not a unitary sensory phenomenon, but one of complex sensory and affective components, is consistent with Sternbach's (1968) position (see earlier discussion of the adequate stimulus in this section).

While the theory provides an adequate framework of specific proposals for investigation, subsequent research has been sometimes contradictory to earlier findings and continues to be attended by considerable controversy. The mechanism by which pain is mediated is by no means a settled issue.

## Threshold measurements

### *Spatial parameters*

The increase of sensation as the area of stimulation is increased is not as consistent for pain as it is for vibrotaction or temperature. Thresholds for pricking pain did not change as the stimulated area was increased from 0.5 to 28 cm$^2$ (Hardy, Wolff, & Goodell, 1952). Later experiments showed, however, that if the area of stimulation is kept small, the pain threshold does display spatial summation (Greene & Hardy, 1958). Spatial summation of pain caused by conducted heat can be shown if the differences in stimulator area are sufficiently large (Benjamin, 1968).

*Temporal parameters*

Temporal summation is an important characteristic of pain sensitivity. Indeed, the rationale for the intensive definition of pain rests upon the summation of impulses over time. The repetition rate of electrical charges applied to the skin determines the threshold for pain, and the painfulness of the stimulus increases as a function of the repetition rate (Heinbecker, Bishop, & O'Leary, 1933). Collins, Nulsen, and Shealy (1966) were able to show that single impulses conducted over *C* fibers elicit no pain sensations in conscious human subjects. However, pain was consistently reported when the rate was raised to three or more impulses per second.

It had been thought that the intensity of pain does not decrease over prolonged durations until Strauss and Uhlmann (1919) demonstrated not only that one adapts to painful pressure but also that adaptation time varies as a function of pressure. Numerous studies have since demonstrated adaptation for painful sensations caused by needles (Wells & Hoisington, 1931), radiant heat (Neisser, 1959; Stone & Dallenbach, 1934), and cold (Edes & Dallenbach, 1936). The importance of the intensity of the painful stimulus was demonstrated by Greene and Hardy (1962), who showed that adaptation to pain could not be achieved near the threshold for pain (45° C). Reports of "very hot" and "painful" were intermittent for up to 38 minutes, after which a continuous pain reaction was evoked. Hardy (1962) reported that the intensity of heat needed to elicit pain actually decreases with duration; that is, the pain increased with time.

The many contradictions concerning adaptation to pain led Hardy and Stolwijk (1966) to attribute the lack of adaptation to thermal pain at temperatures of 43° C to 46° C to the action of an "inactivated protein complex" that is the result of a thermally induced breakdown of tissue proteins. Their theory uses temperature coefficients and rates of protein destruction and repair to predict pain over time and intensity. The view that substances released in the breakdown of tissue activates pain endings is similar to that of Benjamin (1968), Lim (1968), and Rosenthal (1968).

Common experience tells us that pain sometimes persists and sometimes goes away in the presence of a continuous painful stimulus. The experimental evidence suggests that currently undetermined combinations of durations and intensities may explain these experiences.

**Suprathreshold measurements**

*Intensity scaling*

Investigation of the relationship between stimulus intensity and the subjective magnitude of pain was delayed for many years by measurement difficulties. Mechanical devices that were adequate for determining pain thresholds produced injuries when above-threshold measurements were attempted. The determination of pain scales is further complicated because the intensity range between the pain threshold and unbearable pain is extremely narrow; for radiant heat the ratio is about 2:1, compared to a ratio of 2000:1 for the range from the warmth to the pain threshold.

Hardy, Wolff, and Goodell (1947, 1948) partially solved the problem of cutaneous injury by constructing an instrument, the *dolorimeter,* which utilized radiant heat focused on the skin to produce pain. They were able to construct a scale for pain using the methods of just noticeable differences (jnd's) and fractionation (see Chapter 2). They proposed the name *dol,* from the Latin *dolor* (pain), as the unit of pain intensity. The dol is equal to two successive jnd's. Because the jnd measurements were considered statistically crude, this scale has not been widely utilized. Adair, Stevens, and Marks (1968) determined that the growth of pain is a power function of the intensity of thermal irradiation on the forehead and forearm. Although their method (magnitude estimation) differed from that of Hardy et al., the results were strikingly similar between the threshold and a level 6 dols above threshold. Within this range the slope of the power function was 1.0 in both studies. Swartz (1953) also found that subjective pain was directly proportional to the intensity of the stimulus when he stimulated tooth pulp with electrical current and asked subjects to adjust the stimulus intensity in a series of *bisections*. The upper limits of the pain scale have not been investigated in great detail because of the problem of tissue destruction. Hardy (1956) showed that once tissue damage begins there is no further change in the perceived magnitude of the pain.

*Referred pain*

Pathology within the abdominal or thoracic cavities often gives rise to pain that is poorly localized or even localized to the body surface, a phenomenon called *referred* pain. The clinician has long used the knowledge of reference sites as an important diagnostic tool for locating diseased or malfunctioning organs. Another type of referred pain is that felt at one site on the skin while the stimulus is being applied to some other, distant site. The reports of such phenomena are not uncommon and are well documented in the medical literature (Sinclair, 1967). It was once thought that the sites of the referred pain and the stimulus were always within the same *dermatome,* the area of skin served by the same spinal nerve, but this is no longer held to be a necessary condition for referred pain (Sinclair, 1949).

A number of hypotheses have been advanced to explain referred pain (Rosenthal, 1968), some of which involve the confluence of visceral and cutaneous nerve fibers within synaptic pools of the spinal cord (Weddell, 1957). Others emphasize physiochemical changes within the nervous system. However, the reason for feeling pain in one part of the body in response to stimulation of another part has no adequate explanation.

## SUMMARY AND CONCLUSIONS

The surface of the skin constitutes the largest sensory system of the body. It is a complex system since it has the capacity to mediate more than a single sense modality, including touch, temperature, and pain. The variety of sensations originating in the skin has led to many theories concerning the neural mechanisms that make this possible. Principal among these are the *receptor specificity theory,* which states that each modality has morphologically distinct end-organs with specific nerve tracts to conduct impulses centrally; and the *pattern theory,* which contends that each nerve ending responds to all forms of stimulation, the different sensations arising from the spatio-temporal pattern of impulses arriving at the brain. Attempts have been made to reconcile the two theories by combining selected features of both. There is insufficient evidence at this time to resolve the conflict conclusively, but current research appears to favor the specificity position.

Sensory experiences from the skin may be broadly categorized as *mechanoreception, thermoreception,* and *pain.* Mechanoreception includes those sensations such as touch, vibration, and pressure that result from the mechanical distortion of cutaneous tissue. The adequate stimulus is most likely the *displacement* of tissues immediately below the skin's surface. Displacements as small as 0.001 mm (0.00004 inch) are sufficient to arouse a sensation of touch at 250 Hz. There are at least two distinct systems of receptors involved in mechanoreception. One system can summate energy over space and time; that is, sensitivity increases as the area of stimulation increases or as the frequency or duration of the stimulus is increased. The end-organ of this system is the Pacinian corpuscle. The other system is unable to summate in the same way; that is, no decrease in threshold is produced by increasing area, frequency, or duration. Most of the research on mechanoreception uses sinusoidal vibrations. The practical limits for *vibrotaction* lie between 20 and 1000 Hz. Stimuli below 20 Hz are not felt as vibrations, and stimuli above 1000 Hz cannot be felt at all.

The subjective intensity of vibration is related in an orderly fashion to the physical intensity of the stimulus, just as it is for hearing and vision. This relationship is called the *power law* because the perceived intensity increases as a power function of the intensity of the stimulus. This law is one of the firmly established principles of sensory measurement.

Although the vibrotactile systems do not discriminate pitch as well as the auditory system, some discriminations can be made, especially at frequencies below 40 Hz. At higher frequencies a rather large difference between two frequencies is required in order to distinguish a difference between them.

The information concerning threshold as a function of frequency, intensity functions, and frequency discrimination has a practical aspect. There has been an increasing effort to utilize the skin as an alternate or surrogate channel of communication for vision and hearing to compensate for blindness and deafness. It becomes immensely important to know the functional characteristics of cutaneous sensation if adequate, practical devices are to be developed that can aid the blind and the deaf.

Thermoreception refers to the ability to perceive temperature changes on the skin. When the temperature is lowered we say it is "cool" or "cold"; when the temperature is raised we say it is "warm" or "hot." The sensation that we report is most directly dependent upon three factors: (1) the temperature of the skin, (2) the size of the area stimulated, and (3) the rate of change in skin temperature. The sensation of temperature is also closely related to the temperature to which the skin has become adapted. A temperature which might be considered "warm" on a cold day may be perceived as "cool" on a hot day. This phenomenon is embodied in the concept of *physiological zero,* which is very important in research relating to temperature sensitivity. Physiological zero refers to that skin temperature at which no thermal sensation is perceived. The *neutral zone* is a narrow range of temperatures above and below physiological zero within which temperatures can change without producing a detectable change in sensation.

Temperatures not too different from physiological zero, when applied for a sufficient period of time, will result in a reduction of thermal sensation. This experience is called *adaptation,* a phenomenon common to all sensory systems. The rate at which adaptation occurs and the intensity limits that can be tolerated have been extensively investigated, but they have yielded a wide variety of results that are not readily summarized.

Suprathreshold measurements of thermal sensitivity are of great practical importance to industries concerned with the control of indoor temperatures for purposes of comfort and health. The scaling methods used in vibrotaction are also used extensively to measure the growth of thermal sensations as a function of the temperature of stimuli applied to the body. This research indicates that people prefer temperatures that are slightly above or below a temperature at which no thermal sensation at all is experienced.

Pain presents a unique problem to the investigator since there are no adequate definitions of what pain is or what the adequate stimulus is to produce pain. Pain is a more private experience than sight, hearing, or touch. It depends more heavily on such nonsensory factors as personality, past experience, and current environment. The most simple and direct definition for pain is that it is a sensation of hurt. It is generally conceded that pain is mediated by free nerve endings of very small diameter and carried over a variety of pathways to the brain. The immediate stimulus for pain at the nerve ending is probably a chemical reaction brought about by damage to the surrounding tissues. A great many theories have been propounded to explain pain, but none is completely adequate. Because of the nature of the experience itself, the amount of laboratory research on pain is meager. Most of the research has been conducted in a clinical setting without adequate experimental controls. There have been more speculation and theorizing about the nature and mechanisms of pain than about any other sense modality originating from the skin, which is not surprising considering the urgency with which most of us try to alleviate or eliminate the experience.

The aim of this chapter has been to present a brief overview of our knowledge about the skin, with emphasis on its role as a sensory system. An attempt has been made to integrate current material from diverse but related fields of research, such as anatomy, electrophysiology, and psychophysics. When compared to vision and hearing, progress in skin research has been slow and the total number of basic principles is small indeed. However, the pace of research into the precise response characteristics of the various types of nerve fibers and receptors that innervate cutaneous tissue has been greatly accelerated in the past decade. There has been an important trend toward the investigation of basic functions and the integration of knowledge derived from different research disciplines. It is clear that progress in our understanding of the functions and capacities of skin as a sensory system will be accomplished only by a close liaison among these disciplines. And lastly, it is imperative that the phenomena underlying our sensory experiences be conceptualized as coherent, functional *systems,* and not merely as a conglomeration of parts somehow working together. It is the proper analysis of these systems that will lead ultimately to an understanding of the sensory experience.

# REFERENCES

**Adair, E. R., Stevens, J. C., & Marks, L. E.** Thermally induced pain, the dol scale, and the psychophysical power law. *American Journal of Psychology,* 1968, **81,** 147–64.

**Alrutz, S.** Untersuchungen über die Temperatursinne. *Zeitschrift für Psychologie,* 1908, **47,** 161.

**Bach-y-Rita, P.** *Brain mechanisms in sensory substitution.* New York: Academic Press, 1972.

**Bagh, K. von.** Quantitative Untersuchungen auf dem Gebiet der Berührungs- und Druckempfindungen. *Zeitschrift für Biologie,* 1935, **96,** 153–77.

**Bazett, H. C.** Temperature sense in man. In *Temperature, its measurement, and control in science and industry.* New York: Van Nostrand Reinhold, 1941. Pp. 489–501.

**Bazett, H. C., McGlone, B., Williams, R. G., & Lufkin, H. M.** Sensation: I. Depth, distribution and probable identification in the prepuce of sensory end-organs concerned in sensations of temperature and touch; thermometric conductivity. *Archives of Neurology and Psychiatry,* 1932, **27,** 489–517.

**Beecher, H. K.** *Measurement of subjective responses: Quantitative effects of drugs*. New York: Oxford University Press, 1959.

**Beecher, H. K.** Increased stress and effectiveness of placebos and "active" drugs. *Science*, 1960, **132**, 91–92.

**Békésy, G. von.** Über die Vibrationsempfindung. *Akusticheski Zhurnal*, 1939, **4**, 316–34.

**Békésy, G. von.** Microphonics produced by touching the cochlear partition with a vibrating electrode. *Journal of the Acoustical Society of America*, 1951, **23**, 29–35.

**Békésy, G. von.** Direct observation of the vibrations of the cochlear partition under a microscope. *Acta Oto-Laryngologica*, 1952, **42**, 197–201.

**Békésy, G. von.** Human skin perception of traveling waves similar to those on the cochlea. *Journal of the Acoustical Society of America*, 1955, **27**, 830–41.

**Békésy, G. von.** Sensations on the skin similar to directional hearing, beats, and harmonics of the ear. *Journal of the Acoustical Society of America*, 1957, **29**, 489–501. (a)

**Békésy, G. von.** Neural volleys and the similarity between some sensations produced by tones and by skin vibrations. *Journal of the Acoustical Society of America*, 1957, **29**, 1059–69. (b)

**Békésy, G. von.** Funneling in the nervous system and its role in loudness and sensation intensity on the skin. *Journal of the Acoustical Society of America*, 1958, **30**, 399–412.

**Békésy, G. von.** Synchronism of neural discharges and their demultiplication in pitch perception on the skin and in hearing. *Journal of the Acoustical Society of America*, 1959, **31**, 338–49. (a)

**Békésy, G. von.** Neural funneling along the skin and between hair cells of the cochlea. *Journal of the Acoustical Society of America*, 1959, **31**, 1236–49. (b)

**Békésy, G. von.** Neural inhibitory units of the eye and skin. Quantitative description of contrast phenomena. *Journal of the Optical Society of America*, 1960, **50**, 1060–70.

**Békésy, G. von.** Can we feel the nervous discharges of the end organs during vibratory stimulation of the skin? *Journal of the Acoustical Society of America*, 1962, **34**, 850–56. (a) Figure 1, p. 851, reproduced by permission of the American Institute of Physics.

**Békésy, G. von.** Synchrony between nervous discharges and periodic stimuli in hearing and on the skin. *Annals of Otology, Rhinology and Laryngology*, 1962, **71**, 678–92. (b)

**Bell, C.** *Idea of a new anatomy of the brain: Submitted for the observation of his friends*. London: Privately printed, 1811. Also in *Journal of Anatomy and Physiology*, 1869, **3**, 154–57.

**Benjamin, F. B.** The release of intracellular potassium as a factor in pain production. In D. R. Kenshalo (Ed.), *The skin senses*. Springfield, Ill.: Charles C Thomas, 1968. Pp. 466–79.

**Benussi, V.** Versuche zur Analyse taktil erweckter Scheinbewegungen. *Archiv für die gesamte Psychologie*, 1916, **36**, 59. Cited by C. E. Sherrick, Studies of apparent tactual movement. In D. R. Kenshalo (Ed.), *The skin senses*. Springfield, Ill.: Charles C Thomas, 1968. Pp. 331–44.

**Bishop, G. H.** Neural mechanisms of cutaneous sense. *Physiological Reviews*, 1946, **26**, 77–102.

**Bishop, G. H.** Relation of pain sensory threshold to form of mechanical stimulator. *Journal of Neurophysiology*, 1949, **12**, 51–57.

**Bliss, J. C.** A relatively high-resolution reading aid for the blind. *IEEE Transactions. Man-Machine Systems*, 1969, **MMS-10**, 1–8.

**Bliss, J. C. (Ed.)** Tactile displays conference, special issue. *IEEE Transactions. Man-Machine Systems*, 1970, **MMS-11**, 1–122.

**Bliss, J. C., Crane, H. D., Mansfield, P. K., & Townsend, J. T.** Information available in brief tactile presentations. *Perception & Psychophysics*, 1966, **1**, 273–83.

**Blix, M.** Experimentelle Beiträge zur Lösung der Frage über die specifische Energie des Hautnerven. *Zeitschrift für Biologie*, 1884, **20**, 141–56.

**Boring, E. G.** *Sensation and perception in the history of experimental psychology*. New York: Appleton-Century-Crofts, 1942.

**Brecher, G. A.** Die untere Hör- und Tongrenze. *Pflügers Archiv für die gesamte Physiologie des Menschen und der Tiere*, 1934, **234**, 380–93.

**Burnett, N. C., & Dallenbach, K. M.** The experience of heat. *American Journal of Psychology*, 1927, **38**, 418–31.

**Chambers, M. R., Andres, K. H., Duering, M. V., & Iggo, A.** The structure and function of slowly adapting type II mechanoreceptors in hairy skin. *Quarterly Journal of Experimental Physiology*, 1972, **57**, 417–45.

**Chambers, M. R., & Iggo, A.** Slowly adapting cutaneous mechanoreceptors. *Journal of Physiology*, 1967, **192**, 26–27.

**Cohen, L. H., & Lindley, S. B.** Studies in vibratory sensibility. *American Journal of Psychology*, 1938, **51**, 44–63.

**Collins, W. F., Nulsen, F. E., & Randt, C. T.** Relation of peripheral nerve fiber size and sensation in man. *Archives of Neurology*, 1960, **3**, 381–85.

**Collins, W. F., Nulsen, F. E., & Shealy, C. N.** Electrophysiological studies of peripheral and central pathways conducting pain. In R. S. Knighton & P. R. Dumke (Eds.), *Pain*. Boston: Little, Brown, 1966, Pp. 33–45.

**Cosh, J. A.** Studies on the nature of vibration sense. *Clinical Science*, 1953, **12**, 131–50.

**Craig, J. C.** Vibrotactile spatial summation. *Perception & Psychophysics*, 1968, **4**, 351–54.

**Dallenbach, K. M.** Pain: History and present status. *American Journal of Psychology*, 1939, **52**, 331–47.

**Donaldson, H. H.** On the temperature sense. *Mind*, 1885, **10**, 399–416.

**Edes, B., & Dallenbach, K. M.** The adaptation of pain aroused by cold. *American Journal of Psychology*, 1936, **48**, 307–15.

**Eijkman, E. G. J.** Adaptation of the senses of temperature and touch. Unpublished doctoral dissertation, University of Nijmegen, The Netherlands, 1959.

**Eijkman, E. G. J., & Vendrik, A. J. H.** Dynamics of the vibration sense at low frequency. *Journal of the Acoustical Society of America*, 1960, **32**, 1134–39.

**Eskildsen, P., Morris, A., Collins, C. C., & Bach-y-Rita, P.** Simultaneous and successive cutaneous two-point thresholds for vibration. *Psychonomic Science*, 1969, **14**, 146–47.

**Fletcher, H., & Munson, W. A.** Loudness, its definition, measurement, and calculation. *Journal of the Acoustical Society of America*, 1933, **5**, 82–108.

**Franzén, O.** On summation: A psychophysical study of the tactual sense. In *Quarterly Progress and Status Report*. Speech Transmission Laboratory, Royal Institute of Technology, Stockholm, Sweden, January 15, 1966. Pp. 14–25.

**Frey, M. von.** Beiträge zur Physiologie des Schmerzsinnes. *Akademie der Wissenschaften Leipzig. Mathematisch-Naturwissenschaftlich Klasse Berichte*, 1894, **46**, 185–96.

**Frey, M. von.** Beiträge zur Sinnesphysiologie der Haut: III. *Akademie der Wissenschaften Leipzig. Mathematisch-Naturwissenschaftlich Klasse Berichte*, 1895, **47**, 166–84.

**Frey, M. von.** Untersuchungen über die Sinnesfunktionen der menschlichen Haut: Druckempfindung und Schmerz. *Abhandlungen der Sächsischen Akademie der Wissenschaften Leipzig,* 1896, **23,** 175–266. (a)

**Frey, M. von.** Beiträge zur Sinnesphysiologie der Haut: IV. *Akademie der Wissenschaften Leipzig. Mathematisch-Naturwissenschaftlich Klasse Berichte,* 1896, **48,** 462–68. (b)

**Frey, M. von, & Goldman, A.** Der zeitliche Verlauf der Einstellung bei den Druckempfindungen. *Zeitschrift für Biologie,* 1915, **65,** 183–202.

**Frey, M. von, & Kiesow, F.** Über die Function der Tastkörperchen. *Zeitschrift für Psychologie,* 1899, **20,** 126–63.

**Frey, M. von, & Metzner, R.** Die Raumschwelle der Haut bei Successivreizung. *Zeitschrift für Psychologie,* 1902, **29,** 161. Cited by C. E. Sherrick, Studies of apparent tactual movement. In D. R. Kenshalo (Ed.), *The skin senses.* Springfield, Ill.: Charles C Thomas, 1968. Pp. 331–44.

**Gagge, A. P., & Stevens, J. C.** Thermal sensitivity and comfort. In D. R. Kenshalo (Ed.), *The skin senses.* Springfield, Ill.: Charles C Thomas, 1968. Pp. 345–67. Figure 16–7, p. 359, Courtesy of Charles C Thomas, Publisher, Springfield, Illinois.

**Gault, R. H.** Touch as a substitute for hearing in the interpretation and control of speech. *Archives of Otolaryngology,* 1926, **3,** 121–35.

**Geldard, F. A.** Adventures in tactile literacy. *American Psychologist,* 1957, **12,** 115–24.

**Geldard, F. A.** Some neglected possibilities of communication. *Science,* 1960, **131,** 1583–88.

**Geldard, F. A.** Cutaneous channels of communication. In W. A. Rosenblith (Ed.), *Sensory communication.* New York: Wiley, 1961. Pp. 73–87.

**Geldard, F. A.** *Virginia cutaneous project, 1948–1962.* Final Report to the Office of Naval Research, Psychological Laboratory, University of Virginia, Charlottesville, Va., 1962.

**Geldard, F. A.** Cutaneous coding of optical signals: The optohapt. *Perception & Psychophysics,* 1966, **1,** 377–81.

**Geldard, F. A.** Pattern perception by the skin. In D. R. Kenshalo (Ed.), *The skin senses.* Springfield, Ill.: Charles C Thomas, 1968. Pp. 304–21.

**Geldard, F. A., & Sherrick, C. E.** Multiple cutaneous stimulation: The discrimination of vibratory patterns. *Journal of the Acoustical Society of America,* 1965, **37,** 797–801.

**Geldard, F. A., & Sherrick, C. E.** The cutaneous "Rabbit": A perceptual illusion. *Science,* 1972, **178,** 178–79.

**Gerard, R. W.** The physiology of pain: Abnormal neuron states in causalgia and related phenomena. *Anesthesiology,* 1951, **12,** 1–13.

**Gertz, E.** Psychophysische Untersuchungen über die Adaptation im Gebiet der Temperatursinne und über ihren Einfluss auf die Reiz- und Unterschiedsschwellen. *Zeitschrift für Sinnesphysiologie,* 1921, **52,** 1–51, 105–56.

**Gescheider, G. A.** Resolving of successive clicks by the ears and skin. *Journal of Experimental Psychology,* 1966, **71,** 378–81.

**Gescheider, G. A.** Auditory and cutaneous temporal resolution of successive brief stimuli. *Journal of Experimental Psychology,* 1967, **75,** 570–72.

**Gibson, R. H.** Requirements for the use of electrical stimulation of the skin. In L. L. Clark (Ed.), *Proceedings of the International Congress on Technology and Blindness.* Vol. II. New York: American Foundation for the Blind, 1963. Pp. 183–207.

**Gibson, R. H.** Electrical stimulation of pain and touch. In D. R. Kenshalo (Ed.), *The skin senses.* Springfield, Ill.: Charles C Thomas, 1968. Pp. 223–61.

**Gilmer, B. von H.** The measurement of the sensitivity of the skin to mechanical vibration. *Journal of General Psychology,* 1935, **13,** 42–61.

**Gilmer, B. von H.** The relation of cold sensitivity to sweat duct distribution and the neurovascular mechanisms of the skin. *Journal of Psychology,* 1942, **13,** 307–25.

**Gnudi, M. T., & Webster, J. P.** *The life and times of Gaspara Tagliacozzi, surgeon of Bologna, 1545–1599.* New York: H. Reichner, 1950.

**Goff, G. D.** Differential discrimination of frequency of cutaneous mechanical vibration. *Journal of Experimental Psychology,* 1967, **74,** 294–99. Figure 3, p. 297, Copyright © 1967 by the American Psychological Association, and reproduced by permission.

**Goldscheider, A.** Die spezifische Energie der Temperaturnerven. *Monatshefte für praktische Dermatologie,* 1884, **3,** 198–208.

**Goldscheider, A.** Neue Thatsachen über die Hautsinnesnerven. *Archiv für Physiologie,* 1885, Suppl. Bd., 1–110.

**Gray, J. A. B., & Sato, M. J.** Properties of the receptor potential in Pacinian corpuscles. *Journal of Physiology,* 1953, **122,** 610–36.

**Greene, L. C., & Hardy, J. D.** Spatial summation of pain. *Journal of Applied Physiology,* 1958, **13,** 457–64.

**Greene, L. C., & Hardy, J. D.** Adaptation of thermal pain in the skin. *Journal of Applied Physiology,* 1962, **17,** 693–96.

**Grindley, G. C.** The variation of sensory thresholds with the rate of application of the stimulus: I. The differential threshold for pressure. *British Journal of Psychology,* 1936, **27,** 86–95. (a)

**Grindley, G. C.** The variation of sensory thresholds with the rate of application of the stimulus: II. Touch and pain. *British Journal of Psychology,* 1936, **27,** 189–95. (b)

**Hahn, J. F.** Vibrotactile adaptation and recovery measured by two methods. *Journal of Experimental Psychology,* 1966, **71,** 655–58.

**Hardy, J. D.** The nature of pain. *Journal of Chronic Diseases,* 1956, **4,** 22–51.

**Hardy, J. D.** The pain threshold and the nature of pain sensation. In C. A. Keele & R. Smith (Eds.), *International symposium on assessment of pain in man and animals.* Edinburgh: Livingstone, 1962. Pp. 170–201.

**Hardy, J. D., & Oppel, T. W.** Studies in temperature sensation: III. The sensitivity of the body to heat and spatial summation of the end-organ responses. *Journal of Clinical Investigation,* 1937, **16,** 533–40.

**Hardy, J. D., & Stolwijk, J. A. J.** Tissue temperature and thermal pain. In A.S.V. deReuck & J. Knight (Eds.), *CIBA Foundation symposium on touch, heat, and pain.* London: Churchill, 1966. Pp. 27–56.

**Hardy, J. D., Wolff, H. G., & Goodell, H.** Studies on pain: Discrimination of differences in intensity of a pain stimulus as a basis of pain intensity. *Journal of Clinical Investigation,* 1947, **26,** 1152–58.

**Hardy, J. D., Wolff, H. G., & Goodell, H.** Studies on pain: An investigation of some quantitative aspects of the dol scale of pain intensity. *Journal of Clinical Investigation,* 1948, **27,** 380–86.

**Hardy, J. D., Wolff, H. G., & Goodell, H.** *Pain sensations and reactions.* Baltimore: Williams & Wilkins, 1952.

**Harrington, T., & Merzenich, M. M.** Neural coding in the sense of touch. *Experimental Brain Research,* 1970, **10,** 251–64.

**Head, H.** *Studies in neurology.* London: Keegan Paul, 1920.

**Hebb, D. O.** *The organization of behavior.* New York: Wiley, 1949.

**Heinbecker, P., Bishop, G. H., & O'Leary, J.** Pain and touch fibers in peripheral nerves. *Archives of Neurology and Psychiatry,* 1933, **29,** 771–89.

**Hellman, R., & Zwislocki, J.** Monaural loudness function at 1000 cps and interaural summation. *Journal of the Acoustical Society of America,* 1963, **35,** 856–65.

**Hensel, H.** Temperaturempfindung und intracutane Wärmebewegung. *Pflügers Archiv,* 1950, **252,** 165–215.

**Hensel, H.** Physiologie der Thermoreception. *Ergebnisse der Physiologie,* 1952, **47,** 166–368.

**Hensel, H., Ström, L., & Zotterman, Y.** Electrophysiological measurements of depth of thermoreceptors. *Journal of Neurophysiology,* 1951, **14,** 423–39.

**Hensel, H., & Witt, I.** Spatial temperature gradient and thermoreceptor stimulation. *Journal of Physiology,* 1959, **148,** 180–87.

**Hensel, H., & Zotterman, Y.** Action potentials of cold fibers and intracutaneous temperature gradient. *Journal of Neurophysiology,* 1951, **14,** 377–85.

**Herget, C. M., & Hardy, J. D.** Spatial summation of heat. *American Journal of Physiology,* 1942, **135,** 426–29.

**Holm, K. G.** Die Dauer der Temperaturempfindung bei konstanter Reiztemperatur. *Skandinavishes Archiv für Physiologie,* 1903, **14,** 242–58.

**Holway, A. H., & Crozier, W. J.** The significance of area for differential sensitivity in somesthetic pressure. *Psychological Record,* 1937, **1,** 178–84.

**Hugony, A.** Über die Empfindung von Schwingungen mittels des Tastsinnes. *Zeitschrift für Biologie,* 1935, **96,** 548–53.

**Jenkins, W. L.** Studies in thermal sensitivity: 4. Minor contributions. *Journal of Experimental Psychology,* 1938, **22,** 178–85.

**Jenkins, W. L.** Somesthesis. In S. S. Stevens (Ed.), *Handbook of experimental psychology.* New York: Wiley, 1951. Pp. 1172–90.

**Jenkins, W. L., & Karr, A. C.** Paradoxical warmth: A sufficient condition for its arousal. *American Journal of Psychology,* 1957, **70,** 640–41.

**Kenshalo, D. R.** Improved method for the psychophysical study of the temperature sense. *Review of Scientific Instruments,* 1963, **34,** 883–86.

**Kenshalo, D. R., Decker, T., & Hamilton, A.** Spatial summation on the forehead, forearm, and back produced by radiant and conducted heat. *Journal of Comparative and Physiological Psychology,* 1967, **63,** 510–15.

**Kenshalo, D. R., & Gallegos, E. S.** Multiple temperature-sensitive spots innervated by single nerve fibers. *Science,* 1967, **158,** 1064–65.

**Kenshalo, D. R., Holmes, C. E., & Wood, P. B.** Warm and cool thresholds as a function of rate of stimulus temperature change. *Perception & Psychophysics,* 1968, **3,** 81–84. Figure 1, p. 83, reproduced by permission.

**Kenshalo, D. R., & Nafe, J. P.** A quantitative theory of feeling: 1960. *Psychological Review,* 1962, **69,** 17–33.

**Kenshalo, D. R., Nafe, J. P., & Brooks, B.** Variations in thermal sensitivity. *Science,* 1961, **134,** 104–5. Figure 1, p. 104, Copyright © 1961 by the American Association for the Advancement of Science, and reproduced by permission.

**Kenshalo, D. R., & Scott, H. A., Jr.** Temporal course of thermal adaptation. *Science,* 1966, **151,** 1095–96. Figure 1, p. 1095, Copyright © 1966 by the American Association for the Advancement of Science, and reproduced by permission.

**Kietzmann, O.** Zur Lehre vom Vibrationsinn. *Zeitschrift für Psychologie,* 1927, **101,** 377–422.

**Knudsen, V. O.** "Hearing" with the sense of touch. *Journal of General Psychology,* 1928, **1,** 320–52.

**Korte, A.** Kinematoskopische Untersuchungen. *Zeitschrift für Psychologie,* 1915, **72,** 193–296.

**Lele, P. P.** Relationship between cutaneous thermal thresholds, skin temperature and cross-sectional area of the stimulus. *Journal of Physiology,* 1954, **126,** 191–205.

**Lewis, G. P.** Active polypeptides derived from plasma proteins. *Physiological Reviews,* 1960, **40,** 647–76.

**Lewis, G. P.** Pharmacological actions of bradykinin and its role in physiological and pathological reactions. *Annals of the New York Academy of Sciences,* 1963, **104,** 236–49.

**Lewis, T.** *Pain.* New York: Macmillan, 1942.

**Lewis, T., & Pochin, E. E.** The double pain response of the human skin to a single stimulus. *Clinical Science,* 1937, **3,** 67–76.

**Lim, R. K. S.** Cutaneous and visceral pain, and somesthetic chemoreceptors. In D. R. Kenshalo (Ed.), *The skin senses.* Springfield, Ill.: Charles C Thomas, 1968. Pp. 458–64.

**Lindblom, U., & Tapper, D. N.** Terminal properties of a vibrotactile sensor. *Experimental Neurology,* 1967, **17,** 1–15.

**Linvill, J. G., & Bliss, J. C.** A direct translation reading aid for the blind. *IEEE Proceedings,* 1966, **54,** 40–51.

**Livingston, W. K.** *Pain mechanisms.* New York: Macmillan, 1943.

**Loewenstein, W. R.** On the "specificity" of a sensory receptor. *Journal of Neurophysiology,* 1961, **24,** 150–58.

**Loewenstein, W. R., & Skalak, R.** Mechanical transmission in a Pacinian corpuscle: An analysis and a theory. *Journal of Physiology,* 1966, **182,** 346–78.

**Mark, V. H., Ervin, F. R., & Yakovlev, P. I.** Stereotactic thalamotomy: III. The verification of anatomical lesion sites in the human thalamus. *Archives of Neurology,* 1963, **8,** 528–38.

**Mark, V. H., & Yakovlev, P. I.** A note on problems and methods in preparation of a human stereotactic atlas: Including a report of measurements of posteromedial portion of the ventral nucleus of the thalamus. *Anatomical Record,* 1955, **121,** 745–52.

**Marks, L. E., & Stevens, J. C.** Perceived warmth and skin temperature as functions of the duration and level of thermal irradiation. *Perception & Psychophysics,* 1968, **4,** 220–28.

**Meissner, G.** Untersuchungen über den Tastsinn. *Zeitschrift für rationelle Medicin,* 1859, **7,** 92–119.

**Melzack, R., & Casey, K. L.** Sensory, motivational, and central control determinants of pain. In D. R. Kenshalo (Ed.), *The skin senses.* Springfield, Ill.: Charles C Thomas, 1968. Pp. 423–43.

**Melzack, R., & Wall, P. D.** On the nature of cutaneous sensory mechanisms. *Brain,* 1962, **85,** 331–56.

**Melzack, R., & Wall, P. D.** Pain mechanisms: A new theory. *Science,* 1965, **150,** 971–79.

**Merzenich, M. M., & Harrington, T.** The sense of flutter-vibration evoked by stimulation of the hairy skin of primates: Comparison of human sensory capacity with the responses of mechanoreceptive afferents innervating the hairy skin of monkeys. *Experimental Brain Research,* 1969, **9,** 236–60.

**Mountcastle, V. B.** Some functional properties of the somatic afferent system. In W. A. Rosenblith (Ed.), *Sensory communication.* New York: Wiley, 1961. Pp. 403–36.

**Mountcastle, V. B.** Pain and temperature sensibilities. In V. B. Mountcastle (Ed.), *Medical physiology.* Vol. II. (12th ed.) St. Louis: C. V. Mosby, 1968. Pp. 1424–64.

**Mountcastle, V. B., LaMotte, R. H., & Carli, G.** Detection thresholds for stimuli in humans and monkeys: Comparison with threshold events in mechanoreceptive afferent nerve fibers innervating the monkey hand. *Journal of Neurophysiology,* 1972, **35,** 122–36.

**Müller, J.** *Handbuch der Physiologie des Menschen.* Vol. 2. Book V. Coblenz, 1838.

**Nafe, J. P.** The psychology of felt experience. *American Journal of Psychology,* 1927, **39**, 367–89.

**Nafe, J. P.** The pressure, pain and temperature senses. In C. A. Murchison (Ed.), *A handbook of general experimental psychology.* Worcester, Mass.: Clark University Press, 1934. Pp. 1037–87.

**Nafe, J. P., & Kenshalo, D. R.** Stimulation and neural response. *American Journal of Psychology,* 1958, **71,** 199–208.

**Nafe, J. P., & Wagoner, K. S.** The nature of pressure adaptation. *Journal of General Psychology,* 1941, **25,** 323–51.

**Neff, W. S.** A critical investigation of the visual apprehension of movement. *American Journal of Psychology,* 1936, **48,** 1–42.

**Neisser, U.** Temperature thresholds for cutaneous pain. *Journal of Applied Physiology,* 1959, **14,** 368–72.

**Noordenbos, W.** *Pain: Problems pertaining to the transmission of nerve impulses which give rise to pain.* Amsterdam: Elsevier, 1959.

**Pickett, J. M., & Pickett, B. H.** Communication of speech sounds by a tactual vocoder. *Journal of Speech & Hearing Research,* 1963, **6,** 207–22.

**Rhodin, J. A. G.** Fine structure of vascular walls in mammals. In L. Eichna (Ed.), *Symposium on vascular smooth muscle (Physiological Reviews Supplement*), 1962, **5,** 48–87.

**Rogers, R.** Apparent tactual movement: An experimental study. Unpublished senior thesis, Princeton University, 1964.

**Rosenthal, S. R.** Histamine as the chemical mediator for referred pain. In D. R. Kenshalo (Ed.), *The skin senses.* Springfield, Ill.: Charles C Thomas, 1968. Pp. 480–98.

**Sato, M.** Response of Pacinian corpuscles to sinusoidal vibration. *Journal of Physiology,* 1961, **159,** 391–409.

**Schwartz, H. G., & O'Leary, J. L.** Section of the spinothalamic tract at the level of the inferior olive. *Archives of Neurology and Psychiatry,* 1942, **47,** 293–304.

**Sherrick, C. E.** Variables affecting sensitivity of the human skin to mechanical vibration. *Journal of Experimental Psychology,* 1953, **45,** 273–82.

**Sherrick, C. E.** Final report on N.S.F. Project No. G-3366. Psychological Laboratory, University of Virginia, 1959.

**Sherrick, C. E.** Observations relating to some common psychophysical functions as applied to the skin. In G. R. Hawkes (Ed.), *Symposium on cutaneous sensitivity.* Ft. Knox, Ky.: U.S. Army Medical Research Laboratory, 1960. Pp. 147–58.

**Sherrick, C. E.** Studies of apparent tactual movement. In D. R. Kenshalo (Ed.), *The skin senses.* Springfield, Ill.: Charles C Thomas, 1968. Pp. 331–44.

**Sinclair, D. C.** The remote reference of pain aroused in the skin. *Brain,* 1949, **72,** 364–72.

**Sinclair, D. C.** Cutaneous sensation and the doctrine of specific energy. *Brain,* 1955, **78,** 584–614.

**Sinclair, D. C.** *Cutaneous sensation.* London: Oxford University Press, 1967.

**Sinclair, D. C., & Stokes, B. A. R.** The production and characteristics of "second pain". *Brain,* 1964, **87,** 609–18.

**Sternbach, R. A.** *Pain: A psychophysiological analysis.* New York: Academic Press, 1968.

**Stevens, J. C., & Marks, L. E.** Apparent warmth as a function of thermal irradiation. *Perception & Psychophysics,* 1967, **2,** 613–19.

**Stevens, J. C., Marks, L. E., & Gagge, A. P.** The quantitative assessment of thermal discomfort. *Environmental Research,* 1969, **2,** 149–65.

**Stevens, J. C., & Stevens, S. S.** Warmth and cold: Dynamics of sensory intensity. *Journal of Experimental Psychology,* 1960, **60,** 183–92.

**Stevens, S. S.** On the psychophysical law. *Psychological Review,* 1957, **64,** 153–81.

**Stevens, S. S.** Tactile vibration: Dynamics of sensory intensity. *Journal of Experimental Psychology,* 1959, **57,** 210–18.

**Stevens, S. S.** The psychophysics of sensory function. *American Scientist,* 1960, **48,** 226–53.

**Stevens, S. S.** The psychophysics of sensory function. In W. A. Rosenblith (Ed.), *Sensory communication.* New York: Wiley, 1961. Pp. 1–33.

**Stevens, S. S.** Tactile vibration: Change of exponent with frequency. *Perception & Psychophysics,* 1968, **3,** 223–28.

**Stoll, A. M., & Greene, L. C.** Relationship between pain and tissue damage due to thermal radiation. *Journal of Applied Psychology,* 1959, **14,** 373–82.

**Stone, L. J., & Dallenbach, K. M.** Adaptation to the pain of radiant heat. *American Journal of Psychology,* 1934, **46,** 229–42.

**Strauss, H. H., & Uhlmann, R. F.** Adaptation to superficial pain. *American Journal of Psychology,* 1919, **30,** 422–24.

**Strughold, H., & Karbe, M.** Die Topographie des Kältesinnes auf Cornea und Conjunctiva. *Zeitschrift für Biologie,* 1925, **83,** 189–200.

**Sumby, W. H.** An experimental study of vibrotactile apparent motion. Unpublished master's thesis, University of Virginia, 1955.

**Swartz, P.** A new method for scaling pain. *Journal of Experimental Psychology,* 1953, **45,** 288–93.

**Sweet, W. H.** Pain. In J. Field (Ed.), *Handbook of physiology:* Section 1. *Neurophysiology.* Vol. 1. Baltimore: Williams & Wilkins, 1959, Pp. 459–506.

**Talbot, W. H., Darian-Smith, I., Kornhuber, H. H., & Mountcastle, V. B.** The sense of flutter-vibration: Comparison of the human capacity with response patterns of mechanoreceptive afferents from the monkey hand. *Journal of Neurophysiology,* 1968, **31,** 301–34.

**Tapper, D. N.** Stimulus-response relationships in the cutaneous slowly-adapting mechanoreceptor in hairy skin of the cat. *Experimental Neurology,* 1965, **13,** 364–85.

**Vendrik, A. J. H., & Vos, J. J.** Comparison of the stimulation of the warmth sense organ by microwave and infrared. *Journal of Applied Physiology,* 1958, **13,** 435–44.

**Verrillo, R. T.** Investigation of some parameters of the cutaneous threshold for vibration. *Journal of the Acoustical Society of America,* 1962, **34,** 1768–73.

**Verrillo, R. T.** Effect of contactor area on the vibrotactile threshold. *Journal of the Acoustical Society of America,* 1963, **35,** 1962–66. Figures 6, p. 1964, and 7, p. 1965, reproduced by permission of the American Institute of Physics and the author.

**Verrillo, R. T.** Temporal summation in vibrotactile sensitivity. *Journal of the Acoustical Society of America,* 1965, **37,** 843–46. (a) Figure 4, p. 846, reproduced by permission of the American Institute of Physics and the author.

**Verrillo, R. T.** The effect of number of pulses on vibrotactile thresholds. *Psychonomic Science,* 1965, **3,** 73–74. (b)

**Verrillo, R. T.** Vibrotactile threshold and pulse polarity. *Psychonomic Science,* 1965, **3,** 171. (c)

**Verrillo, R. T.** Effect of spatial parameters on the vibrotactile threshold. *Journal of Experimental Psychology,* 1966, **71,** 570–75. (a)

**Verrillo, R. T.** Vibrotactile sensitivity and the frequency response of Pacinian corpuscles. *Psychonomic Science,* 1966, **4,** 135–36. (b)

**Verrillo, R. T.** Taction thresholds for short pulses. *Psychonomic Science,* 1966, **4,** 409–10. (c)

**Verrillo, R. T.** Specificity of a cutaneous receptor. *Perception & Psychophysics,* 1966, **1,** 149–53. (d)

**Verrillo, R. T.** Vibrotactile thresholds for hairy skin. *Journal of Experimental Psychology,* 1966, **72,** 47–50. (e)

**Verrillo, R. T.** The role of the Ruffini ending in vibrotaction. Paper presented at the meeting of the Eastern Psychological Association, Boston, 1967.

**Verrillo, R. T.** A duplex mechanism of mechanoreception. In D. R. Kenshalo (Ed.), *The skin senses.* Springfield, Ill.: Charles C Thomas, 1968. Pp. 139–59.

**Verrillo, R. T.** Vibrotactile intensity scaling at several body sites. In F. A. Geldard (Ed.), *Cutaneous communication systems and devices.* Austin, Tex.: The Psychonomic Society, 1974. Pp. 9–14.

**Verrillo, R. T., & Chamberlain, S. C.** The effect of neural density and contractor surround on vibrotactile sensation magnitude. *Perception & Psychophysics,* 1972, **11,** 117–20.

**Verrillo, R. T., Fraioli, A. J., & Smith, R. L.** Sensation magnitude of vibrotactile stimuli. *Perception & Psychophysics,* 1969, **6,** 366–72. Figures 8 and 10, p. 371, reproduced by permission.

**Volkmann, A. W.** Von der specifischen Reizbarkeit der Nerven. In R. Wagner (Ed.), *Handwörterbuch der Physiologie,* 1844, **2,** 521–26.

**Wall, P. D.** Repetitive discharge of neurons. *Journal of Neurophysiology,* 1959, **22,** 305–20.

**Wall, P. D.** Cord cells responding to touch, damage, and temperature of the skin. *Journal of Neurophysiology,* 1960, **23,** 197–210.

**Wall, P. D., & Sweet, W. H.** Temporary abolition of pain in man. *Science,* 1967, **155,** 108–9.

**Weber, E.** Über den Tastsinn. *Archiv für Anatomie, Physiologie und Wissenschaftliche Medicin,* 1835, 152. Cited by S. Weinstein, Intensive and extensive aspects of tactile sensitivity as a function of body part, sex, and laterality. In D. R. Kenshalo (Ed.), *The skin senses.* Springfield, Ill.: Charles C Thomas, 1968. Pp. 195–222.

**Weber, E.** Der Tastsinn und das Gemeingefühl. In R. Wagner (Ed.), *Handwörterbuch der Physiologie,* 1846, **3,** 481–588.

**Weddell, G.** Somesthesis and the chemical senses. *Annual Review of Psychology,* 1955, **6,** 119–36.

**Weddell, G.** Referred pain in relation to the mechanism of common sensibility. *Proceedings of the Royal Society of Medicine, London,* 1957, **50,** 581–86.

**Weddell, G., & Sinclair, D. C.** The anatomy of pain sensibility. *Acta Neurovegetativa,* 1953, **7,** 135–46.

**Weddell, G., & Verrillo, R. T.** Common sensibility. In M. Critchley, J. L. O'Leary, & B. Jennett (Eds.), *Scientific foundations of neurology.* Philadelphia: F. A. Davis, 1972. Pp. 117–25.

**Wedell, C. H., & Cummings, S. B.** Fatigue of the vibratory sense. *Journal of Experimental Psychology,* 1938, **22,** 429–38.

**Weinstein, S.** Intensive and extensive aspects of tactile sensitivity as a function of body part, sex, and laterality. In D. R. Kenshalo (Ed.), *The skin senses.* Springfield, Ill.: Charles C Thomas, 1968. Pp. 195–222.

**Wells, E. F., & Hoisington, L. B.** Pain adaptation: A contribution to the von Frey–Goldscheider controversy. *Journal of General Psychology,* 1931, **5,** 352–67.

**White, B. W.** Perceptual findings with the vision-substitution system. *IEEE Transactions. Man-Machine Systems,* 1969, **MMS-11,** 54–58.

**Wilska, A.** On the vibrational sensitivity in different regions of the body surface. *Acta Physiologica Scandinavica,* 1954, **31,** 285–89.

**Woodworth, R. S., & Schlosberg, H.** *Experimental psychology.* (Rev. ed.) New York: Holt, Rinehart & Winston, 1954.

**Woolard, H. H., Weddell, G., & Harpman, J. A.** Observations on the neurohistological basis of cutaneous pain. *Journal of Anatomy, London,* 1940, **74,** 413–40.

**Zigler, M. J.** Pressure adaptation time: A function of intensity and extensity. *American Journal of Psychology,* 1932, **44,** 709–20.

**Zotterman, Y.** Thermal sensations. In J. Field (Ed.), *Handbook of physiology:* Section 1. *Neurophysiology.* Vol. 1. Baltimore: Williams & Wilkins, 1959. Pp. 431–58.

**Zwislocki, J.** Theory of temporal auditory summation. *Journal of the Acoustical Society of America,* 1960, **32,** 1046–60.

**Zwislocki, J. J.** On intensity characteristics of sensory receptors: A generalized function. *Kybernetik,* 1973, **12,** 169–83.

# OLFACTION AND TASTE

# 6

**Thomas S. Brown**
**DePaul University**

Olfaction and taste are generally classified as chemical senses in that a stimulus molecule must excite a receptor cell for a sensation to occur. They are considered more primitive than the auditory and visual systems because they presumably evolved earlier. While hard to demonstrate an earlier evolution, support for this position comes by way of analogy. All cells within an organism communicate with each other by means of molecules. Communication comes about when a molecule from one cell acts on the membrane of another cell. The membrane itself is a layer of specifically arranged molecules, phospholipides for the most part. The molecular stimulus initiates its action by binding itself onto a presumed *receptor molecule*, forming a complex of two molecules. The nature of the complex is determined by the stereochemical configurations of both molecules, and by their other physicochemical properties. This broad picture of cellular interaction may, in a general way, be applied to any chemical reaction.

Our chemical senses are probably the result of many years of evolutionary processes that began with the first molecular interaction. Although little or no direct evidence is available, some indirect data suggest the early evolutionary appearance of chemical detector systems. Organisms as primitive and simple as certain bacteria, for example, seem to have a chemical sense since they show chemotactic behavior. Motile bacteria, such as *Escherichia coli,* are attracted to chemicals like sucrose, galactose, and lysine independently of metabolic need (Adler, 1969). Hence, such varieties of *E. coli* represent an early stage in the development of chemical sensory systems.

Dastoli and Price (1966) succeeded in extracting a sweet-sensitive protein molecule from bovine taste buds. This protein forms complexes with sugars and other sweet-tasting substances. Price and Hogan (1969) extended this work and suggested the possibility that this protein, or sweet receptor molecule, evolved from an enzyme.

These reports have two far-reaching implications for understanding the chemical senses. First, they imply a rather early evolutionary development. Second, they suggest that the way an olfactory or taste stimulus affects a receptor cell may become known by research in pharmacology, endocrinology, or any discipline that focuses on how molecules affect membranes. An olfactory or gustatory stimulus may very well act on the receptor cell membrane in the same way that a drug affects a cell or a hormone excites a target organ.

## *OLFACTION*

> A smell is a sensation we perceive when odorous molecules impinge on sensitive nerve endings in our noses. There are three important things about smells. The first is that the nose is the most sensitive chemical detector known; at its best, its threshold of perception is more than one hundred times lower than the best of our gas chromatographs. Secondly, smell sensations are highly specific: most of us can easily distinguish cigarette smoke from cigar smoke or a rose perfume from a violet scent, but an experienced perfumer can do much better, so that, for example, there are men who can not only name the country of origin of a sample of lavender oil, but can even name the farm from which it came. The third important thing is the emotional impact of a smell [Wright, 1966a, p. 551].

This quote from Wright succinctly summarizes the field of olfaction and this chapter takes up his three major points concerning sensitivity, discriminability, and emotionality.

## THE OLFACTORY STIMULUS

Olfaction is initiated by the interaction of odorous molecules and the epithelium containing the receptor cells. The interaction involves both *adsorption* and *desorption*. Adsorption, a process whereby gases or solutes are held to the surface of a solid, refers to the formation of a complex between an odorous molecule and the cell membrane; desorption refers to the separation or breakdown of this complex. These processes take place at the interface between the epithelial layer and the receptor cells. During respiration odorous molecules are continuously brought to and removed from this interface by the air currents in the nasal passages.

The mucous secretion covering the epithelium, called *mucus,* is viscous and colloidal and is an ideal medium for the adsorption and transport of molecules (Beets, 1970). An odorous molecule is adsorbed from the mucus onto the surface membrane of the receptor cell. The degree of affinity between the molecule and the receptor site determines how long the molecule and cell are in contact. The molecule then returns, or is released into the mucus to return, ultimately to the air.

During the period of adsorption, olfactory stimulation occurs. The receptor cell is excited, presumably becomes depolarized, and a nerve impulse passes along its axon (see Chapter 3). The afferent pattern of information then begins to flow toward the brain.

### Properties of odorous molecules

The frequency range of human hearing is from approximately 20 Hz to 20 kHz. The visible spectrum extends from 400 nm to 700 nm. For the chemical senses we do not know the exact physical continuum on which to place the perceivable stimuli. In olfaction, however, *molecular weight* appears to be a meaningful continuum on which to specify the range of adequate stimuli.[1] Humans are not able to detect olfactory stimuli below a molecular weight of about 30 or above about 300. The upper limit is related to the volatility of the substance. Except for the halogens, which are corrosive, most substances of low molecular weight are odorless. Among the hydrocarbons, methane is almost odorless, and compounds such as water and carbonic acid are entirely odorless. Generally, for compounds with low molecular weights, the heavier the molecule the stronger the odor. Also, a number of compounds of low molecular weight—for example, ammonia and formaldehyde—tend to be irritants or evoke activity in the trigeminal nerve.

An interesting relationship exists between the upper limits of olfactory perception and the incidence of *anosmia,* the loss of the sense of smell. The molecules most frequently associated with anosmia are those of the musk family and amber substances. These molecules have weights between 235 and 260, which are close to the normal upper limit. All anosmias tend to be close to this limit (Stoll, 1957).

Molecular weight, however, is only one of a number of factors that apparently contribute to olfactory perception. The majority of odorous substances are compounds of carbon, hydrogen, oxygen, nitrogen, or sulphur. Strongly odorous, but less frequent, are the phosphorous and arsenic compounds. Among the relatively few odorous elements are oxygen, nitrogen, and sulphur.

The shape of the molecule currently appears to be the most important property in smell. Molecular form or some associated factor is likely to be a major determinant of perceived olfactory quality.

[1]The molecular weight of a compound is the sum of the atomic weights of all the atoms in the molecular formula. The *mole* is the molecular weight of a substance expressed in grams. The *molar solution (M)* contains 1 mole of solute per liter of solution.

Its possible role is discussed in the following section.

The adsorption-desorption processes are to some extent statistical in nature. All molecules of a given compound are alike, yet they will be adsorbed onto the receptor cell in a variety of orientations. The relative degree of randomness of the adsorbed patterns depends on factors such as degree of rigidity of the molecule. Molecular rigidity is increased by double bonds between atoms and by circular or ring patterns in the overall shape of the molecule. Generally, more rigid molecules elicit more intense odors.

Although there is general agreement that the odorous molecule must contact the receptor cell, there is little agreement, and thus many theories, as to the exact mechanism by which the molecule stimulates the cell. Several of the current hypotheses will now be considered. One, the stereochemical theory, is considered in more detail than the others simply because more data pertain to it. The earlier theories, and earlier versions of current theories, have been reviewed by Jones and Jones (1953).

## Theories of olfactory stimulation

### *Stereochemical theory*

The theory as initially proposed by Amoore (1952) postulates that the odor of a chemical compound can be correlated with the physical fit of its molecules into certain "sites" on the membrane surface of the receptor cell. Molecules of the same shape fit into the same receptor sites and evoke identical or highly similar odors. Amoore tested this theory by determining correlations between molecular configuration and judgments of perceived similarity by human subjects. As part of this theory, Amoore proposed seven primary olfactory qualities: *ethereal, camphoraceous, musky, floral, minty, pungent,* and *putrid*. For each class Amoore selected a standard odorant given in Table 6.1. To determine the perceived similarity Amoore had a panel of subjects compare unknown odorants to each of the seven known standards. Similarity was rated on an eight-point scale from 0 (not similar) to 8 (extremely similar). All odorants were initially matched for subjective intensity to a standard solution of musk containing one part of musk per million of water.

The molecular configurations of the standards and the presumed membrane sites for five of the proposed qualities appear in Figure 6.1. The qualities of pungent and putrid are not based on molecular shape but rather on the electric charge on the molecule. The molecular silhouettes of each unknown odorant were compared with the corresponding silhouettes of the standard odorants. Similarity was assessed by comparing the corresponding length of radii at every ten degrees of arc around all three views of the molecules. The measure for similarity of shape is $(1/\bar{\Delta}) + 1$, where $\bar{\Delta}$ is the average value of the absolute difference in length between the corresponding radii of the two compounds. Amoore and Venstrom (1967) pre-

**Table 6.1 Primary Odor Standards**

| Code | Primary odor | Standard compound | Solubility in water[a] (ppm[b]) | Odor threshold (ppm[b]) | Matched concentration (ppm[b]) | Ratio: matched/ threshold |
|---|---|---|---|---|---|---|
| A | Ethereal | 1,2-Dichloroethane | 6900 | 29 | 800 | 28 |
| B | Camphoraceous | 1,8-Cineole | 3800 | 0.012 | 10 | 830 |
| C | Musky | 15-Hydroxypentadecanoic acid lactone | 1.1[c] | 0.0007 | 1[d] | 1430 |
| D | Floral | *d,l*-β-Phenylethylmethylethyl carbinol | 1200[c] | 6.4 | 300 | 47 |
| E | Minty | *d,l*-Menthone | 780 | 0.17 | 6 | 35 |
| F | Pungent | Formic acid (90%) | ∞ | 1500 | 50,000 | 33 |
| G | Putrid | Dimethyl disulfide | 2800[c] | 0.0012 | 0.1 | 83 |

[a]At 20–25°C; literature values except where indicated.
[b]Parts per million of water; concentrations are volume/volume, except for the musk, which is weight/volume.
[c]Observed approximately in this work.
[d]Warm the water to about 40°C to melt the musk, then shake vigorously to dissolve.

(From Amoore & Venstrom, 1966.)

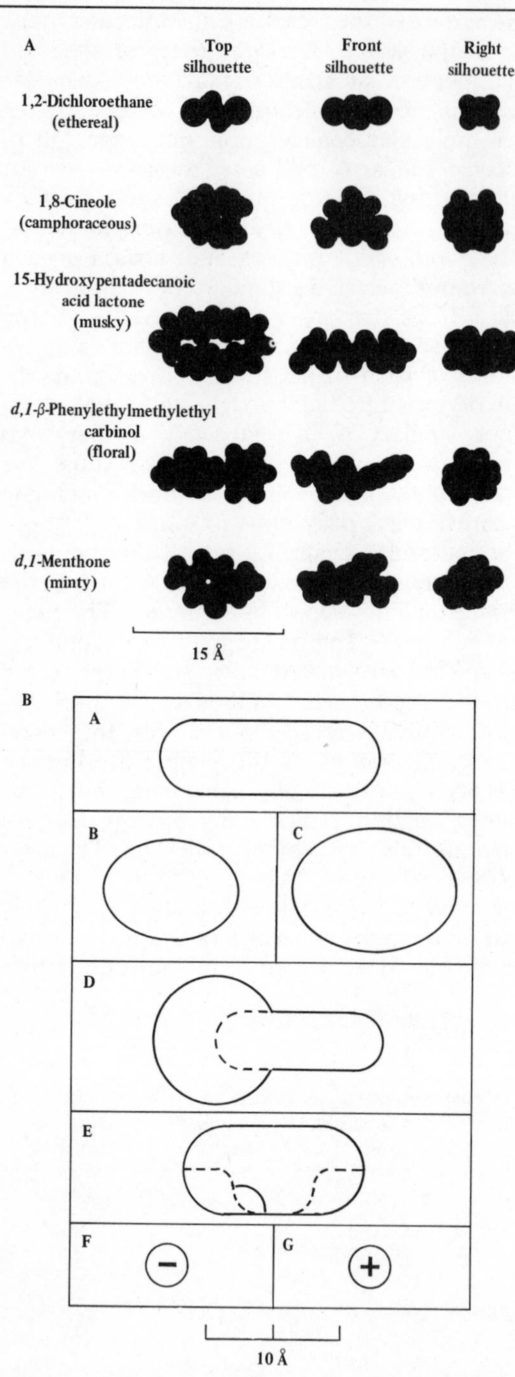


**Figure 6.1** Panel A: Molecular model silhouettes of the five standard odorants. (From Amoore & Venstrom, 1967.) Panel B: The presumed human olfactory receptor sites corresponding to the seven primary odors. A, ethereal; B, camphoraceous; C, musky; D, floral; E, minty; F, pungent; G, putrid. (From Amoore, 1952.)

sented the results of similarity judgments and shape similarity for 107 compounds. Table 6.2 contains the data for the standard odorants and a somewhat random selection of other odorants from their list of 107. The molecular similarity data for the pungent and putrid standards are not presented because their molecular shape is not related to olfactory quality. The standards were also presented as unknown odorants so that the subject would experience maximum similarity. The scores of judged similarity when the standards and unknowns were the same appear in parentheses. Thus, 1,2-Dichlorethane, the standard for the ethereal class, received an average similarity rating of 6.25. A score of 6.0 was considered as very similar, 4.0 was judged as moderately similar, and 2.0 was judged as slightly similar (Amoore & Venstrom, 1966). The nonstandard compounds were put into two sets. The compounds in one subset were judged highly similar to one of the standards and also had a similar molecular shape. An example from this subset is *d,l*-Camphor. The compounds in the second subset were either like phenylacetic acid and were not very similar to any of the standards, or they were like isopulegol and were judged similar to one standard but had a molecular shape like that of another.

The correlation coefficients that Amoore and Venstrom (1967) report for each class are 0.516 for minty, 0.543 for floral, 0.621 for musky, 0.599 for camphoraceous, and 0.660 for ethereal, based on an $n$ of 106 compounds. All are highly significant ($p < 10^{-9}$) and indicate a positive and rather strong relation between molecular configuration (size and shape) and odor. That the correlations are not perfect is to be expected when one considers the arbitrariness of the approach—for example, selection of the primary qualities, selection of the standards for each quality, the rating scale method for the similarity judgments, the silhouette of the molecule rather than some other property. Improvements in methodology should push the correlations closer to 1.00.

More recently, Amoore (1967, 1969) sharpened the relationship of olfactory quality and molecular configuration by the intense study of *specific anosmia*. This little-known phenomenon occurs when persons having a generally good sense of smell lack the ability to perceive the odor of a certain substance. For example, one individual in a thousand does not notice the butyl mercaptan odor of the skunk (Patterson & Lauder, 1948).

Amoore (1967) studied specific anosmia for isobutyric acid. He first determined threshold con-

**le 6.2 Organoleptic Analyses and Stereochemical Assessments. The first five compounds are the standard odorants for the ethereal (ETH), camphoraceous (CAM), musky (MUS), floral (FLO), and minty (MIN) classes. The other classes are pungent (PUN) and putrid (PUT). The second five compounds are examples of high similarity scores and shape correlations. The last six compounds have low similarity scores or mismatches between odor and shape.**

| Compound | Matched concentration (ppm) | Similarity of odor to standards | | | | | | | Similarity of shape to standards | | | | |
|---|---|---|---|---|---|---|---|---|---|---|---|---|---|
| | | ETH | CAM | MUS | FLO | MIN | PUN | PUT | ETH | CAM | MUS | FLO | MIN |
| ,2-Dichlorethane | 800 | (6.25) | 1.09 | 0.54 | 0.87 | 1.09 | 0.30 | 0.08 | (1.0) | 0.484 | 0.398 | 0.463 | 0.484 |
| ,8-Cineole | 10 | 0.82 | (5.23) | 1.00 | 1.21 | 2.25 | 0.18 | 0.06 | 0.484 | (1.0) | 0.503 | 0.534 | 0.628 |
| 15-Hydroxypentadecanoic acid lactone | 1, w/v | 0.52 | 0.77 | (5.66) | 2.27 | 1.11 | 0.22 | 0.03 | 0.397 | 0.500 | (1.0) | 0.559 | 0.546 |
| d,l-B-Phenylethylmethylethyl carbinol | 300 | 0.43 | 1.23 | 1.63 | (6.32) | 1.53 | 0.09 | 0.04 | 0.463 | 0.531 | 0.553 | (1.0) | 0.593 |
| d,l-Menthone | 6 | 0.61 | 1.23 | 0.61 | 1.82 | (6.60) | 0.16 | 0.00 | 0.484 | 0.628 | 0.546 | 0.593 | (1.0) |
| Acetone | 30,000 | 4.42 | 1.04 | 0.63 | 0.70 | 1.83 | 0.37 | 0.27 | 0.687 | 0.460 | 0.378 | 0.429 | 0.453 |
| d,l-Camphor | 40, w/v | 1.60 | 5.42 | 1.29 | 0.90 | 2.27 | 0.32 | 0.18 | 0.469 | 0.662 | 0.466 | 0.488 | 0.558 |
| Cyclopentadecanone | 2.5 w/v | 0.35 | 0.42 | 5.46 | 2.52 | 0.96 | 0.12 | 0.14 | 0.411 | 0.527 | 0.793 | 0.588 | 0.579 |
| Geraniol | 40 | 0.88 | 1.80 | 2.18 | 4.38 | 2.08 | 0.28 | 0.04 | 0.466 | 0.529 | 0.509 | 0.633 | 0.558 |
| -Carvone | 25 | 0.82 | 1.78 | 0.81 | 2.10 | 4.60 | 0.13 | 0.17 | 0.514 | 0.586 | 0.524 | 0.599 | 0.664 |
| Benzonitrile | 8 | 1.14 | 2.54 | 1.32 | 2.16 | 1.35 | 0.09 | 0.26 | 0.640 | 0.506 | 0.431 | 0.478 | 0.509 |
| Coumarin | 100 w/v | 0.89 | 1.87 | 1.96 | 2.36 | 1.47 | 0.17 | 0.17 | 0.586 | 0.507 | 0.483 | 0.511 | 0.542 |
| sopulegol | 17 | 0.61 | 1.20 | 0.48 | 4.18 | 2.11 | 0.21 | 0.17 | 0.499 | 0.632 | 0.583 | 0.603 | 0.764 |
| l-Limonene | 5,000 | 0.98 | 1.34 | 0.95 | 3.22 | 1.92 | 0.20 | 0.00 | 0.495 | 0.619 | 0.505 | 0.581 | 0.634 |
| Phenylacetic acid | 150, w/v | 0.75 | 0.96 | 1.98 | 1.75 | 1.05 | 1.08 | 0.98 | 0.565 | 0.575 | 0.488 | 0.575 | 0.587 |
| Salicylaldehyde | 10 | 1.82 | 2.07 | 0.97 | 0.85 | 1.55 | 0.53 | 0.83 | 0.618 | 0.517 | 0.453 | 0.487 | 0.520 |

(After Amoore & Venstrom, 1967.)

centrations for a large number of individuals. Each subject was presented with five flasks, two of which contained highly purified, undiluted acid and the other three an odorless liquid. The subject's task was to distinguish the odorous from the odorless flasks. The acids were diluted to one-half the concentration on each succeeding trial until the subject could no longer distinguish the odor. Thus measured, the mean threshold for 97 normal subjects was 16.8 binary dilution steps. A specific anosmic was arbitrarily defined as an individual whose sensitivity was at least 3 binary dilution steps below the normal mean. By this criterion, 10 persons were classified as specifically anosmic to isobutyric acid, with a mean threshold of 11.2 dilution steps. The threshold for a different odorous substance, isobutyl isobutyrate, was then determined for both groups. The group mean thresholds differed by only 1.2 steps.

Threshold measurements were also made with compounds chosen to assess the relative importance of molecular size, molecular shape, and functional groups. Molecular size was examined by measuring thresholds with a series of normal aliphatic carboxylic acids containing from one to ten carbon atoms. The largest effects were from those compounds having from four to seven carbon atoms, as shown in Figure 6.2. *Structural isomers* of valeric acid (which has five carbon atoms) were investigated next. Isomers are compounds composed of the same number and kinds of atoms but in different arrangements. The branched-chain isovaleric acid gave the greatest difference in dilution steps between the specific anosmics and the controls. This was slightly larger than the difference for isobutyric acid. Changing the *functional group,* the group of atoms causing the characteristic behavior of the compound, significantly reduced the threshold differences between the anosmic and the control subjects. These are the data points in Figure 6.2 marked aldehyde, alcohol, and ester. These experiments led Amoore to accept the hypothesis of Guillot (1948) that each type of specific anosmia may be caused by a defect in the corresponding primary odor detector. Amoore (1967) views isovaleric acid as a primary odor, and the corresponding primary olfactory quality is *sweaty*. The odor detector for this primary is specialized to react to the carboxylic acid group and, though sensitive to normal acids having from

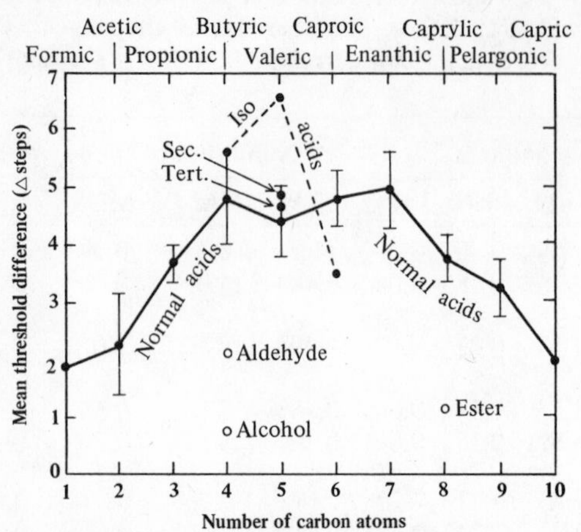


**Figure 6.2** Specific anosmia to a series of carboxylic acids. Mean threshold differences in binary dilution steps is shown between control and specific anosmic subjects. The normal acid series is shown as a solid line (the vertical line through each point indicates its standard error). Isomeric forms for butyric, valeric, and caproic acids are shown as a dotted line. The largest mean difference was for isovaleric acid ($\Delta = 6.6$ steps). The alcohol, aldehyde, and ester data points are for isobutyl derivatives. (From Amoore, 1967.)

one to ten carbon atoms, it is tuned more to molecules of from four to seven carbons. It has a distinct preference for certain branched-chain acids—for example, isovaleric. Amoore considers this the first experimental demonstration of a primary odor, and it is interesting that this primary was not in his original classification of olfactory qualities. Amoore (1967) proposed that there may be as many as twenty to thirty primaries based on the reported types of specific anosmia. He suggested that each instance of specific anosmia be systematically investigated, as he has done for butyric acid anosmia. Research of this kind would certainly provide much needed data concerning the relationship between molecular structure and olfactory quality. One cautionary consideration is that specific anosmics are only relatively anosmic. They can detect the given odor, but only at higher intensities than most other people.

### *Penetration and puncturing theory*

This theory (Davies, 1962, 1965, 1969, 1971) proposes that olfactory stimulation occurs when a sharp hole in the receptor cell membrane is made by one or several adsorbed odorous molecules. The hole could be made when the molecules desorb from the lipide membrane of the cell or when the molecules diffuse through the membrane and thus penetrate the cell. Through this hole, potassium and sodium ions may interchange momentarily. A nerve impulse is initiated if sufficient time elapses before the membrane flows back to its undisturbed position. The time it takes for the hole to close depends on a number of physical variables, such as surface pressure, rigidity, and viscosity of the lipide film. Once the hole has closed, the cell is ready to initiate another impulse. This theory requires only that the odorous molecule make a hole large enough to allow ionic transfer to occur for a period long enough to stimulate the cell.

Although there is little direct evidence for this theory, Davies (1962) presented some data that indirectly support it. (On the other hand, Cherry, Dodd, and Chapman, 1970, presented some negative evidence.) The first line of support comes from *hemolysis,* in which the membrane of the red blood cell ruptures, releasing hemoglobin. Odorous molecules have weak hemolytic properties, but they do act as accelerators for hemolysis by saponin, a water soluble glucoside and commonly used hemolysin (Davies & Taylor, 1954). The odorous molecules weaken the membrane, thus facilitating the penetration by saponin. By analogy, those odorous molecules with the greatest accelerating power should have the lowest olfactory thresholds because they can more easily puncture the receptor cell membrane. Such correspondence has been reported (Davies & Taylor, 1954). Whereas this theory accounts for intensity functions by the molecule's ability to penetrate the cell, it explains olfactory qualities by a combination of membrane and molecule properties. Davies (1965) assumes that the nerve membranes vary with respect to their resistance to puncturing by molecules of odorous substances and to the speed, depending on their fluidity, with which they close the hole. The odorous molecules differ in their capability to penetrate; factors such as the cross-sectional area of the molecule are important here.

### *Other theories*

*Pigment theory.* This theory, advanced by Rosenberg, Misra, and Switzer (1968), postulates that the pigments in the cell membranes of the olfactory receptors constitute the receptor sites. The odorous molecule forms a weakly bound complex with the pigment molecule, thereby increasing the conductivity of the membrane and depolarizing the cell which initiates a nerve impulse. Stimulus threshold and intensity functions are determined by the nature of the complexes that are formed. Olfactory quality depends on the strength of the complex and the type of pigment at the various receptor sites. Although no psychological and physiological data are yet available, this theory does postulate a precise mechanism and thus is testable. The interested reader may want to consult Moulton's (1971) review of the composition, location, and possible functional role of the olfactory pigment.

*Molecular vibration theory.* A molecule vibrates in various ways whenever energy is applied to it, as when molecules collide. Wright (1966b) proposes that the vibratory motion of the molecule determines olfactory quality. He presents this theory as a refinement of or a complement to Amoore's stereochemical theory. For example, molecules of toluene and benzaldehyde have closely similar shapes but very different odors. They are highly correlated (with regard to molecular shape) and so should fit the same receptor site and have similar odors. The difference in their odors could be accounted for by the differences in the vibration frequency of the molecules. Adding the dimension of vibratory motion to those of molecular shape or profile may permit better predictions of perceived olfactory quality.

All the theories discussed are alike in assuming that the odorous molecule comes into contact with the receptor cell mosaic. The theories differ with respect to just how the molecule and receptor cell interact. The diversity of opinion clearly indicates that a real understanding of olfactory transduction is yet to come. Present theories stress molecular shape as the key property of the olfactory stimulus. However, in addition to determining how the key fits the lock, we must also discover how the key turns the lock. Both questions remain unanswered.

## Classification of olfactory qualities

Although systems for classifying the primary olfactory qualities are usually associated with Zwaardemaker (1895) and Henning (1916a), many others before and after them have also developed such systems. Linnaeus, the great Swedish botanist, seems to have proposed the first system in 1752. He developed it to describe the odors of plants. He suggested seven classes: *aromatic* (carnation), *fragrant* (lily), *ambrosial* (musky), *alliaceous* (garlic), *hircine* (valerian), *repulsive* (certain insects), and *nauseous* (carrion). Between the time of Linnaeus and Zwaardemaker, at least eight other attempts were made to classify the olfactory qualities (see Boring, 1942). Zwaardemaker accepted the system of Linnaeus and added two new classes, *ethereal* (fruity) and *empyreumatic* (burnt). Zwaardemaker's total, including many subclasses, was about thirty.

Table 6.3 presents a number of schemata, including those of Zwaardemaker and Henning. Included also are the reports of incidences of specific anosmia collated by Amoore. As mentioned earlier, Amoore (1969) proposed that specific anosmia reflects an absence of an ability to detect one of the primary qualities. Presumably this deficit is related to the absence of a receptor site for that primary. Based on the number and kinds of specific anosmias, Amoore now suspects that there may be as many as twenty to thirty primary qualities, a number coincidentally close to that proposed by Zwaardemaker.

As suggested by Wright (1968), following Hainer, Emslie, and Jacobson (1954), one approach to the question concerning primary olfactory qualities is to ask how many odors can be distinguished. The answer appears to be very large, probably in the millions. Professional perfumers profess that two odorous substances seldom, if ever, smell exactly alike.

Neurons and olfactory receptor cells respond yes or no; that is, nerve impulses are elicited or they are not (see Chapter 3). If there were only one kind of receptor, there would be two types of molecules, those which excite the receptors and those which do not. With two receptors, 4 odors could be detected. With twenty receptors, 1,048,576 odors could be detected. With thirty receptors, 1 billion odor patterns could be discriminated. Thus, it would be possible that a system having from twenty to thirty primary receptors and qualities could account for all possible odors that a human can discriminate.

This approach, of course, gives no information about the type of receptor, whether it be a cell or a molecule. Nor does it specify the relation between the primary odor and the receptor. The effects of stimulus and physiological variables such as intensity and adaptation would have to be incorporated. For now it can be assumed that there are between twenty and thirty primary olfactory qualities. For each quality there may be a specific receptor element.

## Table 6.3 Clues to the Olfactory Code

| | | General Odor Classifications | | | | | | | | | Specific Anosmia Analyses | | | | | |
|---|---|---|---|---|---|---|---|---|---|---|---|---|---|---|---|---|
| LINE NO. | | ZWAARDEMAKER 1895 30 (SUB) CLASSES | LINNAEUS 1756 7 CLASSES | HENNING 1915 6 CLASSES | CROCKER & HENDERSON 1927 4 CLASSES | AMOORE 1952 7 CLASSES | SCHUTZ 1964 9 CLASSES | WRIGHT & MICHELS 1964 8 CLASSES | HARPER ET AL. 1968 44 CLASSES | MISCEL-LANEOUS ADDITIONAL | REPUTED SPECIFIC ANOSMIAS | | | | ESTABLISHED PRIMARY ODORANT | PROBABLE PRIMARY ODOR |
| 1 | | FRUITY | | | | | | HEXYL ACETATE | FRUITY | | γ-UNDECA LACTONE | | | | | |
| 2 | | WAXY | | | | | | | SOAPY | | | | | | | |
| 3 | | ETHEREAL | | | | ETHEREAL | ETHERISH | | ETHERISH; SOLVENT | | ETHYLENE DICHLORIDE | TRICHLORO-ETHYLENE | BENZENE | METHYL-CYCLOPROPYL KETONE | | |
| 4 | | CAMPHOR | | | | CAMPHOR | | | CAMPHOR; MOTHBALLS | | 1.8-CINEOLE | NAPHTHALENE | p-DICHLORO-BENZENE | ADAMANTANE | | |
| 5 | | CLOVE | AROMATIC | | | | | | AROMATIC | | EUGENOL | BENZYL ALCOHOL | ANISOLE | | | |
| 6 | | CINNAMON | | SPICY | | | | SPICE | SPICY | | CINNAM-ALDEHYDE | SALICYL ALDEHYDE | | | | |
| 7 | | ANISEED | | | | | | BENZO-THIAZOLE | | | | | | | | |
| 8 | | MINTY | | | | MINTY | | | MINTY | | MENTHONE | MENTHOL | TERT-BUTYL CARBINOL | | | |
| 9 | | THYME | | | | | | | | | THYMOL | | | | | |
| 10 | | ROSY | | | | | | | | | GERANIOL | PHENYL-ETHANOL | | | | |
| 11 | | CITROUS | | FRUITY | | | | CITRAL | CITROUS | | GERANIAL | | | | | |
| 12 | | ALMOND | | | | | SPICY | | ALMOND | | HYDROGEN CYANIDE | ISOBUTYR-ALDEHYDE | | | | |
| 13 | | JASMINE | | FLOWERY | | FLORAL | | | FLORAL | | PEME CARBINOL | | | | | |
| 14 | | ORANGE-BLOSSOM | FRAGRANT | | FRAGRANT | | FRAGRANT | | FRAGRANT | | | | | | | |
| 15 | | LILY | | | | | | | | | | | | | | |
| 16 | | VIOLET | | | | | | | | | IONONE | FARNESOL | | | | |
| 17 | | VANILLA | | | | | SWEET | | VANILLA; SWEET | | VANILLIN | BENZYL SALICYLATE | ANISIC ALDEHYDE | CYCLOTENE | | |
| 18 | | AMBER | | | | | | | ANIMAL | | | | | | | |
| 19 | | MUSKY | AMBROSIAL | | | MUSKY | | | MUSK | | MACROCYCLIC MUSKS (4) | ANDROSTENOL | MUSK XYLOL | VERSALIDE | | |
| 20 | | LEEK | ALLIACEOUS | | | | | | GARLIC | | ALLYL ISO-THIOCYANATE | PHENYL ISO-THIOCYANATE | ALLICIN | PROPENYL-SULFENIC ACID | | |
| 21 | | FISHY | | | | | | | AMMONIA; FISHY | | HEXYLAMINE | | | | | |
| 22 | | BROMINE | | | | | | | | | IODOFORM | | | | | |
| 23 | | BURNT | | BURNT | BURNT | | BURNT | AFFECTIVE | BURNT | | | | | | | |
| 24 | | PHENOLIC | | | | | | | CARBOLIC | | | | | | | |
| 25 | * | CAPROIC | HIRCINE | | CAPRYLIC | | | | SWEATY | | ISOBUTYRIC ACID | PHENYLACETIC ACID | CAPROIC ACID | | ISOVALERIC ACID | SWEATY |
| 26 | — | CAT-URINE | | | | | | | | | | | | | =25? | — |
| 27 | | NARCOTIC | REPULSIVE | | | | | | | | PHENYL-ISOCYANIDE | | | | | |
| 28 | | BED-BUG | | | | | | | | | | | | | | |
| 29 | | CARRION | NAUSEOUS | | | | | | SICKLY | | PUTRESCINE | | | | | |
| 30 | | FECAL | | | | | | | FECAL | | SKATOLE | INDOLE | | | | |
| 31 | | | | RESINOUS | | | | RESINOUS | RESINOUS; PAINT | | | | | | | |
| 32 | | | | FOUL | | PUTRID | SULFUROUS | UNPLEASANT | PUTRID; SULFUROUS | | MERCAPTANS (3) | DIMETHYL DISULFIDE | THIOPHANE | | | |
| 33 | | | | | ACID | | | | ACID | | FORMIC ACID | ACETIC ACID | | | | |
| 34 | | | | | | | OILY | | OILY | | | | | | | |
| 35 | — | | | | | | RANCID | | RANCID | | | | | | =25? | — |
| 36 | | | | | | | METALLIC | | METALLIC | | | | | | | |
| 37 | | | | | | | | | MEATY | | | | | | | |
| 38 | | | | | | | | | MOLDY | | 2-HEPTANONE | | | | | |
| 39 | | | | | | | | | GRASSY | | | | | | | |
| 40 | | | | | | | | | BLOODY | | | | | | | |
| 41 | | | | | | | | | COOKED-VEGETABLE | | METHIONAL | | | | | |
| 42 | | | | | | | | | | SANDAL | CEDRYL ACETATE | | | | | |
| 43 | | | | | | | | | | WATERY | | | | | | |
| 44 | | | | | | | | | | URINOUS | ANDROSTA-DIENONE | | | | | |
| (NON-OLFACTORY) | | | | | | (PUNGENT) | | (TRIGEMINAL) | (PUNGENT; & 5 OTHERS) | | | | | | | |

(From Amoore, 1969.)

**Stimulus control in olfaction**

The problem of precise stimulus control is a major factor that has retarded experimental investigation of olfaction. Historically, the most noted instrument for this purpose has been Zwaardemaker's *olfactometer,* which permitted a quantification of olfactory stimuli in units he called *olfacties*. One olfactie is the amount of stimulus material that must be exposed to give a barely perceptible odor.

One totally unsuccessful instrument was developed by Komuro (1921). The *camera inodorata* was essentially a large glass box into which the subject placed his head, thereby preventing the inclusion of any background odors. Of course, controls had to be used to eliminate any odor from the subject himself. To insure this, the subject had to shave his head and coat his face with petroleum jelly. Imagine trying to get subjects for that experiment today.

At the other extreme is the *olfactorium,* developed by Foster, Scofield, and Dallenbach (1950), which is a room and antechamber constructed of glass and stainless steel. This construction insures that thorough steam cleaning can be carried out, and the subject wears a plastic parka which can also be thoroughly cleaned. Air is forced into the room after it has passed through appropriate filters, heaters, and washers, at a specified temperature and humidity. The stimuli are delivered by adding known quantities to the airstream. This is essentially a flow-meter olfactometer, and most research conducted with olfactory stimuli today use some variation of it, usually without the olfactorium chamber. For descriptions of typical olfactometers see Cain (1969), Grundvig, Dustman, and Beck (1967), Johnston and Sandoval (1960), Schneider, Costiloe, Vega, and Wolf (1963), Stone and Bosley (1965), and Tucker (1963). Many studies simply use a method whereby the subject holds a stimulus source next to his nose (e.g., a test tube or cotton swab) and inhales. Although this latter procedure is useful for determining relative intensity or quality judgments, it would clearly not be a suitable method for taking threshold measurements.

## OLFACTORY PSYCHOPHYSICS

### Threshold and intensity functions

Boring (1942) mentions that the first determination of the absolute threshold for smell was made by Fischer and Penzoldt (1886), who released a known stimulus amount into a standard chamber and could thereby determine its concentration. Table 6.4 presents some of the reported olfactory thresholds.

Olfactory thresholds, like most other sensory limens, are based on external stimulus measures; the concentration of molecules at the entrance to the nostril can be known, but the concentration or exact number at the receptor epithelium has never been measured. It is estimated that of all the molecules that enter the nose, only 2 percent reach the epithelium. Moreover, since the exact stimulus mechanism is not yet determined, the relative importance of the various molecular properties is not known. For example, applying his puncturing theory Davies (1962) calculated approximate thresholds from two basic parameters. The first is the partition coefficient of a substance between air and a water-oil interface. In simpler terms, this is the ratio of the number of odorous molecules in air to the number in the water-oil liquid (the mucous layer in this instance) at equilibrium. It would determine the number of molecules that collect on the receptor surface. The second parameter is the cross-sectional area of the odorous molecule, which would determine the relative ease with which each molecule punctures the cell membrane.

A number of reports have examined relationships between thresholds and various physicochemical properties of the stimulus. Tucker (1963), recording the electrical responses from small branches of the olfactory nerve of the tortoise, found that variations in ionic strength, pH, or

**Table 6.4 Reported Representative Olfactory Thresholds of Humans**

| Substance | Thresholds Mg/liter of air |
|---|---|
| Artificial musk | .00004 |
| Butyric acid | .009 |
| Carbon tetrachloride | 4.533 |
| Chloroform | 3.300 |
| Ethyl acetate | .686 |
| Ethyl ether | 5.833 |
| Ethyl mercaptan | .046 |
| Methyl salicylate | .100 |
| Propyl mercaptan | .006 |
| Valeric acid | .029 |
| Amyl acetate | .039 |

(After Allison & Katz, 1919.)

osmotic pressure of the stimulus had no effect on the receptor responses. He also found that relative humidity had no effect. The influence of temperature was absent between 20° and 30°C. At lower temperatures, down to 10°C, and at higher temperatures, up to 35°C, the magnitude of the response was a monotonic, slowly decreasing function of temperature. A similar and greater effect of temperature was reported by Grundvig, Dustman, and Beck (1967). Measuring olfactory thresholds, they found that between 15° and 45°C, log threshold is a linear function of temperature; threshold increases with temperature. This rise in threshold was related to increments in the vapor pressure of the stimulating odorant, and was interpreted by the authors as supporting an adsorption-vaporization model of olfaction. As such, the results are in accord with the theoretical position of Davies (1962). Similar effects for temperature have been reported by Bocca and Battiston (1964).

Other studies have examined the change in detection thresholds in series of homologous compounds. These compounds are of the same chemical type, but differ by a fixed increment in certain atoms. Figure 6.3 shows the thresholds for a series of n-aliphatic alcohols obtained from the rat. It indicates that detectability tends to increase logarithmically as the number of carbon atoms in the molecule is increased. Highly similar results were obtained for n-aliphatic acetates (Moulton, 1960) and n-aliphatic acids (Moulton, Ashton, & Eayrs, 1960). Recognition thresholds and magnitude estimations of intensity have also been determined in human subjects for four of the n-aliphatic alcohols: n-propanol (three carbon atoms), n-butanol (four carbons), n-hexanol (six carbons), and n-octanol (eight carbons). Cain (1969) found that threshold concentrations decreased as a function of chain-length. The exponents of the power functions also decreased systematically as molecular chain-length increased, as shown in Figure 6.4.

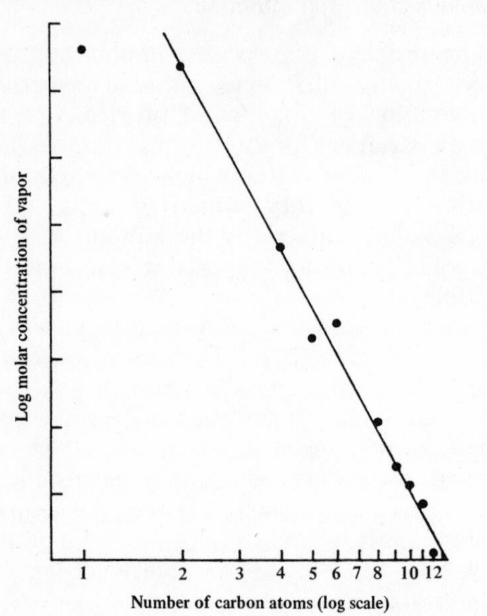


**Figure 6.3** Median threshold concentration of homologous series of alcohols, expressed as log molar concentration of vapor, as a function of the number of carbon atoms in the chain. The aberrant value for methanol (one carbon atom) has been excluded from the computation of the regression line. (From Moulton & Eayrs, 1960.)

### Olfactory adaptation

Adaptation is characteristic of all sensory systems. Prolonged unchanging stimulation results in a decrement of the perceived intensity. Adaptation is generally considered to be fairly rapid for olfactory stimuli. Anecdotal evidence frequently suggests that a person who enters a room containing a noticeable or strong odor soon becomes unaware of the odor. However, few studies have been performed to systematically examine how intensity and duration of exposure affect odor detection. One exception to this is a paper by Berglund, Berglund, Engen, and Lindvall (1971). These authors examined the ability of human subjects to detect a weak odor (hydrogen sulphide) following prior exposure to the same odor which varied in both duration and intensity. The proportion of successful recognitions was lower, the higher the concentration of the adapting stimulus. Thus, there was a clear adaptation effect for the intensity of the adapting stimulus. However, the ability to detect the presence of the test stimulus was independent of the duration of the adaptation period. This independence suggests that the sense of smell is more stable than is usually believed.

Adaptation provided the experimental basis for Zwaardemaker's classification of odors. Two odors from the same class would cause marked fatigue effects on each other, whereas odors from two different classes would have small fatigue effects on each other.

An extensive comparison of adaptation by similar and dissimilar odorant pairs was reported by Moncrieff (1956). Odorants selected with dissimilar odors were acetone, isopropanol, n-butanol, diacetone alcohol, cellosolve, and methanol; each odorant was paired with every other one. Pairs of similar odors were n-butanol and sec-butanol; n-propanol and isopropanol; amyl acetate and butyl acetate; benzaldehyde and nitrobenzene. The stimulus was presented by having the subject take one breath when a 200-ml, wide-neck bottle containing 20 ml of the adapting solution was placed just below the nose. This constituted the adaptation period. The bottle was removed while the subject breathed out. Then another bottle containing the test solution was placed under the nose, and the subject inhaled once more. He reported whether or not he detected the test odorant.

Moncrieff (1956) found that self-adaptation, in which the adapting and test odorants are the same, is much greater than cross-adaptation, in which the adapting and test odorants differ. Very little cross-adaptation occurred, possibly due, in part, to the brief (one breath) adaptation period. However, if cross-adaptation is minimal, then it would appear that the grouping of odors into a small number of primary qualities is virtually impossible. Moncrieff found that only two odorants with very similar odors mutually cause a high degree of adaptation. However, since perceived odor apparently was the only criterion used by Moncrieff in selecting the odorants, this procedure may have minimized the cross-adaptation effects. He also noted an asymmetry in adaptational effects. The effect on odorant B of prior adaptation to odorant A may be different from the effect on A of adaptation to B. This asymmetry has been noted by other investigators (Cain, 1970; Engen, 1963; Engen & Bosack, 1969).

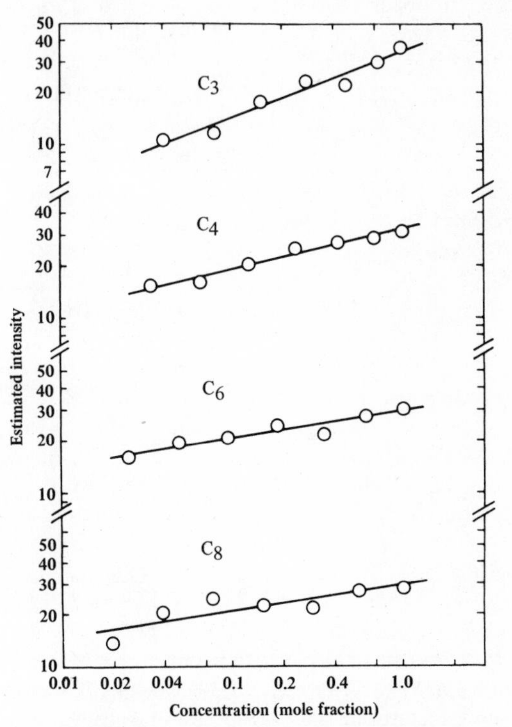


**Figure 6.4** Magnitude estimation as a function of concentration for four aliphatic alcohols: n-propanol ($C_3$), n-butanol ($C_4$), n-hexanol ($C_6$), and n-octanol ($C_8$). The functions were fitted by the method of least squares. (From Cain, 1969.)

Cain and Engen (1969) demonstrated that self-adaptation and cross-adaptation for propanol ($C_3$) and pentanol ($C_5$) cause the psychophysical function to become steeper and generally concave downward in log-log coordinates as shown in Figure 6.5. Cross-adaptation effects for propanol and pentanol were asymmetric. Propanol had a very small effect on pentanol, whereas pentanol had a large effect on propanol. This asymmetry is distinctly visible in Figure 6.5B. It also can be noted that both self-adaptation and cross-adaptation have generally the same effect on the psychophysical functions. This similarity suggests that they may be two aspects of the same effect.

Cain and Engen (1969) have shown that an interpolated standard in the testing procedures alters the exponent of the power law. Figure 6.6 shows psychophysical power functions for amyl acetate with and without the use of a standard. Because the interpolated standard was presented to the subject immediately before each test stimulus, it therefore served not only as a reference point to the subject but also induced some adaptational effects. The steepening of the power function in Figure 6.6 parallels the change in slope of the psychophysical measures for various adaptation conditions given in Figure 6.5.

An important point made by Cain and Engen (1969) is that odorants may differ in their adapting effectiveness because they are not psychophysically equivalent. Odorous substances at equal concentrations almost always differ in subjective intensity. Also, the rate of growth of subjective intensity as a function of concentration differs among odorants. Thus, what may appear to be different adaptation effects could really be differences in their subjective intensity. Cain and Engen (1969) found that the self-adaptation effects of n-propanol

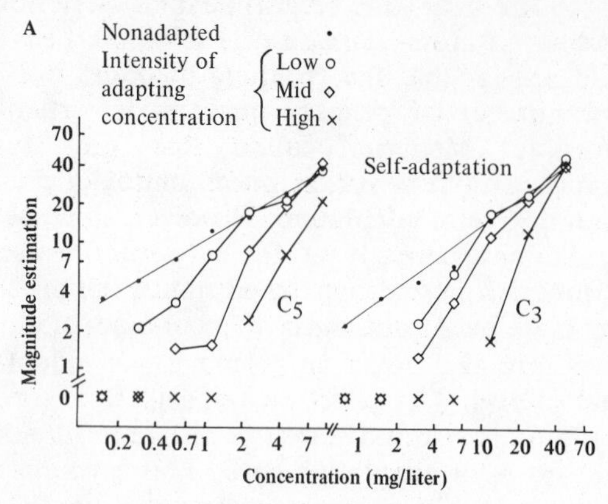


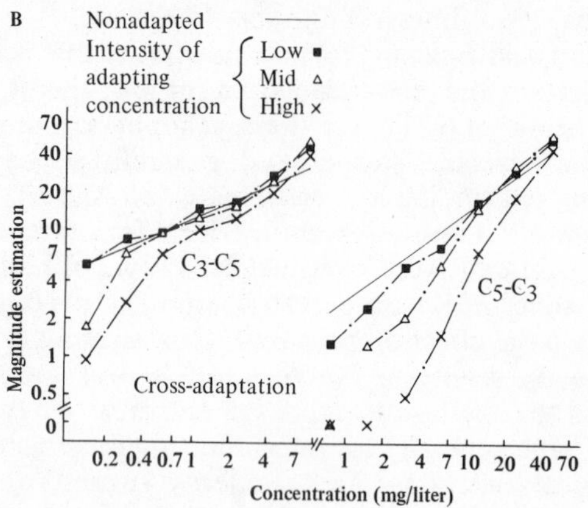


**Figure 6.5** Panel A: Psychophysical functions of pentanol ($C_5$) and propanol ($C_3$) obtained under different levels of self-adaptation. Each adapting concentration was presented for three breaths. The straight lines are the power functions fitted to the magnitude estimations obtained under non-adaptation conditions. Panel B: Psychophysical functions obtained under different levels of cross-adaptation. The straight lines are the power functions fitted in panel A to the magnitude estimations obtained under nonadaptation conditions. (From Cain & Engen, 1969.)

and n-pentanol were identical when their respective concentrations were matched for subjective intensity. The psychophysical functions measured by magnitude estimation were virtually identical. Referring back to Figure 6.5, one can see that without adaptation the exponents of the functions for n-propanol and n-pentanol differ, indicating that their physical differences are psychophysically significant under that condition. It remains to be determined whether or not the similarity of adaptation effects for psychophysically equivalent stimuli applies to all or even large classes of odorants.

The data on cross-adaptation are still extremely limited. Beets (1970) reviewed the earlier work of Le Magnen (1948). When benzonitrile is used as an adapting stimulus, the odor of benzaldehyde is described as safrole-like. An adapting mixture of benzonitrile and safrole renders the odor of benzaldehyde reminiscent of indole. Benzaldehyde is perceived as benzene-like after an adapting mixture of safrole and indole. Similar relations were found in a series of camphoraceous odorants.

## OLFACTORY CUES AND BEHAVIOR: PHEROMONES

Olfactory stimuli are generally associated with moderate to strong emotional experiences. The perfume and deodorant industries recognize and exploit this connection. The allure of the female threads its way through evolution from moth to man. Television brings to our attention that the male, in order to mate successfully, must not be detected with bad breath. This is also true for the moth (Birch, 1970).

In many respects the study of olfactory cues and

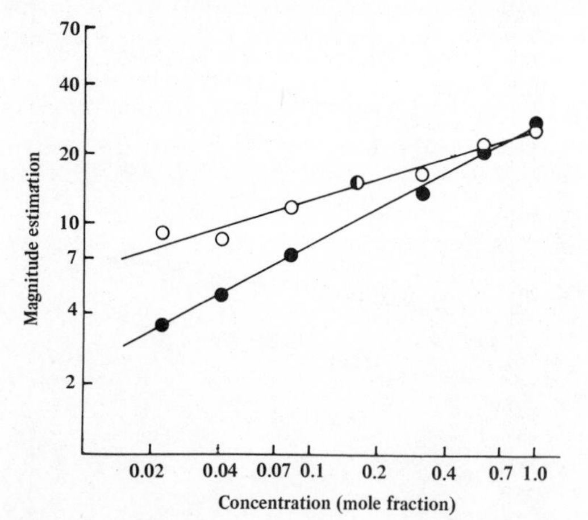


**Figure 6.6** The psychophysical power functions for amyl acetate obtained when the middle concentration was presented only at the beginning of the session (unfilled circles) and when it was presented immediately before each of six test concentrations (filled circles). The half-filled circle represents the judgment of the standard concentration in both conditions. (From Cain & Engen, 1969.)

behavior is the study of the role of *pheromones,* which are substances produced by one individual that convey information to other individuals of the same species (Karlson & Lüscher, 1959). Some pheromones are called *releasers* because they release a specific behavioral response; an example is the female sex attractant. Other pheromones are considered to be *primers* or triggering substances that initiate endocrine or metabolic activities.

The most intensively studied pheromones are those produced by insects, especially the female sex attractants. The olfactory receptors, or *sensilla,* are primarily on the antenna. While olfactory receptors account for the majority of cells, receptors for taste, temperature, humidity, and mechanical stimulation are also located there. For example, the branched part of the giant antenna of the male polyphemus moth (*Tela polyphemus*) bears more than 60,000 sensilla containing 150,000 cells. Between 60 and 70 percent of these cells, nearly 100,000, are specialized receptors for the female sex attractant, 20 percent respond to other odors, and the rest serve other modalities (Schneider, 1969). The female polyphemus moth has no receptors for sex odors, and its antenna shows no neural response to its own attractant.

Other moth species employ both female and male attractants before mating. The female attractants have long-range effects, being carried downwind when released. Generally, but not always, males respond only to attractants from females of their own species. Male moths proceed upwind in search of the female. Upon finding the female, the male releases his own attractant and the female either accepts or rejects the potential mate. Priesner (1969) has shown that the female sex attractants or pheromones are not unique to each species. Closely related species are fully receptive to each other's attractants, which may even be identical. Other factors must be involved in protecting the integrity of a species. Birch (1970) indicated that the male scent is also not unique to each species. For example, three varieties of the wainscot moth (*Levcania impura, L. pallens,* and *L. conigera*) appear to have the same male scent (benzaldehyde/isobutyric acid). All three species are found in the same locality and have similar feeding habits, but each species has different periods of peak activity during the night. The temporal features of behavior contribute toward the maintenance of species differentiation. The concentration of the sex attractant is also a factor in reproductive isolation. Two closely related species of noctuid moths (*Trichoplusia ni* and *Autographa californica*) utilize the same pheromone, Cis-7-dodecenyl acetate, for mating purposes. Females of the *T. ni* species, however, release the pheromone at a higher rate than females of *A. californica*. Traps releasing various amounts of the pheromone attract males of only one of the species depending on the rate of release (Kaae, Shorey, & Gaston, 1973).

Sometimes the sex pheromone's specificity does act as an isolating mechanism in reproduction. The female sex attractant of one species may inhibit the approach response of another closely related and closely existing species (Roelofs & Comeau, 1969).

Pheromones are also important in communication among social insects like bees and ants. Wilson (1965) suggests that pheromones provide the chief channels of communication in insect societies. One example of this is the inhibitory pheromone referred to as the *queen substance*. When the queen is removed from a honey-bee hive, worker bees begin within a few hours to alter one or two worker cells into emergency queen cells from which a new queen will emerge. Also, within two days, some workers begin to have increased ovarian development. Both of these effects are normally inhibited by the presence of the queen substance.

**Pheromones in mammals**

Evidence is growing that pheromones are not restricted to insects and fish, but are also important in many mammalian species, including the primates.

The role of olfactory pheromones is well documented in the reproductive behavior of many rodents, especially mice. This area of research has been reviewed by Whitten and Bronson (1970). The housing of females together in groups brings about a mutual disturbance in their estrous cycles (Lee & Boot, 1955). In small groups of approximately four or fewer members, pseudopregnancies occur. In larger groups containing approximately thirty members, estrous cycles become highly irregular, and many of the females have long anestrous periods. Those effects can be prevented by excision of the olfactory bulbs (Lee & Boot, 1956) and are rapidly reversible when a stud male is introduced into the group (Whitten, 1956). After a male is introduced, the mating tends to become synchronous, with the largest number of matings occurring on the third night. More estrous synchrony occurs if females are housed in groups prior to the introduction of the male than if housed singly. However, if the females are exposed to the males for two days without physical contact, then a higher proportion of copulations occurs on the first night (i.e., the third night after exposure to the male).

This effect appears to be mediated by a substance secreted in the urine of the male, and it affects the female by way of the olfactory receptors. Females that had their olfactory bulbs removed do not show estrous synchrony. Grouped females that are exposed to just male urine for two days prior to pairing show a high degree of estrous synchrony on the first and second nights after the introduction of a male. Other groups of females that are exposed to female urine or receive no treatment exhibit their largest amount of estrous synchrony on the third night after the male has been introduced (Marsden & Bronson, 1964). Exposure to the male urine consisted of placing one drop (0.05 ml) on the general area of the external nares four times a day during the two days prior to pairing. Thus, estrous synchrony seems to depend on the odor of male urine, but unlike the sex attractants in insects the chemical identification has yet to be made. Further support for the olfactory role of the urine was shown by the fact that female mice housed downwind from a cage of male mice exhibited synchrony of estrous cycles, whereas those housed upwind did not (Whitten, Bronson, & Greenstein, 1968).

Olfactory cues can also block pregnancy, an effect first described by Bruce (1959). If a newly mated female is removed from her stud male and exposed to other (strange) males of the same strain as her mate or to males of a different (alien) strain, pregnancy and pseudopregnancies (the expected result of an infertile mating) are usually blocked. Actual contact between the sexes is not necessary. The blocking still occurs if the female is housed inside a box in the cage containing the strange or alien males (Bruce, 1959) or if she is housed on nesting material previously used by alien males (Bruce, 1960). Recently mated females whose olfactory bulbs have been excised do not have the pregnancy block in the presence of strange males (Bruce & Parrott, 1960). The period of susceptibility lasts four days after mating, and the exposure to the males must last about two days (Bruce, 1961). As with the synchrony effect, the pheromone appears to be the urine of the alien male (Dominic, 1964), but its chemical composition is unknown. Application, three times a day, of 0.25 cc of fresh urine from alien males produces an effect identical with that described by Bruce (1961); see also Dominic (1966).

Removal of the olfactory bulbs in various rodent species may affect other behaviors that are generally related to reproduction. For example, the removal of the olfactory bulbs has been reported to eliminate both maternal behavior (Gandelman, Zarrow, Denenberg, & Myers, 1971) and nest building (Zarrow, Gandelman, & Denenberg, 1971) in the mouse. Olfactory bulb removal also eliminates mating behavior in both naïve and experienced male golden hamsters (Murphy & Schneider, 1970). Rats without olfactory bulbs fail to show habituation across test sessions in an open-field measure (Klein & Brown, 1969). This last finding indicates that in addition to being involved in reproductive behaviors, olfactory cues are involved in the processes necessary for habituation of exploratory behavior. Schultz and Tapp (1973), who reviewed the literature concerning the utilization of olfactory cues by rodents, concluded that research efforts should be directed toward analysis of normal behaviors in natural social contexts in order to understand the complex and rich olfactory world of the rodent species.

Michael and Keverne (1968) provided evidence that sexual excitation and activity in male rhesus monkeys are sometimes mediated by a hormone-dependent, olfactory pheromone of vaginal origin. These authors demonstrated that male monkeys will learn to press a bar in order to have access to a female that is recognizably receptive. A male will not work at the bar when the female is not in a receptive state or when his nasal passages are blocked. The cue used by the males is clearly an olfactory pheromone that indicates the endocrine status of the female. In a more recent paper, Michael, Keverne, and Bonsall (1971) isolated the pheromone and demonstrated that short-chain aliphatic acids are responsible for eliciting the sexual behavior of male rhesus monkeys. The presence and importance of such pheromones in human reproductive behavior are not clearly understood, but this finding by Michael et al. should encourage comparative studies.

Nonsexual behavior can also be influenced by pheromones, such as alarm substances, trail substances, and scents used for delineation of territory (see Gleason & Reynierse, 1969). Though not directly related to reproductive behavior, some of these signals (e.g., pheromones for territoriality) do affect behavior during reproduction and rearing of the offspring.

## *TASTE*

The study of taste as a pure sensory system is virtually impossible under normal feeding conditions because at the same time that the taste receptors are stimulated so are tactual receptors for temperature and pressure and so are olfactory receptors. The texture and temperature of foods are part of a complex stimulus array that tells us we are eating graham crackers and not ice cream. In addition, the gustatory system is part of the larger system that regulates all food and water intake. At a still more complex level, consideration must be given to an individual's past history and cultural background and their effect on his food preferences and eating habits.

A distinction will be made between flavor and taste to facilitate the discussion. The distinction is similar to that made in Chapter 1 between perception and sensation. *Flavor* will be used broadly to include all oral sensations such as taste, temperature, texture, and others that occur when food is eaten. *Taste* will refer only to sensations that result from stimulation of the specialized taste receptors. (See Chapter 3 for discussion of the anatomy and physiology of taste receptors.)

## TASTE QUALITIES

Four basic taste qualities are commonly accepted: sweet, salty, bitter, and sour. Henning (1916b) proposed this scheme in his taste tetrahedron, shown in Figure 6.7. This model is the result of his own testing of chemical series and his summarizing of the previous attempts at classifying the taste qualities. For want of a better plan, it has remained the preferred one. The problem here is similar to that in olfaction: The nature of the taste stimulus is unknown.

It is often asserted that the four taste qualities are mediated at different places on the surface of the tongue. Who has not heard or read something like the following passage?

> The tip of the tongue is particularly sensitive to sweet, i.e., the thresholds are lower in this region than in other areas. The base of the tongue is especially sensitive to bitter. The sides show the lowest thresholds for sour. These taste qualities can be evoked by stimulation in other areas but the thresholds are higher. Salt is apparently about as easily sensed in one area as in another [Wenger, Jones, & Jones, 1956, p. 138].

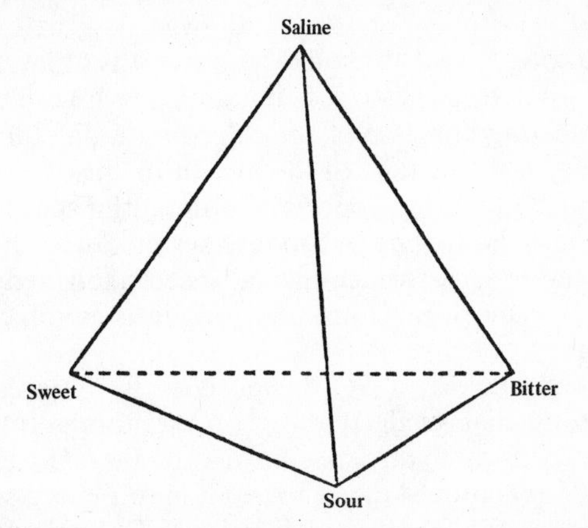


**Figure 6.7** Taste tetrahedron proposed by Henning (1916b). The four principal qualities of taste are shown. Intermediate qualities lie along the edges or on the surfaces.

These general statements came originally from the data of Shore (1892) and were repeated by Hänig (1901).

Taste buds exist, however, not only on the tongue but also on the hard and soft palate, as well as on the epithelial surface of other areas in the oral cavity and in the pharynx. In the human newborn, for example, estimates indicate that over 2500 taste buds are located over the oral and pharyngeal areas, exclusive of the tongue (Lalonde & Eglitis, 1961). It appears that these taste buds are also important in the perception of taste. An anecdotal bit of evidence concerning the role of the palatal region is the frequently noted report of patients who have been fitted with a full upper denture plate that covers and tightly fits against the roof of the mouth. These patients often complain of a loss of taste. Moreover, experiments have shown that their thresholds for sour and bitter are significantly elevated (Henkin & Christiansen, 1967a). In a more extensive investigation, Henkin and Christiansen (1967b) studied the relative roles of the tongue, palate, and pharynx in taste perception. Detection and recognition thresholds for the four basic taste qualities were determined separately before and after the tongue, palate, or both, were anesthetized. These authors reported that detection thresholds for salty and sweet increased by 25-fold after the tongue was anesthetized and were unaffected after the palate was anesthetized. Thresholds for sour and bitter were unaffected when the tongue was anesthetized, but recognition thresholds increased 5-fold after the palate was anesthetized. These results show that sensitivity for salty and sweet is greatest on the tongue, but for sour and bitter it is greatest on the palate. These investigations, while clearly indicating the important role of the palatal and pharyngeal regions of the mouth for taste, do not negate the earlier reports of differential sensitivity on just the tongue. A modern systematic mapping of the tongue surface has not been published, but clearly more than just the tongue is involved in taste.

Von Békésy (1966) reported the interesting finding that single papillae on the human tongue are sensitive to one specific taste quality. He developed techniques that allowed him to place a small droplet of fluid on a single papilla. To avoid adaptation effects, the stimuli were presented only once every 10 minutes. Papillae were stimulated with chemicals normally associated with each of the four basic taste qualities. The quality of the sensation was not changed by increasing the concentration of the solution when a single papilla was stimulated. Extensive mapping of the tongue was not carried out, but data for the tip of the tongue (presumably most sensitive to sweet) indicated that specific papillae for each quality are about equally distributed (see Figure 6.8).

This finding is difficult to integrate with the data related to regional differences within the oral cavity for the various taste qualities. Logically one would expect more sweet-sensitive papillae at the tip of the tongue. This finding is also difficult to reconcile with the neurophysiological finding that individual receptor cells respond to all four basic qualities (Kimura & Beidler, 1961). Stimulation of a single human fungiform papilla would excite several hundred receptor cells. It is unlikely that all of these cells are specific in their response to a single quality. Yet, according to von Békésy, taste perception implies a papilla specificity—that is, each papilla senses one quality and not the others.

Two other experiments failed to find the specificity of the papilla response that von Békésy (1966) reported (Harper, Jay, & Erickson, 1966; McCutcheon & Saunders, 1972). Both studies used suprathreshold stimuli and rather short interstimulus intervals (e.g., 1 minute for McCutcheon & Saunders, 1972). Von Békésy (1966), in addition to using threshold concentrations, noted that at least a 10-minute interval between stimulus presentations is necessary to overcome adaptation effects, with shorter intervals tending to produce unreliable effects. Taken all together, the three studies indicate that, whereas single papillae are specific to single taste qualities at threshold stimulation, the specificity disappears with more intense stimuli.

The results can be summarized as follows: Individual taste receptor cells respond to all four taste qualities, but the fungiform papillae of the human tongue are specific in the taste they mediate at stimulus threshold. There appears to be a random distribution of the various qualities across the tongue, at least at the tip. When larger areas of the tongue are stimulated, regional specificities also appear to exist. The classical report indicates sweet at the tip, bitter at the back, sour at the sides, and salty all over the tongue. A recent extension of this picture is that sweet and salty are most effective when applied to the tongue, and sour and bitter are most effective when applied to the hard and soft palates.

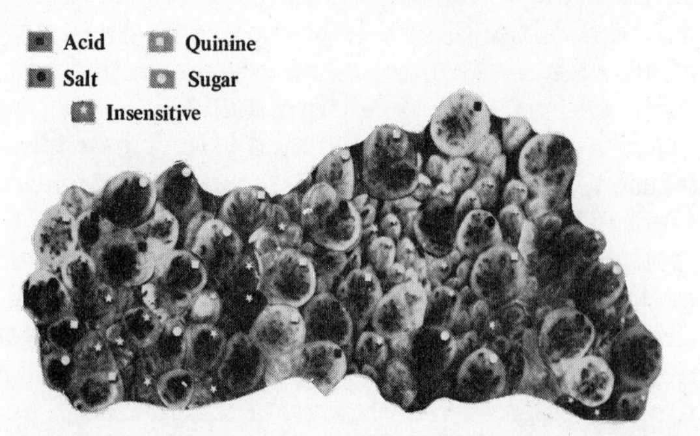


**Figure 6.8** Microphotograph of the surface of the tip of the tongue showing the various taste papillae. The sensation quality of each papilla is shown by the appropriate symbol. (From von Békésy, 1966.)

## THE TASTE STIMULUS

The adequate stimulus for taste is not completely known, but taste sensations are initiated by the molecules that act on the membranes of the receptor cells. The four primary taste qualities can be considered as resulting from the action of different kinds of molecules. For example, sweet-tasting substances, such as the various sugars, have several $CH_2OH$ groups. Common table salt (NaCl) gives a typical salt taste. Salts of low molecular weight *cations* (positively charged ions), such as $Na^+$, $Li^+$, and $NH_4{}^+$, taste salty, whereas cations of high molecular weight, such as $Ca^{++}$ and $Mg^{++}$, taste bitter. Yet the same salt (e.g., potassium chloride) can elicit different tastes at different concentrations. The sour taste seems to be mainly a function of hydrogen ion concentration. Bitter tastes are elicited by alkaloids such as quinine and strychnine, as well as by other substances such as picric acid. Since a number of the alkaloids are toxic, organisms that can readily detect them in their diets have a better chance of survival.

The molecular characteristics on which taste depends are only vaguely understood. Acids tend to be sour, salts are usually salty, and a large number of organic compounds may be bitter or sweet. The relation between chemical structure and perceived sensory quality does not appear to hold for taste as well as it does for olfaction. Moreover, the action of the taste molecules on the cell membrane is virtually unknown. A recent finding, however, does offer a potential clue about this important relationship.

Dastoli and Price (1966) isolated from homogenates of bovine tongue epithelium a protein fraction that forms complexes with sugars. They postulated that this protein is the taste receptor's molecule for sweet compounds and referred to it as the *sweet-sensitive protein*. It was later purified and found to have a molecular weight of about 150,000 (Dastoli, Lopiekes, & Price, 1968). Several specific findings support Dastoli and Price's suggestion that they had isolated a taste-receptor molecule: It is derived from bovine taste buds; the protein has an extraordinary tendency to form complexes with sweet-tasting compounds; the relative strength of the complexes which it forms with sugars parallels the relative sweetness of the sugars.

One hypothesis of taste sensitivity proposes that *thiols* (sulphur-containing compounds) and metals are in dynamic equilibrium in the metabolic net. Thiols normally have an inhibitory role (i.e., they elevate taste thresholds), whereas metal ions lower taste thresholds (Henkin & Bradley, 1969; Henkin, Graziadei, & Bradley, 1969). These authors proposed that conformational changes of the protein molecules lining the pores of the taste bud are regulated by thiols and metals. The conformational changes control the diameter of the taste pores and thereby the ease with which taste molecules affect the receptor cells. The chemical reactions are hypothesized to cause the protein to unfold and decrease taste sensitivity if thiols are increased or metals are decreased; these reactions may cause the protein to refold and return taste sensitivity to normal if thiols are decreased to normal or metals are increased. Through these biochemical steps, taste sensitivity is regulated, but taste quality would depend on the interaction between the molecule and the receptor cell membrane.

## TASTE PERCEPTION

### Intensity

Stevens (1969) reported a number of measurements of taste intensity. The subjective intensity was scaled by the method of magnitude estimation in which observers assign numbers to designate the apparent strength of stimulus concentrations (see Chapter 2). For aqueous solutions of each substance, taste intensity was found to increase as a power function of concentration by weight, as shown in Figure 6.9. Some approximate exponents were sucrose, 1.3; sodium chloride, 1.3; and quinine sulphate, 1.0.

Moskowitz (1970) developed scales for a series of sixteen different sugars. For all sugars except mannose, the intensity of sweetness grows as a power function of concentration with an exponent of about 1.3, thus replicating the data of Stevens (1969).

The afferent taste nerves from the anterior two-thirds of the tongue leave the lingual nerve as a separate strand. This strand is called the *chorda tympani nerve* because it runs through the middle ear close to the tympanic membrane, or eardrum (see Chapter 3). Its location makes it more readily accessible than other sensory nerves, and its responses have been studied on a number of human patients during middle ear surgery. Recording from the human taste nerve affords the opportunity to compare the psychophysical judgment to the neural response to taste stimuli of varying intensities. Borg, Diamant, Ström, and Zotterman (1967) made such a comparison. Two days prior to middle ear surgery, patients made magnitude estimations of the subjective intensities of citric acid, sodium chloride, and sucrose as taste stimuli. The same stimuli and the same random order of presentation were used in the electrophysiological measurements during the surgery. While stimuli were flowed over the tongue of the anesthetized patient, the summated activity evoked in the entire chorda tympani bundle was measured. The mean neural and psychophysical responses to citric acid and sucrose from two patients are plotted on a log-log scale in Figure 6.10.

The close correspondence between these two measures in Figure 6.10 clearly indicates, as Borg et al. note, that the responses reflect a fundamental congruity between the early neural

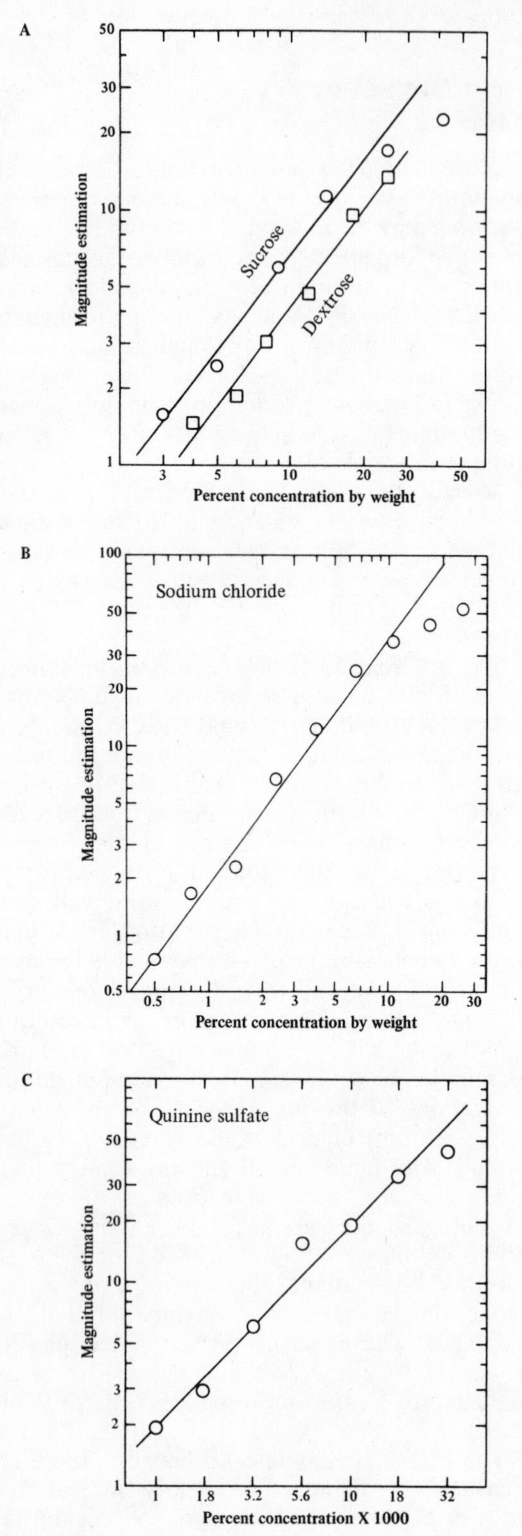


**Figure 6.9** Psychophysical functions for sweetness (A), saltiness (B), and bitterness (C). The sweetness data are the geometric means of fourteen subjects. The vertical displacement of the two lines through the data suggests that sucrose is about 1.5 times as sweet as dextrose. For NaCl, each point is the geometric mean of twenty judgments, two by each of ten subjects. The slope of the line indicates that the exponent of the power function is 1.3. The bitterness function is based on nine subjects and has an exponent of about 1.0. (From Stevens, 1969.)

response and perceptual intensity. Such a congruity implies that the relationship between neural and stimulus intensity is maintained throughout the afferent pathway. Data are not available for the entire pathway of taste for any species, but Doetsch, Ganchrow, Nelson, and Erickson (1969) have shown that such a neural intensity code is transmitted across the synapse where the chorda tympani axons terminate, and the neural response is amplified by a factor of almost five in the process. It appears reasonable from this result and the combined evidence from other sensory systems that some such relation is maintained throughout the system and that it forms the substrate for the psychophysical judgments (see Chapters 1 and 2).

## Intensity-quality interactions

In the previous discussion of intensity discrimination, it was assumed that any taste stimulus evokes the same quality of sensation regardless of

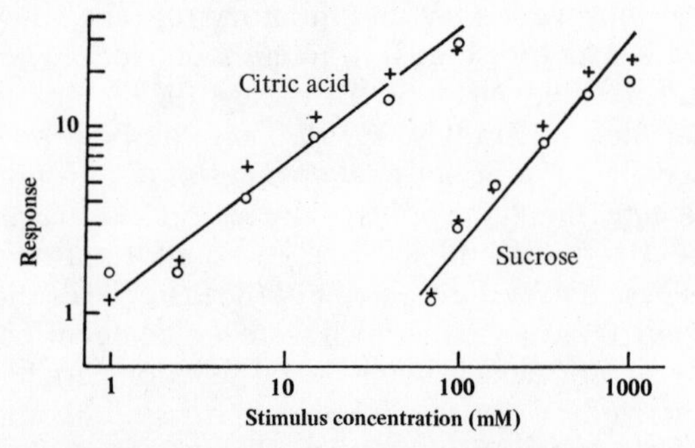


**Figure 6.10** Mean values of neural response (unfilled circles) and of subjective response (crosses) from two patients plotted against molarity of citric acid and sucrose solution. (From Borg, Diamant, Ström, & Zotterman, 1967.)

its intensity. However, changes in stimulus intensity can change the quality of the sensation.

Early workers (e.g., Höber & Kiesow, 1898; Renqvist, 1919) did report changes in taste quality as a function of stimulus strength (cited by Dzendolet & Meiselman, 1967). For example, potassium chloride (KCl) evokes a sweet sensation at low concentrations (0.009 M). With increasing stimulus intensity, sweet gradually gives way first to bitter and finally to salty at a concentration of 0.3 M. Dzendolet and Meiselman (1967) reinvestigated this problem and studied taste quality of lithium chloride (LiCl), lithium sulphate ($Li_2SO_4$), and potassium sulphate ($K_2SO_4$) over a wide range of strengths. Each subject sipped all of a 10-ml solution and held it in his mouth for 3 seconds. He then spit out the solution and reported its quality. Responses were limited to salty, bitter, sour, sweet, and no taste. Figure 6.11 shows the percentage of responses in each category as a function of concentration for lithium chloride and potassium chloride. Both salts were called sweet at the lowest concentrations. As the concentrations increased, the percentage of sweet responses declined and the number of sour responses increased for LiCl, and the number of bitter responses increased for KCl. The responses to KCl progressed from sweet to bitter to salty with increasing stimulus intensity.

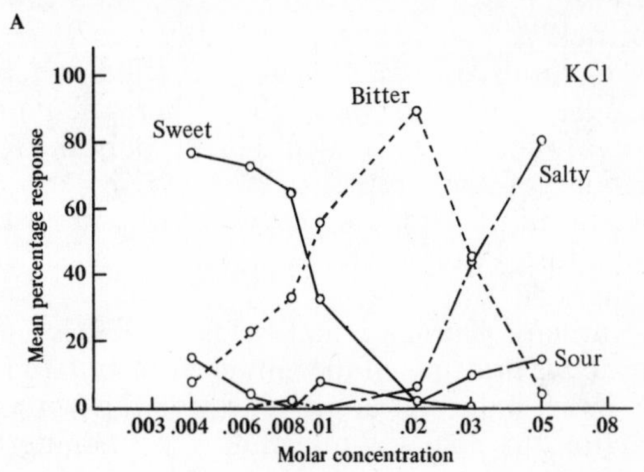


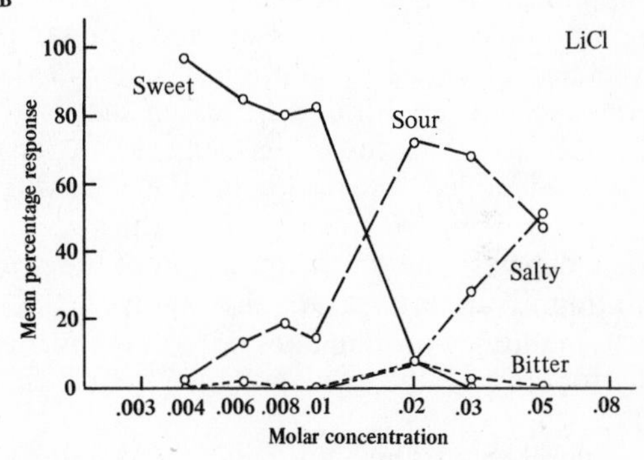


**Figure 6.11** A quantitative indication of the change in taste quality with increase in concentration for KCl (A) and LiCl (B). KCl changes from sweet to bitter to salty, whereas LiCl changes from sweet to sour to salty. Results are given for four subjects. (From Dzendolet & Meiselman, 1967.)

### Interactions among taste qualities

The sequence in which stimuli are presented may significantly affect taste quality; eating one substance usually affects the quality of substances eaten after it. The interaction can be easily experienced by reversing the order in which grapefruit and cereal are eaten at breakfast. In the laboratory the phenomenon is generally studied with a group of substances referred to as *taste modifiers.* Two such modifiers are the fruit of the shrub *Synsepalum dulcificum* and the leaves of the plant *Gymnema sylvestre.* The fruit of the *Synsepalum dulcificum,* known as *miracle fruit,* changes sour to sweet. The leaves of the *Gymnema sylvestre,* which taste bitter, completely suppress the sweet taste of sugar taken afterwards.

Shore (1892) studied this effect of the *Gymnema sylvestre* plant as part of his investigation of regional differences in the sensitivity of the tongue. He demonstrated that the sweet taste of glycerine could be entirely prevented by the previous application of a decoction of the sodium salt of gymnemic acid for 20 seconds. Early workers like Shore found that the gymnemic acid also suppressed the bitter taste of quinine sulphate. This suppression was probably due to cross-adaptation between the two substances. If one prevents cross-adaptation, then the active principle of the *Gymnema sylvestre* plant does not suppress bitter substances and is specific for sweet tastes. The suppression of sweet tastes has been demonstrated physiologically by the reduction of the response of the chorda tympani nerve to sweet stimuli (Diamant, Oakley, Ström, Wells, & Zotterman, 1965).

As previously noted, weak concentrations of salt solutions taste sweet. Distilled water can also taste sweet when preceded by adaptation to citric acid, hydrochloric acid, or quinine hydrochloride (Bartoshuk, 1968; Bartoshuk, McBurney, & Pfaffmann, 1964). The sweet taste is abolished after exposure to an aqueous decoction of *Gymnema sylvestre* leaves (Bartoshuk, Dateo, Vandenbelt, Buttrick, & Long, 1969).

The shrub *Synsepalum dulcificum,* which is native to West Africa, bears a small red berry about the size of an olive. Daniell (1852) published an account of the properties of the red berry, or miracle fruit. After it is chewed, sour foods like grapefruit taste sweet, and lemons taste like oranges.

Kurihara, Kurihara, and Beidler (1969) isolated the active principle of the miracle fruit and studied its sweet-inducing effectiveness. Subjects were required to hold a 5-ml solution containing the active principal, a protein, in their mouths for 5 minutes and then spit it out. They then rinsed their mouths with distilled water and compared the sweetness of a 0.02-M solution of citric acid to a series of sucrose solutions. From ten sucrose solutions (0.1 to 1.0 M) the subjects chose the one that most resembled the acid in the intensity of sweetness. Figure 6.12 shows how the sweetening effect depends on the concentration of the protein solution. Kurihara et al. also showed that the taste-modifying protein does not affect the threshold for any of the taste qualities, even that of sour.

A number of other inorganic and organic acids have been tested and all found to have sweet-inducing potency. The sweet-inducing potency of an acid is closely associated to its degree of sourness. Further studies of the taste modifiers should provide data that will help elucidate the mechanism of taste itself. In some ways this research is analogous to that on specific anosmia in olfaction.

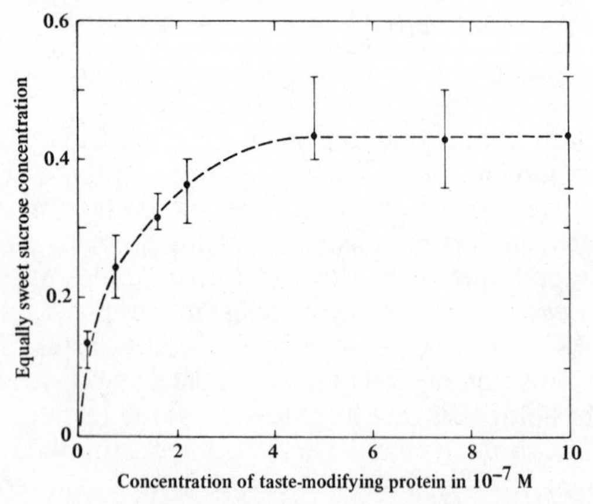


**Figure 6.12** The sweetening effect as a function of the concentration of the taste-modifying protein. The sweetening effect on 0.02 M citric acid was assayed after the different concentrations of the protein were held in the mouth for 5 minutes. (From Kurihara, Kurihara, & Beidler, 1969.)

## Taste adaptation

Although it is often assumed that sensory adaptation reflects the exhaustion or fatigue of the receptor cells, the evidence suggests that fatigue is usually not the cause. Prolonged stimulation can affect a sensory system such as taste in a number of ways other than merely to reduce sensitivity. Cross-adaptation is one example, and a change in the just noticeable difference (jnd) is another. Cross-adaptation occurs when a steady stimulus raises the threshold for a chemically different stimulus. As in olfaction, such an effect is evidence that the two stimuli share a common receptor mechanism.

The receptor cells in the mouth are adapted to the environmental conditions of the oral region, mainly to the chemicals present in saliva. Sodium is one component of saliva, and therefore adaptation to it should affect the detection threshold for sodium chloride. Adaptation of the tongue to water does lower the threshold for NaCl considerably, whereas adaptation to NaCl raises the threshold to a value just above the adapting concentration (McBurney, 1966). McBurney's subjects rated the subjective intensity of NaCl solutions which ranged from water to 1.0 M following adaptation to one of four different NaCl concentrations. The minimum subjective intensity occurred at the adapting concentration.

In a later experiment (Smith & McBurney, 1969), subjects tasted twelve salts after 1 minute of adaptation to distilled water and also after adaptation to 0.1 M solution of sodium chloride. Prior to the experiment, the twelve test stimuli had been equated in overall subjective intensity to the 0.1 M NaCl solution. The adapting stimuli were flowed over the tongue for 1 minute before each test stimulus. The subjects made magnitude estimations of the overall intensity of the test stimuli and were asked to divide these estimates appropriately among the four primary taste qualities. After adaptation to NaCl, the saltiness of all twelve salts fell below threshold, while their bitterness generally increased. Although all twelve test stimuli were salts, and therefore chemically similar, the adaptation effects of NaCl varied among them. Sourness increased for the salts with sulphate *anions* (negatively charged ions). Overall subjective intensity was less for eight salts, but was greater for the other four, all of which had either a sulphate or a nitrate anion. Cross-adaptation effects have also been found for sweet (McBurney, 1972) and sour and bitter compounds (McBurney, Smith, & Shick, 1972).

Ordinarily water has little or no taste. The taste quality of water, and quite likely the taste qualities of all substances, is affected by the prior adaptation of the mouth and hence by the composition of the fluids bathing the receptor cells. Bartoshuk, McBurney, and Pfaffmann (1964) studied the effect of adapting the tongue to either a 0.003 M or a 0.03 M concentration of NaCl on the taste quality of water and of sodium chloride. Ten test solutions were used: nine concentrations of NaCl from 0.001 M to 0.1 M, and water. Test solutions that were above the adapting solution were called salty by the subjects. At the adapting concentration, stimuli were predominantly labeled as tasteless. Subadapting concentrations were either bitter, sour, or tasteless. Judgments of tastelessness decreased in frequency with increasing difference between the adapting concentration and stimulus. The subjects were quite surprised to learn that only water and NaCl solutions had been used as test stimuli. The flat taste of water becomes bitter when the tongue has been adapted to NaCl. Does the taste of water change if the tongue is adapted to other taste stimuli? Probably, yes. Bartoshuk (1968) adapted the tongue to solutions of NaCl, quinine hydrochloride (QHCl), sucrose, and hydrochloric acid (HCl). Adaptation to moderate concentrations of these solutions generally produced magnitude estimations of zero at the adapting concentrations and increasing values for higher and lower (subadapting) concentrations. At the lower concentrations, adaptation to NaCl and sucrose produced bitter tastes, and adaptation to HCl and QHCl produced sweet tastes.

Adaptation also affects the jnd. McBurney, Kasschau, and Bogart (1967) found that the jnd for a standard 0.1 M solution of NaCl was 0.018 M when the tongue was adapted to water, and only 0.0009 M when adapted to a 0.1 M solution of NaCl. As noted by McBurney (1969), this change in the jnd is perhaps the strongest evidence that adaptation is not exclusively a diminution of sensory capacity. In fact, the results which have been reviewed in this section indicate that adaptation probably has more than one underlying physiological process. What those processes may be remains to be determined.

**Taste preferences and aversions**

Taste psychophysics is replete with examples of power functions between physical and perceived magnitudes—for example, between sucrose concentration and sweetness. The straight-line functions of taste are not, however, paralleled by corresponding functions for hedonic intensity. Scales of hedonic value, preference-aversion or acceptance-rejection, are typically biphasic or curvilinear. Preference, as defined by Young (1966) is an "evaluative concept implying that Response A is more acceptable, more desirable, more esteemed, more valued, better liked, more pleasant than Response B [p. 60]."

Figure 6.13A plots the preference curves measured on rats for the four types of taste qualities. Preference is indicated by the rat's intake of the stimulus at each concentration. These behavioral preference curves either decrease as stimulus intensity increases or are curvilinear with a peak at some optimal concentration. As the stimulus value moves away from the hedonic high point for sucrose and NaCl, the relative intake decreases; for quinine and HCl, however, intake decreases over the entire range of concentrations used so that only the aversion slope of a presumed preference-aversion curve is seen. In contrast, Figure 6.13B shows that for all four taste qualities and in both the chorda tympani and glossopharyngeal nerves, the neural response grows monotonically with stimulus intensity. Obviously, taste preference in rats is not related in any simple way to the magnitude of the afferent nerve response.

In addition to measuring preference as a function of stimulus intensity, research workers have sought to determine curves of equal hedonic value for various gustatory stimuli. Such curves are called *isohedons* (Guilford, 1939). All stimulus combinations along an isohedon are equally preferred, just as all sounds along an equal-loudness contour are equally loud (see Chapter 4). Young (1966, 1968) developed isohedons for a number of taste stimuli.

Figure 6.14 shows the isohedonic curves obtained with two different standards, one a 4% solution of sucrose and the other a 16% solution. The ordinate shows how many grams of sucrose and the abscissa how many grams of NaCl must be mixed together to give a compound solution equal in preference or hedonic value to the standard solution. For example, a standard of 4% sucrose is isohedonic to a compound solution which

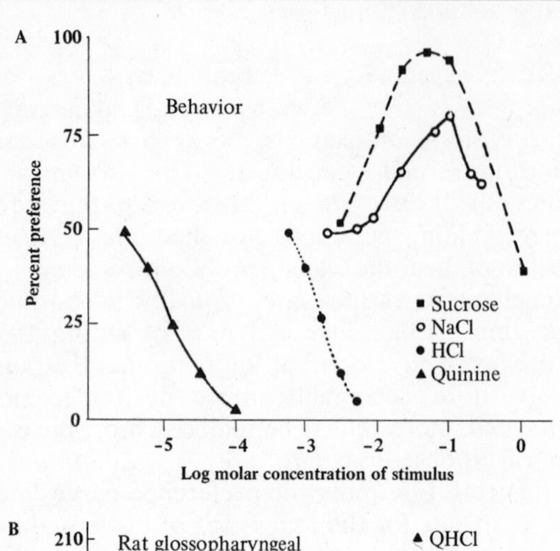


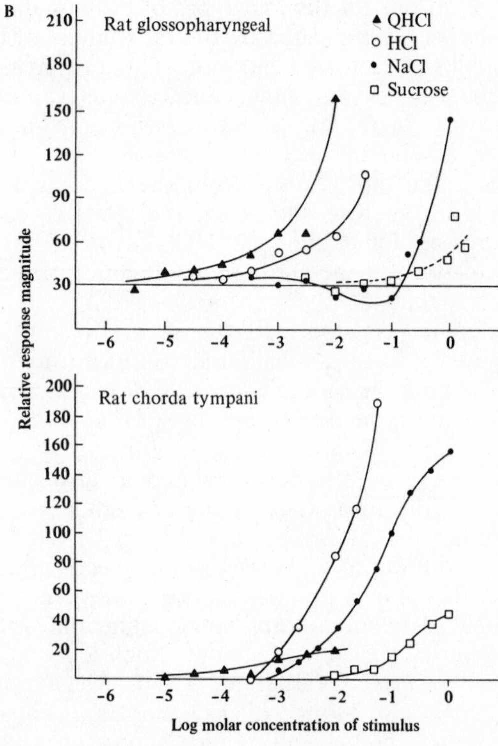


**Figure 6.13** Panel A: Percentage preference as a function of stimulus concentration in the rat. (From Pfaffmann, 1960.) Panel B: Comparison of the relative response magnitudes of rat glossopharyngeal and chorda tympani nerves. Responses were equated at 1.0 M NaCl. (From Pfaffmann, Fisher, & Frank, 1967.)

contains 2 grams of NaCl and approximately 6.33 grams of sucrose. In other words, one must add 6.33 grams of sucrose to a 2% solution of NaCl to make it equal in preference to the standard.

To obtain the data points along the isohedon, animals were offered a choice between pairs of solutions. For example, one member of the pair was the 4% sucrose standard. The other member of the pair was the compound solution that always contained 2% NaCl and some variable amount of sucrose. The sucrose concentration in the compound solution was varied up and down from trial to trial. Four to six different concentrations separated by equal log units were used. The choice made by the rat on each trial determined the value of the compound solution on the next trial. If the rat selected the standard solution, the comparison was made sweeter on the next trial; if it selected the comparison, the comparison was made less sweet on the next trial and so on up and down from trial to trial.

The determination of hedonic equalities for compound taste solutions has been largely neglected by psychologists. Yet such determinations would provide important evidence, perhaps not directly on the stimulus mechanism of taste, but on the entire psychology of eating. For example, the precise seasoning of foods has always been the goal of the gourmet chef, while a pinch of salt in your beer and a dip of mustard on your pretzel greatly enhance an evening of conversation at the tavern.

One example from the laboratory clearly demonstrates the dramatic synergistic action that can occur between taste substances. Valenstein, Cox, and Kakolewski (1967) reported that normal rats consumed excessive quantities of a compound solution containing 3 percent glucose and either 0.25 percent or 0.125 percent saccharin. The average 24-hour intake of water was around 40 ml. In a two-bottle preference test, the rats consistently chose the mixture of glucose and saccharin over a constant alternative which was either 3 percent glucose or 0.25 percent saccharin or water. Female rats consumed each day, on the average, 137 ml of the mixture of 3 percent glucose and 0.125 percent saccharin and 171 ml of the mixture of 3 percent glucose and 0.25 percent saccharin. Male rats consumed 187 ml of the mixture containing 0.125 percent saccharin and 129 ml of the mixture containing 0.25 percent saccharin. The females therefore consumed more of the mixture containing 0.25 percent saccharin and the males more of the

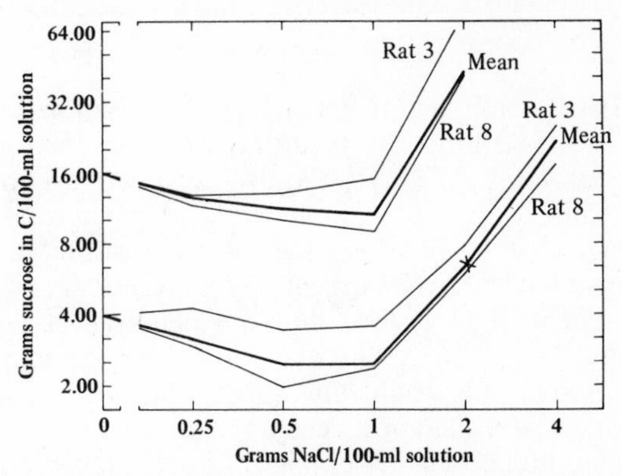


**Figure 6.14** Isohedons for compounds of sucrose and NaCl. For each standard the heavy line represents the mean based on eight rats. Lighter lines record individual isohedons for rats 3 and 8. The data point described in the text is signified by an X. (From Young & Madsen, 1963.)

mixture containing only 0.125 percent saccharin. The increased consumption of the mixture has been verified by Murphy and Brown (1970) and appears to be a very strong effect. To dramatize the excessive consumption by these animals, Valenstein et al. (1967) pointed out that the equivalent consumption by an adult human male weighing 165 pounds would amount to more than 20.8 gallons (80 liters) of fluid per day.

The sex difference in saccharin preference is in accord with the report that mature female rats, which do not drink more water than males, do consume significantly greater quantities of a slightly sweet 3 percent-glucose solution and a very sweet 0.25 percent-saccharin solution. Females also prefer significantly higher concentrations of saccharin than males (Valenstein, Kakolewski, & Cox, 1967). Such sexual differences suggest that hormones play an important role in taste preferences.

Taste preferences are, of course, influenced by a number of factors besides hormones. After the taste quality itself, perhaps postingestional factors have been studied the most. McCleary (1953) has shown that ingestion of glucose solutions by rats is depressed as a function of the osmotic pressures of preload solutions of glucose, NaCl, and urea in varying concentrations. Isohedonic concentrations of sucrose and glucose are equally consumed only in short-term tests. In longer tests, owing to its higher osmotic pressure less glucose is consumed than is a matched sucrose solution. Thus, as Shuford (1959) has shown, the intake curve is determined by two opposing factors: a taste factor that facilitates ingestion, and a postingestional factor that inhibits ingestion. A taste factor related to palatability determines the rate of drinking initially in the test session. A postingestional factor related to the osmotic pressure of the solution subsequently slows the rate of drinking. The higher the osmotic pressure of a solution, the sooner the postingestional factor takes effect, as Shuford (1959) has shown during the first minute or two for a 35 percent-solution of glucose.

A clear separation of the roles of oral and postingestional factors comes from the use of an esophageal fistula. In this preparation, the esophagus is severed and brought out at the neck so that everything the animal takes from the drinking tube flows out of the fistula. A polyethylene tube is inserted into the stomach through the lower end of the esophagus and the same or a different liquid can be pumped into the stomach as the animal drinks. By varying the contents of the drinking tube and the reservoir independently, one can determine the relative influence of taste and postingestional factors on intake. Mook (1963) used this procedure to show that the normal rat's preference for isotonic saline solutions is determined by postingestional factors. A water-deprived animal normally drinks more saline solution than water. However, if only water enters the stomach, the intake of saline decreases to the lower water-drinking level. The taste of isotonic saline alone is not sufficient to elevate saline intake. On the other hand, intake is raised when saline enters the stomach regardless of whether the animal drinks saline or water. This dependence of preference for isotonic saline on postingestional factors also holds for the nondeprived animal (Mook & Kozub, 1968).

By allowing the animal to drink various concentrations of NaCl, glucose, and sucrose, but putting only water into the stomach, Mook (1963) was able to determine the role of the oral responses with the inhibiting postingestional factors held constant. When this is done, the preference for isotonic NaCl disappears as noted. The preference for hypotonic glucose solutions is flattened, but there is an increased intake of hypertonic solutions. Sucrose drinking is a positive, negatively accelerated function of concentration. These findings imply that, once hydrational needs are cared for by letting water flow into the stomach, drinking of various concentrations is almost completely regulated by oral factors, particularly taste.

The importance of taste or oral factors in preference-aversion functions is further demonstrated by the work of Borer (1968). Using Epstein and Teitelbaum's (1962) method of direct intragastric feeding which completely bypasses all of the taste and olfactory receptors, Borer found that in 24-hour tests the animals showed no preference for NaCl, glucose, sucrose, or saccharin in a variety of concentrations when the animals received the solutions intragastrically. When the animals ingested the taste substances orally, intake was the typical nonmonotonic function of concentration. Borer interpreted her results as demonstrating that taste receptors have a primary role in generating spontaneous preference for sweet solutions and preference-aversion for saline. Preferences and aversions are primarily taste functions that, depending on experimental conditions, are modified by postingestional factors.

Taste preferences and aversions are to some extent unique to each species. For example, the rabbit, rat, cow, and human respond positively to sucrose, whereas the cat and chicken are indifferent to it (Kare & Ficken, 1963). Fisher, Pfaffmann, and Brown (1965) compared the taste preferences of the rat, squirrel monkey, and human for two sweetening agents, saccharin and dulcin. Humans responded positively to both, but rats preferred only saccharin and monkeys only dulcin. Other differences have been noted for the rabbit, hamster, and cat (Carpenter, 1956). Although one can cite many more instances of such differences across species, there has not as yet emerged from these results any pattern, either chemical-nutritional, physiological, or otherwise, that would account for the observed differences.

Within a given species, developmental factors are operative in behavioral patterns of acceptance and rejection that appear in the adult organism. For the human being, sociocultural variables are extremely important and most likely are the counterpart of the ecological variables in other species. Consider for a moment the many factors that affect your food intake or preference at any given moment. Obvious ones are the time of day and your dietary habits. Dietary habits themselves are most likely the result of many factors, such as ethnic group, religious convictions, knowledge of nutrition, metabolic needs, and the social meaning of the situation. All of these variables contribute to the psychology of eating.

## SUMMARY AND CONCLUSIONS

In olfaction, it appears that an odorous molecule is adsorbed onto the membrane of the olfactory receptor cell. We do not know, however, just how the adsorption of the molecule evokes neural activity, that is, just how the olfactory stimulus is transduced. Two current hypotheses are the stereochemical theory and the penetration and puncturing theory. The first emphasizes the shape of the stimulus molecule, which must fit into an appropriately shaped receptor site on the membrane, much as a key fits into a lock. Odors have similar olfactory qualities when similar molecular configurations stimulate the same receptor sites. The second hypothesis proposes that the stimulus molecule punctures the cell membrane, creating a hole that allows an exchange of sodium and potassium ions. This exchange depolarizes and excites the receptor cell.

The primary olfactory qualities have not yet been positively identified. Research continues with recent work on specific anosmia (insensitivity to particular odors), providing some fruitful leads as to the primary qualities in human olfaction.

Both animal behavior, especially as influenced by olfactory pheromones, and human psychophysics are currently receiving much attention by olfactory scientists.

Taste, like smell, remains much of a mystery as far as transduction is concerned. We do not know how taste stimuli evoke nervous activity in the gustatory nerve. Recent evidence suggests that specific receptor molecules may form a complex with the stimulus molecules. Whether each of the four recognized taste qualities—sweet, salty, sour, and bitter—has a corresponding receptor molecule remains to be determined. So far only one such receptor molecule, the so-called sweet-sensitive protein, has been isolated.

Meanwhile, the notion that the four taste qualities are mediated in different parts of the mouth may have to be modified. Some new data suggest that this areal division may be very complicated; at the tip of the tongue, an area supposedly concerned mainly with sweet, receptors have been found which are sensitive to the other three taste qualities as well.

The present concern with the long-term effects on health of food additives and substitutes has led to renewed research in the human psychophysics of taste. Attention seems to be concentrated on taste adaptation. Such research will hopefully lead to a better understanding of the taste system, as well as to new and safer foods.

# REFERENCES


**Adler, J.** Chemoreceptors in bacteria. *Science,* 1969, **166,** 1588–97.

**Allison, V. C., & Katz, S. H.** An investigation of stenches and odors for industrial purposes. *Journal of Industrial and Engineering Chemistry,* 1919, **11,** 336–38.

**Amoore, J. E.** The stereochemical specificities of human olfactory receptors. *Perfumery & Essential Oil Record and Flavours,* 1952, **43,** 321–23, 30. Figure 2, p. 322, reproduced by permission of the publishers.

**Amoore, J. E.** Specific anosmia: A clue to the olfactory code. *Nature,* 1967, **214,** 1095–98. Figure 3, p. 1096, reproduced by permission.

**Amoore, J. E.** A plan to identify most of the primary odors. In C. Pfaffmann (Ed.), *Olfaction and taste III.* New York: Rockefeller University Press, 1969. Pp. 158–71. Table II, p. 165, reproduced by permission.

**Amoore, J. E., & Venstrom, D.** Sensory analysis of odor qualities in terms of the stereochemical theory. *Journal of Food Science,* 1966, **31,** 118–28. Table 1, p. 120, Copyright © 1966 by Institute of Food Technologists, and reproduced by permission.

**Amoore, J. E., & Venstrom, D.** Correlations between stereochemical assessments and organoleptic analysis of odorous compounds. In T. Hayashi (Ed.), *Olfaction and taste II.* Oxford: Pergamon Press, 1967. Pp. 3–17. Figure 1, p. 6, and Table 3, pp. 8–11, reproduced by permission of Pergamon Press Ltd.

**Bartoshuk, L. M.** Water taste in man. *Perception & Psychophysics,* 1968, **3,** 69–72.

**Bartoshuk, L. M., Dateo, G. P., Vandenbelt, D. J., Buttrick, R. L., & Long, L., Jr.** Effects of *Gymnema sylvestre* and *Synsepalum dulcificum* on taste in man. In C. Pfaffmann (Ed.), *Olfaction and taste III.* New York: Rockefeller University Press, 1969. Pp. 436–44.

**Bartoshuk, L. M., McBurney, D. H., & Pfaffmann, C.** Taste of sodium chloride solutions after adaptation to sodium chloride: Implications for the "water taste." *Science,* 1964, **143,** 967–68.

**Beets, M. G. J.** The molecular parameters of olfactory response. *Pharmacological Reviews,* 1970, **22,** 1–34.

**Békésy, G. von.** Taste theories and the chemical stimulation of single papillae. *Journal of Applied Physiology,* 1966, **21,** 1–9. Figure 5, p. 5, reproduced by permission of The American Physiological Society.

**Berglund, B., Berglund, U., Engen, T., & Lindvall, T.** The effect of adaptation on odor detection. *Perception & Psychophysics,* 1971, **9,** 435–38.

**Birch, M.** Persuasive scents in moth sex life. *Natural History,* 1970, **79**(9), 34–39.

**Bocca, E., & Battiston, M. N.** Odour perception and environment conditions. *Acta Oto-Laryngologica,* 1964, **57,** 391–400.

**Borer, K. T.** Disappearance of preferences and aversions for sapid solutions in rats ingesting untasted fluids. *Journal of Comparative and Physiological Psychology,* 1968, **65,** 213–21.

**Borg, G., Diamant, H., Ström, L., & Zotterman, Y.** The relation between neural and perceptual intensity: A comparative study on the neural and psychophysical response to taste stimuli. *Journal of Physiology,* 1967, **192,** 13–20. Figure 7, p. 17, reproduced by permission.

**Boring, E. G.** *Sensation and perception in the history of experimental psychology.* New York: Appleton-Century-Crofts, 1942.

**Bruce, H. M.** An exteroreceptive block to pregnancy in the mouse. *Nature,* 1959, **184,** 105.

**Bruce, H. M.** Further observations on pregnancy block in mice caused by proximity of strange males. *Journal of Reproduction and Fertility,* 1960, **1,** 311–12.

**Bruce, H. M.** Time relations in the pregnancy block induced in mice by strange males. *Journal of Reproduction and Fertility,* 1961, **2,** 138–42.

**Bruce, H. M., & Parrott, D. M. V.** Role of olfactory sense in pregnancy block by strange males. *Science,* 1960, **131,** 1526.

**Cain, W. S.** Odor intensity: Differences in the exponent of the psychophysical function. *Perception & Psychophysics,* 1969, **6,** 349–54. Figure 1, p. 350, reproduced by permission.

**Cain, W. S.** Odor intensity after self-adaptation and cross-adaptation. *Perception & Psychophysics,* 1970, **7,** 271–75.

**Cain, W. S., & Engen, T.** Olfactory adaptation and the scaling of odor intensity. In C. Pfaffmann (Ed.), *Olfaction and taste III.* New York: Rockefeller University Press, 1969. Pp. 127–41. Figures 1, p. 128, 2, p. 134, and 8, p. 139, reproduced by permission.

**Carpenter, J. A.** Species differences in taste preferences. *Journal of Comparative and Physiological Psychology,* 1956, **49,** 139–44.

**Cherry, R. D., Dodd, G. H., & Chapman, D.** Small molecule lipid membrane interactions and the puncturing theory of olfaction. *Biochimica et Biophysica Acta,* 1970, **211,** 409–16.

**Daniell, W. F.** On the *Synsepalum dulcificum* or miraculous berry of Western Africa. *Pharmaceutical Journal,* 1852, **11,** 445–48. Cited by Kurihara, Kurihara, & Beidler, 1969.

**Dastoli, F. R., Lopiekes, D. V., & Price, S.** A sweet-sensitive protein from bovine taste buds: Purification and partial characterization. *Biochemistry,* 1968, **7,** 1160–64.

**Dastoli, F. R., & Price, S.** Sweet-sensitive protein from bovine taste buds: Isolation and assay. *Science,* 1966, **154,** 905–907.

**Davies, J. T.** The mechanism of olfaction. *Symposia of the Society for Experimental Biology,* 1962, **16,** 170–79.

**Davies, J. T.** A theory of the quality of odours. *Journal of Theoretical Biology,* 1965, **8,** 1–7.

**Davies, J. T.** The "penetration and puncturing" theory of odor types and intensities of odors. *Journal of Colloid and Interface Science,* 1969, **29,** 296–304.

**Davies, J. T.** Olfactory theories. In L. M. Beidler (Ed.), *Handbook of sensory physiology:* IV. *Chemical senses.* Part 1: *Olfaction.* New York: Springer-Verlag, 1971. Pp. 322–50.

**Davies, J. T., & Taylor, F. H.** A model system for the olfactory membrane. *Nature,* 1954, **174,** 693–94.

**Diamant, H., Oakley, B., Ström, L., Wells, C., & Zotterman, Y.**

A comparison of neural and psychophysical responses to taste stimuli in man. *Acta Physiologica Scandinavica,* 1965, **64,** 67–74.

**Doetsch, G. S., Ganchrow, J. J., Nelson, L. M., & Erickson, R. P.** Information processing in the taste system of the rat. In C. Pfaffmann (Ed.), *Olfaction and taste III.* New York: Rockefeller University Press, 1969. Pp. 492–511.

**Dominic, C. J.** Source of the male odor causing pregnancy block in mice. *Journal of Reproduction and Fertility,* 1964, **8,** 266–67.

**Dominic, C. J.** Observations on the reproductive pheromones of mice: I. Source. *Journal of Reproduction and Fertility,* 1966, **11,** 407–414.

**Dzendolet, E., & Meiselman, H. L.** Gustatory quality changes as a function of solution concentration. *Perception & Psychophysics,* 1967, **2,** 29–33. Figures 1 and 2, p. 31, reproduced by permission.

**Engen, T.** Cross-adaptation to the aliphatic alcohols. *American Journal of Psychology,* 1963, **76,** 96–102.

**Engen, T., & Bosack, T. N.** Facilitation in olfactory detection. *Journal of Comparative and Physiological Psychology,* 1969, **68,** 320–26.

**Epstein, A. N., & Teitelbaum, P.** Regulation of food intake in the absence of taste, smell and other oropharyngeal sensations. *Journal of Comparative and Physiological Psychology,* 1962, **55,** 753–59.

**Fischer, E., & Penzoldt, F.** Über die Empfindlichkeit des Geruchssinnes. *Sitzungsberichte der Physikalisch medizinischen Sozietät in Erlangen,* 1886, **18,** 7–10. Cited by Boring, 1942.

**Fisher, G. L., Pfaffmann, C., & Brown, E.** Dulcin and saccharin taste in squirrel monkeys, rats and men. *Science,* 1965, **150,** 506–507.

**Foster, D., Scofield, E. H., & Dallenbach, K. M.** An olfactorium. *American Journal of Psychology,* 1950, **63,** 431–40.

**Gandelman, R., Zarrow, M. X., Denenberg, V. H., & Myers, M.** Olfactory bulb removal eliminates maternal behavior in the mouse. *Science,* 1971, **171,** 210–11.

**Gleason, K. K., & Reynierse, J. H.** The behavioral significance of pheromones in vertebrates. *Psychological Bulletin,* 1969, **71,** 58–73.

**Grundvig, J. C., Dustman, R. E., & Beck, E. C.** The relationship of olfactory receptor stimulation to stimulus environmental temperature. *Experimental Neurology,* 1967, **18,** 416–28.

**Guilford, J. P.** A study in psychodynamics. *Psychometrika,* 1939, **4,** 1–23.

**Guillot, M.** Anosmies partielles et odeurs fondamentales. *Comptes rendus hebdomadaires des séances de l'Academie des Sciences* (Paris), 1948, **226,** 1307–1309.

**Hainer, R. M., Emslie, A. G., & Jacobson, A.** An information theory of olfaction. *Annals of the New York Academy of Sciences,* 1954, Art. 2, 158–74.

**Hänig, D. P.** Zur Psychophysik des Geschmackssinnes. *Philosophische Studien,* 1901, **17,** 576–623. Cited by Boring, 1942.

**Harper, H. W., Jay, J. R., & Erickson, R. P.** Chemically evoked sensations from single human taste papillae. *Physiology & Behavior,* 1966, **1,** 319–25.

**Henkin, R. I., & Bradley, D. F.** Regulation of taste acuity by thiols and metal ions. *Proceedings of the National Academy of Sciences,* 1969, **62,** 30–37.

**Henkin, R. I., & Christiansen, R. L.** Taste thresholds in patients with dentures. *Journal of the American Dental Association,* 1967, **75,** 118. (a)

**Henkin, R. I., & Christiansen, R. L.** Taste localization on the tongue, palate and pharynx of normal man. *Journal of Applied Physiology,* 1967, **22,** 316. (b)

**Henkin, R. I., Graziadei, P. P. C., & Bradley, D. F.** The molecular basis of taste and its disorders. *Annals of Internal Medicine,* 1969, **71,** 791–821.

**Henning, H.** *Der Geruch,* 1916. (a) Cited by Boring, 1942.

**Henning, H.** Die Qualitätsreibe des Geschmacks. *Zeitschrift für Psychologie,* 1916, **74,** 203–19. (b) Cited by Boring, 1942.

**Höber, R., & Kiesow, F.** Über den Geschmack von Salzen und Haugen. *Zeitschrift für physikalische Chemie,* 1898, **27,** 601–616. Cited by Dzendolet & Meiselman, 1967.

**Johnston, J. W., & Sandoval, A.** Organoleptic quality and the stereochemical theory of olfaction. *Proceedings of the Scientific Section of the Toilet Goods Association,* 1960, **33,** 3–9.

**Jones, F. N., & Jones, M. H.** Modern theories of olfaction: A critical review. *Journal of Psychology,* 1953, **36,** 207–241.

**Kaae, R. S., Shorey, H. H., & Gaston, L. K.** Pheromone concentration as a mechanism for reproductive isolation between two lepidopterous species. *Science,* 1973, **179,** 487–88.

**Kare, M. R., & Ficken, M. S.** Comparative studies on the sense of taste. In Y. Zotterman (Ed.), *Olfaction and taste I.* Oxford: Pergamon Press, 1963. Pp. 285–97.

**Karlson, P., & Lüscher, M.** "Pheromones": A new term for a class of biologically active substances. *Nature,* 1959, **183,** 55–56.

**Kimura, K., & Beidler, L. M.** Microelectrode study of taste receptors of rat and hamster. *Journal of Cellular and Comparative Physiology,* 1961, **58,** 131–39.

**Klein, D., & Brown, T. S.** Exploratory behavior and spontaneous alternation in blind and anosmic rats. *Journal of Comparative and Physiological Psychology,* 1969, **68,** 107–110.

**Komuro, K.** Le minimum perceptible de l'odorat dans une enceinte absolument inodorée. *Archives Néerlandaises de Physiologie,* 1921, **6,** 20–24. Cited by R. S. Woodworth & H. Schlosberg, *Experimental psychology.* New York: Holt, Rinehart & Winston, 1954.

**Kurihara, K., Kurihara, Y., & Beidler, L. M.** Isolation and mechanism of taste modifiers; taste-modifying protein and gymnemic acids. In C. Pfaffmann (Ed.), *Olfaction and taste III.* New York: Rockefeller University Press, 1969. Pp. 450–69. Figure 9, p. 458, reproduced by permission.

**Lalonde, E. R., & Eglitis, J. A** Number and distribution of taste buds on the epiglottis, pharynx, larynx, soft palate, and uvula in a human newborn. *Anatomical Record,* 1961, **140,** 91–95.

**Lee, S. van der, & Boot, L. M.** Spontaneous pseudopregnancy in mice. *Acta Physiologica et Pharmacologica Neerlandica,* 1955, **4,** 442–44.

**Lee, S. van der, & Boot, L. M.** Spontaneous pseudopregnancy in mice: II. *Acta Physiologica et Pharmacologica Neerlandica,* 1956, **5,** 213–15.

**Le Magnen, J.** Analyse d'odeurs complexes et homologues par fatigue. *Comptes rendus hebdomadaires des séances de l'Academie des Sciences* (Paris), 1948, **226,** 753–54. Cited by Beets, 1970.

**Marsden, H. M., & Bronson, F. H.** Estrous synchrony in mice: Alteration by exposure to male urine. *Science,* 1964, **144,** 1469.

**McBurney, D. H.** Magnitude estimation of the taste of sodium chloride after adaptation to sodium chloride. *Journal of Experimental Psychology,* 1966, **72,** 869–73.

**McBurney, D. H.** Effects of adaptation on human taste function. In C. Pfaffmann (Ed.), *Olfaction and taste III.* New York: Rockefeller University Press, 1969. Pp. 407–419.

**McBurney, D. H.** Gustatory cross adaptation between sweet-tasting compounds. *Perception & Psychophysics,* 1972, **11,** 225–27.

**McBurney, D. H., Kasschau, R. A., & Bogart, L. M.** The effect of adaptation on taste jnds. *Perception & Psychophysics,* 1967, **2,** 175–78.

**McBurney, D. H., Smith, D. V., & Shick, T. R.** Gustatory cross-adaptation: Sourness and bitterness. *Perception & Psychophysics,* 1972, **11,** 228–32.

**McCleary, R. A.** Taste and postingestive factors in specific-hunger behavior. *Journal of Comparative and Physiological Psychology,* 1953, **46,** 411–21.

**McCutcheon, N. B., & Saunders, J.** Human taste papilla stimulation: Stability of quality judgments over time. *Science,* 1972, **175,** 214–17.

**Michael, R. P., & Keverne, E. B.** Pheromones in the communication of sexual status in primates. *Nature,* 1968, **218,** 746–49.

**Michael, R. P., Keverne, E. B., & Bonsall, R. W.** Pheromones: Isolation of male sex attractants from a female primate. *Science,* 1971, **172,** 964–66.

**Moncrieff, R. W.** Olfactory adaptation and odour likeness. *Journal of Physiology,* 1956, **133,** 301–316.

**Mook, D. G.** Oral and postingestional determinants of the intake of various solutions in rats with esophageal fistulas. *Journal of Comparative and Physiological Psychology,* 1963, **56,** 645–59.

**Mook, D. G., & Kozub, F. J.** Control of sodium chloride intake in the nondeprived rat. *Journal of Comparative and Physiological Psychology,* 1968, **66,** 105–109.

**Moskowitz, H. R.** Ratio scales of sugar sweetness. *Perception & Psychophysics,* 1970, **1,** 315–20.

**Moulton, D. G.** Studies in olfactory acuity: III. Relative detectability of n-aliphatic acetates by the rat. *Quarterly Journal of Experimental Psychology,* 1960, **12,** 203–213.

**Moulton, D. G.** The olfactory pigment. In L. M. Beidler (Ed.), *Handbook of sensory physiology:* IV. *Chemical senses.* Part 1: *Olfaction.* New York: Springer-Verlag, 1971. Pp. 59–74.

**Moulton, D. G., Ashton, E. H., & Eayrs, J. T.** Studies in olfactory acuity: IV. Relative detectability of n-aliphatic acids by the dog. *Animal Behaviour,* 1960, **8,** 117–28.

**Moulton, D. G., & Eayrs, J. T.** Studies in olfactory acuity: II. Relative detectability of n-aliphatic alcohols by the rat. *Quarterly Journal of Experimental Psychology,* 1960, **12,** 99–109. Figure 1, p. 101, reproduced by permission.

**Murphy, H. M., & Brown, T. S.** Effects of hippocampal lesions on simple and preferential consummatory behavior in the rat. *Journal of Comparative and Physiological Psychology,* 1970, **72,** 404–415.

**Murphy, M. R., & Schneider, G. E.** Olfactory bulb removal eliminates mating behavior in the male golden hamster. *Science,* 1970, **167,** 302–304.

**Patterson, P. M., & Lauder, B. A.** Incidence and probable inheritance of "smell blindness" to normal butyl mercaptan. *Journal of Heredity,* 1948, **39,** 295–97.

**Pfaffmann, C.** Taste and smell. In S. S. Stevens (Ed.), *Handbook of experimental psychology.* New York: Wiley, 1951. Pp. 1143–71.

**Pfaffmann, C.** The pleasures of sensation. *Psychological Review,* 1960, **67,** 253–68. Figure 4, p. 257, Copyright © 1960 by the American Psychological Association, and reproduced by permission.

**Pfaffmann, C., Fisher, G. L., & Frank, M. K.** The sensory and behavioral factors in taste preferences. In T. Hayashi (Ed.), *Olfaction and taste II.* Oxford: Pergamon Press, 1967. Pp. 361–81. Figure 3, p. 368, reproduced by permission of Pergamon Press Ltd.

**Price, S., & Hogan, R. M.** Glucose dehydrogenase activity of a "sweet-sensitive protein" from bovine tongues. In C. Pfaffmann (Ed.), *Olfaction and taste III.* New York: Rockefeller University Press, 1969. Pp. 397–403.

**Priesner, E.** A new approach to insect pheromone specificity. In C. Pfaffmann (Ed.), *Olfaction and taste III.* New York: Rockefeller University Press, 1969. Pp. 235–40.

**Renqvist, Y.** Über den Geschmack. *Skandinavisches Archiv für Physiologie,* 1919, **38,** 97–201. Cited by Dzendolet & Meiselman, 1967.

**Roelofs, W. L., & Comeau, A.** Sex pheromone specificity: Taxonomic and evolutionary aspects in Lepidoptera. *Science,* 1969, **165,** 398–400.

**Rosenberg, B., Misra, T. N., & Switzer, R.** Mechanism of olfactory transduction. *Nature,* 1968, **217,** 423–27.

**Schneider, D.** Insect olfaction: Deciphering system for chemical messages. *Science,* 1969, **163,** 1031–37.

**Schneider, R. A., Costiloe, J. P., Vega, A., & Wolf, S.** Olfactory threshold technique with nitrogen dilution of n-butane and gas chromatography. *Journal of Applied Physiology,* 1963, **18,** 1–4.

**Schultz, E. F., & Tapp, J. T.** Olfactory control of behavior in rodents. *Psychological Bulletin,* 1973, **79,** 21–44.

**Shore, L. E.** A contribution to our knowledge of taste sensations. *Journal of Physiology* (London), 1892, **13,** 191–217.

**Shuford, E. H.** Palatability and osmotic pressure of glucose and sucrose solutions as determinants of intake. *Journal of Comparative and Physiological Psychology,* 1959, **52,** 150–53.

**Smith, D. V., & McBurney, D. H.** Gustatory cross-adaptation: Does a single mechanism code the salty taste? *Journal of Experimental Psychology,* 1969, **80,** 101–105.

**Stevens, S. S.** Sensory scales of taste intensity. *Perception & Psychophysics,* 1969, **6,** 302–308. Figures 3, p. 304, 8, p. 306, and 10, p. 307, reproduced by permission.

**Stoll, M.** Facts old and new concerning relationships between molecular structure and odor. In *Molecular structure and organoleptic quality.* London: Society of Chemistry and Industry, 1957. Pp. 1–12.

**Stone, H., & Bosley, J. J.** Olfactory discrimination and Weber's law. *Perceptual and Motor Skills,* 1965, **20,** 657–65.

**Tucker, D.** Physical variables in the olfactory stimulation process. *Journal of General Physiology,* 1963, **46,** 453–89.

**Valenstein, E. S., Cox, V. C., & Kakolewski, J. W.** Polydipsia elicited by the synergistic action of a saccharin and glucose solution. *Science,* 1967, **157,** 552–54.

**Valenstein, E. S., Kakolewski, J. W., & Cox, V. C.** Sex differences in taste preferences for glucose and saccharin solutions. *Science,* 1967, **156,** 942–43.

**Wenger, M. A., Jones, F. N., & Jones, M. H.** *Physiological psychology.* New York: Holt, Rinehart & Winston, 1956.

**Whitten, W. K.** Modification of the oestrous cycle of the mouse by external stimuli associated with the male. *Journal of Endocrinology,* 1956, **13,** 399–404.

**Whitten, W. K., & Bronson, F. H.** The role of pheromones in mammalian reproduction. In J. W. Johnston, D. G. Moulton, & A. Turk (Eds.), *Advances in chemoreception.* Vol. 1. *Communication by chemical signals.* New York: Appleton-Century-Crofts, 1970. Pp. 309–325.

**Whitten, W. K., Bronson, F. H., & Greenstein, J. A.** Estrusinducing pheromone of male mice: Transport of movement of air. *Science,* 1968, **161,** 584–85.

**Wilson, E. O.** Chemical communication in the social insects. *Science,* 1965, **149,** 1064–71.

**Wright, R. H.** Why is an odour? *Nature,* 1966, **209,** 551–54. (a)

**Wright, R. H.** Odour and molecular vibration. *Nature,* 1966, **209,** 571–73. (b)

**Wright, R. H.** How animals distinguish odours. *Science Journal* (London), 1968, **4**(7), 57–62.

**Young, P. T.** Hedonic organization and regulation of behavior. *Psychological Review,* 1966, **73,** 59–86.

**Young, P. T.** Evaluation and preference in behavioral development. *Psychological Review,* 1968, **75,** 222–41.

**Young, P. T., & Madsen, C. H., Jr.** Individual isohedons in sucrose–sodium chloride and sucrose-saccharin gustatory areas. *Journal of Comparative and Physiological Psychology,* 1963, **56,** 903–909. Figure 1, p. 906, Copyright © 1963 by the American Psychological Association, and reproduced by permission.

**Zarrow, M. X., Gandelman, R., & Denenberg, V. H.** Lack of nest building and maternal behavior in the mouse following olfactory bulb removal. *Hormones and Behavior,* 1971, **2,** 227–38.

**Zwaardemaker, H.** *Die Physiologie des Geruchs.* Leipzig, 1895. Cited by Boring, 1942.

# 7

# VISION

**Leo Ganz**
**Stanford University**

For the experimental psychologist, vision comprises the study of how the lights, colors, and shapes of the subjective world we create with our eyes is related to varying physical conditions in the environment. Generally speaking, a major portion of such study involves the determination of thresholds: What is the least amount of light needed to see a stimulus at all? What is the least difference in light conditions that can be seen? What is the fastest flicker rate that can be seen as fluttering in brightness? How small an object can we recognize? How much of a difference in the wavelength of light is needed to recognize one light as having a different color from another? These are among the classical questions posed in the study of human and animal vision. Although, at first glance they may appear purely technical, of interest only to the specialist, it turns out that complete answers to these queries go a long way toward explaining the laws that underlie the subjective phenomena of visual sensations. Therefore, a large part of this chapter is devoted to acquiring an understanding for the determinants of various thresholds.

## THE THRESHOLD DETECTION OF VISUAL STIMULI

### Light quantum requirements

Science often investigates threshold conditions, the boundary values where a specific effect may be produced. In the study of vision, an obvious boundary exists between seeing and not seeing. Accordingly, the question arises, How many quanta of light, or *photons*, are needed in a stimulus to obtain consistent seeing?[1] The answer to this question has revealed a lot about the operation of the visual system.

To determine the smallest total amount of energy needed for a visual sensation, it is necessary to maximize certain of the experimental parameters: (1) A small spot of light must be used, because when the angular diameter of a source is small enough the energy needed becomes minimal. (2) The stimulus duration must be less than 100 msec, because the energy in a flash of light needed for vision is minimal when

[1]A section is appended at the end of this chapter that describes very briefly some physical aspects of light: its emission, propagation, and absorption, as well as the units of its measurement. It is suggested that the reader go through the chapter initially without undue concern with the units of measurement.

the flash is brief (Graham & Margaria, 1935). (3) The stimulus should be presented not in the center of vision, where it would project to the fovea which is largely composed of cones, but to the periphery of the visual field where it would project to the retinal periphery which is composed of rods. Compared to the cones, the rod receptors contain much larger amounts of visual pigment and are therefore far more likely to absorb light. Because rods are more numerous toward the periphery of the visual field, this differential sensitivity can be maximized by presenting the stimulus at an angle of 20° from the fovea, thereby stimulating the area in which the rods achieve their maximum density per unit of retinal area. (4) The light should be of a wavelength to which the rods are maximally sensitive, namely, about 510 nanometers (nm). (5) The subject should be dark adapted so that his visual receptors contain a maximum amount of visual pigment.

In the classic experiment by Hecht, Shlaer, and Pirenne (1942), the subject was dark adapted for a period of 30 minutes prior to making any observations. Thresholds were determined for a small stimulus, only 10 minutes of arc in diameter, presented to a retinal area 20° from the fovea and flashed for a duration of 10 msec. The stimulus light was a narrow band of wavelengths, centered at 510 nm. The threshold was defined in their experiment as the light energy needed to obtain a correct detection on 60 percent of the trials on which a stimulus was shown. Subjects were trained to give a very low proportion of false positive responses (see Chapter 2). Hecht et al. found that the light energy required to attain a 60 percent frequency of seeing for seven subjects lay between 2.1 and $5.7 \times 10^{-10}$ ergs, which corresponds to 54 to 148 photons. However, these figures represent the number of quanta reaching the cornea, and not the amount absorbed by the receptors. The cornea itself reflects approximately 4 percent of the energy. More energy is lost within the eye, where the vitreous and aqueous humors of the human eye absorb 50 percent of the energy at 510 nm (Ludvigh & McCarthy, 1938). Of the light reaching the retina, only about 20 percent is absorbed by the visual pigment; the rest is absorbed by the dark pigment epithelium and other structures. Thus no more than about 10 percent of the light striking the eye is finally absorbed by the visual receptors. The authors therefore concluded that the minimum number of photons needed to achieve a visual detection rate of 60 percent is 5 to 14, an incredibly small number when it is remembered that light is emitted and absorbed in units no smaller than one photon.

The question then arises as to just how those 5 to 14 photons are distributed among the rods on the retina. Are 5 to 14 photons needed because one rod must absorb two or more photons? The stimulus used by Hecht *et al.* (1942) was focused on the retina as a spot of about .003 $mm^2$, taking diffraction into consideration. Such a retinal area contains about 500 rods. Given that 10 photons impinge on 500 rods, each photon acting independently of the other, the probability that a single rod will absorb two or more quanta is 0.10 (Pirenne, 1956). This probability is too small to account for the subject's threshold detection probability of .60. It follows, therefore, that a visual sensation is initiated when the 10 or more photons are distributed one to a rod receptor. Furthermore, since the photochemical conversion of the rod pigment *rhodopsin* to the succeeding stage has a photon efficiency of 1 (Wald & Brown, 1953), it is probably true that when 1 photon is absorbed in each of some 10 receptors, and each photon changes a single molecule in each of those receptors, this event is sufficient to initiate a visual response. Since the photon is the smallest unit of light that is emitted and absorbed, we see that the rods have achieved the ultimate limit of sensitivity. The limit is imposed by the physics of light production, not by the biological system.

Why, however, is it necessary to activate 5 to 14 receptors to obtain a 60 percent frequency of seeing? Why is it not sufficient to activate merely a single receptor? Hecht (1945) has suggested that a single activated rod would have an effect easily confused with the spontaneous excitation that occurs among the receptors of the retina even in complete darkness. The subject cannot distinguish an effect generated by light in a single rod from the effects of spontaneous excitation. Therefore, he can give a report of a visual sensation significantly beyond chance levels (e.g., a 60 percent frequency of seeing) only if the excitatory effect in his retina is also significantly beyond spontaneous levels. The simultaneous activation in a small retinal area of between 5 and 14 receptors represents an event sufficiently improbable to be discriminable from spontaneous activity or *dark noise*. A more precise formulation of this explanation is given in a later discussion of the discrimination of brightness differences.

### Spectral luminosity

Sensitivity to light depends on the wavelength of the stimulus. Using 22 subjects, Wald (1945) measured the detection threshold for a 1°-diameter stimulus, presented for a period of 40 msec. In some measurements the stimulus disc was presented entirely within the fovea, where the detection was mediated almost entirely by the cones. In the rest of the measurements the disc was presented 8° above the fovea. Here the rods predominate and, since they are more sensitive than the cones to most wavelengths, they alone determine the absolute threshold. Figure 7.1 shows that at some wavelengths the threshold is as much as a million times lower than at other wavelengths. The fovea is most sensitive to wavelengths of about 560 nm, and the periphery is most sensitive to wavelengths of about 500 nm. This shift in maximal sensitivity toward the shorter wavelengths as the stimulus moves from a predominantly cone to a predominantly rod population is closely related to the *Purkinje shift*. As the story is told, Purkinje was watching the display of colors in an oriental carpet at dusk. He observed that the blues and violets became relatively brighter and the oranges and reds relatively darker as daylight gave way to nocturnal illumination. His inference, the so-called Purkinje shift, refers to a shift of the peak of greatest sensitivity in the direction of short wavelengths as one goes from daylight to nighttime levels of illumination.

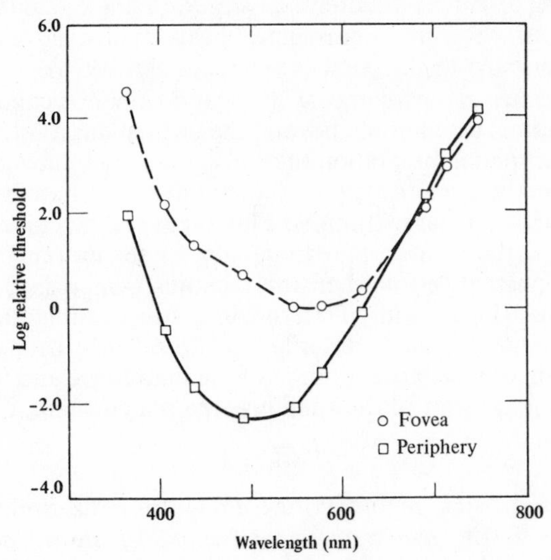


**Figure 7.1** The energy required to detect a 1°-diameter test object as a function of the wavelength of light employed. The dashed line represents foveal viewing; the solid line is obtained when the test object is presented 8° from the fovea, into the periphery of the visual field. Data for 22 subjects are shown. (After Wald, 1945.)

Note in Figure 7.1 that the curve for peripheral stimulation shows much higher sensitivity (lower threshold) to the shorter wavelengths. Thus, with white, blue, or bluish green light a stimulus is effectively detected in the periphery at luminance levels not sufficient for foveal detection. This explains why a dim star will often disappear from view when looked at directly, but will reappear when looked at indirectly since stimulation is once more eccentric. Further, it means that there must be a range of dim stimulation which activates rods but not cones. This range is called the *photochromatic interval*, which is represented for any wavelength by the vertical distance between the two curves in Figure 7.1. When a stimulus of a given wavelength is within that interval it is detected, but it appears colorless.

## Temporal summation

The critical factor that determines the detectability of a very brief flash of light is the mean number of photons delivered to the retina. This observation implies that if the duration of the flash is increased, say by a factor of 10, then the rate of photon delivery can be decreased by the same factor of 10. The rate of photon delivery is equivalent to the intensity of the visual stimulus. Thus, at least for short flashes, the visual response is determined by the product of intensity and time. This relation is known as *Bloch's law* (1885):

$$It = k, \qquad [1]$$

where $I$ is the intensity of the flash, $t$ is the duration of the flash, and $k$ is a constant. The product $It$ is a measure of the total stimulus energy in the flash. An identical principle, known as the *Bunsen-Roscoe law*, applies more widely to all photochemical processes, such as the response of photographic emulsions to flashes of light.

Verifying Bloch's law, measurements of threshold for flashes of different durations have shown that the energy, or $It$, is constant up to durations of about 60 to 70 msec (cf. Blondel & Rey, 1911; Karn, 1936). Within this period, intensity can be proportionately decreased as the flash is lengthened. Over this period the eye summates perfectly the number of impinging photons for a period of time up to 60 to 70 msec. Beyond this duration the eye stops summating, and the duration of the flash is no longer a factor. The flash duration below which the eye integrates perfectly and above which no integration occurs is called the *critical duration*.

Within the critical duration, the distribution of energy or photons is unimportant. As Long (1951) demonstrated experimentally, the threshold for short flashes is the same whether the photons are emitted mostly at the beginning of the flash or mostly at the end. Also, Davy (1952) has shown that the threshold is independent of the number of flashes as long as the total energy is the same, provided that the size of the stimulus is small and the flashes are all presented during an interval of time shorter than the critical duration. Many persons are surprised that they can detect stroboscopic flashes which last only a microsecond. But this should not surprise the reader if it is understood that below the range of 60 to 70 msec it is the number of quanta, not duration that is critical.

Bloch's law can also be demonstrated in the neurophysiological response of simpler organisms. Individual nerve fibers innervate single units, called *ommatidia*, of the compound eye of an arthropod such as *Limulus* (the horseshoe crab). These fibers give action potentials that decrease in latency and increase in number when the intensity of the stimulating flash is increased. Using the latency of the first action potential or the number of discharges elicited as measures of the visual response of that eye, Hartline (1934) showed that Bloch's law does apply in the *Limulus* eye. The nerve fiber studied was a first-order neuron, suggesting that the reciprocal relationship between intensity and time is established in the peripheral portion of the visual system.

### Spatial integration

An analogy can be drawn between temporal and spatial summation. When a flash stimulates only a small area of the retina, the eye can integrate spatially all the impinging photons. Reducing the stimulus area by a specified amount while keeping the luminance the same (i.e., maintaining the same rate of photon emission per unit of stimulus area) has the effect of reducing the total number of impinging photons per second. However, the visual effect on detection threshold will be the same as that produced by the original stimulus flash if the luminance of the smaller stimulus is increased to restore the total number of impinging photons to its original level. As an illustration, suppose a small flash yields a frequency of seeing of 60 percent. If the area of the stimulus is now reduced by a factor of 5, also reducing the stimulated retinal area by a factor of 5, the frequency of seeing will be lowered. The smaller stimulus will have to be increased in luminance fivefold to regain a 60 percent frequency of seeing. This relation describes *Ricco's law* (1877):

$$AI = k, \qquad [2]$$

where $A$ is the area of the stimulus, $I$ is the intensity of the stimulus, and $k$ is some constant visual effect.

A simple transformation of Ricco's law (Equation 2) gives:

$$\begin{aligned} \pi r^2 I &= k \\ \log \pi + 2 \log r + \log I &= \log k \\ k' - 2 \log r &= \log I, \end{aligned} \qquad [3]$$

where $r$ is the radius of the stimulus, $I$ is the intensity of the stimulus, and $k'$ is a constant. It is apparent that for the ranges of stimulus size and intensity within which Ricco's law holds, the function relating $\log I$ to $\log r$ should have a negative slope of $-2$. Experimentally, the $-2$ slope is realized, especially for stimuli presented to the periphery of the visual field, up to a stimulus radius of 100 minutes of visual angle. For larger stimuli the function approaches a slope of 0; the 0 slope indicates that the retina stops integrating spatially when the radius exceeds about 100 minutes of visual angle. Graham and Bartlett (1939) suggested that this critical stimulus size represents the limits of the retinal area served by single ganglion cells. According to this interpretation, total spatial integration is obtained when a stimulus is small enough so that all its photons impinge on receptors all of which ultimately converge on a single ganglion cell. Recent neuroanatomical evidence lends support to this view (see Creutzfeldt, 1970).

Just as in temporal integration the eye cannot summate photons beyond the critical duration, so in spatial integration the eye cannot summate perfectly over the entire retinal surface. Therefore, with very large stimuli the luminance level required to obtain a certain frequency of seeing remains constant, even when the stimulus is increased in size. For stimuli of intermediate size, summation is imperfect and is described by *Piper's law*, according to which the product of the luminance and the square root of the stimulus area is a constant, i.e.,

$$I\sqrt{A} = k. \qquad [4]$$

In the section on theories of brightness discrimination, the *quantum fluctuation model* shows one possible reason for square-root functions in vision.

## LIGHT AND DARK ADAPTATION

As most of us are well aware, the visual sensitivity of a subject is strongly dependent on the light level to which he has just been exposed. Exposed to intense luminances, the subject becomes less sensitive; exposed to very dim luminances, he becomes more sensitive. For example, when entering a movie theater from broad daylight, one cannot at first distinguish filled seats from empty ones. But after a few minutes, more and more details are discernible, and improvement continues for as long as half an hour. This ability to adapt is one of the most remarkable aspects of vision, allowing us to discriminate visual stimuli over an intensity range of some ten billion to one.

A dark-adaptation curve relates the increases in sensitivity to time. Figure 7.2 shows that while the subject is in the dark, threshold for a 2° spot of light projected on the fovea decreases smoothly along a single curve (Hecht, Haig, & Wald, 1935). After 2 or 3 minutes the threshold has declined to a minimum and no longer changes; the subject has achieved maximum sensitivity. The same figure shows that a 2° spot placed at an angular distance of 10° from the fovea yields a dark-adaptation curve with two branches. Sensitivity increases quickly during the first few seconds, then slows down, accelerates again after about 5 to 7 minutes have elapsed, and then slows down once more, approaching asymptote after approximately 30 minutes. The first branch of the curve, because it is present when the stimulus is projected to the fovea, is attributed to dark adaptation of the cones (*photopic* vision). Because the second branch of the dark-adaptation curve is found when the periphery is tested, it is attributed to dark adaptation of the rods (*scotopic* vision). Although the cones never reach the same sensitivity as the rods, they adapt more quickly and thus, during the first few minutes of adaptation, respond to weaker visual stimuli than do the rods. During this period the subject uses exclusively cone receptors for detection. As time passes the rods gain steadily in sensitivity and after 5 to 7 minutes they become more sensitive than the cones; thereafter they are used exclusively for detection. The two branches of the dark-adaptation curve are therefore a reflection of the *duplicity theory,* which states that there are two intermingled visual systems in the human eye, one mediating photopic vision and the other scotopic vision.

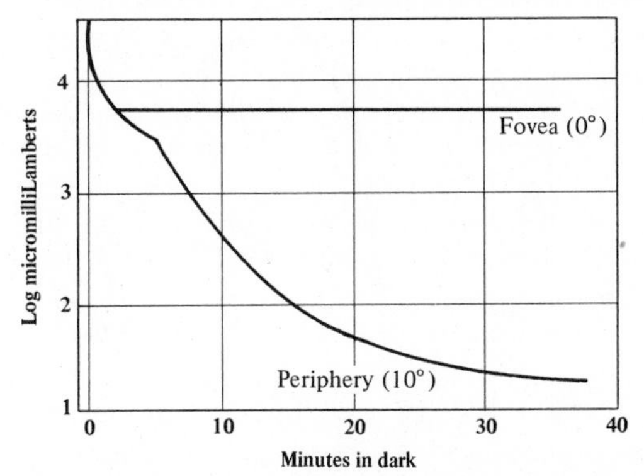


**Figure 7.2** Dark adaptation in the fovea and in the periphery. The stimulus was a white disc. The threshold luminance of the test flash (in micromilliLamberts) is plotted against time since the end of light adaptation. Data for one subject are shown. (After Hecht, Haig, & Wald, 1935.)

The duplicity theory is reflected in another aspect of dark adaptation, which is predictable from the threshold curves in Figure 7.1. Since rods are not more sensitive than cones to light at long wavelengths, only at wavelengths shorter than about 600 nm should we expect rods and cones to yield different dark-adaptation curves, and that is just what we find. When a test stimulus of a longer wavelength is used to measure sensitivity during dark adaptation, only the cone branch appears, producing a curve that is similar to the curve for the fovea in Figure 7.2. The shorter the wavelength of the test stimulus, the more pronounced the second, rod branch of the adaptation curve (Chapanis, 1947).

Because high acuity is mediated exclusively by cone receptors, and acuity improves with increases in target luminance (see later discussion of acuity), it is possible to dissociate the presumed rod and cone branches in yet another way. In an experiment by Brown, Graham, Leibowitz, and Ranken (1953) a thin grid pattern was presented to the subject during dark adaptation. The luminance of the test pattern at which the subject could identify the orientation of the lines diminishes as dark adaptation proceeds. When the grid pattern had an interbar width of about 1 minute of arc, a width so small that the subject had to use his fovea for the task, only the initial, cone branch of the dark-adaptation curve was found. This curve was similar to the fovea curve in Figure 7.2. When the interbar width was increased to approximately 10 minutes of arc so that the rods could be used, a two-branch curve was found, producing a second curve similar to the periphery curve in Figure 7.2.

In dark-adaptation experiments it is customary first to thoroughly dark adapt a subject without testing sensitivity, then to present a flash to light adapt him, and finally to measure visual sensitivity during the recovery from this controlled light adaptation. Mote and Riopelle (1953) showed that increasing either the duration or the intensity of the adapting flash will (a) raise the threshold at the beginning of dark adaptation, (b) give a more pronounced rod-cone break, (c) prolong the cone branch of the curve, and (d) make the rod branch of the curve shallower. With short or dim adapting flashes, the cone branch of the curve is totally absent and the rod branch declines very rapidly. Mote and Riopelle were also able to show that Bloch's law applied: Equal intensity-duration products gave identical dark-adaptation curves.

**The mechanism of dark adaptation**

Until recently, Hecht's (1934, 1937) theory, which attributed the loss in visual sensitivity following the adapting flash entirely to the bleaching of visual pigment by light, seemed sufficient to account for the mechanism of dark adaptation. According to the theory, following light adaptation the receptors would contain substantial quantities of bleached pigment, causing them to reflect more of the light quanta impinging on them and thus to absorb a smaller proportion. The loss in sensitivity then would presumably be due to the receptors' reduced ability to capture light quanta.

Hecht's theory attributes the recovery of sensitivity during dark adaptation to the regeneration of visual pigment while the eye is in darkness. The rod and the cone branches of the dark-adaptation curves yield recovery functions that are exponential because, like other monomolecular chemical reactions, the rate of reconstitution is a fixed proportion of the amount of constituents present. In this case, the constituents necessary for regeneration are the bleached visual pigments. There are two branches to the dark-adaptation curve because rod and cone receptors contain different visual pigments which break down and regenerate at different velocities.

The rate of regeneration of the rod pigment rhodopsin has been measured following light adaptation. The function is not unlike that of the rod branch of the recovery of visual sensitivity during dark adaptation (Wald, 1954). Several discrepancies have emerged, however, which make it virtually certain that the changes in visual sensitivity are only partially due to bleached visual pigment; a significant portion of the changes is attributable to neural events in the retina. Some of this evidence involves an analysis of the electrical response of the eye to light.

**The electroretinogram (ERG)**

If a recording electrode is placed on the cornea of the eye, a flash of light will evoke a series of electrical responses, relative to a reference electrode placed on nonresponding tissue (Riggs, 1965b). The components of the ERG are shown in Figure 7.3. The two components of interest are the initial negative component, or *a* wave, and the second response, or *b* wave.

It is believed that the *a* wave is a manifestation of the transducer activity of the receptors (Brown & Watanabe, 1962). A pulse of light energy is translated by the receptors of the eye into a pulse of electrical activity. This activity in turn evokes the *b* wave, a response of opposite polarity probably originating at the subsequent neural stage, the bipolar cells. Neither the *a* wave nor the *b* wave represents action potentials in axons; rather, they are local, nonpropagated dc-potential shifts (see Chapter 3). However, it is important for our purposes to realize that the visual response of ganglion cells—whose axons comprise the optic nerve—is very closely related to the magnitude of the *b* wave. Therefore, the magnitude of the *b* wave correlates fairly closely with the intensity of the organism's response to a visual stimulus.

In an adaptation experiment in which the *b* wave is measured instead of the subject's psychophysical threshold, the light-adapting flash lowers the size of

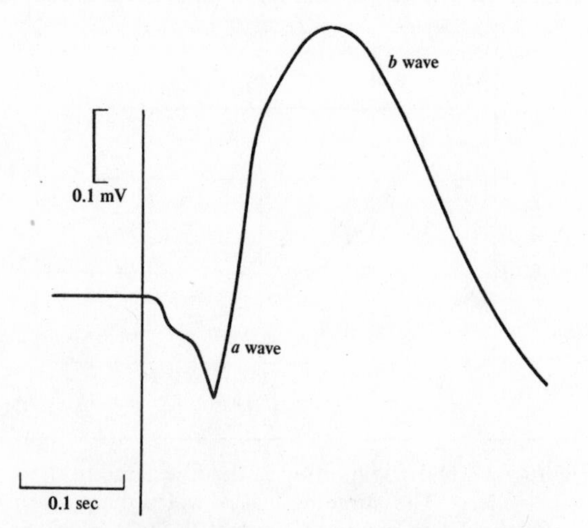


**Figure 7.3** The ERG in the dark adapted human eye. (After Armington, Johnson, & Riggs, 1952.)

the *b* wave. The *b* wave then recovers during dark adaptation (Riggs, 1937). Granit, Holmberg, and Zewi (1938), in a study of the *b* wave of the ERG of the frog, noticed that an adapting flash of moderate intensity greatly decreased the magnitude of the *b* wave. When the visual pigment of these frogs was extracted and measured, it was found not to have bleached noticeably. In other words, the loss in sensitivity was proportionately far greater than the amount of decomposed pigment would lead us to expect. In a related experiment on rats, Dowling and Wald (1960) measured the *b* wave of the ERG during dark adaptation and assessed rhodopsin levels in visual-pigment extracts from the same animals. Again, sensitivity changes were far more extensive than rhodopsin changes. Log sensitivity was approximately proportional to rhodopsin concentration. Brown and Watanabe (1965) were able to dissociate the *b* wave of the ERG from a presumptive receptor potential. (The receptor potential refers to the electromotive force generated by the receptors as a result of stimulation. This potential eventually acts on axons in the nervous system so as to initiate propagated action potentials; see Chapter 3.) Brown and Watanabe have shown that adapting flashes of moderate intensity which induced sizable reductions in the *b* wave nevertheless did not alter the magnitude of the receptor potential. This experiment demonstrates a reduction in visual sensitivity even when the receptors are no less sensitive. Presumably, a neural mechanism reduces the synaptic effects of the receptor potential.

These conclusions are further supported by an experiment by Rushton, Campbell, Hagins, and Brindley (1955) in which both visual threshold and the bleaching and regeneration of rhodopsin were measured in the intact eye of a human subject. It is possible to measure pigment density of the eye by stimulating the eye with light and measuring the amount of light which is reflected out of the eye. The more unbleached visual pigment present, the more light is absorbed by that pigment and the less reflected light emerges from the eye. Thus, by knowing how much light was absorbed, it is possible to estimate how much pigment was in the eye. Rushton et al. found, for example, that after an adapting flash of 280 milliLamberts (mL) was presented for 20 seconds, the rhodopsin level in the eye was at 98 percent of its maximal value. Nevertheless, with only 2 percent of the visual pigment absent, sensitivity was below its preadaptation level by a factor of 10. In other words, sensitivity changes are often much larger than bleaching changes. Some other mechanism appears to be at work.

Current theories must take into account the discrepancy between the amount of rhodopsin bleached by an adapting flash and the magnitude of the consequent sensitivity loss. One approach, Wald's (1954) *compartment theory*, in effect postulates a series of compartments of rhodopsin, all of which must be regenerated before the response of the rods can initiate a visual response. This theory, however, fails to account for the neurophysiological results of Brown and Watanabe (1965) and of Lipetz (1961), which show that it seems most likely that the loss in sensitivity is due to events occurring central to the receptor, perhaps at the receptor-bipolar junction.

Consider the threshold for the detection of an increment of light against a large illuminated background field: The threshold becomes higher as the background is made more intense. Crawford (1947) concluded that immediately following a light-adaptation flash, the subject had an *equivalent background* light in his field of view, even in total darkness. This background reduced his sensitivity to the target spots of light. Similarly, Rushton (1963) suggested that every bleached rhodopsin molecule emits a continuous signal of *dark light* which has the effect of increasing the brightness of the background. This suggestion is related to the familiar positive afterimage. If a bright flash is presented to a subject in a dark room, a bright afterimage will continue long after the stimulus is removed. Rushton is saying simply that we are less sensitive after the flash because we are forced to detect the test flash against the bright background of the positive afterimage. As the rhodopsin molecules regenerate they stop emitting dark-light signals, the positive afterimage decays in brightness, and we regain visual sensitivity. But just how does the brightness of the afterimage decay?

Barlow and Sparrock (1964) obtained a series of measurements of the brightness of positive afterimages as a function of time. The unfilled symbols in Figure 7.4 show their results. The circles represent brightness measurements following a flash that bleaches about 80 percent of the rhodopsin, the triangles represent about 20-percent bleach, and the squares represent about 2-percent bleach. The filled symbols represent the predicted brightness of the afterimage as derived from sensitivity losses following the various degrees of bleaching. The fact that the filled and unfilled symbols fall along the same curve supports the equivalent-background and dark-light hypotheses.

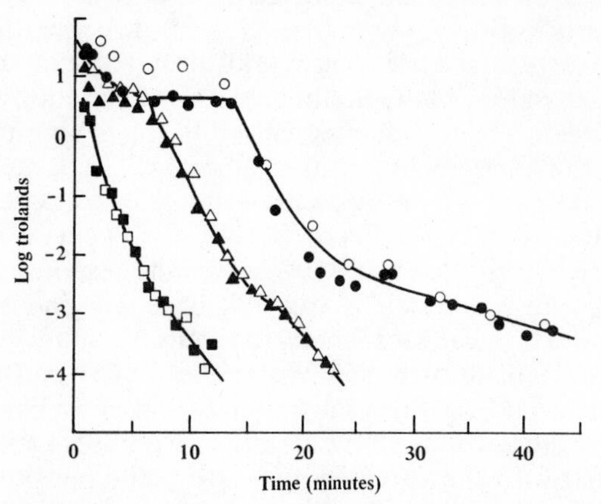


**Figure 7.4** The luminance of a positive afterimage (filled symbols) as a function of time elapsed since the bleaching flash. The unfilled symbols depict the luminance of a veiling light needed to induce a loss in sensitivity equal to that found after such a bleaching flash. The more rightward curves represent the effects of more complete bleaches. (From Barlow & Sparrock, 1964.)

## Light adaptation

When a brightly illuminated field is first viewed steadily by a dark adapted eye, it appears to become progressively darker. One way of measuring this effect is by the *binocular matching technique*, in which one eye is presented with the steadily illuminated field while the other eye is kept in darkness. At periodic intervals, a matching field is briefly presented to the dark adapted eye and the subject varies the luminance of that field until the two fields appear to be of equal brightness. Craik (1940) found that if light adaptation is allowed to proceed for 2 or 3 minutes, then the steadily illuminated field, whatever its objective level of luminance, is equivalent in brightness to a matching field of about 3 footLamberts (ftL). This perfect adaptation holds over the photopic range of 15,000 ftL. Other workers, however, have not obtained such perfect adaptation, except at very high intensities (cf. Stevens & Stevens, 1963).

This finding has an interesting implication. Suppose one fixates steadily a dark bar, 1 ftL in luminance, surrounded by a bright field of 1000 ftL. At first the subjective contrast of the bar against its background will be strong. But since both the bar and its background come to have the same apparent brightness, the contrast will reduce to zero and the bar will disappear from view. Troxler (1804) was probably the first to note that objects that are viewed steadily disappear from sight, particularly in the periphery of the visual field. Like other aspects of light adaptation, the duration of viewing required before objects disappear is independent of the intensity of the stimulus. Such independence must mean that the *Troxler phenomenon* is in large measure not attributable to the bleaching of visual pigment, but to neural factors. In Clarke's (1957) experiment on light adaptation, a 5° stimulus of low contrast, presented 20° from the fovea and viewed steadily, disappeared in about 6 seconds. Pirenne (1962b) calculated from the intensity of the stimulus that disappearance occurred after only 1/12 of the rods received 1 quantum. Thus, since disappearance occurred before most receptors received any light at all, the effect must be in large part neural rather than photochemical.

## The detection of brightness differences between visual stimuli

A basic measurement in vision is the threshold for brightness differences between two spatial loci of the visual field. One way this measurement can be obtained is by having a subject fixate an adapting field on which a smaller disc of light is briefly superimposed. The subject is then asked whether he detected the increment. The size of the increment, that is, the intensity of the smaller disc, is varied.

Representative results of measurements of the incremental brightness threshold are shown in Figure 7.5. As might have been predicted, the frequency of positive responses increases as the energy of the increment, $\Delta I$, increases. The family of curves is obtained by varying the background illuminance, $I$. It is more difficult to detect an increment when the background is brighter, as reflected in the rightward displacement of the ogives as the intensity of the background increases. The effect is a large one. When the log of background intensity $I$ has a value of $-1.45$ (an illuminance of about 1/500 the reference level), then an increment must be $-0.3$ (about 1/5000 trolands). When the log of background intensity $I$ is raised to 4.45, making it 10,000 times more intense, a log increment of $+3.5$ (about 5000 trolands) is needed. Hence the magnitude of the increment ($\Delta I$) is some 3.8 log units greater, or about 10,000 times more energy is needed, against the more intense background than against the dim background.

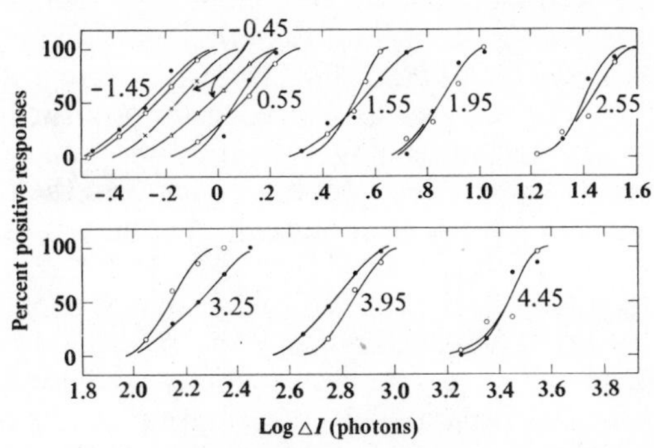


**Figure 7.5** Frequency-of-seeing curves for one subject are shown. Percentage of positive responses as a function of the increment in retinal illuminance. Each cluster of curves is obtained with a background of different luminous intensity (−1.45, −0.45, 0.55 up to 4.45 representing the logarithm of the background luminance). (From Mueller, 1951.)

Note that the relative increase of $I$ and $\Delta I$ is the same.

As discussed in Chapter 2, the observation that the just noticeable difference, or jnd (here $\Delta I$), is proportional to the stimulus magnitude, $I$, led to the formulation of *Weber's law,* which states that

$$\frac{\Delta I}{I} = k. \qquad [5]$$

According to Weber's law, $\Delta I$ is a constant proportion of $I$. To test the law for the data in Figure 7.5, it is convenient to express the equation logarithmically:

$$\log \Delta I - \log I = \log k.$$

For the sets of values given here we have

$$(-0.3) - (-1.45) = \log k$$
$$+1.15 = \log k \text{ at the lower luminance}$$

and

$$(3.5) - (+4.45) = \log k$$
$$+0.95 = \log k \text{ at the higher luminance}$$

Clearly, log $k$ is constant to a first approximation, though not perfectly so.

A better test of the law requires many more combinations of $\Delta I$ and $I$. These values can be obtained by drawing a horizontal line through Figure 7.5 at some particular frequency of seeing, say, 50 percent, to give one point of intersection on each ogive. This point gives the $\Delta I$ value at which the increment against one particular background value $I$ was detected 50 percent of the time. Taking these pairs of values to form the ratio $\Delta I/I$, and plotting log $\Delta I/I$ as a function of log $I$, we obtain Figure 7.6, which is a customary plot of increment threshold data. (Note that the data in this figure are for a different, although similar, set of data than shown in Figure 7.5.) Weber's law predicts horizontal lines, but clearly this is not the case. Rather, the Weber ratio diminishes (the subject becomes relatively more sensitive) as the background intensity increases. Nevertheless, between 2 and 5 log units, the curve is approximately horizontal, and over that range Weber's law remains a useful approximation. Note that as the intensity of the background increases from −4 to −1 log units there is a rapid improvement which then tapers off at about −0.5 log $I$, followed by a second branch of the curve with initially rapid improvement and again a tapering off. Once more the eye's duplex mechanism is at work: The initial branch of the curve applies to very dim backgrounds where vision is mediated entirely by rods, while the rightward branch applies to bright backgrounds where vision is mediated by cones. That the two branches are attributable to rods and cones is apparent from the fact that the two branches appear only when an area outside the fovea is tested; when the increment spot is placed entirely within the fovea, where there are only cone receptors, only the lower branch is found (Steinhardt, 1936; Stiles & Crawford, 1934).

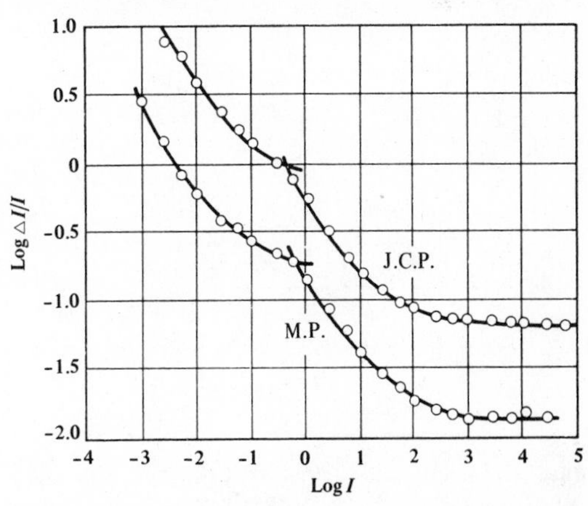


**Figure 7.6** The logarithm of the Weber ratio, $\Delta I/I$, as a function of the logarithm of the background luminance. Data are for two subjects, M.P. and J.C.P. (From Hecht, Peskin, & Patt, 1938.)

*Varying the test increment*

As the level of background illumination is reduced, the measurement of the differential threshold becomes increasingly similar to, and finally identical with, the measurement of the absolute threshold. It is not surprising then to find that parameters such as the duration, size, wavelength, and retinal position of the test patch affect the differential threshold in the same manner as the absolute threshold.

With regard to temporal integration, for example, Graham and Kemp (1938) presented increment flashes of different durations against background fields. Figure 7.7 indicates that for short test-flash durations the product of duration ($t$) and intensity (log $\Delta I$) needed to obtain a particular frequency of seeing is constant. The horizontal portions of the curves represent stimulus ranges wherein Bloch's law applies (i.e., perfect temporal integration). We see that the law applies even when the increment is superimposed on fairly bright backgrounds (log $I = 2.27$), but the critical duration decreases as the background luminance increases. At log $I = -2.73$, the critical duration is nearly 10 msec (log $t = -1.0$); at log $I = +2.27$, the critical duration is about 30 msec. With flashes longer than the critical period, the curves of the product of $t$ and log $\Delta I$ have an upward slope of +1.0. A slope of +1 means there is no temporal integration at all beyond the critical duration. In other words, beyond the critical duration the intensity of the test flash needed for a particular level of detection is independent of duration.

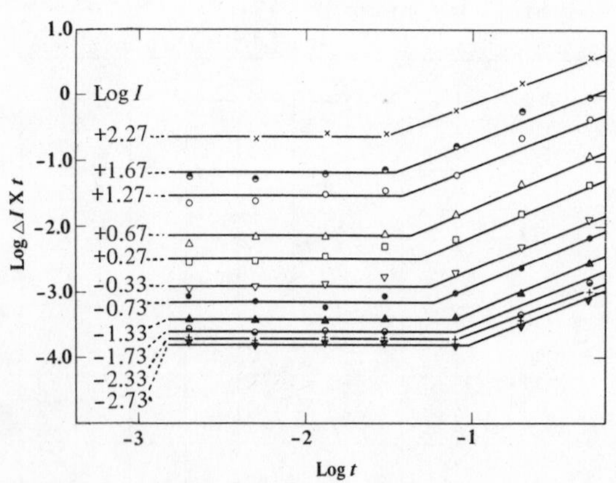


**Figure 7.7** The relationship between the total energy of a threshold test stimulus (the product of $\Delta I$ and exposure time $t$) and its duration ($t$). Each curve represents a different level of background luminance. Where the lines are horizontal, the equation $\Delta I \times t = k$ applies. (From Graham & Kemp, 1938.)

Spatial integration is also a factor, and the size of the test field is an important parameter in the detection of brightness differences. As the size of the test increment flash increases, so does sensitivity to brightness differences. The ratio $\Delta I/I$ gets smaller owing to the eye's ability to integrate information spatially. Representative results are those obtained by Heinz and Lippay (1928), which show that for equal frequency of seeing,

$$\frac{\log \Delta I}{\log \text{diameter}} = k. \qquad [6]$$

This statement is equivalent to Equation 2, indicating that Ricco's law is equally applicable whether the test flash is presented with the subject in darkness, or whether it is superimposed on a bright background.

*Varying the background field*

We have seen that if the intensity of the background field is varied, sensitivity to brightness differences can change over a very wide range. We have dealt thus far only with background fields maintained over relatively long periods of time. How is the detection of brightness differences affected at the moment the background is turned on or off? Presenting a bright background field for 0.5 sec, Crawford (1947) superimposed a 0.01-sec test flash at varying points in time. The test flash could be presented as much as 0.3 sec before the background was turned on, at various intervals nearer the time it was turned on, during the background presentation, at the time it was turned off, or after the background was turned off. Figure 7.8 shows that sensitivity is least (i.e., threshold is highest) during transient conditions, when the background is just being turned on or off.

### Theories of differential brightness detection

Why does absolute sensitivity to brightness differences range so widely? Why does Weber's law apply over the upper range of background intensities? Why are we not always equally sensitive to some absolute increment in quantum impingement regardless of the background field? In other words, why isn't $\Delta I = k$? To answer these questions, a knowledge of the mechanism of differential brightness detection is needed.

*Photochemical bleach model*

Hecht's (1937) theory ascribed the reduction in absolute sensitivity at high levels of background illumination to photochemical bleaching and explained why there is less photopigment in the receptors of the eye when the subject views such a bright background. According to Hecht, a light will be detected when it causes at least a minimum amount of decomposition of visual pigment. High-intensity background fields, however, bleach so much photochemical pigment that much of the entering target light fails to be absorbed by the receptors. Hence, more light is needed to attain the minimum level of bleaching required for detection, and the subject is therefore less sensitive, in absolute terms, to the detection of brightness differences.

When the intensity of the background field is high in the photopic range, Hecht's theory is important because considerable bleaching of visual pigment does occur. For example, Rushton (1958) measured the amount of visual pigment in the living human eye and demonstrated that with background fields of high intensity the amount of visual pigment is considerably reduced. But, as we shall see, it is not a sufficient model even in the upper intensity ranges.

Hecht's theory fails more severely in the lower and middle ranges of background intensities. Pirenne (1962a) calculated that with a background field of an intensity high enough to just begin to involve cones, bleaching occurs at a rate of only 1.5 percent of visual pigment per hour. This rate is hardly sufficient to support Hecht's theory.

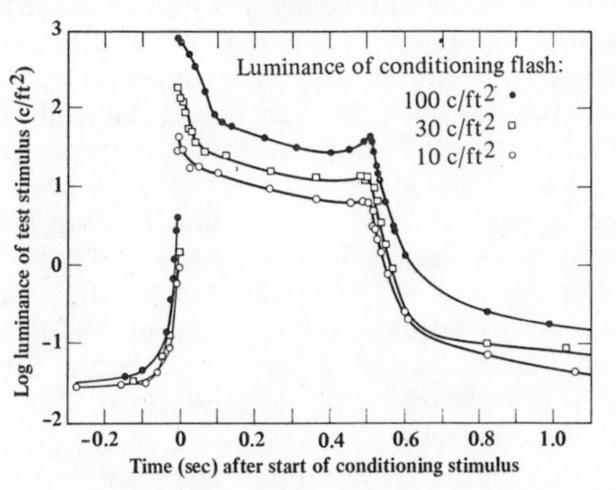


**Figure 7.8** The effect of a 0.5-second presentation of an adapting (conditioning) luminance on the detection of a brief test flash. (From Crawford, 1947.)

*Quantum fluctuation model*

This model as applied to brightness discrimination attempts to explain some of the facts of sensitivity to differences in luminance on the basis of the physical properties of light (Barlow, 1958; Barlow & Sparrock, 1964; DeVries, 1943; Rose, 1942, 1948). Such an explanation applies equally to the human eye and to physical photodetectors. As explained in the appendix, light is emitted and absorbed in photons. Each emission or absorption of a photon is a probabilistic event that is independent of all other emissions and absorptions. When one sets the intensity of a lamp, one actually determines the average rate of photon emission by the source and the average rate of photon impingement on the retina. Since at any moment a single emission or a single photon impingement is probabilistic, the actual number of photons impinging on the retina at any moment can vary considerably from the average rate. The probability distribution is a Poisson distribution which, in turn, is approximated by a normal distribution with a standard deviation equal to the square root of the average rate. We will assume for the present argument that if the intensity of the source is such as to cause an average rate of $X$ quanta to impinge on the retina, then the distribution of moment-to-moment impingements will be a normal distribution with a mean of $X$ and a standard deviation of $\sqrt{X}$.

In Figure 7.9A the subject's task is to detect increments in light $\Delta I$ presented against a large background of luminance $X$. We want to consider what happens when the intensity of the background changes. Values along the abscissa represent the number of photons impinging on the retina at any moment, and the ordinate values represent the frequency with which these events occur. Let us consider a catch trial (labeled *N trial* in the figure), in which the subject views the background disc and the experimenter does not deliver a stimulus. The subject's task is to say whether a flash was or was not presented. The *N*-trial distribution shows that on the average $X$ photons are impinging on the retina every second. The distribution is normal and has a standard deviation of $\sqrt{X}$. Thus, from what

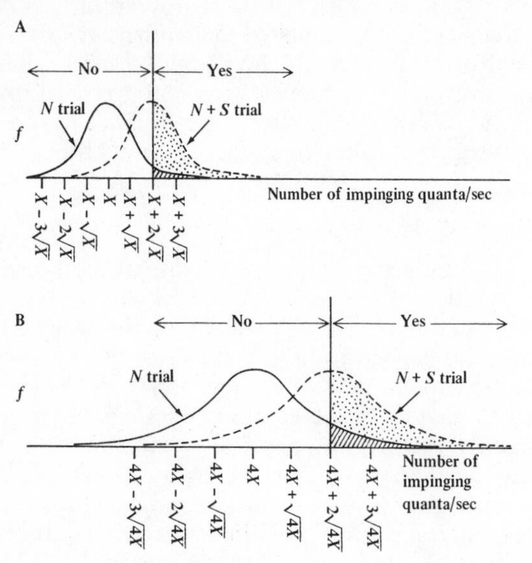


**Figure 7.9** Quantum fluctuation model. The effect of background luminance on the distribution of the rate of impinging quanta. See text for discussion.

we know about the area under the normal curve, 50 percent of the time $X$ or more photons will have impinged during 1 second; about 15 percent of the time (1 standard deviation above the mean) more than $X + \sqrt{X}$ photons will have impinged during 1 second; about 2.3 percent of the time (2 standard deviations above the mean) more than $X + 2\sqrt{X}$ photons will have impinged during 1 second, and so on. Since the effects of random fluctuations are indistinguishable from the effects of actual experimental stimuli, no matter how cautious the subject is he must sometimes say that a visual stimulus was presented on the catch trial (i.e., give a yes response). If the subject says yes whenever he has a visual sensation equivalent to one elicited by $X + \sqrt{X}$ photons or more, then he will make errors of the *false positive* type 15 percent of the time. The subject wanting to make fewer false positive errors can do so by requiring a more intense visual sensation before he says yes. If the subject decides he will say yes only when he experiences a visual sensation equal to the effect of $X + 2\sqrt{X}$ impinging photons per second, then he will give false positives only 2.3 percent of the time. The value $X + 2\sqrt{X}$ is the criterion level set by the hypothetical subject illustrated in Figure 7.9A.

On a trial where signal plus noise is presented ($N + S$ *trial*) this subject will give a 50 percent frequency of seeing when the experimenter presents a visual stimulus with an intensity of $2\sqrt{X}$, as shown by the stippled area under the $N + S$ curve in Figure 7.9A. The distribution $N + S$ depicts the frequency of different numbers of photons impinging on the retina when a light stimulus is actually presented. With a stimulus of $2\sqrt{X}$, the subject will say no 50 percent of the time when the experimenter did in fact present a stimulus (unshaded area under the $N + S$ distribution). Without changing the subject's criterion level, the experimenter can, of course, guarantee a higher proportion of yes responses merely by raising the intensity of stimulation. For example, if the experimenter presents a stimulus $3\sqrt{X}$ average photons per second, then the subject will say yes 85 percent of the time.

If the subject wants to reduce his false positives, perhaps because some penalty is attached to saying yes incorrectly, he can do so by requiring a more intense sensation before saying yes. But the penalty paid is a loss of apparent sensitivity. For example, if the subject will tolerate only a 0.2 percent rate of false positives, then his criterion level must be 3 standard deviations above the mean of the noise distribution. In turn, he will achieve only a 50 percent frequency of seeing when the experimenter uses a stimulus of intensity $3\sqrt{X}$. To achieve the same frequency of seeing as that before he changed his criterion level, the subject will now require a stimulus 50 percent more intense than previously. In other words, the subject who becomes more conservative about saying yes makes fewer false positive errors but now makes more *false negative* errors by more frequently saying that a visual stimulus was not presented on the last trial, when in fact a stimulus was presented. A more complete analysis of the strategies of perceiving has been presented by Swets, Tanner, and Birdsall (1961) and is also discussed in Chapter 2.

We are now ready to consider the effect of increasing background intensity on the detection of light flashes. The situation is described in Figure 7.9B. For illustrative purposes we show a fourfold increase in background intensity. In the absence of any momentary flash, photons from the steady background of intensity $4X$ impinge on the subject's retina. Thus, the mean of the $N$ distribution is displaced to the right (compared to panel A) in order to depict a higher total effective rate of impinging photons. This displacement is less crucial, however, than the broadening of the $N$ distribution. The standard deviation has increased to $\sqrt{4X}$. The effect of this increase is that the subject who will tolerate only a 2.3-percent level of false positives must still place his detection criterion 2 standard deviations above the mean of the *no signal* ($N$) distribution. Thus the subject's criterion level is now at $4X + 2\sqrt{4X}$ photons per second, so that the experimenter must use a stimulus ($\Delta I$) which will deliver $2\sqrt{4X}$ quanta per second.

The effect of introducing a brighter background field should now be clear. With background illumination of $X$ quanta per second a subject whose criterion level results in 2.3 percent false positives will have a 50 percent frequency of seeing when the stimulus intensity ($\Delta I$) is $2\sqrt{X}$ quanta per second. The same subject with the same criterion level but with a background field impinging an average of $4X$ quanta per second on his retina will need a stimulus that averages $2\sqrt{4X}$ impinging quanta per second to achieve the same 50 percent frequency of seeing. Since $\sqrt{4X}$ is larger than $\sqrt{X}$ it is clear that the quantum fluctuation model predicts a drop in absolute sensitivity as the intensity of the background field is increased. More specifically, since $\sqrt{4X} = 2\sqrt{X}$, we see that a fourfold increase in background intensity leads to a twofold increase in the intensity of an incremental stimulus necessary to maintain criterion level. More generally, we see the quantum fluctuation model predicts a square-root law:

$$\frac{\Delta I}{\sqrt{I}} = k. \qquad [7]$$

Barlow (1957) isolated some of the conditions under which the quantum fluctuation model operates (giving a square-root law, $\Delta I/I^{1/2} = k$) and those under which Weber's law operates (giving $\Delta I/I = k$). Figure 7.10 shows that on a graph plotting log $\Delta I$ against log $I$, the quantum fluctuation model predicts a slope of +0.5, while Weber's law predicts a positive slope of +1.0. The data points reveal first that at very low levels of background luminance, 3 log units or less, neither model is appropriate because the slopes are horizontal; that is, at low levels of background brightness, the threshold is independent of the background. Then there is a middle range of background intensities, 3 to 7 log units, where the threshold for a short and small $\Delta I$ flash (filled circles) is closely predicted by the quantum model; the threshold for a long and large $\Delta I$ flash (unfilled circles) is, however, better predicted by Weber's law. Finally, at a range of background intensities above 7 log units, Weber's law operates no matter how brief or small $\Delta I$ is.

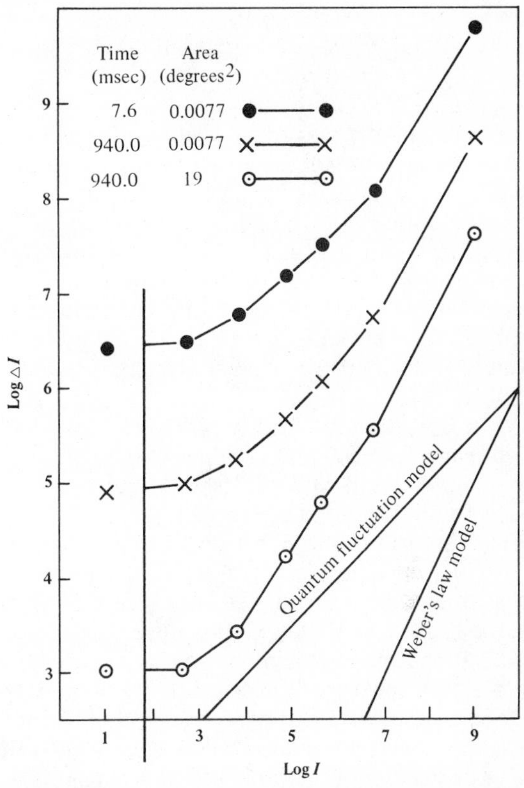


**Figure 7.10** The differential brightness threshold (log $\Delta I$) as a function of the intensity of the background on which the flash is superimposed. Filled circles indicate a small test stimulus of short duration; crosses indicate a small test stimulus of long duration; and unfilled circles indicate a large test stimulus of long duration. Lines at the lower right-hand corner indicate the slopes predicted from a quantum fluctuation model and from a Weber's law model. Data for one subject are shown. (From Barlow, 1957.)

Let us consider the first empirical deviation from the quantum fluctuation model. Why should $\Delta I$ become independent of background intensities when the background is made dim? Suppose that within the eye a certain amount of *visual noise* is generated that is indistinguishable from activity generated by a light stimulus. This visual noise could arise from random quanta generated within the eye, since the eye is a *black-body radiator* at 96.4° F, or from spontaneous breakdowns of visual pigments such as rhodopsin, or even from spontaneous action potentials generated within the axons of the visual system. Whatever the source, this internally generated noise is formally identical to the external background described in the quantum fluctuation model, except of course that it is not under the control of the experimenter. Fechner (1860), in a similar vein, spoke of an *Augengrau,* and thus anticipated the notion that it is intrinsic retinal noise that places a lower limit on the absolute threshold. We have an explanation, now, for the empirical fact that more than 1 quantum is required for above-chance levels of seeing in an absolute threshold experiment (Hecht, Shlaer, & Pirenne, 1942).

Note that Barlow's (1957) experiment provides us with an actual estimate of what the magnitude of this "equivalent dark light" should be: It should correspond in luminance to the brightest background intensity at which the three functions in Figure 7.10 are horizontal, roughly a little under 3 log units. Barlow estimated that this dark light, internally generated in the human eye, has a value equal to the impingement on the retina of 1000 quanta (at a wavelength of 507 nm) per second per degree$^2$ of visual angle. It is interesting that Kuffler, Fitzhugh, and Barlow (1957) noted considerable activity in the optic nerve fibers of a cat in darkness.

The second deviation from the quantum fluctuation model appears with either long or large $\Delta I$ flashes or with intense background luminances. Under these conditions, Weber's law operates.

*Weber's law model*

We have seen that under photopic conditions the increment threshold is proportional to the intensity of the background:

$$\frac{\Delta I}{I} = k. \qquad [5]$$

A number of models have been proposed to predict Weber functions (e.g., Koenderink, van de Grind, & Bouman, 1970; Sperling & Sondhi, 1968). Although it is not possible to discuss these theories here in satisfactory detail, they can be characterized as follows. It is usually assumed that the visual system includes a decision stage where an impact of specified size must be registered before the subject will say that he sees the $\Delta I$ increment. The effect of a short $\Delta I$ flash on the visual system is as if the increment were divided by the steady-state background intensity on which it is superimposed. The general idea, then, is quite simple: Weber's law involves the division of $\Delta I$ by $I$ to obtain a constant; the visual system works like an analog computer to perform an analogous internal division operation. The proposed mechanisms usually involve inhibitory feedback networks (Fuortes & Hodgkin, 1964; Koenderink et al., 1970). The anatomical studies of the retina suggest many possible locations for such networks, but interest has been focused on the most peripheral connections, those at the receptor-bipolar junctions.

Recent neurophysiological evidence supports the surmise that the Weber function is generated within the visual receptors themselves (Boynton & Whitten, 1970). They used Brown and Watanabe's (1962) technique to isolate a receptor potential from monkey photoreceptors. Basically, a very small electrode is introduced in the eye of an anesthetized monkey and positioned so that it records electrical activity from surrounding photoreceptors. Then the circulation of blood to bipolars and ganglion cells is cut off so that only photoreceptors are left operating. Now when a light flash impinges on the retina, it probably generates electrical activity (receptor potential) solely in the photoreceptor. The voltage generated by these photoreceptors—specifically, foveal cones—is generally thought to be directly related to the generation of a neural response in succeeding stages of the visual system. In their experiment, Boynton and Whitten closely followed the incremental threshold paradigm: The eye tested was adapted to a particular background intensity. Then a brief incremental flash was presented and the voltage generated by the photoreceptor at the electrode was measured. The intensity of the incremental flash was increased until the receptors gave a standard response of 10 microvolts. This procedure was repeated over a wide range of background intensities. One set of results is shown by the filled circles in Figure 7.11. Note that the diagonal linear portion of the curve has a slope of +1 on a log-log plot. This means that Weber's law originates within or among individual photoreceptors, within the very mechanism that generates the receptor potentials.

The unfilled circles in Figure 7.11 show the results obtained when Boynton and Whitten substituted a human subject for the monkey photoreceptors and measured incremental thresholds with various background intensities. They obtained a similar function.

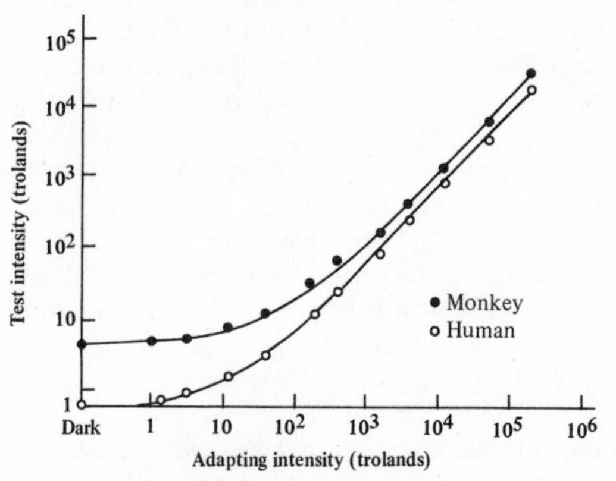


**Figure 7.11** Filled circles indicate the log intensity of a test flash necessary to obtain a standard response (10 microvolts) from the late receptor potential from the cones of a monkey's eye. The horizontal axis plots the log intensity of the background against which the flash was presented. The unfilled circles depict the results of an identical experimental paradigm applied to a human subject, except that the standard response is the subject's psychophysical threshold. In both cases, a steady background light was presented to the eye, allowing sufficient time for a stable voltage to be reached. Then, incremental flashes 150-msec long were added. The monkey data represent means from six subjects. (From Boynton & Whitten, 1970.)

As shown in Figure 7.12, the output of a cone photoreceptor increases as stimulus intensity increases about 2 log units. Beyond that, the receptor saturates and its output no longer increases. This is shown in the horizontal slopes of the functions in Figure 7.12. Therefore, without negative feedback the receptors would not transmit information about the environment beyond 2 log units. In other words, by effectively dividing the $\Delta I$ increment by the steady-state background, as the Weber's law function implies, the receptor is once more affected by the $\Delta I$ flash on the sensitive portion of its dynamic range. The effect of negative feedback operating on the cone photoreceptor is to allow the visual system to work sensitively over an enormous dynamic range, using sensory transducers of more limited range. Presumably, that is the reason for Weber's law.

To summarize, brightness discrimination obeys at least two laws, but neither one alone is sufficient to explain the whole range of phenomena. With fairly dim backgrounds and with test flashes short enough and small enough so that essentially perfect spatial and temporal integration holds, the quantum fluctuation model applies. Beyond these limits, where cone photoreceptors play an increasing role, the eye becomes progressively less efficient in utilizing the full amount of energy entering the eye during the flash. Through a range of such upper values, Weber's law appears to hold. Weber's law seems to result from negative feedback mechanisms operating at the photoreceptors themselves.

## Apparent brightness

How bright is an object? Although a seemingly simple question, scientifically it is a question fraught with methodological pitfalls. All the visual phenomena discussed here (with the exception of color naming described briefly later in this chapter) can in principle be reduced to a situation in which a subject is unable to make a visual discrimination involving a simple yes or no response. The reader should satisfy himself, after a bit of thought on the matter, that this applies to absolute thresholds, differential thresholds, and to color mixtures. But asking a subject to estimate subjective brightness cannot be so reduced because we are not testing the subject's visual capacity. We are requesting the subject to give an arithmetical opinion regarding his sensation. We assume that his arithmetical responses constitute a scale methodologically equiv-

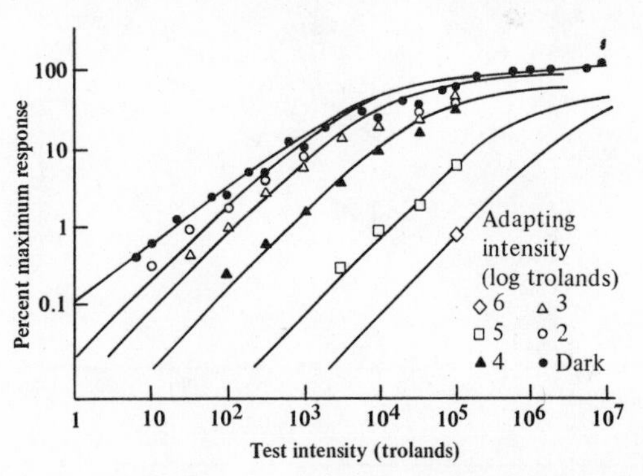


**Figure 7.12** Same experiment represented by filled circles in Figure 7.11. The relative magnitude of the receptor potential as a function of the intensity of the flash is shown. Each curve depicts a different level of background intensity. The drawn curves are theoretical. (From Boynton & Whitten, 1970.)

alent to a yardstick, which is a very substantial assumption. For example, in one such study the psychophysical method of magnitude estimation was used (Stevens & Stevens, 1963; see also Chapter 2). Subjects were presented a standard patch of light (−3.6 log lamberts in luminance) to their left eye, and were told that this stimulus had a subjective brightness arbitrarily equal to 10 units. Then test stimuli that varied in physical intensity were shown to their right eye. The subjects assigned numbers to these test stimuli, using the stimulus to the left eye as a standard. Subjects can do this without great difficulty. Pooling the results of a number of subjects in two different studies yielded a plot such as that shown in Figure 7.13. The ordinate represents the logarithm of the subjects' magnitude estimations. The abscissa represents log intensity of the stimulus.

The main finding from these two independent studies is that the points fall along a straight line on a log-log plot, with a slope of about +0.33. To judge from these results, subjective brightness grows as a *power function* of the stimulus:

$$\Psi = k(L - L_0)^{0.33}, \qquad [8]$$

where $\Psi$ is the estimated strength of the visual sensation (in units of *brils*), $k$ is a constant, $L$ is the luminance of the stimulus in question, and $L_0$ is the luminance of the stimulus at threshold.

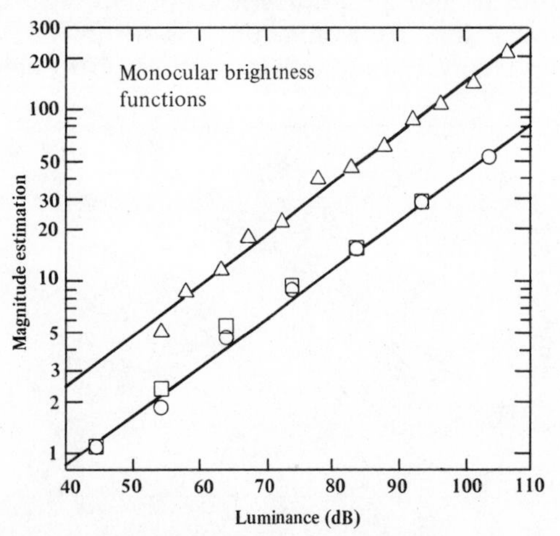


**Figure 7.13** Subjective brightness functions obtained by a direct magnitude estimation procedure. The triangles are from an experiment by Onley (cited in Stevens & Stevens, 1963) and the circles and squares were obtained from Stevens and Stevens' (1963) experiment. The procedure is described in the text. (From Stevens & Stevens, 1963.)

Suppose, as an expert in vision, you were consulted by an industrial firm. Reporting the luminance of a working surface—say, a metal lathe—to be $L_1$ mL, they want the surface to be psychologically or subjectively twice as bright to the lathe operator. Must they raise the physical energy twice as much in order to accomplish this goal? Let us use the power function. The original brightness, $\Psi_1$, is given by

$$\Psi_1 = k(L_1 - L_0)^{0.33}.$$

Then the surface that is twice as bright, $\Psi_2$, is given by

$$\Psi_2 = 2\Psi_1 = k(L_2 - L_0)^{0.33},$$

where $L_2$ is the quantity we seek, the physical energy of the brighter surface. Combining the two equations gives us

$$2k(L_1 - L_0)^{0.33} = k(L_2 - L_0)^{0.33},$$

which simplifies algebraically to

$$2^3 = 8 = \frac{L_2 - L_0}{L_1 - L_0}.$$

In other words, where $L_1$ and $L_2$ are large with respect to the threshold luminance $L_0$, we must raise the physical intensity by a factor of 8 in order to double the apparent brightness. More generally, the exponent of 0.33 in the power function means we must raise physical intensity to the third power of the subjective change we desire. If we want to increase a sensation 5 times, we must raise physical intensity 125 times.

There are several reasons why Stevens' power function has gained increasing acceptance by researchers in vision, even though the data on which it is based are highly subjective. First of all, the results are surprisingly simple. Simple, orderly functions inspire scientific confidence. Second, a variety of procedures have been used besides magnitude estimation and they yield essentially the same results. Third, it has been found that the receptor potential generated in the eye also follows a power function of stimulus intensity over certain ranges (Stevens, 1970). Such was the case in the measurements of Boynton & Whitten (1970) mentioned earlier. However, whereas the exponent of the power function for human subjects is 0.33, the exponent derived from photoreceptor potentials in the monkey is 0.70. Does this mean subjects in their verbal responses underestimate strong sensations and overestimate weak ones? Or is it too much to expect subjective judgments to be related to the stimulus in just the same way as single-unit responses in the sensory system? (See Chapters 1 and 2 for further discussion.)

### The effect of a contour on brightness discrimination

It is more difficult to see one brightness discontinuity when it is brought near another brightness discontinuity. Fry and Bartley (1935) tested the detection of a bright flash superimposed on a large background field. When they surrounded the test spot by a dark annulus, the detection of the spot became more difficult. The closer the annulus was brought to the test spot, the higher the detection threshold. Generally when a spot of light is brought near an edge between a light and a darker figure, the spot becomes more difficult to detect.

### Simultaneous contrast

How would one arrange a situation so as to see the darkest black color? Since we see the brightest white when exposed to a bright flash, one might conclude that the darkest black is seen in a darkroom where one is exposed to the minimum quantity of light. In fact, in a room as totally devoid of light quanta as is practical to arrange, we do not see a good dark black at all, but a gray. That, of course, is the phenomenological correlate of the *Augengrau* we have inferred theoretically in our discussion of the absolute and differential threshold. As most painters know, the best way to obtain a deep black is to place dark pigment very near white pigment. Black is the color we see when a strongly illuminated patch of retina exerts an inhibitory effect on an adjoining patch not as intensely illuminated; we see deep black only as a result of *simultaneous contrast*.

Contrast is usually measured by presenting two stimulus fields, the test field and the matching field, as far away from each other as feasible. The subject adjusts the luminance of the matching field until the two fields look equally bright. Frequently, the two fields are presented one to each eye in order to minimize their effects on one another. The *dichoptic* presentation assures little retinal interaction between the two. Then, contrast is created by surrounding the test field with a bright field called the *inducing field*. As a result, the test field looks dimmer. The amount of brightness contrast can be estimated by how much the subject diminishes the intensity of the matching field to regain a brightness match with the test field. The results of such an experiment (Heinemann, 1955) are shown in Figure 7.14. Each line represents a single test-field luminance. The abscissa depicts the luminance of the inducing field, and the ordinate depicts the luminance of the comparison field when set equal in brightness to the test field. Considering the rightmost curve, a test field of 1.55 log luminance (mL), we see that increasing the log luminance of the inducing field from $-\infty$ to 0 has

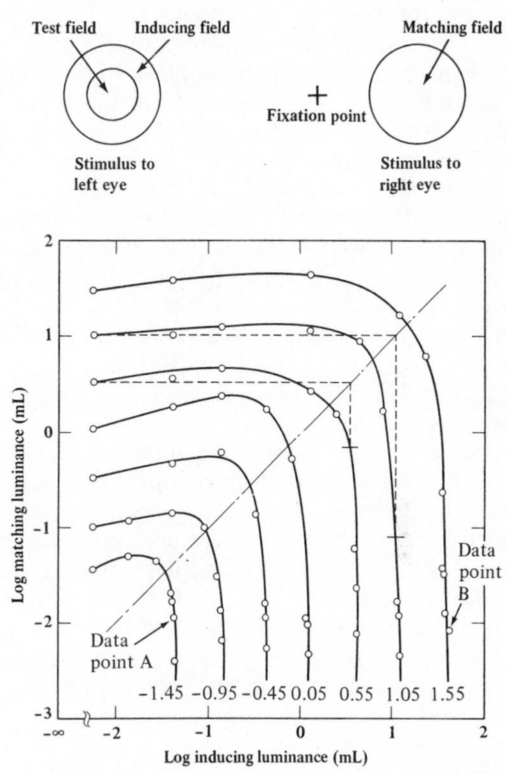


**Figure 7.14** Simultaneous contrast. A disc test field is surrounded by an annulus, here called the inducing field. The two are presented to different eyes. When the inducing field, which surrounds the test field, is made more intense, it makes the test field look dimmer. The physical intensity of the matching field must then be decreased to obtain a match with the test field. The figure depicts these changes in the luminance of the matching field as a function of increases in the luminance of the inducing field. (After Heinemann, 1955.)

little effect on the brightness of the test field except perhaps to enhance it slightly. But when the inducing-field luminance approaches and then exceeds the luminance of the test field, the apparent brightness of the latter diminishes precipitously.

As has been found in other studies, Figure 7.14 shows no dimming effect on the test field until the inducing field exceeds the test field in brightness (cf. Diamond, 1953). Expressed a bit differently, bright patches cause dimmer ones to look even dimmer (data points below the diagonal), but dim patches do not dim bright ones (data points above the diagonal); the contrast effect is asymmetrical.

Another interesting aspect of the data in Figure 7.14 has to do with the appearance of pairs of stimuli of some given luminance ratio. If we take a test field of −1.45 log luminance (the leftmost curve in Figure 7.14) and place near it an inducing field of −1.35 (1/10 log unit added luminance), the test field appears to equal the brightness of a −2.5 matching field. In other words, making the inducing field only 1/10 log unit brighter dims the test field by one whole log unit. Furthermore, the precipitous drop at higher inducing-field luminances means that tiny differences in the ratio between the inducing field and the test field lead to very large differences in appearance. Contrast enhances the psychological effect of edges and contours in our visual field.

But there is an even more surprising fact that can be gleaned from Heinemann's (1955) data. Take, for example, the two data points A and B, which are listed in Table 7.1 after being converted from log milliLamberts to actual milliLamberts. In the A condition a .0355 mL luminous disc is surrounded by an inducing-field annulus 1.25 times more intense. The test disc appears dimmer and is equated to a .01 mL comparison field. In the B condition the luminous disc is 100 times more intense than in A (3.55 mL) and is surrounded by an annulus 1.25 times more intense. This disc looks no brighter than the one in A; it also is matched to a .01 mL comparison field. In other words, we reach the surprising conclusion that within certain ranges the apparent brightness of an object is independent of its absolute luminance level, if only the ratio of intensities of that object to its surround is kept constant. Phrased differently, we can state that within certain ranges *brightness constancy* holds: The apparent brightness is a function of the luminance ratios between an object and its surround.

**Table 7.1**

| | Data points (mL) | |
|---|---|---|
| | A | B |
| Test field (mL) | 0.0355 | 3.55 |
| Inducing field (mL) | 0.0447 | 4.47 |
| Inducing-field–test-field ratio | 1.25 | 1.25 |
| Luminance of the comparison field (mL) when it matches the test field cited at top of column | 0.01 | 0.01 |

It is easy to see why brightness constancy is a very adaptive mechanism for the visual system. Using vision, we are more often interested in recognizing external objects than in appraising the level of illumination. Constant external objects present us with constant luminance ratios. Take for example a man who is wearing a black tie that reflects 10 percent of the impinging light and a white jacket that reflects 90 percent. He will be projected onto an observer's retina as, among other things, a pair of light patches with a 1 to 9 illumination ratio. This ratio remains invariant with all changes in the absolute amount of illumination (twilight, sun moving behind a cloud, etc.). Because of brightness constancy, his appearance will also remain constant despite large changes in illumination.

Brightness constancy is, no doubt, a manifestation of the same mechanism that causes simultaneous contrast. A considerable amount of neurophysiological research has been devoted to its elucidation (cf. Ratliff, 1965).

## ACUITY

When we ask what is the smallest object we can see, or the thinnest, or the smallest displacement of one object relative to another, we are asking about the resolving power, or *acuity*, of the visual system. Figure 7.15 shows, for example, that subject A can recognize the letter *C* at least 50 percent of the time when it has a gap of size *W* at distance *D*. The visual angle of the gap is equal to the arc tangent, $W/D$. If the letter *C* is 240 inches (20 feet) away and the gap is .07 inches, the tangent $W/D = .00029$. The visual angle is equal to the arc tangent of 0.0003 which is 1 minute of arc. Subject B needs a larger *C* with a correspondingly larger gap in order to make correct recognitions at least 50 percent of the

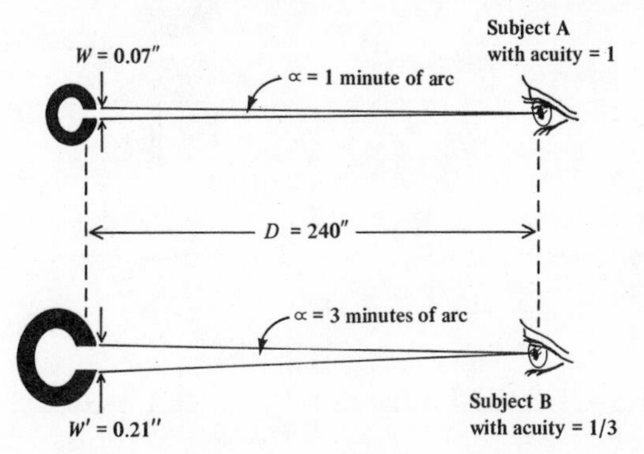


**Figure 7.15** A schematic drawing of the measurement of acuity using a Landolt *C*. The *C* is presented with the gap up, down, left, or right. A subject who can recognize the orientation of the gap in the *C* correctly 50 percent of the time when the gap is 1 minute of arc in width ($\alpha$) has an acuity of 1.0. The subject who needs a gap of 3 minutes of arc to attain a 50-percent rate of recognition has an acuity of 1/3.

time. If he needs a gap of .21 inches when the *C* is 20 feet away, then the tangent $W'/D = .0087$ and the visual angle is 3 minutes of arc. It seems reasonable to say that his acuity is three times poorer. Phrased differently, acuity is the reciprocal of the visual angle; that is, acuity = 1/arc tangent [$W/D$]. Hence, Subject A in Figure 7.15 has an acuity of 1 and Subject B has an acuity of 1/3.

Optometrists and ophthalmologists express acuity differently. Subject B recognizes an object at 20 feet with a gap of .21 inches (3 minutes of arc); a normal subject recognizes this same object when it is placed 60 feet away (arc tan [.21 inches/720 inches] = 1 minute of arc). The acuity of Subject B is therefore expressed as 20/60.

The particular value obtained in any acuity task is to a large extent determined by the nature of the task set for the subject. The four usual classes of acuity tasks are detection, recognition, resolution, and vernier acuity.

## Detection

In detection the subject reports whether a test object was present or absent during some specified interval of time. We have already considered the detection of a small, bright object on a dark surround.

Ricco's law states that for small targets, detection frequency remains constant as long as the product of area and intensity is held constant. In other words, as long as the mean number of photons impinging on the retina from the test object is kept constant, the size of the test object is immaterial. There is therefore no lower limit to the size of a bright object which we can detect. For example, many easily detected stars represent visual objects of infinitesimally small visual angles. The ones that appear larger are delivering more quanta more rapidly to our eyes, but they are not necessarily of larger visual angle. Conversely, those that are just detectable are not necessarily the smaller ones, but may be delivering only the few quanta needed at the absolute threshold of vision. In fact, in the appendix it is shown that a pinpoint of light is projected onto the retina as a disc, and that because of diffraction all very small dim objects are about 1.5 minutes of arc at the retina when the pupil is 3 mm wide.

If the task calls for the detection of a dark object on a white surround the results are quite different. No matter how black the object or how bright the background, there is a lower limit to the size of an object that can be detected. This phenomenon is attributable to diffraction.[2] Figure 7.16A illustrates how an opaque edge presented against an illuminated background is projected as a shadow on the retina. Note that the sharp geometrical light distribution in the stimulus is projected onto the retina as a gradient of light whose intensity decreases from nearly 100 percent to nearly 0 percent in approximately 2 minutes of arc (actually a distance of 10 microns on the retina, or $10^{-5}$ meters). The retinal image is spread out because of diffraction.

If, instead of an edge, the target is a wide black line, as in Figure 7.16B, then there are two gradients (one from each edge) which sum. Thus, if we could view the retina we should see a blurred shadowlike line with its darkest part in the center and with very blurred sides. In panels C and D the depth of the shadow diminishes as the black line is made thinner (even though the line stimulus is still quite as opaque). Note, however, that an object can be thinner than a single cone—as in panels C and D—and still throw a shadow on the retina that blurs across several cones. We can, in fact, see black lines against white surrounds even when they are surprisingly thin: We can detect a single dark line only 0.5 second of arc wide (Hecht & Mintz, 1939). This width corresponds to about .67 micron ($10^{-6}$

[2]See the Appendix to this chapter for further explanation.

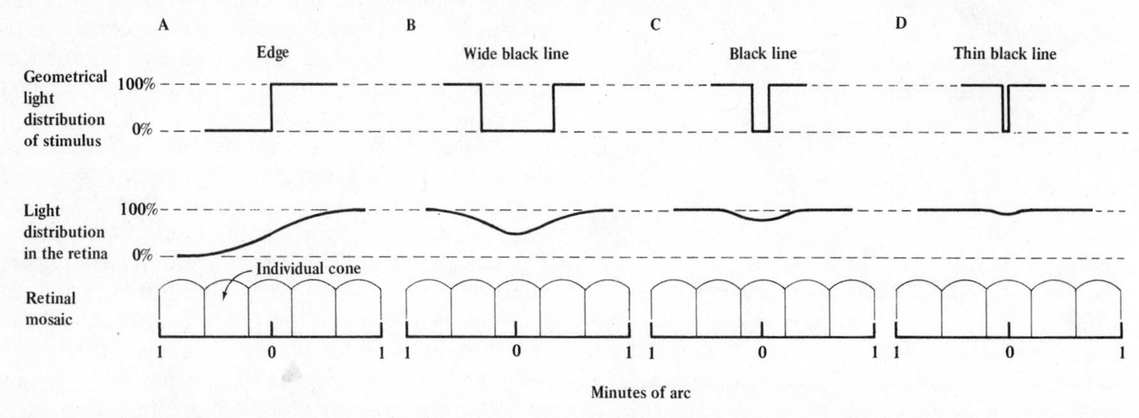


**Figure 7.16** Top: Distribution of luminance in the stimulus target of an edge or a black line against a white background. Bottom: Distribution of illumination in the retinal image of an edge or a black line against a white background. In B, C, and D, the black line is made increasingly thinner. The ordinate is the ratio of the intensity of light falling on a particular point within the target image to the intensity falling on points in the uniform background region surrounding the target image. The abscissa is the distance, in minutes of arc, from the center of the line image.

meters) at a distance of 25 cm, the width of some microorganisms, such as the anthrax bacillus, or a 1/4″-wide wire a mile away. It has been shown that a target of this width projects a thin shadow over an array of cones (Byram, 1944b; Hecht & Mintz, 1939). A cone over which the shadow passes will be illuminated only 1 percent less than a laterally adjoining cone over which the shadow does not pass. Considering the array of slightly more illuminated cones as the edge of a bipartite field (as in a brightness discrimination task), we see that 1 percent represents a Weber ratio, $\Delta I/I$, of 1/100. This ratio is just about the value obtained in the detection of a brightness difference in a large bipartite field under optimal conditions. The similarity in the value of the Weber ratio is the basis for believing that there is essentially no difference between the detection of a fine black line against a white surround and brightness discrimination. Therefore, the models of brightness discrimination previously described presumably account for detection acuity.

## Recognition

Recognition tasks are usually the most familiar because of their adoption for clinical determinations of acuity as in the Snellen chart of letters or the Landolt *C* (Cowan, 1928). With the Landolt *C* chart, the subject is faced with rows of *C*s in which the break in the circle can be either in the upper, lower, left, or right portion of the circle. The *C*s and their gaps get smaller in the lower rows. Under optimal conditions, a gap of 22 seconds of arc can be recognized with a frequency of 50 percent (Shlaer, 1937). What determines this lower limit? The lower limit may be set by the size of the cone receptors in the foveal region of the human retina. Consider a black *C* against a white background, where there is a white gap in the ring surrounded by the dark arms of the *C*. It has been argued that the smallest gap in the *C* that can be recognized is one that will illuminate a single foveal cone, the dark arms illuminating adjoining cones less strongly. A foveal cone is about 1.5 microns in diameter. In the human eye, a cone 1.5 microns thick subtends a visual angle of about 20 seconds of arc. Shlaer's results suggest 22 seconds of arc as the limit, so the acuity limit is about the same size as the diameter of a cone. Further support for the role of cone size or, more precisely, cone density of the retina, on recognition acuity comes from an experiment comparing the acuity for a Landolt *C* target at various distances from the center of fixation (Jones & Higgins, 1947). With greater distances from the center of the fovea, acuity becomes rapidly poorer. The curve relating cone density per area of retina with distance from the center of the fovea follows a similar drop.

The question of the limits of recognition resolution has also been approached from a consideration of light quantum requirements. Acuity, including measurements obtained with a Landolt *C* task, improves considerably when the luminance of the background is increased. This is probably quite obvious to anyone who has tried to read the fine type of a newspaper either by moonlight or by the light of early dawn and found it a frustrating task. Figure 7.17 illustrates the improvement in acuity as background luminance increases (Pirenne & Denton, 1952). In this task the test object, a Landolt *C*, was presented for long exposures. Acuity increased 10,000-fold over the entire range of practical ambient illumination conditions. There is a clear rod-cone break in these curves, with the cone receptors entering into the acuity task at a background level slightly lower than the illumination under the full moon.

In the experiment described in Figure 7.17, the subject could use whatever portion of his retina seemed most effective, changing fixation until the *C* appeared clearest to him. Subjects reported using moderately peripheral fixation when the background levels were dimmest, and more and more foveal fixation as the intensity of the background was increased. One theory of acuity is that the gap in the *C* must be large enough so that it delivers sufficient photons to lead to detection of the gap's presence (Pirenne, Marriott, & O'Doherty, 1957). One can think of the gap as a luminous object delivering photons at a rate determined entirely by the background luminance, since the gap and background have the same luminance. Reducing the intensity of the background lowers the rate of photon impingement on the retina per unit area. Therefore, the rate of photon impingement must be raised somehow so as to bring it to a level where detection is again possible. One way of doing this is to increase the area of the gap. Thus, when the background luminance is lowered, the subject requires a larger gap to attain the same level of correct recognitions; that is, recognition acuity becomes poorer when background luminance is lowered. Specifically, the photon formulation is

$$k = \frac{I}{A},$$

where $k$ equals some total number of photons hitting the retina each second at the place where the gap is projected, $I$ is the intensity of the background luminance, and $A$ is the dimension of the gap in square meters (m$^2$). In logarithmic form this equation becomes

$$\log I = k' + \log m^2$$
$$\log I = k' + 2 \log m. \qquad [9]$$

This formulation predicts that the curve in Figure 7.17 will be linear, with a slope of +2.0, and while clearly oversimplifying the facts it does account for a considerable proportion of the variance. At least two factors complicate matters. At very low background intensities, very large *C* targets have to be used to insure that area *A* delivers sufficient photons. These areas (of the order of 300 × 300 minutes of arc$^2$) are clearly larger than the retina's limit for perfect spatial summation. Since spatial summation is poor, more photons are needed. The subject needs a larger *C* than predicted by Equation 9. Poor summation may be the reason why the curve in Figure 7.17 dips down in the lower left-hand corner. At the upper extreme of background intensity, increases in luminance are less and less effective because the receptors are saturated with light and are therefore less efficient in capturing additional photons. The horizontal portion of the curve then reflects the operation of Weber's law: The background is increased in intensity, and $\Delta I$ increases proportionately. Therefore, the area of the gap stays constant and a horizontal slope is obtained. Again we see that acuity and the differential brightness threshold are closely related.

The photon formulation also predicts other facts. The luminous area *A* should never deliver fewer photons than the minimum flux detectable in the periphery of the retina (100 to 150 photons per second; see the earlier discussion of light quantum requirements). Calculations by Pirenne et al. (1957)

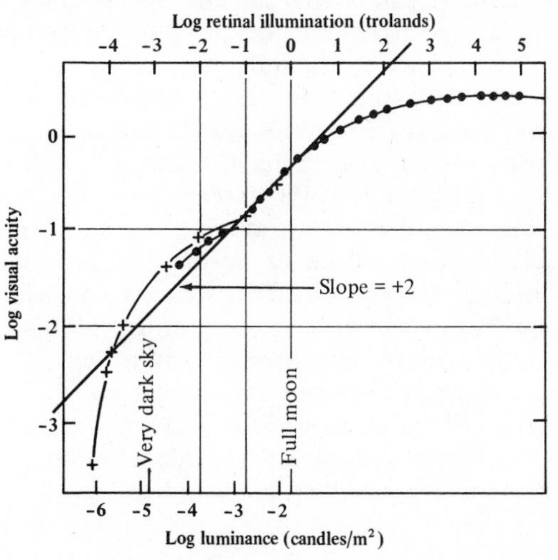


**Figure 7.17** Variation in acuity for a black Landolt C test object as a function of the luminance of the field. (After Pirenne & Denton, 1952.)

show that a gap of 24 minutes of arc in visual angle requires the least total photon flux. At the recognition threshold, such a gap is delivering 140 photons per second and is clearly not below the photon limitations of the absolute threshold.

## Resolution

This term refers to the ability to discern a gap separating one object from another. Acuity is related to the reciprocal of the size of the gap. For example, two stars against a dark background of a night sky can just be resolved as two stars rather than one when they are separated by 1 minute of arc (Helmholtz, 1866). One technique of measuring resolution uses a grating, a series of black and white stripes, such as in Figure 7.18. If the separation between the bars of the grating is small enough, the grating appears to the subject as a homogeneous gray, and at that point the subject will no longer be able to report on the orientation of the stripes. For example, if the reader places himself sufficiently far from Figure 7.18, the visual angle separating the bars will fall below threshold. At that point he should be unable to report the orientation of the grid if it is presented to him at random orientations from trial to trial. Most of the early experimenters (reviewed in Senders, 1948) obtained thresholds in the range of about 1 minute of arc of interbar separation. A more recent experiment indicated a threshold of about 40 seconds of arc (Keesey, 1960).

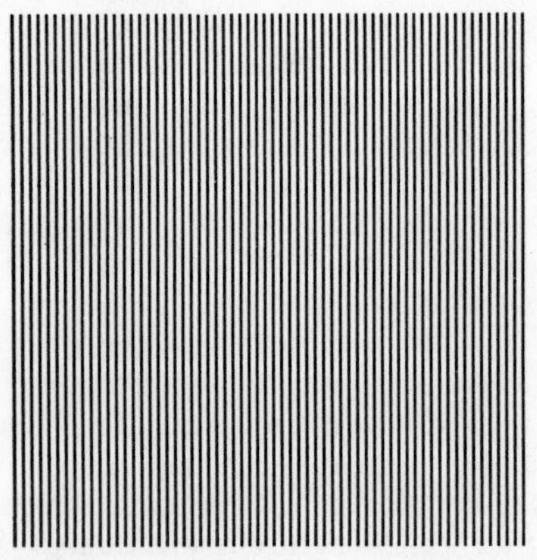

**Figure 7.18** Resolution grid for testing visual acuity. When viewed from a short distance the lines are clearly resolved and their orientation can be perceived, but not when viewed from a long distance.

What are the factors limiting our ability to resolve fine details? Classically, the limits of resolution have been thought to reside in the size of the cone receptors. The cones are very small in diameter, especially in the central fovea (approximately 1.5 $\mu$ or 22 seconds of arc). Helmholtz (1866) postulated that the finest grating that could be resolved would be one in which the white bar projects on one row of receptors, the adjoining black bar on a different row, the white bar adjoining that one on still a third row, and so on. Note that this would predict a threshold of a grating of twice 22 seconds of arc, or 44 seconds of arc. That value is quite close to the one Keesey (1960) obtained. It is necessary to have one row of cones clearly less stimulated than its neighbor in order to discriminate the orientation of the grid.

A bit of thought will reveal that it is not at all clear why Helmholtz' criterion is such a good predictor. If the stripes are narrower than a cone, say 2/3 or even 1/3 the diameter of a cone, it is still true that one row of cones will be less stimulated than an adjoining row. For example, assume that the width of the strips is exactly 1/3 the diameter of the foveal cones. If one row of cones had projected on it a black stripe flanked by the two adjoining white stripes, then the next row would have a white stripe flanked by two black stripes. The rate of photon impingement on these two rows would not be the same. Why can't the subject detect this difference?

Approaching the problem a bit differently, we note that we can as well ask how fine a separation between two lights can be resolved by a camera or telescope as by the human eye. The resolving power of optical instruments is ultimately limited by the effects of diffraction which occurs whenever light passes an edge in the instrument (see discussion of diffraction in the appendix). It is not surprising that diffraction also sets a limit to the resolving power of the human eye. The pupil is one such edge in the eye. Let us see why this should be so. No matter how small, a source of light will be projected by any optical system as a bright central disc, called *Airy's Disc,* surrounded by a number of concentric dark and light rings (see Figure 7.34 in the appendix). The disc contains 84 percent of the light and has a radius

$$\propto = \frac{1.22\lambda}{d_0}, \qquad [10]$$

where $\lambda$ is the wavelength of the light from the point, and $d_0$ is the diameter of the lens system that forms the disc image.

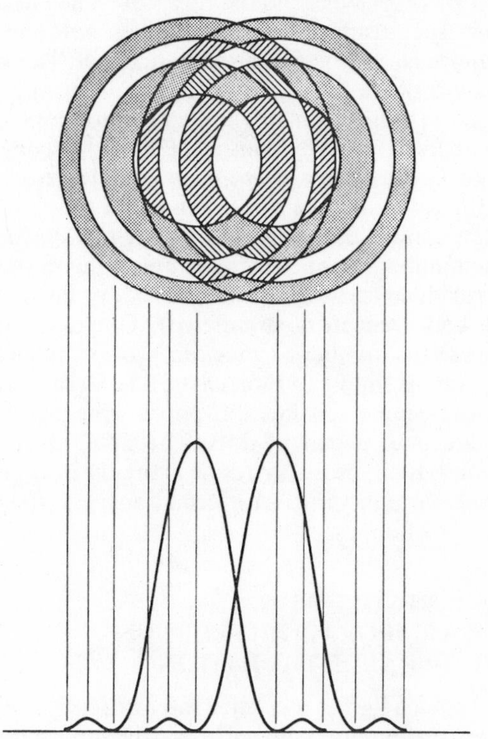

**Figure 7.19** An illustration of the Rayleigh criterion for the resolution of two bright points. At the top is shown the diffraction rings arising from two point sources of light passing through an optical system such as the eye. The bottom of the figure shows the amount of light that would impinge at various points on the retina. (From Jacobs, 1943.)

Figure 7.19 shows how two neighboring points of light produce two superimposed distributions. Added on the retina, these two distributions would yield two peaks of light with a shadow between them. Presumably, a subject reports two point sources, instead of one, provided he detects the shadow between the two peaks. Thus the task is once again, basically, brightness discrimination. What happens if two points of light are brought close together? Figure 7.16 shows that the depth of the shadow becomes less pronounced as the points are brought together. The subject stops seeing two dots and reports only one when the shadow is so slight that it is less than a jnd, that is, when the shadow's brightness is not noticeably different from its surround.

One suggested criterion for the limits of resolution is that two bright points are resolved when, as shown in Figure 7.19, the bright peak resulting from one of the pinpoints is superimposed on the first dark ring resulting from the second pinpoint. This is called the *Rayleigh limit*. There is, in fact, no rationale for choosing just this point. Rayleigh's limit is an arbitrary one, but assuming it holds for the human visual system we can compare its predictions to actual measurements. According to this assumption, the separation, in minutes of arc, of two points of light that can just be detected is equal to $\propto$ in Equation 10. In other words, acuity = $1/\propto$. The diameter, $d_0$, of the lens system that forms the disc image is simply taken as the diameter of the pupil. If the diameter of the pupil increases, acuity should improve. More specifically, the function of acuity as a function of pupil diameter should be linear with a zero intercept since Equation 10 is linear. Riggs (1965c), drawing on a number of different experiments, has shown that acuity does increase with pupillary diameter, in the manner predicted by assuming Rayleigh's limit. This is shown in Figure 7.20. However, the acuity is better than predicted; subjects can discriminate points closer than those set by the Rayleigh limit (a finding also reported by astronomers and microscopists). A more serious discrepancy is that acuity stops increasing when the pupillary diameter is 1.5 mm, or one-fourth its maximum diameter, which is nearly 6 mm. Acuity seems to reach a maximal value above which the optical advantages of a larger pupil are offset by other factors. One such offsetting factor is the increase in optical aberration of the human eye when the size of the pupil is

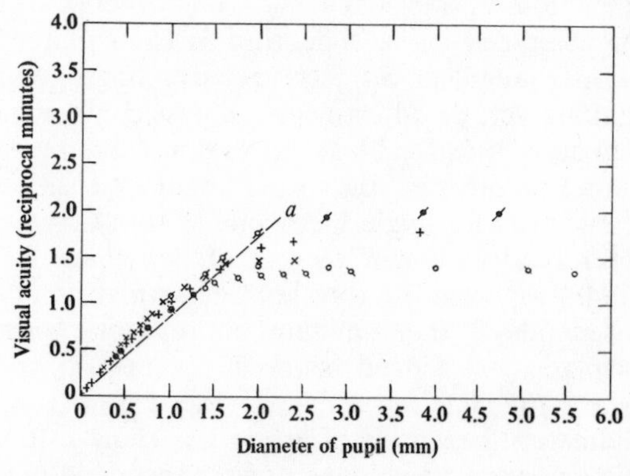


**Figure 7.20** The effect of pupillary diameter on visual acuity. The points are experimental data from a number of different studies. Line *a* represents a predicted acuity limit based on the Rayleigh criterion. (From Riggs, 1965c.)

increased. With a larger pupil, light rays that affect the receptors are refracted by the edges of the lens. At these edges the departures of both the corneal and lenticular surfaces from a spherical contour introduce optical aberrations.

Acuity for grating targets probably does not involve simply the discrimination of a series of linear shadows against a bright field. When, in place of a grating with its series of parallel and closely spaced lines, the target is a single black thread suspended in a bright field, acuity increases 120-fold. Whereas each line in the grating must have a width subtending 1 minute of arc, the single thread is detected when it subtends only 1/120 of a minute of arc. In other words, we are much better at detecting a single black thread than at resolving a grating of many lines. The reason for this difference is probably related to the difficulties in detecting a test object that is near a contour in the visual field, as discussed earlier. Each contour (line edge) of the grating lies near a large number of contours which, in the immediate vicinity, becomes even larger as the interbar distance is diminished. Thus, conditions are created that maximize the interference of one line with the detection of another.

### Vernier acuity

This type of acuity refers to a sensitivity to the displacement of one object relative to another. In a typical vernier task the subject adjusts two halves of an interrupted vertical line until he perceives the two portions as aligned, one above the other, forming one continuous line. The school child comparing the length of an object against a mark on a ruler, the machinist reading a micrometer, or the engineer reading a slide rule, is each making a vernier judgment. Subjects are surprisingly good at making vernier adjustments, almost as good as at detecting a single black line against a white surround. In other words, we are about as sensitive to the width of a single black line as to a very small lateral displacement of one of two lines. Berry (1948) reported the threshold of vernier acuity at 2 seconds (1/30 of a minute) of arc. This is a small displacement indeed, since in the central fovea, where the cone receptors are only 1.5 microns in diameter, 2 seconds of arc is less than 1/10 the diameter of a single cone. It would seem, intuitively, that the smallest detectable displacement of an object would be one cone diameter, or about 25 seconds of arc. How can the eye possibly detect whether an object has been displaced 1/4, 1/2, or 3/4 of the way across the receptor? The answer is that the displaced line stimulates not one, but hundreds, and even thousands, of cones. The visual system pools the information regarding the position of the line from this larger receptor population (Andersen & Weymouth, 1923). In accordance with *Laplace's law of large numbers*, the statistical estimate of the line's position on the retina should then come closer and closer to its real position as the number of cones in the sample is increased (the error decreasing as the square root of the number of cone receptors stimulated). One way to decrease the number of cone receptors stimulated by the line is simply to shorten the line. Vernier acuity does become considerably poorer when the line is reduced to a pair of dots. The limits of vernier acuity, then, probably reside in the central nervous system's ability to pool information from elongated arrays of cones.

## THE RESOLUTION OF TEMPORAL DIFFERENCES IN VISUAL STIMULATION

When a light is presented intermittently so that it slowly alternates with darkness, the subject reports seeing each phase in a clearly separate manner. As the frequency of intermittence is increased to about 8 to 10 Hz, the light part of the cycle becomes brighter and, to some, peculiarly unpleasant with a hypnotic quality. At higher frequencies, the alternation becomes less and less marked until only a faint tremulous appearance remains. Finally, at high speeds of alternation above the *critical flicker frequency (CFF)*, the subject reports seeing a perfectly steady light which he is unable to distinguish from a stimulus that is steadily illuminated and matched in color and brightness to the physically intermittent light. A good example is the light bulb over your desk that is flickering at a rate of 60 Hz but appears quite steady.

Before we consider various aspects of the perception of flicker, it should be noted that the eye does a surprisingly poor job of analyzing intermittence. Consider a television picture, for example, in which a single small dot of light, varying in intensity, traverses the screen. The entire screen is covered in 1/24 second by one still frame, followed in the next 1/24 second by another. We see, of course, a total picture with objects in motion. Yet, at any moment in time, there is only a solitary point on the entire screen.

In various topics discussed earlier, we have seen

that the sensitivity of the visual system is often limited by the characteristics of light itself, such as quantum considerations. In the case of intermittence, this statement clearly does not apply; the eye stops resolving intermittence at about 60 Hz, while a beam of light can be flickered a great many orders of magnitude more frequently. The limit of temporal resolution in single nerve fibers of the nervous system is much higher than CFF, being in the neighborhood of 1000 Hz, and bundles of nerve fibers can probably exceed this limit (see Chapter 4). Apparently the eye, and not the properties of light or nerve fibers, sets the limit of CFF. Perhaps, as a transducer of energy, the eye is biased to respond better to low frequencies. One can make an analogy between the eye and an electronic filter. If the filter is set to pass only high frequencies, then it will do a poor job in detecting very low-level signals of long duration in the presence of noise. If the filter is set to pass only low frequencies, then it will do a poor job in resolving fine temporal variations, although it may be sensitive to low-level signals of relatively longer durations. As is shown in the next section, the low-pass filter analogy turns out to be appropriate for the eye.

## Parameters of temporal resolution

One traditional manner of studying intermittence is to present a light to a subject through a sectored disc which periodically interrupts the light beam, thereby creating an on-phase when the beam passes through an open-sectored portion of the disc and an off-phase when the beam is totally interrupted. A major variable determining CFF is light intensity. Figure 7.21 shows that flicker can be resolved at frequencies of on-off alternation as high as 50 to 60 Hz when more intense illuminance is used during the on-phase (Hecht & Smith, 1936). At very low illuminances a flicker frequency as low as 4 to 5 Hz is seen as a steady light. Figure 7.21 also shows how the size of the intermittent stimulus affects the dependence of CFF on illuminance. With large stimuli, 6° and 19° of visual angle, CFF levels off as illuminance increases to between about −1 and 0 log illuminance; then above about 0.5 log retinal illuminance, CFF again increases before leveling off a second time at about 4 log units. Once more the rod-cone duplicity theory seems to apply. The lower portion of each curve represents the response of the more sensitive rods and the upper portion represents that of the cones. When the stimulus size is reduced to 2° and 0.3°, and the

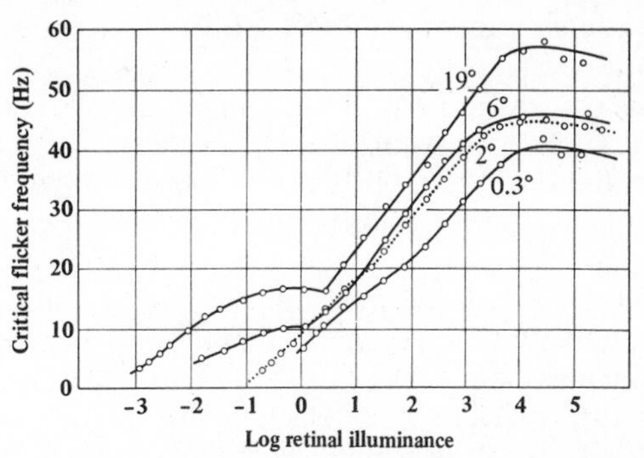


**Figure 7.21** Critical flicker frequency and the intensity of the flickering light. Each curve is obtained with a test object of different diameter, in degrees of visual angle. (From Hecht & Smith, 1936.)

center of the target is fixated, only the cones of the fovea are stimulated, and so the lower rod portion of the curve with its plateau is not present. The relationship between CFF and illuminance means that the most sensitive visual receptors, namely, the rods, which are tapped by the low-intensity light, have the slowest response. Conversely, the least sensitive visual receptors, the cones, which are only tapped at the higher illuminances, have the quickest response to the on-off alternation. Over the upper portion of the curve in Figure 7.21, CFF rises linearly as a function of log illuminance, and the *Ferry-Porter law* applies:

$$\text{CFF} = k \log I. \qquad [11]$$

The relationship between CFF and the retinal receptors is even clearer when CFF is measured for a small spot of light presented to different areas of the retina. Hecht and Verrijp (1933) found that a 2° disc of low-intensity flickering light had a higher CFF when presented 15° into the periphery of the visual field than in the central fovea (0°). Since the fovea is devoid of rods, it responds poorly to a low-intensity stimulus. A high-intensity flickering light shows the opposite relationship, with a much higher CFF in the fovea because the cones are mediating temporal resolution of high-intensity stimuli. At 15° in the periphery there is a near maximum density of rod receptors. Since CFF is lower at 15°, we must assume that the rods' ability to follow high flicker frequencies is poor. These results confirm our interpretation of the curves of Figure 7.21 for the 19° and 6° stimuli as composite curves. The lower branch represents rod-mediated

CFF for low-intensity stimuli; the upper branch represents cone-mediated CFF for high-intensity stimuli.

Hecht and Smith's results in Figure 7.21 show still another relationship. With larger areas of stimulation, larger CFF values are obtained; that is, CFF increases as the stimulus grows in size from 0.3° to 19° in visual angle. Over a range from 10° to about 50°, other investigators found that CFF is proportional to log area (Granit & Harper, 1930; Kugelmass & Landis, 1955). This relationship might be puzzling to the reader at first glance, since at the absolute threshold Ricco's law states that the product $I \times A$ is a constant, not $I \times \log A$. In flicker perception, however, it is the circumference or perimeter of the stimulus figure that appears to be the determining factor. For example, Roehrig (1959), using central fixation and a large stimulus (50°), could darken large portions of the center of the stimulus without lowering CFF. If CFF is proportional to the circumference, then by simple geometry it can be shown that CFF is proportional to 1/2 log area.

## Talbot-Plateau law

When CFF is exceeded, a flickering light appears perfectly steady. Its brightness is easily determined by matching it to a steadily illuminated stimulus. If the flickering light has intensity $I$ a proportion $p$ of the time, and the light is completely off a proportion $1 - p$ of the time, then it will be as bright as a steady stimulus of intensity $pI$. Helmholtz (1924) described the phenomenon as follows: "If a point of the retina is excited by a light which undergoes regular and periodic variations, and which has the duration of its period sufficiently short, it produces a continuous impression equal to that produced if the light emitted during each period were distributed uniformly throughout the duration of the period [vol. 2, p. 174]." This principle, called *Talbot's law* (1834) or sometimes the *Talbot-Plateau law*, has been used to advantage in photometry. For example, a simple and precise method of diminishing the intensity of a light beam to 1/10 its value is accomplished by passing the beam through a rapidly rotating (above 100 Hz, or 6000 rpm) sectored disc, whose open sector is 1/10 the disc's area, or 36 degrees. Suppose the disc is rotating at 100 Hz. Then one revolution takes 1/100 sec. During that 1/100 sec the eye collects energy. The open sector will allow light through during 1/10 of that time, or 1/1000 sec; the beam of light will be blocked during 9/1000 sec. Therefore, the sectored disc sends a beam of light that looks steady and equal in brightness to one of 1/10 the physical energy. The Talbot-Plateau law, which implies perfect temporal integration, holds whenever CFF is exceeded.

## Systems analysis

This approach conceptualizes the subject as a black box to which is applied an input (the stimulus) and out of which comes an output (the response). The organism is assumed to process the input signal by a set of linear transformations. An important property of a system with linear transformations is that if the input is a sinusoidal wave of some particular frequency then the output is also a sinusoidal wave with the same frequency, though possibly different in amplitude. We shall see how closely this applies to the temporal properties of vision.

Earlier, the visual system's response to periodic stimuli was compared to the action of a filter which passes some frequencies and blocks others. We will now pursue this analogy a bit further.

With the techniques developed by Fourier it is possible to analyze any periodic phenomenon into a series of sine-wave functions of different amplitudes and singular phase relations (see Chapter 4). A flickering stimulus going periodically from completely on one-half the time to completely off one-half the time can be thought of as a square-wave periodic function. The sine wave of lowest frequency is called the *fundamental*. The modulation amplitude indicates how high the peak of the sinusoid is above the mean amplitude. For example, suppose a light flickers sinusoidally, that is, its luminous intensity fluctuates smoothly like a sine wave. If the average intensity is 50 mL which increases to a maximum of 100 mL ($\Delta I = 50$ mL) and decreases to a minimum of 0 mL, the modulation amplitude ($r\%$) is 100 percent. A source flickering at 10 Hz with 100 percent modulation would be seen as a markedly flickering light. If the average intensity of the light is 50 mL, but it flickers very, very slightly increasing to a maximum of 50.5 mL ($\Delta I = 0.5$ mL) and decreasing to a minimum of 49.5 mL, then the modulation amplitude is 1 percent. In other words, percent modulation is given by the equation

$$r(\%) = \frac{\text{max mL} - \text{min mL}}{\text{max mL} + \text{min mL}} \times 100, \qquad [12]$$

where *max* refers to the luminance level of the peak of the sine wave, and *min* refers to the trough's luminance level. Note the resemblance between modulation amplitude and the Weber ratio. As the reader might guess, if the modulation amplitude of a flickering light (e.g., 10 Hz) is gradually reduced, a point is reached where the light is seen as steadily on. The more sensitive we are to the flicker, the lower the modulation amplitude (and the lower the Weber ratio) at which flicker is still seen. Figure 7.22 shows the results of a flicker experiment analyzed in terms of modulation amplitude (de Lange, 1958). Note that the onset and offset of the light was varied in four different ways. For example, wave shape 3 differs from wave shape 1 in that the duration of the on-period is shorter in shape 3. In shape 4 the onset and offset are more gradual than in shape 1.

At any particular frequency of on-off alternation, all these wave shapes have the same *fundamental frequency;* but they differ in the amount of energy devoted to the higher frequencies. Wave shape 3 probably has the greatest proportion of higher frequencies. Several aspects of the perception of intermittence are clear from Figure 7.22. Most fundamental is the fact that the different symbols are found to fall along one curve, as long as mean retinal illuminance is constant. This coincidence indicates that the wave shape is not a very significant variable. Or, stated differently, as first demonstrated by Ives (1922) the most important variable that governs flicker perception is the modulation amplitude ($r\%$) of the fundamental frequency. (Exceptions to this rule occur if the fundamental frequency is very low.) The steep drop of the curve at higher frequencies again means that high-frequency components are minor determinants of flicker perception.

There is one additional point of interest in Figure 7.22. The 430-troland curve has a peak at 9 Hz, meaning that flicker of a moderately bright source is more easily seen at 9 Hz than at either higher or lower frequencies. This peak has been replicated in a study by Kelly (1959), who accentuated the resonance by using a flickering stimulus that was in effect edgeless: It was bright in the center and imperceptibly diminished in intensity away from the center. Such a peak implies that the visual system filters out both low and high frequencies, and resonates at a frequency of between 8 and 20 Hz.

It is probably significant that a flickering stimulus looks much brighter than predicted by Talbot's law; at a flicker rate of 8 to 10 Hz it is even brighter than a steady stimulus of the same luminance (Bartley, 1938). This is the same range of frequencies as the resonant frequency in de Lange's (Figure 7.22) and in Kelly's experiments. Moreover, the alpha rhythm of the electroencephalogram (i.e., brain waves), which is very strong when recorded from electrodes near the visual cortex (except in the congenitally blind), also predominates at 8 to 10 Hz.

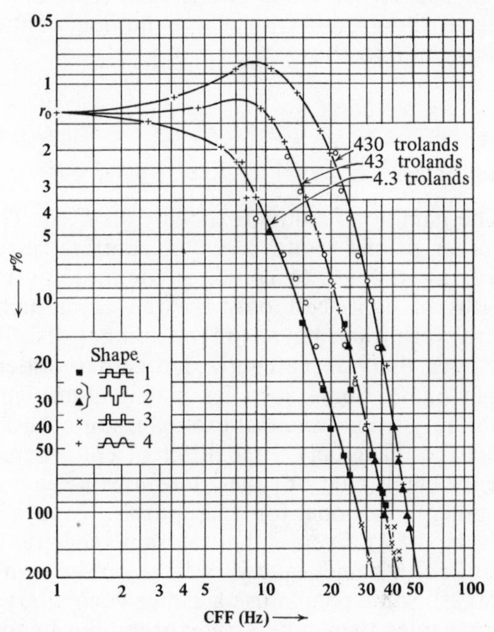


**Figure 7.22** The modulation amplitude of the fundamental sinusoidal component at the point of critical flicker fusion. The three curves represent three levels of mean luminous intensity of the flickering test object. Each symbol stands for a different wave shape. The peak of the 430-troland curve at a frequency between 7 and 11 Hz probably reflects a resonance quality in the temporal response of the visual system. (From de Lange, 1958.)

Why do these two phenomena resonate at the same frequency? Are they related? The peak sensitivity to visual flicker originates peripherally, probably at the photoreceptors themselves, whereas EEG resonance appears quite independently within thalamic nuclei (Eccles, 1965). A number of authors, over the years, speculated that the EEG plays a role in quantizing perceptual experience into 1/10 sec time bins (see Harter, 1967, for a review). Were this true, it would be reasonable that the independent EEG resonance would evolve into a temporal frequency domain (8 to 10 Hz) very similar to the peak sensitivity of the eye itself. An alternative explanation is that the visual system is composed of numerous filters, each with its own peak sensitivity, and with a larger number of filters peaking at 8 to 10 Hz.

## COLOR

### Color names

The naming of colors is socially dictated. That is, other people reinforce us for emitting certain words in response to certain predominant wavelengths of light. Not only are the color names entirely arbitrary, but so are the number of different hues that are categorized together under a single name. Some societies classify hues quite differently from ours. For example, some Australian tribes have only three different color names: one for black, blue, or violet; one for white, yellow, or green; and one for red, purple, or orange (Rivers, 1901). Even within the same society, the use of color names may vary from one person to another. Some people use a richer vocabulary of color names than others. One example of names used in our society has been presented by Judd (1940), who pooled data from a number of studies to arrive at the following average wavelength settings for ten different color names:

| Color name | Nanometers |
|---|---|
| purplish blue | 439 |
| blue | 472 |
| blue-green | 495 |
| green | 512 |
| greenish yellow | 566 |
| yellow | 577 |
| yellowish orange | 589 |
| orange | 598 |
| red | no single wavelength; the complement of 521 nm, a mixture of deep orange (615 nm) with purplish blue (435 nm) |

One version of the *Whorfian hypothesis* states that when you have more names assigned to some portion of a sensory continuum such as color, then you become more sensitive in that portion. According to the Whorfian hypothesis, reality is perceived differently in different linguistic communities and these differences are caused by differences in the structure of language in diverse cultures (Whorf, 1956). Brown and Lenneberg (1959) found that the codability of colors (involving agreement in naming, response latency of naming, and other measures) was positively correlated with accuracy of recognition memory. However, a later study has examined the structure of the perception of color and of color memory using multidimensional scaling techniques (Heider & Olivier, 1972). Structure here refers to the perception of similarity and dissimilarity among colors. This was studied in a group of Americans and in a group of New Guinea Dani; the latter categorize colors verbally in only two groups: bright colors (including light and "warm" colors) and dark colors (including dark and "cold" colors). Yet, the structure of the perceptions and memories of these colors in the two groups was highly similar. This finding suggests that there is a perception and memory for color that is purely visual, as it were, and not affected by verbal codes. The earlier studies can be reinterpreted to mean that a subject's recognition of color will be affected by the structure of his language in tasks emphasizing verbal coding. But subjects have available to them nonverbal codes that are unaffected by linguistic structure.

### Discrimination of colors

Color discrimination, rather than color naming, is the fundamental measure with which color vision researchers have primarily concerned themselves. Color discrimination is usually tested with a bipartite field like the one used to measure brightness discrimination. A light that has a narrow band of wavelengths centered on wavelength $\lambda$ illuminates one half of the field, and a light centered on a slightly different wavelength, $\lambda + \Delta\lambda$, illuminates the other half. The two halves of the field must be carefully matched in luminance; otherwise, the subject continues to see a difference between the two fields even after the wavelength difference between the two is reduced to zero. If most of the light energy is concentrated within a range of a few nanometers, then the source is considered *monochromatic light*. Special techniques are needed to give a light with such a narrow bandwidth.

Figure 7.23 shows how the just noticeable difference in wavelength, $\Delta\lambda$, varies as a function of the wavelength, $\lambda$, at the center of the source's narrow band of light. Clearly, sensitivity to wavelength change is not evenly distributed over the spectrum. We seem to be most sensitive in those portions of the spectrum where hue changes fastest as a function of wavelength. For example, in the yellow portion of the spectrum (580 nm), hue changes toward green if the wavelength is reduced, and toward red if the wavelength is increased. Sensitiv-

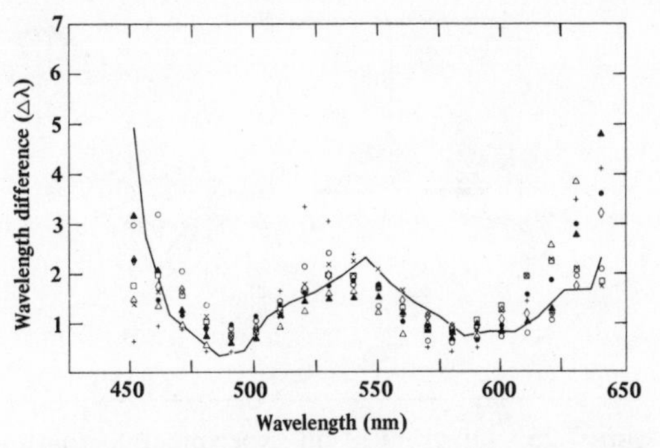


**Figure 7.23** The hue discrimination threshold ($\Delta\lambda$) as a function of the wavelength of the test light, in nanometers. The data come from eight experiments on color-normal subjects. (From Judd, 1932.)

ity to wavelength change is high in this portion of the spectrum, that is, the difference threshold is small. In contrast, in the red region (650 nm) neither small increases nor decreases in wavelength cause much change in hue. In this portion of the spectrum sensitivity to wavelength change is low ($\Delta\lambda$ is large).

## Saturation

Suppose a field is illuminated with a monochromatic light, $L_\lambda$, of wavelength $\lambda$. Superimposing white light $L_w$ would then make the hue appear weakened, desaturated, or "washed out." If $L_w$ is made more and more intense, and $L_\lambda$ is made weaker and weaker, the color will eventually appear white. Conversely, as the white light is made weaker, the hue becomes deeper and more saturated.

As indicated in Chapter 1, it is possible to keep saturation constant while changing brightness and hue. Hence, saturation is the name of a distinct attribute that is varied when white light is added, thereby changing the appearance of a color from one that is deeply hued to one devoid of hue. The stimulus dimension that corresponds most closely to the psychological attribute of saturation is called *colorimetric purity*. Purity ($p$) is defined as follows:

$$p = \frac{L_\lambda}{L_\lambda + L_w}, \qquad [13]$$

where $L_\lambda$ is the luminance of a monochromatic light of wavelength $\lambda$, and $L_w$ is the luminance of the added white light. An unadulterated spectral color has a purity of 1.0; white has a purity of 0.0.

Sensitivity to purity is measured by means of a bipartite field, both sides of which are white at the start. Small amounts of the spectral color, $L_\lambda$, are added until the subject begins to report color consistently in one of the half-fields. The value of $L_\lambda$ at which color is reported at some criterion frequency is then inserted into Equation 13 to give the *minimum colorimetric purity,* some fairly representative values of which are given in Figure 7.24. Purity threshold is highest around 570 nm to 580 nm (yellow), which means we are relatively insensitive to a small addition of the spectral color, 570 nm, to white. On the other hand, the purity threshold is small at the extremes of the visible spectrum; the normal subject can detect relatively small additions of either short or long wavelengths to a white field.

## Laws of color mixing

Because the ear analyzes a musical chord into its components, there are seldom two ways of achieving the same sound. Different chords or tone com-

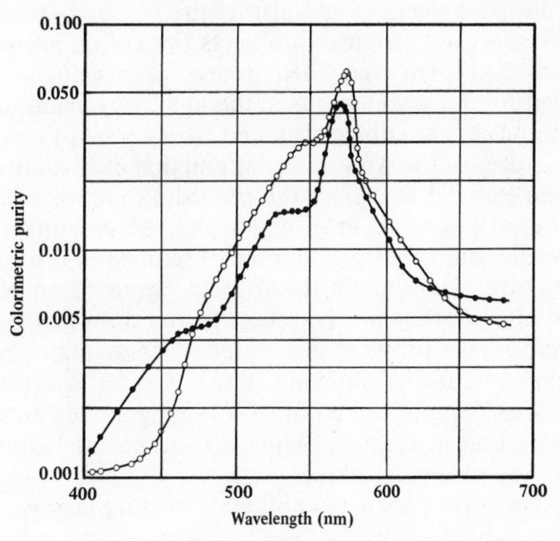


**Figure 7.24** The log colorimetric purity of a hue just perceptibly different from white at various wavelengths of the hue for two subjects. The threshold is lower—a less pure hue is needed for detection—at the short and long extremes of the spectrum. The threshold is highest at about 570 nanometers. (Data from Priest & Brickwedde, 1938.)

binations sound different. But with respect to color, the eye can be fooled. The same yellow can be made up of either a single monochromatic light of 580 nm or a mixture of 570 nm and 590 nm in roughly equal proportions. Still another way to get the same yellow color is to mix monochromatic lights of 560 nm and 600 nm. It should be stressed that these three yellows can be made to look entirely indistinguishable. The eye does not analyze a given color field into all its component wavelengths. If it did, the three yellows would never look alike, since the distribution of energy in each of the three yellow lights is quite different. Apparently the eye analyzes light along only three dimensions. We speak of normal color vision as being *trichromatic.* This tridimensionality becomes evident in color mixing.

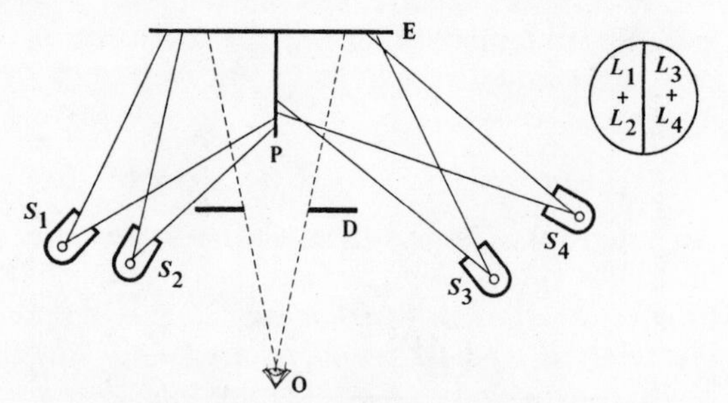


**Figure 7.25** Diagram of an experimental situation used for color mixing. Light sources $S_1$ of luminance $L_1$ is projected onto the left half of the screen E. The luminance $L_2$ from the light source $S_2$ is added to the left half of the screen E. On the right side, the luminances from light sources $S_3$ and $S_4$ are combined. The observer 0 views the screen through a circular aperture D. (From Le Grand, 1957.)

### *Empirical laws of color mixing*

For the laws of color mixing to hold, certain conditions must be met. The stimulus must be small (a few degrees of arc at most) and viewed foveally. The luminance level must be well within the photopic range, but not so high that glare is a problem. The stimulus must be a *film color* or *aperture color,* which cannot be identified as an object. Presenting colored objects would distort the results because we tend to attribute to objects the colors appropriate to them even when these colors are not justified by the wavelengths in the light. For example, suppose that subjects looked at a series of color pictures of the American flag and that each picture had less red in it than the preceding picture until the stripes were gray and white. Some subjects would still report some trace of redness in the last picture even though the stripes contained no red at all. In other words, object colors show *memory color.* This problem is avoided in color-matching experiments by showing film colors or aperture colors (simply the color of a homogeneous luminous hole in a surface) which do not seem to belong to any particular object.

One of the basic laws of color mixture is *Abney's law,* which states that the luminances add, whatever their color (Le Grand, 1957). To demonstrate this law, at least four light sources of different colors are needed. Sources $S_1$ and $S_2$, with luminances $L_1$ and $L_2$, are projected on one half of a screen, and sources $S_3$ and $S_4$, with luminances $L_3$ and $L_4$, on the other half of the screen. Figure 7.25 illustrates how the apparatus is arranged and how the bipartite field is seen by the subject. If the luminances are set so that the sum of $L_1$ and $L_2$ is algebraically equal to the sum of $L_3$ and $L_4$, then, according to Abney's law, the two sides of the screen will look equally bright, even though they are different colors. Actually, the law is only approximately true. Abney's law can be wrong by as much as 34 percent when the luminances of complementary colors are added (Piéron, 1939).

With the same stimulus conditions, it is possible to obtain a color match as well as a brightness match. If the colors of the four sources are chosen correctly, the following equation holds:

$$L_1(S_1) + L_2(S_2) \equiv L_3(S_3) + L_4(S_4). \quad [14]$$

The sign $\equiv$ means that the two sides of the bipartite field are completely indistinguishable by the human subject. This is called a *metameric match.* Equation 14 is not a mathematical equation, but is simply a statement of a psychological match. Nevertheless, *Grassmann's laws* (1854), which follow, state that the quantities can be manipulated like mathematical quantities.

1. *The additive law:* Given that a color match is obtained, adding the same quantity ($L_5$) of still another source ($S_5$) to both sides of the field will leave the two sides still matched:

$$L_1(S_1) + L_2(S_2) + L_5(S_5) \equiv L_3(S_3) + L_4(S_4) + L_5(S_5) \quad [15]$$

Of course, the field may look different as a result of the addition, but the two sides will remain matched.

2. *The multiplicative law:* Given that a color match is obtained, changing the intensity of the two sides equally will leave the bipartite field matched:

$$k[L_1(S_1) + L_2(S_2)] \equiv k[L_3(S_3) + L_4(S_4)] \quad [16]$$

An intensity change will alter the appearance of both sides of the bipartite field, making them either brighter or dimmer, but the two sides will remain identical to each other in appearance. This law holds over a wide range of photopic intensities, but breaks down once intensities in the scotopic range are reached.

3. *The associative law:* Two different light combinations that look like a third combination will look like each other. If

$$L_1(S_1) + L_2(S_2) \equiv L_3(S_3) + L_4(S_4),$$
and
$$L_3(S_3) + L_4(S_4) \equiv L_5(S_5) + L_6(S_6),$$
then
$$L_1(S_1) + L_2(S_2) \equiv L_5(S_5) + L_6(S_6). \quad [17]$$

4. *The adaptation law:* If the two sides of the bipartite field match, they will remain matched over wide ranges of adaptation. For example, if a subject views a blue field for several minutes and then turns to the previously matched field, it will look yellower but will remain matched.

It should be stressed that Grassmann's laws are the empirical results of color matching. They were derived from the data and not from any preconceived notions about how the visual system operates.

*Complementary colors*

Colors, when added, may neutralize each other to give a white light. Two such colors, $S_1$ and $S_2$, are called *complementary colors* if the following relationship is true:

$$L_1(S_1) + L_2(S_2) \equiv L_w(W),$$

where $L_w$ is the luminance of the resultant white light, $W$. The following colors form complementary pairs: yellow and violet-blue, red and blue-green, and orange and blue. The greens, corresponding to wavelengths in the middle of the spectrum, have no monochromatic complementary. The greens form white when mixed with purple, which is not a monochromatic color but is obtained by mixing wavelengths near the extremes of the spectrum (e.g., 400 nm, violet, and 700 nm, red). The wavelength of a purple light is usually specified by the wavelength of its green complementary (e.g., 500 nm).

*The trivariant law of color matching*

The basic empirical facts of color matching (Le Grand, 1957) can be expressed most generally as:

$$L_A(S_A) + L_B(S_B) \equiv L_w(W) + L_\lambda(S_\lambda). \quad [18]$$

This trivariant law states that the effect of any two colored sources of light, $S_A$ and $S_B$, when added together can always be matched by, at most, a single monochromatic color $S_\lambda$ plus some white light $W$. The color $S_\lambda$ is called the dominant wavelength of the $S_A + S_B$ mix. In accordance with this equation, color vision is said to be trivariant because the $S_A + S_B$ mix—which can be the sum of any two colors –can be specified by three numbers:

1. $\lambda$, the dominant wavelength,
2. $L_\lambda$, the quantity of the dominant wavelength,
3. $L_w$, the quantity of white light.

Given these three values, the variable half of a bipartite field can be made to look the same in every respect as the half composed of the $S_A + S_B$ mix.

The $S_A + S_B$ mix can be treated as a single light source $S_{AB}$ with an intensity $L_{AB}$. To this complex light source a new source $S_C$ can be added. Equation 18 would then read as follows:

$$L_{AB}(S_{AB}) + L_C(S_C) \equiv L_w(W) + L_\lambda(S_\lambda)$$
or
$$L_A(S_A) + L_B(S_B) + L_C(S_C) \equiv L_w(W) + L_\lambda(S_\lambda).$$

This equation means that the sum of any three colors can be matched to white light plus a certain amount of the dominant wavelength. By induction, an infinite number of light sources can appear on the left side of Equation 18. Hence, any light source whatsoever can be perfectly matched by white light plus one monochromatic light.

According to one convention of color matching, the value of $L_\lambda$ in Equation 18 may sometimes be negative. The negative sign means that the complementary of $L_\lambda$, not $L_\lambda$ itself, is added to the white light on that side of the bipartite field or, equivalently, that $L_\lambda$ is added to the $S_A + S_B$ mix on the other side of the field.

It can be shown without difficulty (Le Grand, 1957) that when Grassmann's laws are used, Equation 18 is equivalent to the following formulation:

$$L_s(S) = L_1(\lambda_1) + L_2(\lambda_2) + L_3(\lambda_3). \quad [19]$$

This equation states that any color ($S$) can be matched exactly to the sum of three monochromatic lights $\lambda_1$, $\lambda_2$, and $\lambda_3$, whose quantity is specified by $L_1$, $L_2$, and $L_3$.

## Color theories

Color theories attempt to explain comprehensively yet parsimoniously Grassmann's laws, the trivariance of color mixing, and the discrimination of wavelengths. The theories postulate the physiological mechanisms that underlie color vision.

### *The trichromatic theory of Young and Helmholtz*

Under dim illumination, when our vision is mediated by a single pigment, rhodopsin, wavelength discrimination is not possible and different colors are not seen. Rhodopsin absorbs light maximally at about 500 nm; thus a spot of light of 500 nm will appear brighter than one of 400 nm. If, however, the 400-nm spot is made more intense, it will affect rhodopsin as much as the 500-nm spot, and the two spots will look identical. Mixing the two spots together would simply result in a brighter spot with no change in color, that is, the mix would still be gray. When only a single pigment is functional, the results of color mixing vary along a single dimension and any color can be matched by any other wavelength as long as its intensity can be varied. Indeed, in scotopic vision when only rhodopsin is functional, humans see all objects as gray, white, or black.

Suppose daylight vision were mediated by two visual pigments, one that absorbed best in the blue region and one that absorbed best in the green region. Suppose, too, that we place a 500-nm light in the left half of a bipartite field and a 450-nm light in the right half. The 500-nm light will affect the green-pigment cones much more than it will the blue-pigment cones, whereas the 450-nm light will affect the cones in the opposite manner. Therefore, the two lights will never look alike to the two-pigment observer, regardless of the intensities at which the two colors are set. Only by adding a color of a second wavelength, for example 550 nm, to the 450-nm light can a match be achieved. The quantity of each of the two lights in the mixture can be separately adjusted so that their combined effect on both cones will be the same as the effect of the single 500-nm light. Thus with two visual pigments, any color can be matched by a combination of two wavelengths whose intensities are properly adjusted. (It must also be permissible to have negative values where one wavelength is added to the sample to be matched, as in the trivariant system described in the preceding section.)

From this line of reasoning, we infer by induction that the trivariance of normal color vision mixture data implies three visual pigments. Young (1807) arrived at essentially the same conclusion using deductive reasoning. First, Young pointed out that we can see very small spots of color for many colors. Therefore, tiny portions of the retina can mediate a full range of color vision. Young reasoned further that such tiny areas cannot hold thousands of different color receptors, that is, one for each hue we see, since there is not enough space on the retina. Next, Young considered the fact that printers need three colors to match any color sample. He concluded that this implied three types of *particles* on the retina, each maximally sensitive to a different color.

Dalton (1798) had recently made the first observation of color blindness. It had been known, at least since the seventeenth century, that some people confused colors that the rest of the population discriminated easily. But it was Dalton who made the first scientific observations. He claimed he could see only two hues which he called yellow and blue. His yellow included the red, orange, yellow, and green of normal subjects; his blue covered the blue and violet. Young (1807) therefore attributed the color blindness to the absence of the postulated red-sensitive particle. Helmholtz (1866) came to essentially the same conclusions, arguing that the trivariance of color-mixing data implied the existence of three visual pigments in the cones. The bivariance of color-mixing data in certain forms of color blindness was then attributed to the absence of one of the three pigments. Helmholtz described the absorption characteristics of one possible set of visual pigments, which is shown in Figure 7.26. Note especially that the three pigments have considerable overlap. The Young-Helmholtz theory, very briefly, states that a light of a particular wavelength affects all three pigments but to varying extent. Such a light will appear as a highly saturated color if it affects one of the three pigments much more than the others. When the green- and red-absorbing pigments are equally affected while the blue is affected very little, the subject will report a color equivalent to a stimulus of 570 nm (yellow). If all three pigments are equally affected, the subject will report a totally unsaturated color, white. Color is determined by the proportion of activation of the three photopigments. The Young-Helmholtz theory provides the simplest explanation of the most surprising and conspicuous fact of color vision: trivariance. More recent experiments have added considerable support to the theory (e.g., Brindley & Willmer, 1952; Rushton, 1959).

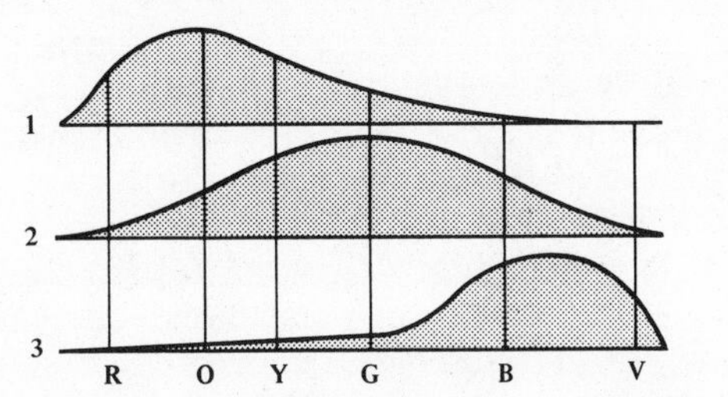


**Figure 7.26** Helmholtz' diagrammatic representation of Young's trichromatic theory. The relative response of each of the three hypothesized receptors or pigments is plotted as a function of light wavelength. Note especially that a light of any wavelength in the range of visible light is assumed to elicit some response from all three receptors. (From Helmholtz, 1866.)

Some of these experiments are based on the fact that light entering the eye is partly absorbed in visual pigment, partly absorbed elsewhere, and partly reflected back out of the eye. If we know how much light of some wavelength goes into the eye and how much comes out again by reflection, then the difference between these two quantities will tell us how much was absorbed. Brindley and Willmer (1952) first used this ophthalmoscopic technique to estimate the density of pigmentation in the fovea. Rushton (1959) used it with a number of technical improvements to identify the visual pigments of the cones in the living, human fovea. He has identified two different foveal pigments in a subject having normal color vision. One pigment, which Rushton called *chlorolabe,* is maximally sensitive to wavelengths of 540 nm (i.e., it is green absorbing), while *erythrolabe*, the second pigment, is maximally sensitive to 590 nm (i.e., it is orange absorbing). Rushton has thus far been unable to identify a blue-sensitive pigment in any subject, probably because of limitations inherent in the technique.

Rushton extended these measurements to color-blind subjects, some with *protanopia,* some with *deuteranopia*. Protanopes need only two colors to match any other color (as described in the preceding theoretical example). They confuse reds and greens and, in addition, are less sensitive to red light than are normal subjects. It is commonly thought that they are missing a red-absorbing pigment, and Rushton confirmed this by measuring visual pigments with the ophthalmoscopic technique in two protanopic subjects. He identified the same chlorolabe pigment with a peak at 540 nm (in fact, protanopes seem to have twice as much chlorolabe as normals), but was unable to find any erythrolabe. Deuteranopes also display two-dimensional (bivariant) color mixing. They also confuse reds and greens, but, in contrast to protanopes, the deuteranopes show no losses in sensitivity anywhere on the spectrum. Following Fick (1879), it has been widely thought that deuteranopes have all three pigments but that either: (a) all the red-absorbing cones and the green-absorbing cones are tied together neurally so that they sum their activities onto the nerve cells to which they connect, or (b) the red and green visual pigments are mixed together in each cone. In either case, the two visual pigments, though differentially bleached by lights of different wavelengths, lose that information and transmit a message to the nerve cells of the subsequent stage in the visual pathways (specifically, the bipolar cells) which represents the action of a hypothetical pigment halfway between green and red. Rushton has given Fick's idea support by finding both erythrolabe and chlorolabe in the eyes of deuteranopes.

More recently it has been found possible to measure the absorption characteristics of the pigment of single human cones by focusing a beam of light as a very small spot, 2 microns in diameter, onto a single cone in a small piece of retina dissected from near the foveal region (Brown & Wald, 1964; Marks, Dobelle, & MacNichol, 1964). The diameter of the light-spot is approximately equal to that of a single cone. As in the ophthalmoscopic technique, the reflected light is measured and this measurement is used to estimate the absorption characteristics of single cones. In these experiments, an *absorption difference spectrum* is obtained by first measuring the absorption characteristics of the dark-adapted cone to various wavelengths, then bleaching the photopigment with a standard amount of light, and again measuring absorption. The difference between pre- and postbleach absorption at each wavelength is proportional to the sensitivity of the pigment to that wavelength. The experiment pushes measurement to its ultimate limits: the quantum nature of light absorption. Because the light that is used to measure the absorption characteristics bleaches the cone's pigments in substantial amounts, only very small amounts of light can be used. The results, so far, point to the existence of three cone pigments with absorption peaks at about 445, 535, and 570 nm, as shown in Figure 7.27.

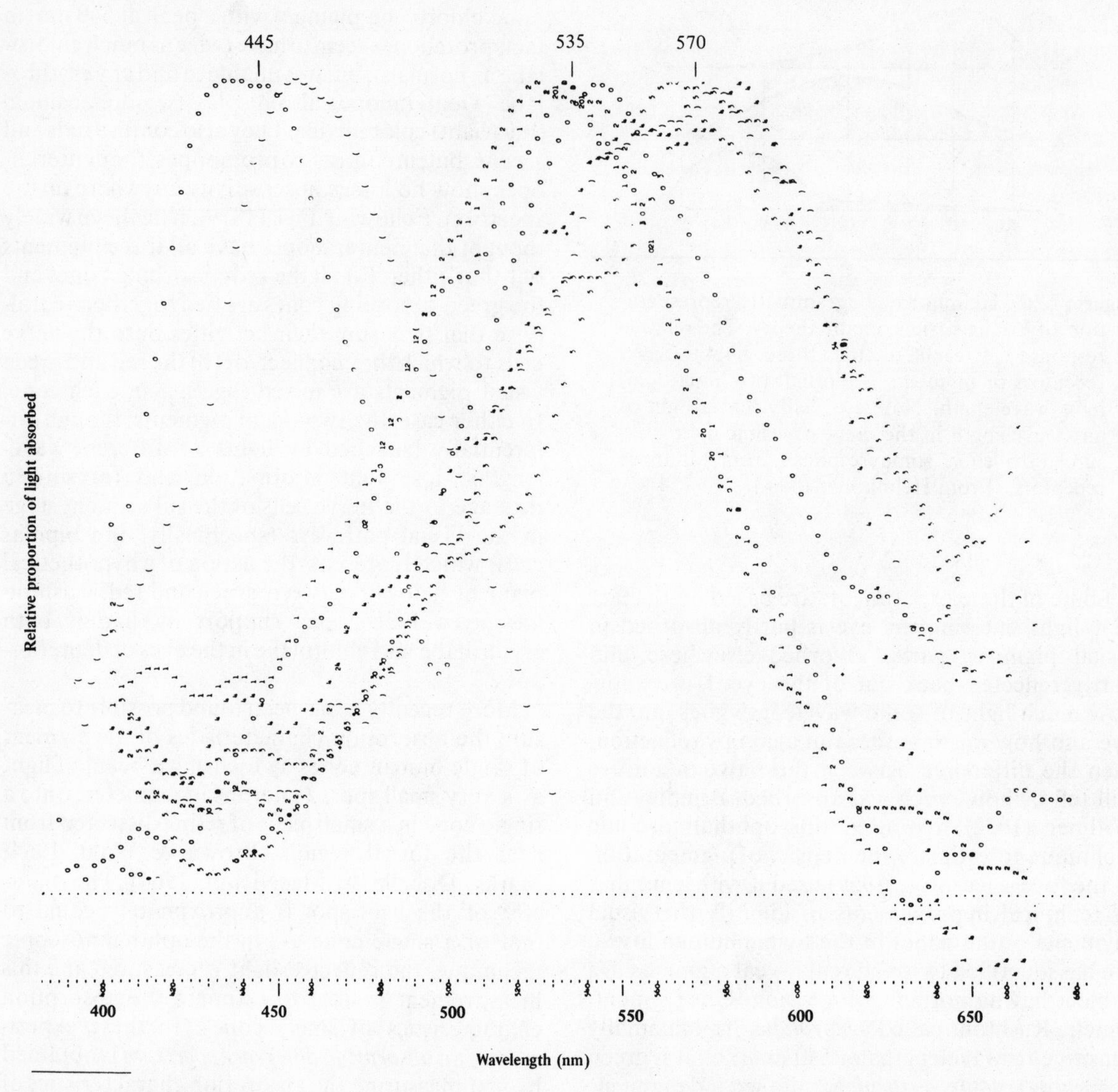


**Figure 7.27** Absorption difference spectra from individual primate cones. (From Marks, Dobelle, & MacNichol, 1964.)

*The opponent-colors theory of Hering and Jameson and Hurvich*

The Young-Helmholtz theory accounted for the fact that all colors can be matched by only three physical lights on the basis of three different pigments in cone photoreceptors. However, several aspects, especially phenomenological aspects, of color vision remained unexplained. For example, blue-green appears to be a mixed color, whereas blue, green, yellow, and red appear to be phenomenologically pure. Why do four pure colors result from three pigments? Moreover, several observations suggest that yellow and blue constitute a single system, green and red another, and white and black a third system. For example, when stimulus size is progressively diminished, yellow and blue discrimination becomes very poor long before red and green (see Hurvich & Jameson, 1955; Jameson & Hurvich, 1955, for references). In addition, Helmholtz had postulated that white is seen when all three cone systems are equally activated. Yet *white* as a sensation often appears independent of the other color systems, when stimulus size, light adaptation, and the number of pigments activated are varied.

Another phenomenon which required explanation was the Bezold-Brücke phenomenon, in which monochromatic lights change in apparent color when their brightness is increased. For example, colors near yellow, such as yellow-green and orange, become yellower as they become more intense; colors near blue, such as violet and blue-green, become bluer as they are made brighter. Yellow (about 580 nm) and blue (about 475 nm) then are two wavelengths that remain invariant in apparent hue as intensity is increased. This association of yellow and blue requires theoretical explanation. Hering's (1878) opponent-colors theory postulated three retinal systems: white-black, yellow-blue, and red-green. Yellow (about 570 to 580 nm) and red (above 600 nm) lights initiated *catabolic* processes in their respective systems, whereas darkness, blue (450 to 470 nm), and green (about 500 nm) initiated *anabolic* processes in their respective systems. Catabolism referred to a breakdown of some unspecified biochemical substance, whereas anabolism referred to its buildup. The actual details of these biochemical processes have not proved to be correct, yet Hering's concept that there are three pairs of processes (white-black, yellow-blue, red-green), with mutual antagonism within each pair, has found both psychological and physiological support.

Jameson and Hurvich (1955), working within the framework of Hering's opponent-colors model, set out to measure by psychological techniques how much each wavelength of monochromatic light affects the postulated yellow-blue and red-green systems. Their work derives from the notion of cancellation in a paired antagonist system. For example, a yellow field of some standard intensity is presented to a subject. Then a light of wavelength $x$ is added and the amount of energy needed at that wavelength to completely cancel the yellow sensation is determined. If little energy is needed, then the antagonist of yellow, namely, the blue sensitive part of the yellow-blue system, is very sensitive to $x$ nm. Similar cancellation measurements are then made, where possible, over the entire range of visible wavelengths, thus yielding the blue functions of Figure 7.28. The yellow functions are generated by canceling a blue sensation by various wavelengths.

An analogous procedure is used to measure the red-sensitive and green-sensitive responses of the red-green system. The red curves in Figure 7.28 indicate that the red-sensitive component is sensitive to both short and long wavelengths. A schematic of one opponent-colors model of Hurvich and Jameson (1957) is shown in Figure 7.29. The three color pigments, $\alpha$ (short wavelength sensi-

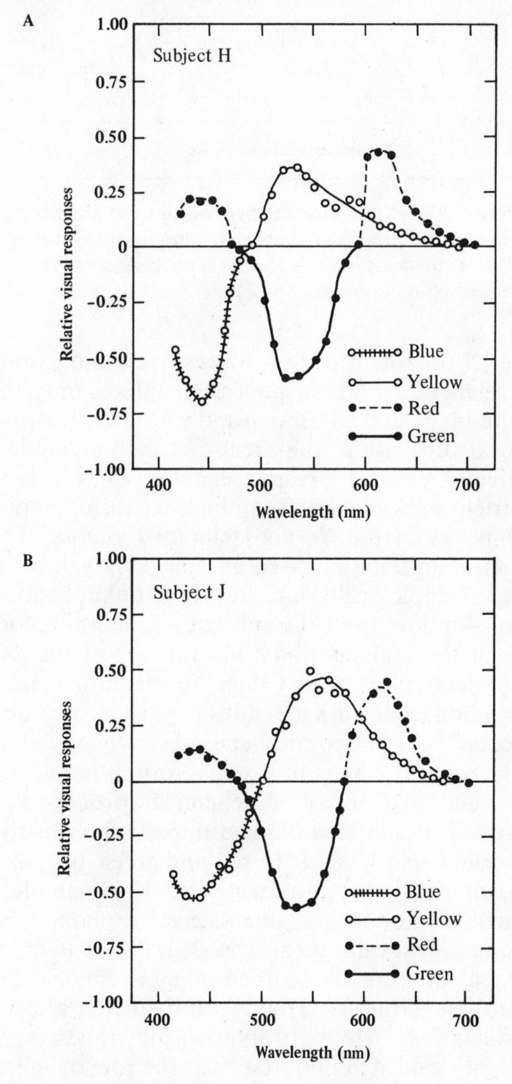


**Figure 7.28** Chromatic response functions for equal energy spectrum for two subjects. (From Jameson & Hurvich, 1955.)

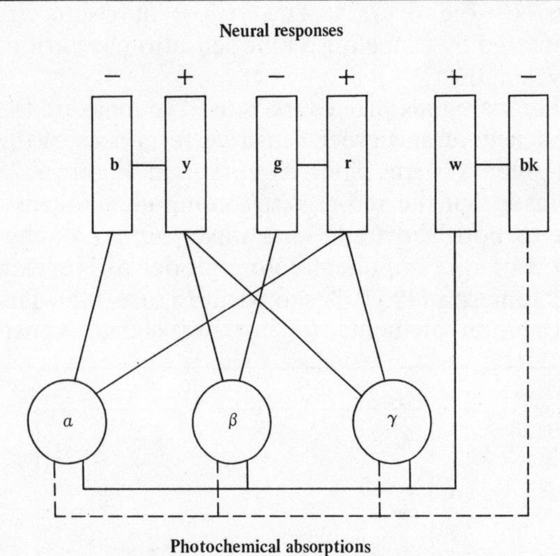


**Figure 7.29** An opponent-process model showing how the three photopigments might feed three pairs of antagonistic neural processes. (From Hurvich & Jameson, 1957.)

tive), $\beta$ (middle wavelength sensitive), and $\gamma$ (long wavelength sensitive), pool their effects onto the white-black system. Both $\alpha$ and $\gamma$ arouse a positive neural response in the green-red system, while $\beta$ activates a negative response, and so on. The laws of trichromacy follow from the three different pigments, as in the Young-Helmholtz theory. The other manifestations—color contrast, yellow as phenomenologically pure, Bezold-Brücke phenomenon—follow from the subsequent neural recoding of the tridimensional information. Thus, the opponent-colors theory does not dispute Young-Helmholtz, but rather refines it so as to include a broader range of color phenomena.

Hering's theory in its original form is not generally accepted today. Biochemical processes of catabolism and anabolism differentially sensitive to yellow and blue, or to red and green, probably do not exist in the photoreceptors. For example, a cone receptor with a green-sensitive pigment responds identically to all wavelengths of light, as long as the rate of absorbed quanta remains constant. Nevertheless, Hering's insight that sensory systems code in terms of antagonistic processes has steadily gained in importance as the role of lateral inhibition in sensory neurophysiology has become better understood. For example, using very thin electrodes, De Valois, Abramov, and Jacobs (1966), recorded the activity of single neurons in the lateral geniculate body, a nucleus within the main pathway of the visual system, of unanesthetized monkeys while they were stimulated by various wavelengths of light. Psychophysical studies in the same laboratory had shown that color vision in a rhesus macque monkey was essentially the same as in humans. De Valois et al. found two classes of cells: *nonopponent* and *spectrally opponent* (following Hurvich and Jameson's terminology).

The graphs in Figure 7.30 depict the number of action potentials or *spikes* per second elicited by monochromatic flashes of light of different wavelengths. Each curve represents a different energy

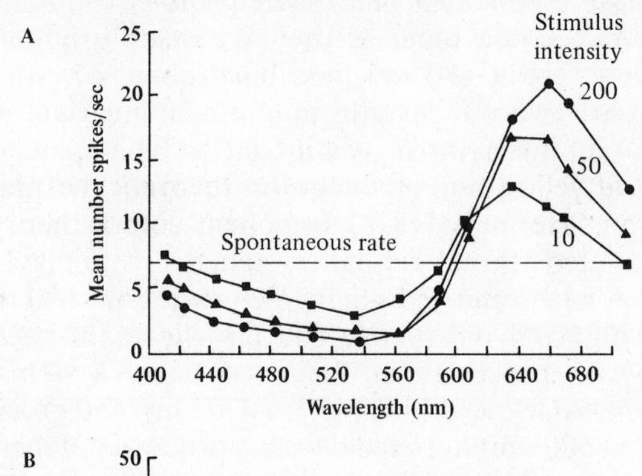


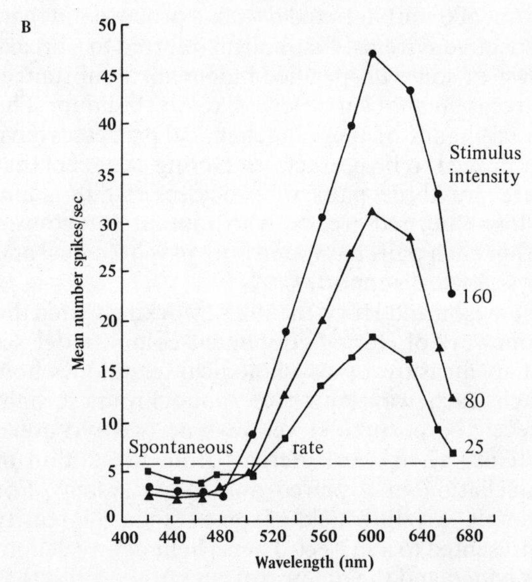


**Figure 7.30** Electrical recording of the activity of single neurons in the lateral geniculate nucleus of a primate. The time rate of action potentials is plotted against the wavelength of the stimulus. Panel A shows an orange (+)–green (−) neuron; panel B shows a yellow (+)–blue (−) neuron. (From De Valois, Abramov, & Jacobs, 1966.)

level. The dashed line represents the spike discharge rate in the absence of any stimulation. For example, Figure 7.30A shows a neuron that is excited by wavelengths around 640 nm and inhibited by wavelengths around 480 to 560 nm, much like an orange (+)–green (–) opponent-colors system. Figure 7.30B shows a neuron excited maximally in the 600-nm range while inhibited in the 460-nm range, much like a yellow (+)–blue (–) opponent-colors system. Although not illustrated here, De Valois et al., as well as other investigators, also found green (+)–red (–) and blue (+)–yellow (–) color-opponent cells. Thus, Hering's conclusion that the visual system takes the trichromatic analysis of color by the photopigments and recodes it into a system of color opponents appears finally to have a solid physiological basis.

What does the visual system accomplish by this recoding? We recall first that over a very wide range of stimulus intensities, covering something like 4 log units, the photoreceptors produce an output which is approximately a logarithmic function of the intensity of the stimulus. The color-opponent cells described in the preceding paragraph seem to operate on the basis of the difference between the activities of cones of one type (say, red-sensitive) and the activities of cones of another type (say, green-sensitive). We know that the difference between two logs is equal to the log of their ratio:

$$\log \frac{r}{g} = \log r - \log g.$$

In other words, when the lateral geniculate cells (or more probably the retinal ganglion cells) extract the difference between the activity of two types of photopigments, they are really computing the ratio of quanta absorption by the two types of cones.[3] The probable purpose of such a computation is to extract constant information about objects in an external world of varying illumination. Illumination levels change constantly, but the ratio of intensities of different wavelengths of light reflected from different aspects of the world (e.g., a red rose against a background of green leaves) remains constant. We see the operation of a simple abstracting device operating at the very periphery of this sensory system.

[3] In reality, the ratio extraction is only approximately constant since the logarithmic transformation of the photoreceptors breaks down at both intensity extremes. The Bezold-Brücke phenomenon presumably results from this departure from a strict logarithmic transformation.

## SUMMARY AND CONCLUSIONS

The experimental psychologist studies the way the colors and shapes of our subjective visual world are related to the physical conditions of our environment. For example, under optimal conditions, we report seeing light when a few quanta of light are absorbed by a few rod receptors in the eye, each rod absorbing a single quantum. Since the quantum is the smallest unit of light that is emitted and absorbed, we conclude that the light receptors of the eye have achieved the ultimate limit of sensitivity.

The human eye really contains two visual systems, a fact which is probably related to our diurnal (night and day) style of existence. The rod receptors form part of a nocturnal system. Being exquisitely sensitive to light, especially in the green region (510 nm), the rods form a visual system that detects light at very low levels, but is poor in acuity, in temporal resolution, and is color blind. The cones form a day-vision system. They are less sensitive than the rods to light, being most sensitive in the yellow-green region (560 nm), and so operate poorly at low illuminances. They form, however, a visual system that is high in acuity, in temporal resolution, and discriminates colors along three dimensions.

Two basic laws of vision concern temporal and spatial summation. Bloch's law states that for a flash of light briefer than 60 to 100 msec, the total number of delivered light quanta, regardless of how they are distributed in time, determines visibility. Ricco's law states that for a flash of light (of fixed duration) whose radius is under 100 minutes of visual angle, the total number of delivered quanta, regardless of how they are distributed over space, determines visibility.

Moving into the dark, our sensitivity to light begins to increase. The resulting dark-adaptation curve has two branches. The first, lasting about 10 minutes, is due to the recovery of the cone receptors. The second, lasting at least 40 minutes, is due to the recovery of the rod receptors. This recovery is clearly related to the dynamic reconstitution of photopigments in the rods and cones. However, the relationship between pigment bleaching and loss of light sensitivity and, conversely, the relationship between pigment regeneration and the recovery of sensitivity is a complex one. A small amount of pigment bleaching causes a large loss in light sensitivity. The proportion of rhodopsin (the rod photopigment) bleached is proportional to the logarithm of the subject's sensitivity. In addition to pigment bleaching, neural effects at synapses in the retina appear to contribute to loss of light sensitivity. It is as if a molecule of bleached rhodopsin keeps on sending neural messages along the optic nerve, thus forming an equivalent background light that makes the test flash harder to see.

Discrimination is relative in vision, as it is in the other senses. We can detect small light changes against dim backgrounds, whereas we can detect only large changes against bright backgrounds. The quantum fluctuation model using statistical decision theory predicts that differential sensitivity will be proportional to the square-root of the background: $k = \Delta I/\sqrt{I}$. This law operates well for dim backgrounds. For bright backgrounds, Weber's law operates: $k = \Delta I/I$. It states that the just detectable change in light intensity is some constant proportion of the background. Recent neurophysiological experiments suggest that Weber's law originates in the most peripheral portions of the visual system, in and among individual photoreceptors. It appears to be the result of negative feedback among photoreceptors. This feedback allows the visual system to function over an enormous dynamic range, despite the limited range of its sensory transducers—the rods and cones.

Brightness grows as a power function of stimulus intensity: $\Psi = k\,(L-L_0)^{0.33}$. To make a surface $x$ times brighter, its physical intensity must be raised to the cube of $x$, namely, $x^3$. Brightness depends not only on intensity, but also on the immediate surround of the stimulus. Contrast enhances the psychological effect of edges and contours in our visual field. A black square looks much darker against a light background than against a dark background. In general, relationships between intensities control responses so thoroughly that a stimulus and its surround continue to look the same as long as the ratio of the two is constant, regardless of how much their absolute levels are changed.

In contrast to the auditory system, the visual system is a poor resolver of temporal changes in the stimulus. The most important variable that governs flicker perception is the modulation amplitude of the fundamental frequency. The visual system seems optimally responsive to a frequency band of 8 to 10 Hz.

Because the ear analyzes a musical chord into its components, there are seldom two ways of achieving the same sound. But with respect to color, the eye can be fooled. Two completely indistinguishable yellows can be created from quite different spectral components. Apparently, the eye analyzes color along only three dimensions. The trivariant law states that the effect of any two colored sources of light, $S_A$ and $S_B$, when added together can always be matched by, at most, a single monochromatic color $S_\lambda$ (in amount $L_\lambda$) plus some white light $L_w$. The three dimensions, in this case, are $\lambda$, $L_\lambda$, and $L_w$. Put succinctly, the Young-Helmholtz theory attributes this three-dimensionality to the existence in the cone receptors of photopigments with maximum sensitivity at three different wavelengths. According to this theory, in certain types of color blindness a person with only a two-dimensional system of color vision (or in rare cases a one-dimensional system) is thought to have been born with only two (or one) cone pigments. Recent measurements on cone pigments in the color blind have added much support to the Young-Helmholtz theory. Even more certain confirmation comes from recent measurements of light absorption by single cones.

From observations such as simultaneous color contrast and from neurophysiological data we know that the visual system recodes the input of the three cone pigments into a set of three pairs of color antagonists: white-black, yellow-blue, and red-green. This neural recoding enables the organism to extract information about the relative absorption of light at different wavelengths by external objects. In this manner, the visual system provides information about the constant properties of objects in the environment, rather than about the ephemeral properties of the light falling on those objects. And so the visual system is less affected by incidental, but normal changes in level of illumination. This ratio extraction may be akin to a simple analog computer performing a simple abstraction at the very periphery of the visual system.

## *APPENDIX*
## LIGHT: THE VISUAL STIMULUS

Light is that small part of the electromagnetic spectrum which is visible (see Figure 7.31). Light exhibits the properties of a finite particle when it is emitted, displays the properties of a wave when it is transmitted in a medium, and acts like a particle once more when it is absorbed in matter.

### Light as a particle

Light quanta, usually referred to as photons, are emitted in two different ways. When electrons in an

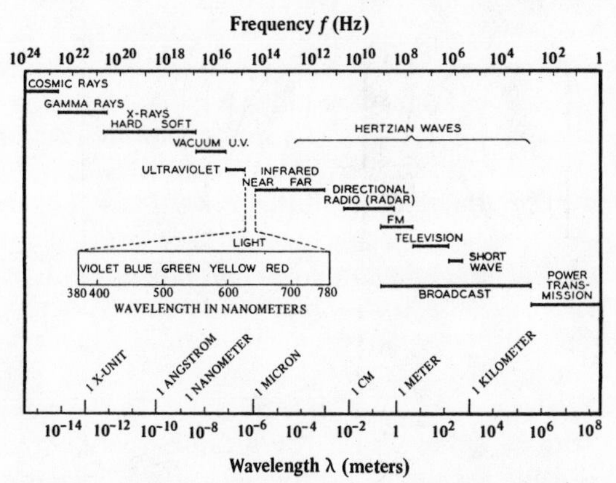


**Figure 7.31** The radiant energy spectrum. The two vertical dashed lines enclose the range of wavelengths of electromagnetic radiation that is visible light. (From Illuminating Engineering Society, 1972.)

atom are excited to the point where they give off photons, we speak of *luminescence*. When molecules are set into rapid motion (such as by heating) and made to give off photons, we speak of *incandescence*.

According to atomic theory (Bohr's model), electrons are distributed around a nucleus in distinct shells, each shell containing electrons at a particular energy level. The inner shells have lower energy levels than the outer shells. If an electron suddenly jumps to a shell of a lower energy level, the difference in energy is made up by the emission of a photon. The frequency of the vibration of that photon is given by Einstein's equation,

$$E = h\gamma, \qquad [20]$$

where $E$ is the energy in ergs of the photon emitted, $h$ is Planck's constant ($6.624 \times 10^{-27}$ erg-sec), and $\gamma$ is the frequency of vibration per second of the emitted photon. If $E_1$ and $E_2$ are the energy levels of the two shells, then

$$h = E_1 - E_2. \qquad [21]$$

Because there are only a few shells surrounding each nucleus, the photons emitted by luminescence will be concentrated at only a few frequencies.

A neon advertising sign is one example of a luminescent source. Electrons, emitted by a negatively charged electrode in a glass tube filled with neon gas, accelerate as they are drawn toward the positively charged anode. If such an electron is traveling rapidly enough, and if it strikes an electron in an inner shell of a neon atom, it may knock the electron to a higher energy level. As the latter leaves the inner shell, one of the electrons in an outer shell jumps in to fill the gap and emits a photon in so doing.

Incandescent sources are solids or liquids heated to a level sufficient to cause the thermal agitation of entire molecules, resulting in the emission of photons. Incandescent sources, rather than emitting photons of only certain vibration frequencies, emit photons over a continuous range of frequencies. The amount of power of the radiation at various frequencies has a distribution which is very similar to *black-body radiation.* A metal container with a small hole in it is a close approximation to a black-body radiator. At low temperatures the hole appears black, but as the temperature of the metal container is raised the hole emits more radiation. Incandescent sources emit most of their radiation outside the visible region. Their mean frequency shifts toward the shorter wavelengths as the temperature is raised; this follows from Einstein's equation since frequency of vibration increases as energy increases. Frequency and wavelengths are reciprocally related: The bunsen burner, which has a rich air mixture, has a relatively cool, yellow (longer wavelength) flame; the acetylene torch has a relatively hot, blue (shorter wavelength) flame.

## Light as a wave

The propagation of light is more conveniently explained by considering its wave properties than its particle properties. Figure 7.31 shows that the dimension of a wave of light is very small, being measured in fractions of a millionth of a meter. The visible wavelengths are longer than X rays and shorter than broadcast wavelengths, but are otherwise essentially similar to all electromagnetic radiations. The velocity of light in a vacuum is about $3 \times 10^8$ meters/sec. In glass, light travels more slowly, having a velocity of $1.9 \times 10^8$ meters/sec. From the frequency of the vibrations and the velocity of the light, the wavelength can be computed. In the equation

$$\lambda_i = \frac{V}{f_i}, \qquad [22]$$

$\lambda_i$ is the wavelength in meters, $V$ is the velocity in meters per second, and $f_i$ is the frequency in cycles per second. Take as an example a light vibration ($i$) at $4.3 \times 10^{14}$ cycles/sec in air:

$$\lambda_i \text{ meters} = \frac{3 \times 10^8 \text{ meters/sec}}{4.3 \times 10^{14} \text{ cycles/sec}}$$

Hence the wavelength is $\lambda_i = .7 \times 10^{-6}$ meters per cycle.

Thus the wavelength in air is .7 microns or 700 nanometers (nm). (The term *nanometer* has recently come to replace millimicron (m$\mu$). Both refer to a length equal to one thousandth of a micron, which itself is one millionth of a meter.) In glass,

$$\lambda_i = \frac{1.9 \times 10^8 \text{ meters/sec}}{4.3 \times 10^{14} \text{ cycles/sec}}.$$

Hence, $\lambda_i = .44 \times 10^{-6}$ meters per cycle, or 440 nm of wavelength.

We see then that light has a shorter wavelength in glass than in air because it travels more slowly in glass but its frequency of vibration is the same. A smaller $V$ in Equation 22 combined with a constant $f_i$ gives a smaller $\lambda$. The shortening of the wavelength explains why light is bent when going from air to glass or from glass to air.

We see in Figure 7.32 various points of a wave front of light ($AA'$) having a frequency of vibration $f$ at time $t = 0$. The wave front is making contact with the glass at point A. When one full cycle of vibration will have elapsed, at time $t = 1/f$, the front, now labeled $BB'$, advanced a distance of one wavelength, $\lambda = V/f$. The length of the wave in air ($\lambda_a$) is longer than the length of the wave in glass ($\lambda_g$). This causes an incident light ray at A to change its angle, reduced from $\theta$ to $\theta'$. The angle of

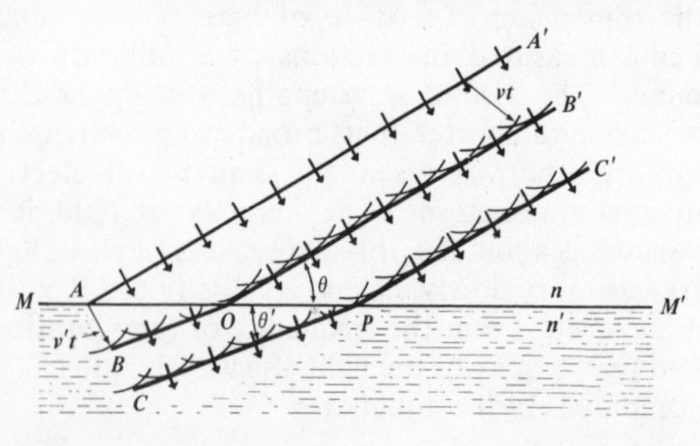


**Figure 7.32** Refraction of a plane wave at a plane surface. (From Richards, Sears, Wehr, & Zemansky, 1960.)

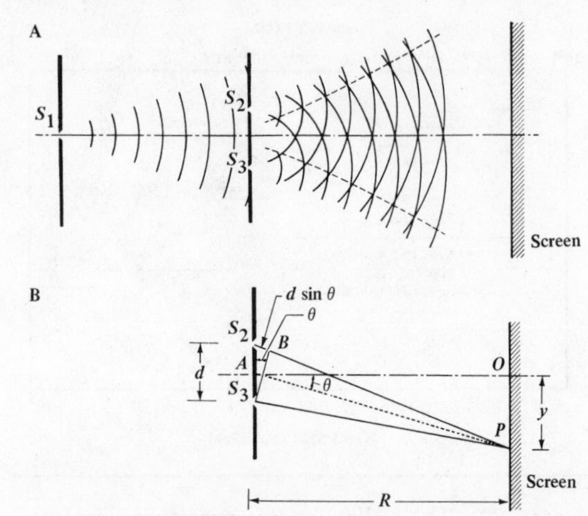


**Figure 7.33** An experiment performed in 1802 by Thomas Young, demonstrating that light can produce interference effects. This study added further evidence to the belief in the wave nature of light. (From Richards et al., 1960.)

incidence ($\theta$) and the angle of refraction ($\theta'$) are related by Snell's law:

$$n \text{ sine } \theta = n' \text{ sine } \theta', \qquad [23]$$

where $n = 1.0$ is the refractive index of air, and $n'$ is the refractive index of the other medium, in this case glass. The refractive index of a material is given by

$$n_g = \frac{1}{V_g}, \qquad [24]$$

where $V_g$ is the velocity of light in that material.

Interference is another of the wave properties of light. Figure 7.33 represents Young's (1802) classic experiment which showed that light can produce interference effects and must therefore have wave properties. A source of light of wavelength $\lambda$ is placed to the left of a slit, $S_1$. The waves that pass through $S_1$ reach slits $S_2$ and $S_3$ at the same instant. From there, two new series of waves continue onto the screen, where, owing to interference, they produce alternating bright and dark bands. Panel B helps explain how these bands arise. Suppose $d$ is the separation between the two slits. Consider a point $P$ which has a longer path to $S_2$ than to $S_3$. If the difference in path lengths ($d$ sine $\theta$) is some integral number of wavelengths, say, $m\lambda$ (where

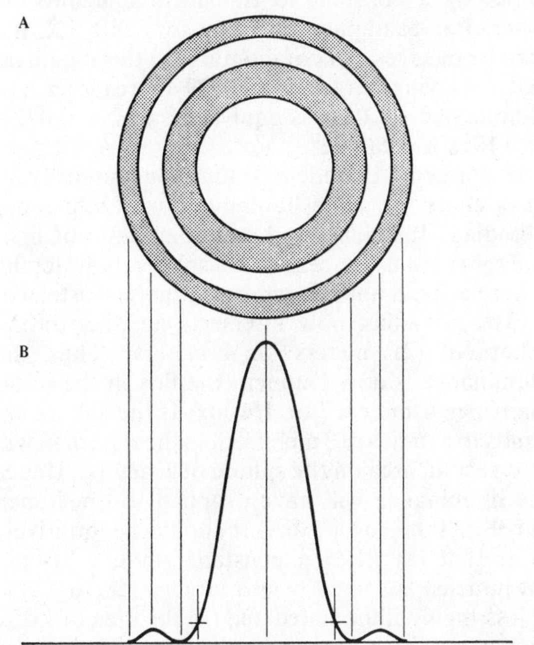


**Figure 7.34** Panel A: Light from an infinitesimally small source, when it passes the edge of an optical system, is diffracted so that it will be imaged as a disc surrounded by a concentric dark ring, which in turn is surrounded by a light ring, etc. The size of the disc does not depend on the size of the source, but on the size of the aperture of the optical system (see Equation 25). The pupil of the eye is such an aperture. Panel B: The relative distribution of light in the image of a point source, as it is imaged by an optical system. It can be seen that most of the light is distributed in the central disc. (From Jacobs, 1943.)

$m = 0, 1, 2, 3$), then the two wavelets arrive at $P$ in phase and reinforce each other, producing a bright band. However, if the difference in length is an integral number of wavelengths plus one-half a wavelength, say, $m\lambda + 1/2\lambda$, then the two wavelengths arrive out of phase and interfere with one another, producing a dark band at $P$. Hence, depending on path length, at different points on the screen bright and dark bands are seen. Interference is important in vision because it occurs whenever light traverses an edge that partially obstructs the waves; the pupil of the eye acts as such an edge.

Figure 7.34 shows the disc and the first concentric band that forms the image of a *point source* after going through a lens system. The angular radius of the first dark ring $\alpha$ is given by the equation

$$\alpha = \frac{1.22\,\lambda}{d}, \qquad [25]$$

where $\lambda$ is the wavelength of light, and $d$ is the diameter of the aperture in the lens system. Note that the size of the disc gets larger when the aperture (the pupil in the case of the eye) gets smaller.

Figure 7.35 shows the diffraction patterns in the image of four point sources. When a very small aperture is used at the lens, the point sources appear as very large discs. Note for example that the discs

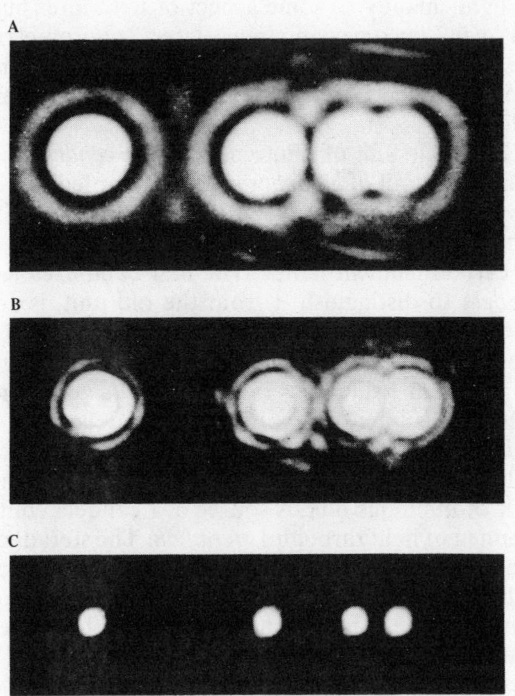


**Figure 7.35** Photographs of the images of four very small points of light as projected by an optical system. The only difference between the three photographs is the size of the lens opening (aperture). In Panel A the opening is extremely small, hence the diffraction patterns are large. Note the disc and the concentric light and dark rings. Note also that such an optical system cannot readily resolve the images of the two dots on the right, which are at Rayleigh's criterion. In Panels B and C increasing the lens opening has the effect of reducing the diffraction pattern, thus increasing the resolution of the optical system. (From Richards et al., 1960.)

farthest to the right in panel A are difficult to resolve into two spots, whereas resolution is easy in panel C. Thus, a small pupil makes resolution poorer. More generally stated, the wave properties of light cause the size of the aperture in a lens system to set certain limits on resolution. The larger the aperture, the smaller the diffraction disc (called *Airy's disc*), and, barring other factors, the better the resolution.

## THE MEASUREMENT OF LIGHT

### Photometry

Photometry is concerned with the measurement of light, mainly of some aspect of light intensity. As will become apparent later, photometric measures are both physical and psychophysical; the physical measures of light are weighted by their effects on vision.

The basic unit of photometry is the *candela (C)*. This is the unit of *luminous intensity* adopted by the Commission Internationale de l'Éclairage (CIE). Until 1948 the *candle* was represented by groups of carbon filament lamps. The new candle, called *candela* to distinguish it from the old unit, is defined as 1/60 of the luminous intensity of 1 $cm^2$ of a black-body radiator at the freezing temperature of platinum (which is 1755° C). *Candlepower (cp)* is luminous intensity expressed in candelas.

*Luminous flux (F)* refers to the rate of flow of light as a function of time. The *lumen (lm)* is the unit of luminous flux. A source of 1 candela emits 1 lumen of light through 1 *steradian.* The steradian is a unit solid angle best defined by a point source of light placed at the center of a sphere with radius of 1 meter. The cone which originates at the center and intersects the sphere so as to cut an area of 1 meter square is the steradian. There are $4\pi$ steradians in the entire sphere. Hence, a 1-candela source emits a total of $4\pi$ lumens.

*Illuminance (E)* is the density of luminous flux falling on a surface. Density equals the total flux divided by the area of the surface. The *lux (lx)* is the unit of illuminance when the square meter is taken as the unit of area. One meter away from a 1-candela light source, a surface receives an illuminance of 1 lux per square meter. When, instead of the square meter, the unit of area is the square foot, then the *footcandle* is the unit of illuminance. If a square centimeter is used as the unit of area, then the *phot* is the unit of illuminance. This proliferation of units is quite confusing. It is helpful to note that the units are all interchangeable; one simply multiplies by a constant to transform one into the other. For example, according to Table 7.2, if a surface receives 1 lux of illuminance this is equivalent to saying it receives 0.0929 footcandles. An illuminance of 2 lux is equivalent to $2 \times 0.0929$, or 0.1858 footcandles.

A source of 1 candela of luminous intensity always emits the same luminous flux, 1 lumen per steradian. Imagine the 1-steradian cone of light emerging from the center of a sphere. Now let the sphere expand until its radius is 2 meters instead of 1. The steradian now intersects an area on the sphere of $(2)^2$ $meters^2$ or 4 $meters^2$. Thus, the illuminance is now 1 lumen (the flux in the steradian) per 4 $meters^2$, or 1/4 lux. If the sphere expands to a radius of 3 meters, then the steradian will intersect an area on the sphere of 9 $meters^2$. Hence the illuminance will have dropped to one lumen per 9 $meters^2$, or 1/9 lux. It should be intuitively clear that (a) when a constant amount of light (of lumens) is spread over a larger area, that area is less highly illuminated and (b) the area of a disc that intersects a cone is inversely proportional to the square of the distance from the point from which the cone emerges. In other words, the inverse-square law applies to illuminance:

$$E = kcp/D^2, \qquad [26]$$

where $E$ is the amount of illuminance on a surface, $cp$ is the candlepower of the source, $D$ is the distance between the source and the surface, and $k$ is a constant. For example, imagine you are in a room with dark walls and a single light bulb illuminating your reading surface. If you bring the bulb five times closer to the reading material, it will be illuminated twenty-five times more.

In addition to a standard light source of 1 candela and the inverse-square law, photometry is based on judgments of equal brightness by human subjects. Suppose, for example, we want to measure the amount of illuminance falling on a test surface. We illuminate another surface similar in color to the first one with our standard source of 1 candela (a 1/60 $cm^2$ surface of platinum at its freezing temperature). Say the human subject views the two surfaces and reports that the one illuminated by the platinum sphere looks brighter. We then move the platinum source farther and farther away until the two surfaces look equally bright when the platinum source is 3 meters away; then by the inverse-square law we know that the platinum source is now illuminating the surface with 1/9 lux, and at the same time we also conclude

**Table 7.2**

Relative Magnitudes of Units of Luminance

| Units | Candle/cm² (stilb) | Lambert | MilliLambert | Candle/in² | FootLambert |
|---|---|---|---|---|---|
| Candle/cm² (stilb) | 1 | 3.142 | 3142 | 6.452 | 2918 |
| Lambert | 0.3183 | 1 | 1000 | 2.054 | 929 |
| MilliLambert | 0.000318 | 0.001 | 1 | 0.00205 | 0.929 |
| Candle/in² | 0.1550 | 0.487 | 487 | 1 | 452 |
| FootLambert | 0.000342 | 0.001076 | 1.076 | 0.00221 | 1 |

Relative Magnitudes of Units of Illuminance

| Units | Lux | Phot | Milliphot | Footcandle |
|---|---|---|---|---|
| Lux | 1 | 0.0001 | 0.1 | 0.0929 |
| Phot | 10,000 | 1 | 1000 | 929 |
| Milliphot | 10 | 0.001 | 1 | 0.929 |
| Footcandle | 10.76 | 0.001076 | 1.076 | 1 |

(From Teele, 1965.)

that the unknown test illuminance must be 1/9 lux.

As the reader may imagine, one does not use platinum heated to its freezing point for field measurements of illuminance. Using the platinum source, one first determines the candlepower of an incandescent bulb when some given amount of electric current goes through it (once more matching brightness and using the inverse-square law), and then uses the incandescent bulb in the field. (For greater details of photometry see Teele, 1965; Walsh, 1958.)

*Luminance*

This photometric measure is closely related to brightness. Luminance refers not to the light falling on a surface, but to the source itself, indicating how much candlepower the source has per unit of its surface. Thus, a very large 1-candela source does not have as much luminance as a very small 1-candela source. Normally, the large source looks dim and the small source looks bright, even though they have the same candlepower. Units of luminance are candles per unit area of the source (the areal density of luminous intensity). A *stilb (sb)* is a unit of luminance of 1 C/cm². (Note that luminance refers to the output of the source relative to the area of the source; the distance between the source and the subject is irrelevant.) There are numerous units of luminance and Table 7.2 shows that they are interchangeable.

*Retinal illuminance*

To determine the amount of illuminance falling on the retina, the aperture of the eye, that is, the area of the pupil, must be taken into account. To a crude first approximation, the entering light is proportional to the pupillary area. The *troland* is a unit that takes pupillary area into consideration: $T = L \times S$, where $T$ is retinal illuminance in trolands, $L$ is the luminance of the stimulus in candles per square meter, and $S$ is the area of the pupil in square millimeters.

## Radiometry

More fundamental than photometry, radiometry is concerned with the measurement of all electromagnetic radiation, only some of which is visible (see Figure 7.31). It is a purely physical system which measures energy without regard to its effect on human subjects. Total radiant energy in *ergs* is given by the sum of the separate energies of all the photons emitted. *Radiant flux* in *watts* is the total energy emitted per unit time in all directions by a radiant source. Other radiometric equivalents of photometric units—*radiant intensity, irradiance, and radiance*—can be derived (Riggs, 1965a).

It is possible to derive the photometric system from the radiometric system if three classes of information are known. First, it is necessary to know $V_\lambda$, the *relative luminosity coefficient*, which represents the relative effectiveness of a wavelength of light in stimulating the eye. This coefficient has been defined by the CIE for a standard subject. Then, we need to know the *luminous efficiency* of the eye. Under daylight conditions of illumination, how much physical energy is required to obtain a particular level of apparent brightness? We know, for example, that at a wavelength of 555 nm, 1 watt of radiant energy (radiometric unit) is the equivalent of 685 lumens of luminous flux (photometric unit). Finally, we need to know how much power (watts) our light source generates at each wavelength. Then,

$$F = 685 \sum_{0}^{\infty} P_\lambda V_\lambda \Delta\lambda \text{ lumens,} \qquad [27]$$

where $F$ is the total luminous flux, $P_\lambda$ is the radiant flux in watts at wavelength $\lambda$, $V_\lambda$ is the relative luminosity coefficient at wavelength $\lambda$, and $\Delta\lambda$ is the band of wavelengths over which radiant flux is summated. Thus it is possible to predict the luminance of any light source without recourse to any new human judgments. However, in practice it is usually more convenient to have subjects make equal-brightness judgments and to use only photometric units.

# REFERENCES


**Andersen, E. E., & Weymouth, F. W.** Visual perception and the retinal mosaic: I. Retinal mean local sign—an explanation of the fineness of binocular perception of distance. *American Journal of Physiology*, 1923, **64**, 561–94.

**Armington, J. C., Johnson, E. P., & Riggs, L. A.** The scotopic A-wave in the electrical response of the human retina. *Journal of Physiology*, 1952, **118**, 289–98. Figure 7, p. 297, reproduced by permission.

**Barlow, H. B.** Increment thresholds at low intensities considered as signal noise discriminations. *Journal of Physiology*, 1957, **136**, 469–88. Figure 2, p. 474, reproduced by permission.

**Barlow, H. B.** Temporal and spatial summation in human vision at different background intensities. *Journal of Physiology*, 1958, **141**, 337–50.

**Barlow, H. B., & Sparrock, J. M. B.** The role of afterimages in dark adaptation. *Science*, 1964, **144**, 1309–14. Figure 4, p. 1313, Copyright © 1964 by the American Association for the Advancement of Science, and reproduced by permission.

**Bartley, S. H.** Subjective brightness in relation to flash rate and the light-dark ratio. *Journal of Experimental Psychology*, 1938, **23**, 313–19.

**Bartley, S. H.** The psychophysiology of vision. In S. S. Stevens (Ed.), *Handbook of experimental psychology*. New York: Wiley, 1951. Pp. 921–84.

**Berry, R. N.** Quantitative relations among vernier, real depth, and stereoscopic depth acuities. *Journal of Experimental Psychology*, 1948, **38**, 708–21.

**Bloch, A. M.** Expériences sur la vision. *Comptes Rendus de la Société Biologique* (Paris), 1885, **37**, 493–95.

**Blondel, A., & Rey, J.** Sur la perception des lumières brèves à la limite de leur portée. *Journal de Physiologie*, 1911, **1**, 530–50.

**Boynton, R. M., & Whitten, D. N.** Visual adaptation in monkey cones: Recordings of late receptor potentials. *Science*, 1970, **170**, 1423–25. Figure 1, p. 1424, Copyright © 1970 by the American Association for the Advancement of Science, and reproduced by permission.

**Brindley, G. S., & Willmer, E. N.** The reflexion of light from the macular and peripheral fundus oculi in man. *Journal of Physiology*, 1952, **116**, 350–56.

**Brown, J. L., Graham, C. H., Leibowitz, H., & Ranken, H. B.** Luminance thresholds for the resolution of visual detail during dark adaptation. *Journal of the Optical Society of America*, 1953, **43**, 197–202.

**Brown, K. T., & Watanabe, K.** Isolation and identification of a receptor potential from the pure cone fovea of the monkey retina. *Nature* (London), 1962, **193**, 958–60.

**Brown, K. T., & Watanabe, K.** Neural stage of adaptation between the receptors and inner nuclear layer of monkey retina. *Science*, 1965, **148**, 1113–15.

**Brown, P. K., & Wald, G.** Visual pigments in single rods and cones of the human retina. *Science*, 1964, **144**, 45–52.

**Brown, R. W., & Lenneberg, E. H.** A study in language and cognition. *Journal of Abnormal and Social Psychology*, 1954, **49**, 454–62.

**Byram, G. M.** The physical and photochemical basis of visual resolving power: I. The distribution of illumination in retinal images. *Journal of the Optical Society of America*, 1944, **34**, 571–91. (a)

**Byram, G. M.** The physical and photochemical basis of visual resolving power: II. Visual acuity and the photochemistry of the retina. *Journal of the Optical Society of America*, 1944, **34**, 718–38. (b)

**Chapanis, A.** The dark adaptation of the color anomalous measured with lights of different hues. *Journal of General Physiology*, 1947, **30**, 423–37.

**Clarke, F. J. J.** Rapid light adaptation of localized areas of the extrafoveal retina. *Optica Acta*, 1957, **4**, 69–77.

**Cowan, A.** Test cards for determination of visual acuity. *Archives of Ophthalmology*, 1928, **57**, 283–95.

**Craik, K. J. W.** The effect of adaptation on subjective brightness. *Proceedings of the Royal Society of London*, Series B, 1940, **128**, 232–47.

**Crawford, B. H.** Visual adaptation in relation to brief conditioning stimuli. *Proceedings of the Royal Society of London*, Series B, 1947, **134**, 283–302. Figure 3, p. 286, reproduced by permission.

**Creutzfeldt, O. D.** Some principles of synaptic organization in the visual system. In F. O. Schmitt (Ed.), *The neurosciences: Second study program*. New York: Rockefeller University Press, 1970. Pp. 630–47.

**Dalton, J.** Extraordinary facts relating to the vision of colors: With observations. *Memoirs of the Manchester*

*Literary and Philosophical Society,* 1798, **5,** 28–45.

**Davy, E.** The intensity-time relation for multiple flashes of light in the peripheral retina. *Journal of the Optical Society of America,* 1952, **42**(12), 937–41.

**de Lange, H.** Research into the dynamic nature of the human fovea-cortex systems with intermittent and modulated light: I. Attenuation characteristics with white and colored light. *Journal of the Optical Society of America,* 1958, **48,** 777–84. Figure 1, p. 778, reproduced by permission of the American Institute of Physics.

**De Valois, R. L., Abramov, I., & Jacobs, G. H.** Analysis of response patterns of LGN cells. *Journal of the Optical Society of America,* 1966, **56,** 966–77. Figures 9 and 10, p. 972, reproduced by permission of the American Institute of Physics.

**De Vries, H.** The quantum character of light and its bearing upon the threshold of vision, the differential sensitivity and visual acuity of the eye. *Physica,* 1943, **19,** 553–64.

**Diamond, A. L.** Foveal simultaneous brightness contrast as a function of inducing and test-field luminances. *Journal of Experimental Psychology,* 1953, **45,** 304–14.

**Dowling, J. E., & Wald, G.** The biological function of vitamin A acid. *Proceedings of the National Academy of Sciences,* 1960, **46,** 587–608.

**Eccles, J. C.** Inhibition in thalamic and cortical neurons and its role in phasing neuronal discharges. *Epilepsia,* 1965, **6,** 89–115.

**Fechner, G. T.** *Elemente der Psychophysik.* Leipzig: Breitkopf und Härtel, 1860.

**Fick, A.** Die Lehre von der Lichtempfindung. In L. Hermann (Ed.), *Handbuch der Physiologie.* Vol. 3. Leipzig: Vogel, 1879. Pp. 139–40.

**Fry, G. A., & Bartley, S. H.** The effect of one border in the visual field upon the threshold of another. *American Journal of Physiology,* 1935, **112,** 414–21.

**Fuortes, M. G. F., & Hodgkin, A. L.** Changes in time scale and sensitivity in the ommatidia of *Limulus. Journal of Physiology,* 1964, **172,** 239–63.

**Graham, C. H., & Bartlett, N. R.** The relation of size of stimulus and intensity in the human eye: II. Intensity thresholds for red and violet light. *Journal of Experimental Psychology,* 1939, **24,** 574–87.

**Graham, C. H., & Kemp, E. H.** Brightness discrimination as a function of the duration of the increment in intensity. *Journal of General Physiology,* 1938, **21,** 635–50. Figure 2, p. 642, reproduced by copyright permission of The Rockefeller University Press.

**Graham, C. H., & Margaria, R.** Area and the intensity-time relation in the peripheral retina. *American Journal of Physiology,* 1935, **113,** 299–305.

**Granit, R., & Harper, P.** Comparative studies on the peripheral and central retina: II. Synaptic reactions in the eye. *American Journal of Physiology,* 1930, **95,** 211–27.

**Granit, R., Holmberg, T., & Zewi, M.** On the mode of action of visual purple on the rod cell. *Journal of Physiology,* 1938, **94,** 430–40.

**Grassmann, H.** On the theory of compound colors. *Philosophical Magazine,* 1854, **7,** 254–64.

**Harter, M. R.** Excitability cycles and cortical scanning: A review of two hypotheses of central intermittency in perception. *Psychological Bulletin,* 1967, **68,** 47–58.

**Hartline, H. K.** Intensity and duration in the excitation of single photoreceptor units. *Journal of Cellular and Comparative Physiology,* 1934, **5,** 229–47.

**Hecht, S.** Vision: II. The nature of the photoreceptor process. In C. A. Murchison (Ed.), *A handbook of general experimental psychology.* Worcester, Mass.: Clark University Press, 1934. Pp. 704–828.

**Hecht, S.** Rods, cones, and the chemical basis of vision. *Physiological Reviews,* 1937, **17,** 239–90.

**Hecht, S.** Energy and vision. In G. A. Baitsell (Ed.), *Science in progress.* Series IV. New Haven, Conn.: Yale University Press, 1945. Pp. 75–97.

**Hecht, S., Haig, C., & Wald, G.** The dark adaptation of retinal fields of different size and location. *Journal of General Physiology,* 1935, **19,** 321–39. Figure 5, p. 335, reproduced by copyright permission of The Rockefeller University Press.

**Hecht, S., & Mintz, E. U.** The visibility of single lines at various illuminations and the retinal basis of visual resolution. *Journal of General Physiology,* 1939, **22,** 593–612.

**Hecht, S., Peskin, J. C., & Patt, M.** Intensity discrimination in the human eye: II. Relation between $\Delta I/I$ and intensity for different parts of the spectrum. *Journal of General Physiology,* 1938, **22,** 7–19. Figure 2, p. 13, reproduced by copyright permission of The Rockefeller University Press.

**Hecht, S., Shlaer, S., & Pirenne, M. H.** Energy, quanta, and vision. *Journal of General Physiology,* 1942, **25,** 819–40.

**Hecht, S., & Smith, E. L.** Intermittent stimulation by light: VI. Area and the relation between critical frequency and intensity. *Journal of General Physiology,* 1936, **19,** 979–89. Figure 2, p. 984, reproduced by copyright permission of The Rockefeller University Press.

**Hecht, S., & Verrijp, C. D.** Intermittent stimulation by light: III. The relation between intensity and critical fusion frequency for different retinal locations. *Journal of General Physiology,* 1933, **17,** 251–65.

**Heider, E. R., & Olivier, D. C.** The structure of the color space in naming and memory for two languages. *Cognitive Psychology,* 1972, **3,** 337–54.

**Heinemann, E. G.** Simultaneous brightness induction as a function of inducing- and test-field luminances. *Journal of Experimental Psychology,* 1955, **50,** 89–96. Figure 3, p. 92, Copyright 1955 by the American Psychological Association, Inc., and reproduced by permission.

**Heinz, M., & Lippay, F.** Über die Beziehungen zwischen der Unterschiedsempfindlichkeit und der Zahl der erregten Sinneselemente: I. *Pflügers Archiv für die Gesamte Physiologie des Menschen und der Tiere,* 1928, **218,** 437–47.

**Helmholtz, H. von** *Handbuch der physiologischen Optik.* Vol. 2. Hamburg & Leipzig: Voss, 1866. (Translation of 3rd ed. by J. P. C. Southall, *Helmholtz's Physiological optics,* Vol. 2. Rochester, N.Y.: Optical Society of America, 1924.)

**Hering, E.** *Zur Lehre vom Lichtsinne.* Vienna: Gerold, 1878. Pp. 107–41.

**Hurvich, L. M., & Jameson, D.** Some quantitative aspects of an opponent-colors theory: II. Brightness, saturation, and hue in normal and dichromatic vision. *Journal of the Optical Society of America,* 1955, **45,** 602–16.

**Hurvich, L. M., & Jameson, D.** An opponent-process theory. *Psychological Review,* 1957, **64,** 384–90. Figure 2, p. 388, Copyright © 1957 by the American Psychological Association, Inc., and reproduced by permission.

**Illuminating Engineering Society.** *I.E.S. Lighting handbook.* (5th ed.) New York: I.E.S., 1972. Figure 2-1, page 2-2, reproduced by permission.

**Ives, H. E.** Critical frequency relations in scotopic vision. *Journal of the Optical Society of America,* 1922, **6,** 254–68.

**Jacobs, D. H.** *Fundamentals of optical engineering.* New York: McGraw-Hill, 1943. Figures 136 and 137, p. 176, Copyright, 1943, by the McGraw-Hill Book Company, Inc. Used with permission of McGraw-Hill Book Company.

**Jameson, D., & Hurvich, L. M.** Some quantitative aspects of an opponent-colors theory: I. Chromatic responses and spectral saturation. *Journal of the Optical Society of America,* 1955, **45,** 546–52. Figures 4, p. 550, and 5, p. 551, reproduced by permission of the American Institute of Physics.

**Jones, L. A., & Higgins, G. C.** Photographic granularity and graininess: III. Some characteristics of the visual system of importance in the evaluation of graininess and granularity. *Journal of the Optical Society of America,* 1947, **37,** 217–63.

**Judd, D. B.** Chromatic sensibility to stimulus differences. *Journal of the Optical Society of America,* 1932, **22,** 72–108. Figure 3, p. 89, reproduced by permission of the American Institute of Physics.

**Judd, D. B.** Hue, saturation, and lightness of surface colors with chromatic illumination. *Journal of Research of the National Bureau of Standards,* 1940, **24,** 293–333.

**Karn, H. W.** Area and the intensity-time relation in the fovea. *Journal of General Psychology,* 1936, **14,** 360–69.

**Keesey, U. T.** Effects of involuntary eye movements on visual acuity. *Journal of the Optical Society of America,* 1960, **50,** 769–74.

**Kelly, D. H.** Effects of sharp edges in a flickering field. *Journal of the Optical Society of America,* 1959, **49,** 730–32.

**Koenderink, J. J., van de Grind, W. A., & Bouman, M. A.** Models of retinal signal processing at high luminances. *Kybernetik,* 1970, **6,** 227–37.

**Kuffler, S. W., FitzHugh, R., & Barlow, H. B.** Maintained activity in the cat's retina in light and darkness. *Journal of General Physiology,* 1957, **40,** 683–702.

**Kugelmass, S., & Landis, C.** The relation of area and luminance to the threshold for critical flicker fusion. *American Journal of Psychology,* 1955, **68,** 1–19.

**Le Grand, Y.** *Light, colour and vision.* London: Chapman & Hall, 1957. Figure 31, p. 130, reproduced by permission.

**Lipetz, L. E.** Mechanism of light adaptation. *Science,* 1961, **133,** 639–40.

**Long, G. E.** The effect of duration of onset and cessation of light flash on the intensity-time relation in the peripheral retina. *Journal of the Optical Society of America,* 1951, **41,** 743–47.

**Ludvigh, E., & McCarthy, E. F.** Absorption of visible light by the refractive media of the human eye. *Archives of Ophthalmology,* 1938, **20,** 37–51.

**Marks, W. B., Dobelle, W. H., & MacNichol, E. F., Jr.** Visual pigments of single primate cones. *Science,* 1964, **143,** 1181–82. Figure 2, p. 1182, Copyright © 1964 by the American Association for the Advancement of Science, and reproduced by permission.

**Maxwell, J. C.** On the theory of compound colours, and the relations of colours of the spectrum. *Philosophical Transactions of the Royal Society of London,* 1860, **150,** 57–84.

**Mote, F. A., & Riopelle, A. J.** The effect of varying the intensity and the duration of pre-exposure upon subsequent dark adaptation in the human eye. *Journal of Comparative and Physiological Psychology,* 1953, **46**(1), 49–55.

**Mueller, C. G.** Frequency-of-seeing functions for intensity discrimination at various levels of adapting intensity. *Journal of General Physiology,* 1951, **34,** 463–74. Figure 2, p. 468, reproduced by copyright permission of The Rockefeller University Press.

**Piéron, H.** La dissociation de l'adaptation lumineuse et de l'adaptation chromatique. *Année Psychologique,* 1939, **40,** 1–14.

**Pirenne, M. H.** Physiological mechanisms of vision and the quantum nature of light. *Biological Review,* 1956, **31,** 194–241.

**Pirenne, M. H.** Liminal brightness increments. In H. Davson (Ed.), *The eye.* Vol. 2. London: Academic Press, 1962. Pp. 159–74. (a)

**Pirenne, M. H.** Light adaptation. In H. Davson (Ed.), *The eye.* Vol. 2. London: Academic Press, 1962. Pp. 198–204. (b)

**Pirenne, M. H., & Denton, E. J.** Accuracy and sensitivity of the human eye. *Nature* (London), 1952, **170,** 1039–42. Figure 1, p. 1039, reproduced by permission.

**Pirenne, M. H., Marriott, F. H. C., & O'Doherty, E. F.** Individual differences in night vision efficiency. *Spec. Rep. Ser. med. Res. Coun.* (London), 1957, **294.**

**Priest, I. G., & Brickwedde, F. G.** The minimum perceptible colorimetric purity as a function of dominant wavelength. *Journal of the Optical Society of America,* 1938, **28,** 133–39.

**Ratliff, F.** *Mach bands: Quantitative studies on neural networks in the retina.* San Francisco: Holden-Day, 1965.

**Ricco, A.** Relazione fra il minimo angolo visuale e l'intensità luminosa. *Memorie della Regia Accademia de Scienze, lettere ed arti in modena,* 1877, **17,** 47–160.

**Richards, J. A., Sears, F. W., Wehr, M. R., & Zemansky, M. W.** *Modern university physics.* Reading, Mass.: Addison-Wesley, 1960. Figures 32-3, 35-2, and 35-22, reproduced by permission.

**Riggs, L. A.** Dark adaptation in the frog eye as determined by the electrical response of the retina. *Journal of Cellular and Comparative Physiology,* 1937, **9,** 419–510.

**Riggs, L. A.** Light as a stimulus for vision. In C. H. Graham (Ed.), *Vision and visual perception.* New York: Wiley, 1965. Pp. 1–38. (a)

**Riggs, L. A.** Electrophysiology of vision. In C. H. Graham (Ed.), *Vision and visual perception.* New York: Wiley, 1965. Pp. 81–131. (b)

**Riggs, L. A.** Visual acuity. In C. H. Graham (Ed.), *Vision and visual perception.* New York: Wiley, 1965. Pp. 321–49. (c)

**Rivers, W. H. R.** Primitive color vision. *Popular Science Monthly,* 1901, **59,** 44–58.

**Roehrig, W. C.** The influence of the portion of the retina stimulated on the critical flicker-fusion threshold. *Journal of Psychology,* 1959, **48,** 57–63.

**Rose, A.** The relative sensitivities of television pickup tubes, photographic films, and the human eye. *Proceedings of the Institute of Electronic and Radio Engineers* (New York), 1942, **30,** 295–300.

**Rose, A.** The sensitivity performance of the human eye on an absolute scale. *Journal of the Optical Society of America,* 1948, **38,** 196–208.

**Rushton, W. A. H.** The kinetics of cone pigments measured objectively upon the living human fovea. *Annals of the New York Academy of Sciences,* 1958, **74,** 291–304.

**Rushton, W. A. H.** Visual pigments in man and animals and their relation to seeing. In *Progress in biophysics and biophysical chemistry.* Vol. 9. London: Pergamon Press, 1959. Pp. 239–83.

**Rushton, W. A. H.** Increment threshold and dark adaptation. *Journal of the Optical Society of America,* 1963, **53,** 104–109.

**Rushton, W. A. H., Campbell, F. W., Hagins, W. A., & Brindley, G. S.** The bleaching and regeneration of rhodopsin in the living eye of the albino rabbit and of man. *Optica Acta,* 1955, **1,** 183–90.

**Senders, V. L.** The physiological basis of visual acuity. *Psychological Bulletin,* 1948, **45,** 465–90.

**Shlaer, S.** The relation between visual acuity and illumination. *Journal of General Physiology,* 1937, **21,** 165–88.

**Sperling, G., & Sondhi, M. M.** Model for visual luminance discrimination and flicker detection. *Journal of the Optical Society of America,* 1968, **58,** 1133–45.

**Steinhardt, J.** Intensity discrimination in the human eye: I. The relation of $\Delta I/I$ to intensity. *Journal of General Physiology,* 1936, **20,** 185–209.

**Stevens, J. C., & Stevens, S. S.** Brightness function: Effects of adaptation. *Journal of the Optical Society of America,* 1963, **53,** 375–85. Figure 3, p. 337, reproduced by permission of the American Institute of Physics.

**Stevens, S. S.** Neural events and the psychophysical law. *Science,* 1970, **170,** 1043–50.

**Stiles, W. S., & Crawford, B. H.** The liminal brightness increment for white light for different conditions of the foveal and parafoveal retina. *Proceedings of the Royal Society of London,* Series B, 1934, **116,** 55–102.

**Swets, J. A., Tanner, W. P., Jr., & Birdsall, T. G.** Decision processes in perception. *Psychological Review,* 1961, **68,** 301–40.

**Talbot, H. F.** Experiments on light. *Philosophical Transactions of the Royal Society of London,* 1834, **3,** 298.

**Teele, R. P.** Photometry. In R. Kingslake (Ed.), *Applied optics and optical engineering.* Vol 1. New York: Academic Press, 1965. Pp. 1–42. Tables 3 and 4, p. 9, by permission.

**Troxler, D.** Über das Verschwinden gegebener Gegenstände innerhalb unseres Gesichtskreises. In K. Himly & J. A. Schmidt (Eds.), *Ophthalmologische Bibliothek,* 1804, **2,** 1–53.

**Wald, G.** Human vision and the spectrum. *Science,* 1945, **101,** 653–58.

**Wald, G.** On the mechanism of the visual threshold and visual adaptation. *Science,* 1954, **119,** 887–92.

**Wald, G., & Brown, P. K.** The molar extinction of rhodopsin. *Journal of General Physiology,* 1953, **37,** 189–200.

**Walsh, J. W.** *Photometry.* (3rd ed.) London: Constable, 1958.

**Whorf, B. L.** *Language, thought and reality.* Cambridge, Mass.: M.I.T. Press, 1956.

**Wright, W. D.** *Researches on normal and defective colour vision.* London: H. Kimpton, 1946.

**Young, T.** On the theory of light and colours. *Philosophical Transactions of the Royal Society of London,* 1802, **92,** 12–48.

**Young, T.** *A course of lectures on natural philosophy.* Vol. 2. London: Johnson, 1807.

8

# POSTSCRIPT

**Bertram Scharf**
**Northeastern University**

Where has sensory psychology been, and where is it going? In this book, we have seen that sensory psychologists have stimulated every part of the human body where a sensory receptor might lie hidden. Pain has been measured on the cornea of the eye, warmth and cold on the prepuce of the penis, vibration on the top and bottom of the tongue. While their studies of the skin show how inquisitive sensory psychologists can be, they have, in fact, concentrated mostly on the eye and ear, using whatever equipment was available—candles and tuning forks one hundred years ago, lasers and computers today—to generate and control specifiable stimuli. Often the stimuli are quite novel, like tones racing up and down in frequency, or cascading sequences of colored lights. In taste and smell, too, novel stimuli have been used—electrical currents that produce a sweet or sour taste, chemicals that make lemons taste sweet. Artificial as they are, such stimuli make possible precise analyses of how our sensory systems function.

On the response side, sensory psychologists have tried to make the observer's task as simple as possible, posing questions like: Which one of two brief time intervals contains the signal? What number corresponds to the perceived magnitude of a stimulus?

With its long history and refined techniques, sensory psychology, more than any other branch of psychology, musters a great many facts and figures on each printed page. The study of thresholds and sensory magnitudes over more than a century has produced countless quantitative relationships between stimuli and responses. In every sensory modality, threshold measurements have shown how the minimum amount of a stimulus needed to elicit a response depends on a variety of stimulus properties and observer conditions. Also in every sensory modality, sensory magnitude has been measured as a function of stimulus magnitude, under a variety of experimental conditions. The problems of threshold and magnitude (which includes the problem of sensory quality) are common to all the senses. What is common about their solutions?

Absolute thresholds for light and sound can be directly related to the transmission properties of the eye and ear plus, in the eye, the absorption characteristics of the visual pigments of the rods and cones. The nose, tongue, and skin have yielded up their secrets more grudgingly, partly because they have received less attention; much is still unknown about how absolute sensitivity in smell, taste, touch, pain, warmth, cold, and so forth depends on the properties of the sensory organ, or even, in the case of the skin, which receptor is involved.

Concerning differential thresholds, Weber's law remains, after nearly a century and a half, the most general statement and, indeed, one of psychology's best known quantitative laws. Over huge ranges of most stimulus magnitudes, the just noticeable difference is proportional to stimulus magnitude: $\Delta I/I = k$. Although still unexplained in physiological terms, Weber's law may yield to a meaningful interpretation in terms of signal detection theory. Meanwhile, signal detection theory has provided a quantitative basis for distinguishing sensitivity from criterion, that is, sensory factors from judgmental factors in the measurement of threshold, and has also fostered powerful, criterion-free procedures for measuring both absolute and differential thresholds.

Sensory psychology's other overriding generalization is the psychophysical law, formerly Fechner's logarithmic version, now Stevens' power law: $S = aI^b$. In every sensory modality, a great many different kinds of experiments have shown that sensory magnitude, *S*, for prothetic continua (but not necessarily for the small class of metathetic continua which includes sensory attributes like pitch and visual position) increases as a power function of stimulus magnitude, *I*. Parameters such as background stimuli, adaptation, duration, and so on, which affect the exponent, *b*, of the power function, have been carefully studied, especially for loudness and brightness. Among the intriguing questions that remain unanswered are: Why does the slope of the power function vary from one sensory continuum to another, from as low as 0.3 for loudness and brightness to at least as high as 3.0 for perceived electric current? Why, within a given continuum, does the slope of the power function vary from individual to individual or, for the same individual, from one session to another? And what of the validity of some of the procedures used in the measurement of sensory magnitude, especially those procedures involving the use of numbers?

These questions and generalizations so far concern mostly stimulus intensity or magnitude. What about those two other primary stimulus properties, time and space? With respect to time, the general rule seems to be that up to about a tenth or twentieth of a second, the longer a given stimulus lasts, the easier it is to detect and the stronger it seems. Most stimuli that last more than a few seconds, however, gradually become subjectively weaker. Adaptation is the prevailing rule for brightness, strengths of odors and tastes, pressure, warmth and cold, and so forth. (Loudness seems to be a major exception: A steady sound just does not become appreciably softer over time.) Physiologically, adaptation seems to occur both in the receptor and in the sensory nervous system.

Time plays another quite different and critical role in sensation. A brief difference in the onset time of a stimulus going to the two ears or the two nostrils or to different parts of the skin or tongue affects the apparent location of the stimulus. Thus, a sound arriving at the left ear before the right ear is heard to come from the left; an odor reaching first the left nostril appears to be on the left. As shown by von Békésy, the onset time differences involved in the various senses are usually under 1 msec. Only in vision are onset time differences unimportant for the location of stimuli. There, onset time differences may result rather in perceived movement of a single light stimulus from one place to another.

While the spatial location of a stimulus is signaled largely by small onset time differences between separated receptors, the size or spatial extent of a stimulus is signaled initially by the number of excited receptor units. But the spatial extent of a stimulus may also directly affect the strength of sensation. As the size of a light stimulus to the eye or pressure or temperature stimulus to the skin increases, sensitivity increases (i.e., intensity threshold goes down) and subjective magnitude increases. For example, a light spot grows brighter as it grows larger, a warm spot grows warmer. However, stimulus size is effective over only a tiny range, beyond which further increases in size have little or no effect on either threshold or magnitude. In hearing, where sound frequency is transformed into a spatial variable, the rules are different and more complex. In taste and smell, little is known about the influence of spatial extent on sensory magnitude.

Has sensory psychology come so far that all that remains is a mopping-up operation? Clearing away a few ambiguities in hearing and seeing and collecting more data about touch, taste, and smell? Yes and no. While we have some solid answers to basic questions, much remains unclear about interactions between stimuli and between paired receptors—between the two eyes, the two ears, and so forth. Modern psychophysical techniques are being applied more and more to these problems of interaction. For example, how does one spot of light affect the brightness or hue of another adjacent or successive light? How does a sound to one ear affect the loudness or locus of a sound to the other ear? How does one flavor affect the magnitude or quality of a flavor presented either simultaneously or successively? How does adapting to one odor affect the perceived magnitude of other odors? These questions are not new; Fechner posed some of them one hundred years ago, but they are getting more attention as modern equipment has made possible the production of complex stimuli under precise control.

Thus, the emphasis in experimental sensory psychology seems to be shifting to a study of interactions between stimuli and between receptors. As the stimulus becomes more complex, the study of sensation becomes more like the study of perception. Therein lies a major direction: the incorporation of the data and theories of sensory psychology with those from the study of perception. A good example is the application of modern psychophysical techniques to the size-weight illusion, a classic perceptual problem in which the perceived heaviness of an object depends on both its physical weight and its perceived size. As noted in the introduction, the distinction between sensation and perception is logically artificial, but in the laboratory the distinction has often been meaningful. However, the laboratory segregation should fade as the basic laws of sensation are mapped out and applied in the interpretation and study of perception.

At the same time that sensory psychology looks at more complex phenomena and stimuli, the field is also becoming more reductionistic as it strives to tie psychophysical data and laws to physiological data. Sensory psychologists have always been keenly aware of the importance of what goes on inside the organism. However, during the past quarter of a century, the physiological data from the receptors and the sensory nervous systems have increased enormously both in quality and quantity. It has thus become possible to map out functional relations between stimulus variables and physiological events occurring in the receptor, in groups of neurons, and in single neurons. These relations can be compared to the stimulus-response relations of traditional sensory psychology.

Although the study of the relation between stimuli and physiological responses is often identified with Fechner's *inner* psychophysics, as contrasted to his *outer* psychophysics, that identification is historically false. By outer psychophysics, Fechner meant the relation between the physical and the sensory, primarily between stimulus magnitude and sensory magnitude. By inner psychophysics, he meant the relation between the sensation and the physiological events triggered by a stimulus. Fechner saw inner psychophysics as the subject of future investigations, since the necessary techniques were not yet available in the nineteenth century. Fechner wanted to study the relation between physiological events and sensation, not between stimuli and physiological responses, which is the main topic of contemporary sensory physiology.

Fechner's definition of inner psychophysics reveals his generation's lack of understanding of sensory transduction and his own pragmatic dualism, according to which the mind and body are two aspects of one world and, as such, parallel one another. For Fechner, inner psychophysics was the ultimate means of getting closer to the boundary between mind and body. However, the physiology has turned out to be much more complex than Fechner envisioned. Perhaps the closest we have come to inner psychophysics is in the direct stimulation of the brains of awake humans who report what they experience. But even that is far from measuring the relation between the physiological events evoked by a normal stimulus and the corresponding sensation.

Stevens favored a more realizable program, a kind of mix between outer psychophysics and middle psychophysics. Middle psychophysics refers to the study of the relations between the stimulus and physiological responses (usually neurelectric) at various levels of the sensory nervous system. These input-output functions, which relate stimuli to physiological responses, are then to be compared to the psychophysical input-output functions, which relate stimuli to responses by intact human observers. For Stevens, the mind-body problem was a pseudoproblem. Given enough input-output functions, one could adequately describe the translation from external stimulus to observable response, and the inferred sensation could be treated as a response variable. For those psychologists, philosophers, and students who feel that the experienced and the personal are real data, this solution is probably unsatisfactory, but the near future seems to hold no other rigorous solution. Perhaps finer analyses of the evoked potentials measured from the brain and other parts of the nervous system will lead to a better understanding of how the sensory systems work and move us closer to a solution of the mind-body problem.

Meanwhile we must rest content with (a) the magnificent techniques developed by psychophysics for unraveling the stimulus-response relations in the sensory domain; (b) the sophisticated analytic tools for dealing with sensory detection provided by signal detection theory; (c) the myriad facts uncovered by sensory physiology about the structure and function of sensory receptors, facts that include more and more subcellular and even molecular events; (d) the many correlations between stimulus variables and both gross and single-unit physiological responses; and (e) the imposing generality of sensory psychology's two great laws: Weber's law of differential sensitivity and Stevens' power law for sensory magnitude.

# NAME INDEX

# SUBJECT INDEX

2 3 4 5 6 7 8 9 10 -KP- 80 79 78 77 76 75